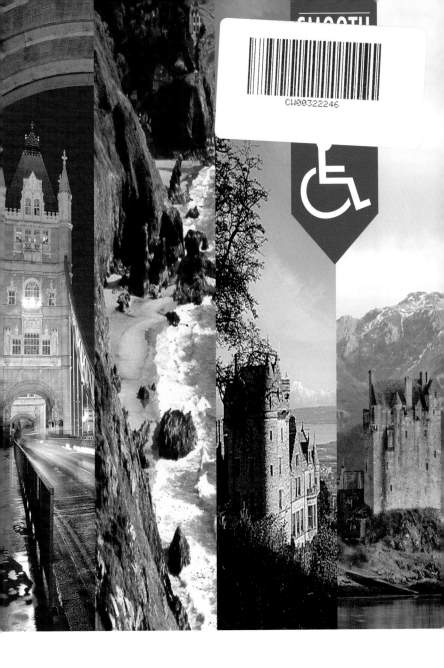

UNITED KINGDOM

FREEWHEELING MADE EASY

SMOOTH RIDE GUIDES
UNITED KINGDOM
By July Ramsey

Researchers: July Ramsey, Ian Wilcox and Liza Grant
Editor: John Bailey
Design: Design 23
Publicity: jrpr
Printed in Great Britain by Richardson Printing,
Lowestoft, Suffolk.

ISBN 0 9521982 8 2

The National Lottery Charities Board aims to meet the needs of those at greatest disadvantage in society and to improve the quality of life in the community.

We are very grateful to the Charities Board for funding this edition of Smooth Ride Guides.

Special thanks to Ian Wilcox and Liza Grant, together with Jo Griffiths, Margaret Hides, Elizabeth Meadows, Lulu Spurling, Jo Tripp and Loraine Wilcox, and to Artsline, Spinal Injuries Association and Tripscope without whose help and support our journey scarcely would have begun.

The contents of this publication are believed correct at the time of going to press, but some details are likely to have changed. The publishers would greatly appreciate comments, criticism and suggestions for the first revision. Please write to: July Ramsey, Smooth Ride Guides, Duck Street Barns, Duck Street, Furneux Pelham, Herts SG9 0LA.

PICTURE CREDITS

We would like to thank the following organisations for kindly allowing us to reproduce the photographs used in this publication.

AMBER VALLEY TOURISM
ASHMOLEAN MUSEUM, OXFORD
ASTLEY HALL MUSEUM
BADDESLEY CLINTON
BEARSTED WINE
BEDE'S WORLD
BEKONSCOT MODEL VILLAGE
BELFAST CONFERENCE AND VISITORS BUREAU
BIRDLAND PARK
BIRMINGHAM BOTANICAL GARDENS
BIRMINGHAM CONFERENCE & VISITOR BUREAU
BIRMINGHAM MARKETING DEPARTMENT
BLACKPOOL TOURISM DEPT.
BRISTOL TOURISM & CONFERENCE BUREAU
BURRELL COLLECTION
CAMELOT THEME PARK
CHATSWORTH HOUSE TRUST
CHESTER CITY COUNCIL TOURISM DEVELOPMENT UNIT
COMPTON ACRES
CORNWALL TOURIST BOARD
COTSWOLD WILDLIFE PARK
COVENTRY & WARWICKSHIRE PROMOTIONS
CUMBRIA TOURIST BOARD
DARTINGTON CRYSTAL
DERBY CITY COUNCIL
DOVER DISTRICT COUNCIL
EARTH CENTRE
EAST OF ENGLAND TOURIST BOARD
ENGLISH WINE CENTRE
ESSEX COUNTY COUNCIL TOURISM SECTION
FITZWILLIAM MUSEUM, UNIVERSITY OF CAMBRIDGE
GUERNSEY TOURISM
HATFIELD HOUSE
HATTON COUNTRY WORLD
HEDGEHOG HOSPITAL
HEREFORDSHIRE TOURISM
HIGHLANDS OF SCOTLAND TOURIST BOARD
HISTORIC SCOTLAND
ISLE OF MAN TOURISM
JERSEY TOURISM
KNOLL GARDENS
LEEDS CASTLE ENTERPRISES
LEEDS CITY COUNCIL
LEEDS DEPARTMENT OF LEISURE TOURISM
LONGTON BRICKCROFT
LONG SHOP STEAM MUSEUM
LOWESTOFT MARITME MUSEUM
MARBLES UK (River & Rowing Museum, Henley)
MARKETING MANCHESTER
MERSEY TOURISM
MUSEUM OF ST. ALBANS
THE NATIONAL TRUST
NATIONAL GALLERY OF SCOTLAND
NATURAL HISTORY MUSEUM
NATIONAL HORSE RACING MUSEUM
NORTHERN IRELAND TOURIST BOARD
NORTH LINCOLNSHIRE COUNCIL TOURISM TEAM
NORTHUMBRIA TOURIST BOARD
NOTTINGHAM CASTLE MUSEUM
PAIGNTON ZOO
ROMNEY, HYTHE & DYMCHURCH RAILWAY
ROYAL BOTANIC GARDENS KEW
ROYAL COLLECTION ENTERPRISES copyright HM Queen Elizabeth II
ROYAL HORTICULTURAL SOCIETY, ROSEMOOR
ROYAL HORTICULTURAL SOCIETY, WISLEY
ROYAL NATIONAL ROSE SOCIETY
SANDRINGHAM ESTATE, by Gracious Permission of HM The Queen
SCOTTISH TOURIST BOARD
SEA LIFE AQUARIUM
SHETLANDS ISLAND TOURISM
SHROPSHIRE TOURISM
SOUTH EAST ENGLAND TOURIST BOARD
SOUTHERN TOURIST BOARD
SOUTH SOMERSET TOURISM & CULTURAL SERVICES
SOUTH WARWICKSHIRE TOURISM
SPOTLIGHT PUBLIC RELATIONS
STOKE-ON-TRENT TOURISM GROUP
SUFFOLK TOURISM
SURREY TOURISM
THRIGBY HALL WILDLIFE GARDEN
UNIVERSITY BOTANIC GARDEN, CAMBRIDGE
UNIVERSITY OF NEWCASTLE MUSEUM OF ANTIQUITIES
WALES TOURIST BOARD
WESTONBIRT ARBORETUM
WHIPSNADE WILD ANIMAL PARK
WIND IN THE WILLOWS ATTRACTION
WORCESTER CITY COUNCIL
YORK TOURISM BUREAU

CONTENTS

INTRODUCTION

This edition of Smooth Ride Guides covering the UK, shows the wide range of activities, attractions, accommodation, and leisure and sporting facilities that are available and accessible to those with mobility difficulties and to the wheelchair bound.

To be included in the guide, organisations have to meet our stringent access criteria and some notable destinations have been omitted because they failed to do so. We are grateful to the many organisations and individuals who have assisted in our research and to those who have modified their facilities as a result of our inspection in order to be included.

To assist us in keeping this guide up to date, a tear-off card for your comments, suggestions, corrections and additions is included at the back of this edition, which we hope you will complete.

Finally, we hope this guide will help you to enjoy a Smooth Ride.

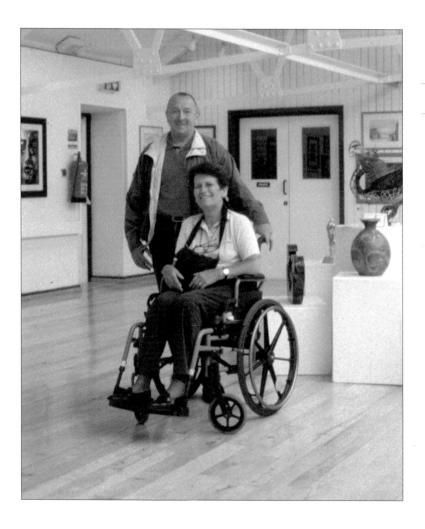

NATIONAL ACCESSIBILITY CRITERIA FOR ACCOMMODATION AND ATTRACTIONS

CATEGORY 1 ♿ Accessible to a wheelchair-user travelling independently.
CATEGORY 2 ♿ Accessible to a wheelchair-user travelling with assistance.
CATEGORY 3 🚶 Accessible to a wheelchair-user or someone with limited mobility, able to walk a few paces and up a maximum of three steps.

The minimum requirements for each of the three categories of accessibility are as follows.

ACCOMMODATION – CATEGORY REQUIREMENTS
PUBLIC ENTRANCE

CATEGORY 3 🚶	CATEGORY 2 ♿	CATEGORY 1 ♿
1. A public entrance must be accessible to wheelchair users from a setting down point or a car park.		
2. If an establishment has a car park, a reservable parking space should be available for a disabled guest on request.		1. If there is a car park, there must be a level reservable space with a minimum width of 3.6m for each bedroom meeting the Category 1 requirements.
3. The route from the parking point or space to the entrance must be sound and free from obstacles. Deep gravel, cobbles or pot-holed surfaces are unlikely to be acceptable.		2. The route from parking point or space to the entrance must be level or ramped.
4. Entrance door must have a clear opening of not less than 70cm.		
5. Where there is no ramp, there must be no more than three steps at any one point to the entrance.	1. Where there is no ramp there must be no more than single steps to the entrance.	3. The threshold at the entrance must be no higher than 2cm.
6. Within the reception area there must be an unobstructed space of not less than 110x70cm.		

INTERIOR GENERAL

CATEGORY 3 🚶

1. Public passageways that lead to a restaurant, dining room, lounge, TV lounge (unless TV is provided in the bedroom), bar, disabled guest's bedroom and bathroom (if other than en suite), should be not less than 75cm wide. The immediate approach to the entrance must include no more than three steps.

2. Doors to the rooms referred to above should have a clear opening of not less than 70cm.

3. There must be no more than three steps at any one point in the corridors a disabled guest will be required to use or at the entrance of the rooms referred to above.

4. If a disabled guest is required to use a lift, the door should have a clear opening of not less than 70cm and the interior of the lift should be not less than 110cm deep by 70cm wide.

3. Have no more than three steps at any point along the route or more than three steps in each 50m.

CATEGORY 2 ♿

1. Public passageways that lead to a restaurant or dining room, lounge, TV lounge (unless TV is provided in the bedroom), bar, disabled guest's bedroom and bathroom (if other than en suite), should not be less than 80cm wide and not less than 120cm opposite the doors to the rooms a disabled guest will be required to use.

2. Doors to the rooms referred to above should have a clear opening of not less than 75cm.

3. There must be no more than single steps at any one point in the corridors or to the rooms a disabled guest will be required to use.

4. In the restaurant or dining room there must be at least one accessible table with a clear underspace of at least 65cm. Blocks to lift the table when required, are acceptable. Where three or more bedrooms meet the requirements for Category 2 or 1, at least two such accessible tables should be provided.

5. If a disabled guest is required to use a lift, the door should have a clear opening of not less than 75cm and the interior of the lift should be not less than 120cm deep by 80cm wide.

CATEGORY 1 ♿

1. All routes to be used by a disabled guest must be level or ramped.

2. Access to a restaurant or dining room, lounge, bar, bedroom, bathroom and WC (where not en suite) must be level or ramped with thresholds that are no higher than 2cm.

3. Where a disabled guest is required to use a lift it must have automatic doors with controls 140cm or less above the floor.

BEDROOM (Only one bedroom should meet these requirements.)

CATEGORY 3 [⚹]	CATEGORY 2 [♿]	CATEGORY 1 [♿]
	1. There must be unobstructed space of not less than 110cm x70cm.	
	2. On at least one side of the bed there must be space of not less than 80cm to allow for lateral transfer.	
		1. The surface of the bed must be between 45-54cm above the floor.
		2. Door handles, light switches, TV controls, curtain pulls, wardrobe rails, etc. should be accessible and not more than 140cm above the floor.
		3. Light switch and telephone (where provided) should be no more than 50cm from the bed.

WC

CATEGORY 3 [⚹]	CATEGORY 2 [♿]	CATEGORY 1 [♿]
1. The WC must be en suite or on the same floor as a disabled guest's bedroom.		
2. Toilet paper must be within reach of the seat.		
	1. There must be a lateral transfer space to the WC of not less than 80cm.	
	2. The rim of the WC seat must be between 45-50cm above the floor.	
	3. There must be a horizontal or angled support rail opposite the transfer space, between 20-30cm above the seat.	
3. Where the WC is separate from the bathroom there must be a washbasin in the same room.	4. If separate from the bedroom, there must be an unobstructed interior space of not less than 100x70cm and a washbasin with clear underspace.	1. The horizontal or angled support rail opposite the transfer space must be no more than 50cm from the centre of the seat.

BATHROOM. Categories 1 and 2. (Only one bathroom, separate or en suite with the bedroom(s) above, should meet these requirements.)

CATEGORY 3	CATEGORY 2	CATEGORY 1
1. The bathroom must be en suite or on the same floor as a disabled guest's bedroom.		1. The door handle and light switch must be 140cm or less above floor level.
	1. There must be an unobstructed interior space, clear of the door swing, of not less than 100x70cm.	2. The horizontal or angled support rail at the far side of the bath must be no more than 30cm above the rim.
2. Where a bath is provided it should have a horizontal or angled support rail on the far side (recommended height is 25cm above the rim).		
	2. Where a bath is provided there must be space alongside of not less than 80cm to allow for lateral transfer.	3. The rim of the bath must be 45-50cm above floor level.
3. Where only a shower is provided, it must have a seat (recommended height 45-50cm above the floor) and a support rail on the far wall (recommended height 25cm above the top of the seat and a maximum of 50cm from the centre of seat).		
	3. Where only a shower is provided, it must have a level entry, i.e. no rim, a lateral transfer space of not less than 80cm, and a seat.	4. Where only a shower is available, the controls must be 140cm or less above floor level.
4. Where there is a step into the shower, it should have a rise of no more than 19cm.		
5. There must be a washbasin within the bathroom or bedroom.	4. The washbasin, either within the bathroom or bedroom, must have sufficient clear underspace and/or lever taps to enable it to be used by someone in a wheelchair.	

KITCHENS (Self-catering-units only.)

CATEGORY 3 🚶	CATEGORY 2 ♿	CATEGORY 1 ♿
		1. There must be a minimum clear floor space of 120cm in front of units and work surfaces.
		2. At least one work surface or table should have a clear underspace between 65-80cm.
		3. The hob should be not more than 80cm high, have a clear underspace below or alongside, and accessible controls.
		4. The oven should have front controls and base between 65cm and 80cm above floor level.
		5. The sink should have level taps and a clear underspace.
		6. The base of wall cupboards and shelves should not be more than 120cm above floor level.
		7. Light switches and door handles should not be more than 140cm above floor level.
		8. Power socket should be unobstructed and not more than 140cm above floor level (extension sockets acceptable).
		9. A fire extinguisher or fire blanket, not more than 140cm above floor level, should be sited between hob and doorway and be accessible.

ATTRACTIONS – CATEGORY REQUIREMENTS

APPROACH

CATEGORY 3 🚶	CATEGORY 2 ♿	CATEGORY 1 ♿
1. A public entrance must be accessible to wheelchair users from either a setting down point or a car park. Any such setting down point must have a firm level surface regardless of whether or not there is a car park.		
2. If an attraction has a car park but no setting down point, two dedicated car parking spaces plus one for every 50 spaces up to a maximum of 20 dedicated spaces should be provided. Dedicated spaces should be as close as possible to the entrance but no farther than 100m.		1. If there is no general car park, there must be at least two dedicated parking spaces, each with a minimum width of 360cm, capable of being reserved in advance.
3. All such dedicated spaces must be clearly signposted and marked using the international wheelchair symbol.		2. If there is a car park, each dedicated space must have a minimum width of 360cm (that may include wheelchair transfer space with an adjoining dedicated space).
4. The car park surface of dedicated spaces and the route to the nearest public entrance must be firm, sound and free from obstacles. Rough grass, deep gravel, cobbles and pot-holed surfaces are not acceptable.		
5. The route to the nearest entrance from dedicated parking spaces must have no more than three steps at any one point and no more than three per 50m. Steps should have risers no greater than 19cm, treads no less than 25cm deep and 75cm wide. Where there are two or more steps a handrail must be provided.	1. The route to the entrance from dedicated parking spaces must be no more than 100m and must have no more than single steps at any one point and no more than three such steps per 50m. Steps may have risers no greater than 19cm, treads no less than 120cm deep and 75cm wide. There must be a clear space not less than 360cm between each step.	3. The route to the entrance must not include steps and must not be steeper than 1:15. Long slopes must have level resting places 150cm long at no more than 10m intervals.

6. Where provided, paths must be not less than 75cm wide and passing places not less than 150cm x 150cm must be provided at intervals of not less than 25m.	2. Where provided, paths must be not less than 90cm wide and passing places not less than 150cm x 150cm must be provided at intervals of not less than 25m.	
7. Slopes on the route must be not steeper than 1:12 at any point and level resting places 150cm long must be provided at 10m intervals on paths or slopes that exceed 15m in length.		
NB: Requirements 4, 5, 6, & 7 may be waived where a regular shuttle transport plies between the car park and the entrance, provided the transport has no more than three steps and is capable of carrying a folded wheelchair.	NB: Category Three waiver applies, provided the vehicle has a wheelchair lift.	NB: Category Two waiver applies

ENTRANCE

CATEGORY 3	CATEGORY 2	CATEGORY 1
1. The immediate approach to the entrance must not have more than three steps.	1. The immediate approach to the entrance must not have more than three single steps with a minimum space of 120cm between each step.	1. The immediate approach to the entrance must be level or ramped with a gradient not exceeding 1:15, with a level landing 120cm deep clear of any door swing, and with level resting places 150cm long at no more than 10m intervals.
2. Thresholds must not exceed 5cm and must be adequately tapered if they exceed 2cm.	2. Ramps must be no steeper than 1:12. The steeper gradient of 1:10 for internal ramps less than 1.5m long is not acceptable.	2. Thresholds must not exceed 2cm.
3. Ramps should be no steeper than 1:12 with level resting places 150cm long at no more than 10m intervals. NB: For internal ramps 1:12 is the preferred gradient except for ramps of less than 1.5m where 1:10 is acceptable. Ramps must be of solid construction, well maintained with a slip-resistant surface.		

4. The entrance door or gate must have a clear opening of not less than 67cm. If the normal entrance is via a turnstile or kissing gate, an alternative nearby entrance with a clear opening of no less than 67cm must be available.

FACILITIES including WCs, retail units, bars. (If an attraction includes one or more of these facilities, at least one or more of each facility must be accessible.)

The route to each accessible facility must

CATEGORY 3	CATEGORY2	CATEGORY 1
1. Have a firm, sound surface, free from obstacles.	1. The route to each accessible facility must have no more than single steps at any point with a minimum space of 120cm between each step and no more than three steps in each 50m.	
2. Contain no incline or ramp steeper than 1:12 except for internal ramps less than 1.5m long where 1:10 is acceptable. Level resting places 150cm long must be provided at no more than 10m intervals on paths or slopes that exceed 15m in length	2. The route to each accessible facility must contain no incline or ramp steeper than 1:12. The steeper gradient of 1:10 for internal ramps less than 1.5m long is not acceptable.	1. The route to each accessible facility must be level or ramped with gradients not exceeding 1:15.
3. Have no more than three steps at any point along the route or more than three steps in each 50m.	3. The route to each accessible facility must have corridors or paths (where present) not less than 90cm wide.	
4. Have corridors or paths (where present) not less than 75cm wide.		
5. Have no doors along the route with clear opening widths of less than 67cm or clear approaches less than 110cm deep.		
6. Have no more than three steps at the entrance. Where there are two or more steps a handrail must be provided.		

13

7. Where the route requires the use of a lift or lifts, their doors should have clear openings of not less than 67cm and internal dimensions of not less than 110cm deep by 70cm wide.		4. Where the route requires the use of a lift or lifts, their doors must have clear opening widths of not less than 75cm and internal dimensions not less than 140cm deep by 110cm wide. Controls for the lift must not be more than 140cm above the floor or landing.
	4. If an attraction has only one WC, it must be an accessible unisex facility.	2. If an attraction contains more than one WC facility, all those located on Category 1 accessible routes must contain an accessible unisex facility.
	5. If an attraction has more than one WC facility, at least 50% of those on Category 2 access routes must be accessible unisex WC facilities.	
	6. Within an accessible WC: a) There must be no more than a single step at the entrance. b) The entrance must not be locked and must have a clear opening width of not less than 75cm and a clear approach not less than 120cm deep. c) There must be unobstructed interior space of not less than 110cm x 70cm. d) There must be a lateral transfer space to the WC of not less than 80cm. e) The rim of the WC seat must be between 45cm and 50cm above the floor. f) A toilet paper dispenser must be within easy reach of the WC. g) There must be a horizontal support rail 65 to 75cm above the floor on the wall opposite the transfer space and positioned between 40 and 50cm from the centre of the seat. h) A hinged support rail must be located on the transfer side. i) There must be a washbasin within the WC with clear underspace to allow access to a wheelchair user. j) A soap dispenser must be located within reach of a wheelchair user at the washbasin. k) A hand dryer and/or paper towel dispenser must be within reach of a wheelchair user at the washbasin.	3. All such accessible WC facilities must be unisex and conform to Part T Building Regulations (Scotland only). Door widths must provide a clear opening width of 80cm.

l) A light switch must not be more than 140cm above the floor.

7. Within an accessible catering outlet and/or bar;
a) There must be no more than a single step at the entrance.
b) The entrance must have a clear opening width not less than 75cm and a clear approach not less than 120cm deep.
c) There must be at least two, plus one in 10, accessible tables with a clear underspace at least 70cm high, 60cm wide and 45cm deep.

8. Within an accessible shop;
a) There must be no more than a single step at the entrance.
b) The entrance must have a clear opening width not less than 75cm and a clear approach not less than 120cm deep.
c) Where there are aisles they must be at least 90cm wide.

FEATURES (Displays, exhibits, rides etc. within an attraction.)

The route to the feature must:

CATEGORY 3 ♿	CATEGORY 2 ♿	CATEGORY 1 ♿
1. Have a firm, sound surface, free from obstacles.		
2. Contain no incline or ramp steeper than 1:12 except for internal ramps less than 1.5m long where 1:10 is acceptable. Level resting places 150cm long must be provided at no more than 10m intervals on paths or slopes that exceed 15m in length.	2. The route to each accessible feature must contain no incline or ramp steeper than 1:12. The steeper gradient of 1:10 for internal ramps less than 1.5m in length is not acceptable.	
3. Have no more than three steps at any point along the route or more than three steps in each 50m.	1. There should be no more than single steps at any one point with a minimum space of 120cm between each step.	1. The route to each accessible feature must be level or ramped with gradients not exceeding 1:15.

4. Have corridors or paths, where present, not less than 75cm wide.	3. There should be no corridors or paths, where present, less than 90cm wide.	
5. Have no doors along the route or at the entrance with clear opening widths of less than 67cm or clear approaches less than 110cm deep.		
6. Have no more than three steps at the entrance. Where there are two or more steps, a handrail must be provided.		3. Entrances and interiors of accessible features must be level or ramped with gradients not exceeding 1:15 and thresholds must be no higher than 2cm.
7. Where the route requires the use of a lift or lifts, their doors should have clear openings of not less than 67cm and internal dimensions of not less than 110cm deep by 70cm wide.		2. Where the route requires the use of a lift or lifts, their doors must have clear opening widths of not less than 75cm and internal dimensions not less than 140cm deep by 110cm wide. Controls for the lift must not be more than 140cm above the floor or landing.

The symbols shown in grey are categories that *Smooth Ride Guides* has devised and have been awarded where appropriate by *Smooth Ride Guides* inspectors.

CODE EXPLANATIONS – ATTRACTIONS

SD = set down
RF = route to facilities
S = shop
G = garden

CP = carpark
L = lift
WC = toilet

E = entrance
C = catering
RFE = route to features

CODE EXPLANATIONS – THEATRES, CONCERT HALLS, SPORTS VENUES

RE = route to entrance
AUD = auditorium

ED = entrance door
SS = stadium seating

INT = interior
B/R = bar or restaurant

FINDING YOUR WAY

AIRPORTS

How to travel by air with a wheelchair.

AIR CARRIER ACCESS RULES

web: www.faa.gov/acr/dat.htm

Usually you can use your own wheelchair so far as the boarding point of the aircraft, where you transfer to a special aisle chair. If you are able to walk a short distance, you should request a seat near the entrance doors. Your own wheelchair will be stored for immediate availability on arrival. You have a choice about preboarding although the airline probably will want to preboard you, so arrive at the airport early.

TYPES OF WHEELCHAIR

1. Normal hand-propelled chairs.
2. Electric wheelchairs, including scooters with wet acid batteries.
3. Electric wheelchairs, including scooters with dry cell or seal gel batteries. Check with the airline if you have type 2 because the battery could be removed and placed in the hold. If so you should be at the airport at least three hours before departure. Most power-operated wheelchairs have safety batteries, but the leads must be disconnected from the terminal and capped to avoid shorting. Pre-boarding may be necessary and there could be a delay on arrival. The airline is responsible for ensuring your battery is reconnected and the chair is working on arrival at your destination. Electric scooter battery requirements are the same as for wheelchairs.

Notes: Wide aisles = more than 90cm wide. High tables = more than 65cm underspace. Trained staff = trained in disability awareness.

ABERDEEN AIRPORT

Dyce AB21 7DU

Tel: (01224) 722331   Fax: (01224) 725751

Setting down point near entrance: 15 non-reservable orange badge spaces, pre-arranged assistance or by telephone in car park from car park to check in. Route to entrance has no lifts: accessible revolving entrance with special controls for wheelchair users and alternative non-automatic side door with level route to check-in. 3 unisex adapted WCs (1 main concourse, 1 main departures, 1 international departures). 2 Restaurants, 4 bars. Ramp down to departure lounge. Shop with ramp, ramp from check-in to departures: First aid at information desk. Wheelchairs available.

ALDERNEY AIRPORT (Channel Islands)

The Blaye, Alderney

Tel: (01481) 822624   Fax: (01481) 623005

Very small airport, setting down point near entrance. No orange badge parking. Level route to entrance, no lifts. Accessible non-automatic door. Route to check-in level, no lifts. 2 separate WCs (150 x 150cm with rail next to WC, not hinged, outward opening door). No bars, restaurants, or shops. Accessible route from check-in to departure. Accessible public phones. No printed information. Medical and first aid available but no trained staff. Wheelchairs available. Can stay in own wheelchair until boarding.

BARRA AIRPORT Western Isles

Eoligarry, Isle of Barra HS9 5UA

Tel: (01871) 890212   Fax: (01871) 890220

Setting down point near entrance. No Orange badge parking. Informal assistance given. Level route to accessible entrance and check-in, no lifts. 1 unisex adapted WC (300 x 300cm, support rail next to WC, hinged rail, outward opening door). Restaurant with high tables. 1 accessible shop, no aisles. Accessible route from check-in to departures. No wheelchairs possible on board. Accessible public phones. No printed information. Medical and first aid available but no trained staff. No wheelchairs available. Can stay in own wheelchair until boarding.

BELFAST CITY AIRPORT
Sydenham By-Pass, Belfast BT3 9JH
Tel: (02890) 457745   Fax: (02890) 738455

Setting down point near entrance. 8 non-reservable orange badge spaces. Assistance by prior arrangement. Accessible non-automatic entrance route to check-in level. Level route from check-in to departure. Level entrance to arrivals. Ramped entrance to departures (less than 1:12, slip resistant, 200cm wide), no steps. 4 unisex adapted WCs (1 departure area, 1 boarding lounge, 1 arrival hall, 1 arrivals waiting, 200 x 180cm, support rail next to WC, hinged support rail, 2 with outward opening doors). 3 Restaurants, 3 bars all with level access and low tables, but not low counters. Accessible shops with wide aisles. Ambulift available, but generally carried. Public phones not accessible. No printed information. First aid trained staff. Wheelchairs available. Can stay in own wheelchair until boarding.

BELFAST INTERNATIONAL AIRPORT
Belfast BT29 4AB
Tel: (02894) 484848/484313
Fax: (02894) 423883

Setting down point near entrance. 16 non-reservable orange badge spaces. 24hr. porterage. Level route to entrance, no steps. Accessible entrance with automatic door, level route to check-in. 8 accessible lifts. 11 separate WCs all over airport (5ft^2), support rails, hinged support rails, outward opening doors. 2 restaurants, 6 bars, all accessible, 1 with ramp, high tables. Accessible shops with wide aisles. Accessible route from check-in to departures via lift. Alternative, 6 gates with bridge, Ambulift and chairlift. Accessible public phones. Printed information available. Medical and first aid available, trained staff. Wheelchairs available. Can stay in own wheelchair until boarding. Information supplied by member of Transport Advisory Committee of Disability Action for Northern Ireland.

BIRMINGHAM INTERNATIONAL AIRPORT
Birmingham B26 3QJ
Tel: (0121) 7678275   Fax: (0121) 7677357

Setting down point near entrance.

Unreservable orange badge spaces. Bus from long-stay car park. Level route to entrance. Accessible, automatic door. Level route to check-in. 22 lifts conform to specs. 23 adapted unisex WCs (measurements unavailable, both supports, outward opening doors). 5 bars, 9 restaurants (table height unavailable). Shops with level access. Accessible route to check-in, sometimes via lift. Accessible public phones. Printed information available. Medical and first aid available. Staff trained in disability awareness, some special staff employed. Wheelchairs available. Can stay in own wheelchair until boarding.

BOURNEMOUTH INTERNATIONAL AIRPORT
Christchurch, Dorset BH23 6SE
Tel: (01202) 364000/364170
Fax: (01202) 364179

Setting down point near entrance. 5 non-reservable orange badge spaces. Assistance provided, minibus available. Level route to entrance. Automatic accessible main entrance door. Level route to check-in, no lifts. 3 unisex adapted WCs (smallest 165 x 235cm, support rail, hinged support rail, outward opening doors. 2 bars, 1 restaurant with high tables. Shops with wide aisles. Accessible route from check-in to departure. Lifts for boarding. Accessible public phones, will lower other phones. Printed information available. Medical and first aid available, trained staff. Wheelchairs available. Can stay in own wheelchair until boarding.

BRISTOL INTERNATIONAL AIRPORT
Bristol BS49 3DY
Tel: (01275) 474444   Fax: (01275) 474767

New terminal completed January 2000. Setting down point near entrance. 76 non-reservable orange badge space. Full assistance from car park to entrance by prior notice. Level route to entrance. Automatic accessible main entrance door. Level route to check-in. 1 accessible lift. 4 unisex adapted WCs (smallest 162 x 172cm support rail next to WC, no hinged support rail, inward opening door). 1 restaurant, 3 bars, main restaurant has high tables. Shops with wide aisles. Accessible route from check-in to departures. Boarding via lifts. Accessible public phones. Printed information available. Medical and first aid available. Staff disabled-aware. Wheelchairs available. can stay in own wheelchair until boarding. Bristol International Flyer; dedicated bus from Bristol Temple Meads railway station and bus station.

CARDIFF INTERNATIONAL AIRPORT
Vale of Glamorgan CF62 3BD
Tel: (01446) 711111   Fax: (01446) 711675

Setting down point near entrance. Some orange badge spaces. Assistance provided on request through travel agent. Level route to entrance. No lifts. Accessible automatic entrance door. Level route to check-in. 4 lifts (104 x 134cm, controls 130-150cm above floor and **not accessible** but to be addressed). 4 adapted unisex and separate WCs (standard sizes, both support rails, outward opening doors). 2 restaurants, 2 bars, all with high tables. Shops with wide aisles. Accessible route from check-in to departure. Boarding via airbridges or lifts. Accessible public phones. Printed information. Medical and first aid available. Most staff are trained. Wheelchairs available. Special staff employed. Can stay in own wheelchair until boarding.

CARLISLE AIRPORT
Carlisle CA6 4NW
Tel: (01228) 573641   Fax: (01228) 573310

Setting down point near entrance. No orange badge spaces. Assistance provided. Level route to entrance. No lifts. Automatic accessible entrance door. Level route to check-in. No lifts. No adapted WCs. 1 bar/restaurant with high tables. No shops. Accessible route from check-in to departure. No airbridges or lifts. 8 accessible public phones. No printed information. Medical and first aid available. Staff trained in disability awareness. No special staff. Wheelchair available. Can stay in own wheelchair until boarding.

DUNDEE AIRPORT
Riverside Drive, Dundee DD2 1UH
Tel: (01382) 643242   Fax: (01382) 641263

Setting down point near entrance. 2 non-reservable orange badge spaces, tel: 01382 641263 with arrival time for assistance.

Level route to entrance. Automatic accessible main entrance door. Level route to check-in. No lifts. 3 unisex-adapted WCs to part M (1 landside, 1 airside departures, 1 baggage reclaim, with support rail next to WC, hinged support rail, outward opening doors). No bars, restaurants or shops. Accessible route from check-in to departures. Accessible public phones. No printed information. Trained staff. Wheelchairs available. Can stay in own wheelchair until boarding.

EAST MIDLANDS AIRPORT
Castle Donnington, Derbyshire DE74 2SA
Tel: (01332) 852852/852885
Fax: (01332) 852899

Setting down point near entrance: 30 reservable orange badge spaces. Phone information desk for assistance from car park to check-in. Level route to entrance, no steps. Automatic accessible main entrance door. Level route to check-in. 2 accessible lifts. 9 adapted unisex WCs, varying sizes, none less than 140cm, all with both support rails, most with outward opening doors. 4 bars, 2 restaurants. Shops accessible, but not all with wide aisles. Accessible route from check-in to departures. Pre-boarded by ambulift. 20 accessible public phones. Printed material available. Medical and first aid available, trained staff. Wheelchairs available. Can stay in own wheelchair until boarding. On site taxi firm can provide wheelchair-accessible transport.

EDINBURGH AIRPORT
Edinburgh EH12 9DN
Tel: (0131) 3331000   Fax: (0131) 3333181

Setting down point near entrance. 10 non-reservable orange badge spaces. No assistance from car park to check-in. Route level to entrance (low, wide, slip-resistant ramp over road). Automatic accessible entry door. 4 accessible lifts. 3 unisex adapted WCs conforming to BAA specs, support rail, hinged support rail, outward opening doors. 2 bars, 3 restaurants with high tables. Accessible shops with wide aisles. 4 accessible phones. Check-in to departure via lift. Boarding by airbridges where necessary.

No printed information. First aid available. Wheelchairs available. No trained staff. Can stay in own wheelchair until boarding.

EXETER AND DEVON AIRPORT
Exeter, Devon EX5 2BD
Tel: (01392) 367433   Fax: (01392) 445539

Assistance provided from set-down point into terminal with slip-resistant ramp. 7 reservable orange badge parking spaces. Level automatic entrance door. Level route to check-in. 3 adapted unisex WCs (1 check-in, 1 arrivals, 1 departures), 140 x 240cm with support rail, hinged support rail, outward opening doors. 1 restaurant, 1 bar with high tables. Level shops with wide aisles. Accessible route from check-in to departure. Specially designed lift-on. Accessible phones. First aid available. No trained staff. Wheelchairs available. Can remain in own wheelchair until boarding.

GLASGOW PAISLEY AIRPORT
Paisley PA3 2ST
Tel: (0141) 8484255/8484778
Fax: (0141) 8484354

Setting down point near entrance. 34 non-reservable orange badge spaces. Fax in advance for assistance (0141) 8484354. Level route to entrance. 2 unisex-adapted WCs 240 x 175cm with supports rails, hinged support tail and outward opening doors. 4 restaurants, 3 bars, all with high tables. Shops with wide aisles. Accessible route from check-in to departures via lift and/or ramp. Boarding by airbridge or Ambulift. Accessible public phones. Printed information available. Medical and first aid available. Staff trained. Wheelchairs available. Can stay in own wheelchair until boarding.

GLASGOW PRESTWICK INTERNATIONAL AIRPORT
Aviation House, Prestwick KA9 2PL
Tel: (01292) 479822/511234
Fax: (01292) 511010

Setting down point near entrance. 30 non-reservable orange badge spaces. Prior notice for assistance recommended. Ramped entrance (1:50, slip-resistant, 250cm wide), no steps or lifts. Automatic accessible entrance door. Level route to

check-in. Lift if arriving by train, 2 lifts at rail station (car interiors 97 x 133cm, controls 130cm high). 1 WC in concourse confirming to spec, 6 unisex and separate WCs to part M, 200 x 200cm, support rail next to WC, hinged support rail, outward opening or sliding doors. 2 bars, 2 restaurants with high tables. Shops with wide aisles. Accessible route from check-in to departures. Boarding via specially adapted vehicle if necessary. Public phones not accessible. No printed information. Medical and first aid available. Wheelchairs available Staff not trained, but aware. Can stay in own wheelchair until boarding. This airport is used every year by those making pilgrimages to Lourdes, it handles large numbers of passengers with mobility difficulties, and is recognised for its sensitive, friendly handling.

STATES OF GUERNSEY AIRPORT
Channel Islands
La Villiaze, Forest, Guernsey
Tel: (01481) 37766/37267
Fax: (01481) 39595

Setting down point near entrance: 3 non-reservable orange badge spaces. Staff available for assistance. Level route to entrance. Automatic accessible door. Level route to check-in. No lifts. 1 unisex-adapted WC, 280 x 170cm, support rail next to WC, hinged support rail, inward opening door. 1 bar, 1 restaurant with high tables. Shops with wide aisles. Accessible route from check-in to departures. Manually lifted on board. Public phones not accessible. No printed information. Medical and first aid available. Staff not trained. Wheelchairs available. Can stay in own wheelchair until boarding. New terminal anticipated during the next three years when better access facilities will be considered.

HUMBERSIDE INTERNATIONAL AIRPORT
Kirmington, Lincolnshire DN39 6YH
Tel: (01652) 688456   Fax: (01652) 680524

Setting down point near entrance. 6 non-reservable orange badge spaces. Assistance preferably pre-arranged. Level route to entrance. No steps or lifts. Automatic accessible entrance door. 4 unisex-adapted WCs, smallest 170 x 133cm, all with support rails next to WC, hinged support rails and outward opening doors. 1 bar, 1 restaurant with some high tables. Shops with wide aisles. Accessible route from check-in to departures. Boarding by Ambulift. Accessible public phones. Printed information available. Medical and first aid available. Trained staff. Wheelchairs available. Can stay in own wheelchair until boarding.

INVERNESS AIRPORT
Inverness, Scotland IV1 2JB
Tel: (01463) 232471 Fax: (01667) 462041
Setting down point near entrance. 2 non-reservable orange badge spaces. Contact airline for assistance. Level route to entrance. Automatic accessible main entrance door. No lifts. 1 unisex-adapted WC, 300 x 200cm, both support rails, outward opening doors, on ground floor. 1 bar, 1 restaurant with high tables. Shops with wide aisles. Level route from check-in to departure. Boarding via Ambulift. Accessible public phones. No printed information. First aid available. Wheelchairs available. Trained staff. Can stay in own wheelchair until boarding.

ISLE OF MAN AIRPORT
Ballasalla, Isle of Man IM0 2AS
Tel: (01624) 821603 Fax: (01624) 821611
web: www.iom-airport.com
Setting down point near entrance. 10 non-reservable orange badge spaces. No assistance from car park to entrance. Ramped route to entrance (less than 1:12, slip resistant, 200cm wide, no steps, no lifts). Accessible entry door. 4 lifts, all conform to specs. 4 adapted WCs, 150 x 205cm, both support rails, outward opening door. 2 bars, 2 restaurants with high tables. Shops with wide aisles. Check-in to departure via lift. Boarding by lift, Ambulift, airline staff assist PRM. Accessible public phones. Printed information available. First aid. Some staff trained. Wheelchairs available. Staff prefer passenger to transfer to airport chairs. Major refurbishment in 1999.

ISLES OF SCILLY AIRPORT
St. Mary's, Isles of Scilly, Cornwall TR21 0NG

Tel: (01720) 422677 Fax: (01720) 423302
Setting down point near entrance. No orange badge spaces. Duty crew available for assistance. Ramp to entrance (1:10, not slip resistant, 112cm wide, no steps, no lifts). Automatic accessible main entrance door. No lifts in terminal. 1 unisex-adapted WC, 240 x 150cm, both support rails, inward opening door. 1 bar/restaurant with high tables. Short ramp between lounge and buffet area. No shops. Accessible route from check-in to departure. Accessible public phones. No printed information. First aid available. No trained staff. Wheelchairs available. Can stay in own wheelchair until boarding.

JERSEY STATES AIRPORT Channel Islands
St. Peter, Jersey JE1 2BY
Tel: (01534) 492266/490999
Fax: (01534) 498084
Setting down point near entrance. 6 non-reservable orange badge spaces. Assistance through customer service agents. Level route to entrance. Automatic accessible main entrance door. 2 lifts conforming to specs. 5 adapted unisex WCs, 162 x 140cm, both support rails, outward opening doors. 2 bars, 2 restaurants with high tables. Shops with wide aisles. Level route from check-in to departures. No airbridges or Ambulifts. Accessible public phones. No printed information. Limited first aid available Sat/Sun. Staff not trained, but special staff employed.

KIRKWALL AIRPORT
Orkney, Scotland KW15 1TH
Tel: (01856) 872421 Fax: (01856) 871252
Small split-level airport. New terminal under consideration but no decision taken when inspected in May 1999. Set-down point near entrance. 1 non-reservable orange badge space. No assistance. Level route to entrance. Accessible automatic entrance door. No lifts in terminal. 1 unisex-adapted WC, 330 x 140cm, support rail next to WC, no hinged support rail, inward opening door. 1 restaurant with high tables. No shops. Route from check-in to departures not accessible inside, requires exit and re-entry to building. Boarding via Ambulift. Accessible public phones. No

printed information. Limited first aid. No trained staff. Wheelchairs available. Can stay in own wheelchair until boarding.

LANDS END AERODROME
St. Just, Penzance, Cornwall TR19 2BL
Tel: (01736) 788771
Very small airport with limited facilities. Setting down point near entrance. No designated parking. Level entrance. Non-automatic door. Level route to check-in. No lifts. No adapted WC. 1 unisex WC 75 x 130cm without handrails in Skybus lounge. 1 restaurant, level access, low tables. No shops. Level route from check-in to departure. Accessible public phones. Limited first aid available. Some staff are trained. Wheelchairs available.

LEEDS BRADFORD INTERNATIONAL AIRPORT
Leeds, West Yorks LS19 7TU
Tel: (0113) 2509696   Fax: (0113) 2505426
Setting down point near entrance. 30 non-reservable orange badge spaces. Assistance available. Level route to entrance. Automatic accessible entry door. Level route to check-in. 3 lifts conforming to specs. 5 unisex adapted WCs, 245 x 2175cm, both support rails, outward opening doors. 2 restaurants, 3 bars with high tables. Shops with wide aisles. Accessible route from check-in to departures. Boarding via airbridge and lifts. Accessible public phones. No printed information. First aid available. Trained staff. Wheelchairs available. Special company Airway to assist special needs passengers. Can stay in own wheelchair until boarding.

LERWICK SUMBURGH AIRPORT
Uirkig, Shetland, Scotland
Tel: (01950) 460204   Fax: (01950) 460218
Set-down point near entrance. 5 reservable orange badge spaces. Assistance provided. Level route to entrance. Accessible automatic entrance door. No lifts in terminal. 1 adapted unisex WC to part M, outward opening door. 1 bar, 1 restaurant. Shops with wide aisles. Level route from check-in to departure. Boarding via Ambulift. No accessible public phones. No printed information. First Aid. No trained staff. Wheelchairs

available. Can stay in own wheelchair until boarding.

LERWICK TINGWALL AIRPORT
Toll Clock, Lerwick, Shetland ZE1 0PE
Tel: (01595) 744872   Fax: (01595) 744869
Set-down point near entrance. No orange badge spaces. Assistance by airline staff. Level route to entrance. Non-automatic accessible entrance door. No lifts. 1 unisex adapted WC, 148 x 242cm, both support rails, outward opening door. No bars or restaurants. No shops. No public phones. No printed information. No trained staff. No wheelchairs available. Tingwall is the base for an inter-island service via Loganair using a seven-seater B/N Islander aircraft that also is used as an air ambulance.

LIVERPOOL AIRPORT
Liverpool, Merseyside L24 1YD
Tel: (0151) 2884000   Fax: (0151) 2884120
Setting down point near entrance. 3 non-reservable orange badge spaces near entrance, 6 in NCP 100m. away, under review, request assistance when booking flight. Ramped entrance, gradient unknown, no steps, no lifts. Automatic accessible main entrance door. Level route to check-in. 1 lift conforming to specs. 3 unisex-adapted WCs, both support rails, outward opening door. 2 restaurants, 2 bars with high tables. Shops with wide aisles. Accessible route from check-in to departures. Boarding by Ambulift. Some accessible public phones. First aid available. Fire service have trained staff. Wheelchairs available. Can stay in own wheelchair until boarding. In 1998 this airport was nominated for an Ease award for services to disabled passengers judged on public response.

LONDON CITY AIRPORT
Royal Docks, London E1
Tel: (020) 7 6460092/6460088
Fax: (020) 7 4745747
Setting down point near entrance. 6 non-reservable orange badge spaces. No assistance provided from car park to check-in. Level route to entrance. Accessible automatic entrance door. Level route to check-in. No lifts. 5 unisex

adapted WCs (146 x 200cm, both support rails, outward opening doors). 2 bars, 2 restaurants with high tables. Shops with wide aisles. Accessible route from check-in to departures via lift. Board by lift. Accessible public phones. No special information. Some special staff. First aid available. Wheelchairs available. Can stay in own wheelchair until boarding.

LONDON GATWICK AIRPORT
Crawley, West Sussex RH6 0NP
Tel: (01293) 503124   Fax: (01293) 504177
Setting down point near entrance. More than 100 non-reservable orange badge spaces. Help points to request assistance. Route to main entrance with automatic door is level. Slip-resistant ramps elsewhere. Lifts to some entrances. Route to check-in varies by terminal entrance. More than 70 lifts all confirming to specs. Many unisex-adapted WCs of varying sizes, most with both support rails and outward opening doors. Many bars and restaurants, all with accessible tables. Shops with wide aisles. Routes from check-in to departures are accessible. Lift for route to UK departures in South Terminal. Boarding via Ambulifts and airbridges. Printed information available. Medical and first aid available. Key operational staff trained. Wheelchairs available. Can stay in own wheelchair until boarding. Annual accessibility audits.

LONDON HEATHROW AIRPORT
Heathrow Travel-Care, Room 1308, Queens Building, Heathrow Airport, Hounslow, Middlesex TW6 1BZ
Tel: (020) 8 7457495   Fax: (020) 8 7454161
Minicom: (020) 8 7457565
This organisation provides social work and counselling at LHR and produces Travellers' Information Guide – Special Needs Edition, a comprehensive guide to all aspects of LHR. It covers getting to and from the airport, parking, arrival, terminal layouts, checking-in, security check, connections, in the air, useful phone numbers and contacts. We strongly recommend a copy be obtained from: Passenger Relations, Public Affairs, Heathrow Airport Ltd. Heathrow Point, 234 Bath Road, Harlington, Middlesex

UB3 5AP, tel: (01233) 211207. SRG is always happy to answer specific queries, call us on (01279) 777966.

LONDON STANSTEAD AIRPORT
Stansted, Essex CM24 1QW
Tel: (01279) 662041/662039
Fax: (01279) 662066
Minicom: (01279) 663725
Setting down point near entrance. 24-hour short stay and 104 long stay unreservable orange badge spaces. Assistance provided on request from help point. Level and ramped route to entrance. Lifts to entrance level. Automatic accessible door. Level and ramped route to check-in desks. Several lifts all conforming to specs. 14 adapted unisex WCs conform to Part M (both supporting rails, outward opening doors). 5 bars, 8 restaurants, all with accessible tables. Accessible shops. Route from check-in to departures accessible, sometimes via lift. Boarding via airbridge and lifts. Accessible public phones. Printed information available. Some tactile/Braille

Stansted offers the finest of facilities for disabled people.

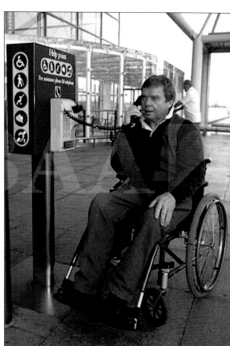

signage. Medical and first aid available. Some staff trained. Wheelchairs available. Some special staff employed. Buses from long-stay car parks are low floor.

MANCHESTER AIRPORT
Manchester M90 1QX
Tel: (0161) 4893000
Fax: (0161) 4893813/3647

Setting down point near entrance. Non-reservable orange badge spaces. Phone for assistance. Level route to entrance. Also lifts to entrance level. Automatic accessible main entrance door. Level route to check-in. 6 lifts conform to specs. Unisex-adapted WCs, number unknown. More than 20 restaurants and bars with high tables. Shops with wide aisles. Accessible route from check-in to departures, one route via lift. Boarding via airbridges and lifts. Accessible public phones. No printed information. Medical and first aid available. No trained staff. Wheelchairs available. Can stay in own wheelchair until boarding, special staff.

NEWCASTLE AIRPORT
Newcastle upon Tyne NE13 8BZ
Tel: (0191) 2144444/2143451
Fax: (0191) 2143351

Setting down point near entrance 50 non-reservable orange badge spaces. Phone from car park for assistance. Level route to entrance. Automatic accessible entrance door. 4 lifts conform to specs. 9 separate WCs, 220 x 140cm, both support rails, outward opening doors. 2 restaurants, 2 bars with high tables. Shops with wide aisles Accessible route from check-in to departures. Boarding by airbridge or lift. Accessible public phones. Printed information available. First Aid available. Trained staff. Wheelchairs available. Can stay in own wheelchair until boarding.

NEWQUAY CORNWALL AIRPORT
c/o Plymouth City Airport Ltd, Roborough House, Crownhill, Plymouth, Devon PL6 8BW
Tel: (01752) 209571/772752
Fax: (01752) 774885

Set-down point near entrance.

Designated non-reservable orange badge spaces. No assistance provided. Level route to entrance. Automatic accessible main entrance. No lifts. 2 adapted unisex WCs to part M, 174 x 146cm, both support rails, outward opening doors. 1 bar/restaurant with high tables. No shops. Accessible route from check-in to departure. Boarding by lift. Accessible public phones. No printed information. First aid available. No trained staff. Wheelchairs available. Can stay in own wheelchair until boarding.

NORWICH AIRPORT
Amsterdam Way, Norwich NR6 6JA
Tel: (01603) 420650/411923
Fax: (01603) 487523

Set-down point near entrance. 30 non-reservable orange badge spaces, assistance available if previously arranged with duty airport manager. Level route to entrance. Accessible entrance door. Level route to check-in, no lifts. 2 unisex-adapted WCs, both support rails, outward opening doors. 2 bars, 2 restaurants with high tables. Shops with wide aisles. Accessible route from check-in to departures. Boarding by lifts. No printed information. First aid available. Trained staff. Wheelchairs available. Passengers must transfer to airport wheelchair at check-in. Terminal on one level and very user-friendly.

PLYMOUTH CITY AIRPORT
Roborough House, Crownhill, Plymouth PL6 8BW
Tel: (01752) 772752
Fax: (01752) 774885

Setting down point near entrance. 4 non-reservable orange badge spaces. Assistance from car park to check-in available on request. Level route to entrance, then one step to accessible automatic entrance door. Level route to check-in, no lifts. 1 adapted unisex WC at check in, conforming to part M, 280 x 167cm with both support rails and outward opening doors. 1 bar, 1 restaurant with high tables. No shops. Accessible route from check-in to departure. Accessible public phones. First aid available. Wheelchairs available. Can stay in own wheelchair until boarding.

SOUTHAMPTON INTERNATIONAL AIRPORT
Southampton, Hants SO18 2NL
Tel: (02380) 620021/627099
Fax: (02380) 629300

Setting down point near entrance. 16 reservable orange badge spaces: Assistance provided on request. Level route to entrance. No lifts. Accessible automatic entrance door. Level route to check-in. 1 lift conforms to all specs. 4 adapted unisex WCs conforming to Part M (both support rails, outward opening doors). 2 bars/2 restaurants with high tables. Accessible shops. Accessible route from check-in to departure. Boarding by lift. Accessible public phones. Printed information available. First aid available. Special staff employed. Staff training in disability awareness. Wheelchairs available. Can stay in own wheelchair until boarding.

SOUTHEND AIRPORT
Southend on Sea, Essex SS2 6YF
Tel: (01702) 340201   Fax: (01702) 331715

Setting down point near entrance. 6 non-reservable orange badge spaces. Assistance by prior request. Level route to entrance. Manual accessible entrance door, no lifts. 1 adapted unisex WC, support rail next to WC, no hinged support rail, outward opening door. 1 bar, 1 restaurant with high tables. No shops. Accessible route from check-in to departures. Boarding by carry-on. Accessible public phones. First aid available. No trained staff. Wheelchairs available. Can stay in own wheelchair until boarding.

STORNOWAY AIRPORT
Stornoway, Isle of Lewis, Western Isles, Scotland HS2 0BN
Tel: (01851) 702256   Fax: (01851) 705090

Setting down point near entrance. No orange badge spaces. Assistance available. Main entrance ramped (1:10, slip-resistant, 1500cm wide, 1 step, no lift). Alternative accessible entrance. Level route to check-in. No lifts in terminal. 1 unisex-adapted WC, 240 x 130cm, support rail next to WC, no hinged support rail. 1 bar, 1 restaurant with high tables. Shops with wide aisles.

Accessible route from check-in to departures. Boarding by lift. No accessible public phones. First aid available. Trained staff. Wheelchairs available. Can stay in own chair until boarding. New terminal planned with more disability facilities.

TEESSIDE INTERNATIONAL AIRPORT
Darlington, North Yorks DL2 1LU
Tel: (01325) 332811 Fax: (01325) 332810

Setting down point near entrance. 12 non-reservable orange badge spaces. Prior notice for assistance. Level route to entrance with ramped kerbs. Accessible main entrance door. Level route to check-in. No lifts in terminal. 3 unisex, 2 separate WCs, 146 x 196cm, both support rails, outward opening doors. 1 bar, 1 restaurant with high tables. Shops with wide aisles. Accessible route from check-in to departures. Boarding by lift. Accessible public phones. First aid available. No trained staff. Wheelchairs available. Can stay in own wheelchair until boarding.

TRESCO HELIPORT Isles of Scilly
Tresco, Isle of Scilly, Cornwall TR24 0QQ
Tel: (01720) 422970   Fax: (01720) 422807

Tresco is a small island without buses, lorries, cars etc. Heliport is small but can accommodate electric wheelchairs, as can the helicopter. Most of terminal building is level but where stepped, staff will come to a passenger, e.g. at check-in. No lifts, public phones, WCs, restaurants or bars. Wheelchairs are taken from the terminal on tractors or by road.

WICK AIRPORT
Wick, Caithness, Scotland KW1 4QP
Tel: (01955) 602215   Fax: (01955) 605946

Very small airport. Setting down point near entrance. 2 non-reservable orange badge spaces. Assistance available. Level route to entrance. Automatic accessible entrance door. No lifts. 1 unisex adapted WC to part M, 165 x 165cm, both support rails, outward opening doors: 1 café with high tables. No shops. Accessible route from check-in to departures. No accessible public telephones: 1 wheelchair available. No trained staff. Can stay in own wheelchair until boarding.

AIRLINES

AER LINGUS
Tel: (0353) 1 7052222
Fax: (0353) 1 7053832
Minicom: (0353) 1 8863666
e-mail: aerweb@aerlingus.ie
web: www.aerlingus.ie

UK ROUTES
City of Derry – Birmingham, Blackpool, Bristol, Channel Islands, Exeter, Glasgow, Isle of Man, London Gatwick, Manchester.
Subscribes to Carefree Journeys & Holidays guide for disabled people, with several pages detailing trip tips for passengers with special needs.
Also information sheet for Passengers Requiring Special Assistance available in Aer Lingus offices and travel agencies.
Medical Form required. Advise reservations staff when booking of nature/degree of disability. Check-in 1 hour prior to departure. Wet-cell batteries cannot be carried.
Special seat allocation:
A330-rows 12-16 and 27-29 AC-HK
A321-row 3 DEF and Economy aft row 20
B737-400/500-row 3 DEF and last row
Fokker 50-row 2 and 10AC
BAE146-row 2ABC and 19AC
These seats have moveable armrests and seat belt extensions only.
With prior notice, special medical apparatus can be offered if compatible with safety regulations. Details to be given through reservations staff to medical centre at airport. A330 aircraft has specially designed WC. Meals for special dietary and medical requirements are available.

AURIGNY AIRLINES
Tel: (01481) 822804
Fax: (01481) 823670
Routes: Southampton to Jersey via Alderney and all inter-island hops: Stansted-Guernsey, Manchester-Guernsey.
No literature for disabled travellers.
Medical Form not required. Advise reservations staff when booking of nature/degree of disability because type of aircraft may preclude travel. Check-in minimum 30 minutes prior to departure.

Wheelchairs provided for transfer from check-in to aircraft. Transporting of personal electric chairs not possible. Special seat allocation. No moveable armrests, leg rests, seat belt extensions, harnesses. No clinical air pumps/Stoma masks. No specially designed WC. No aisle wheelchairs. No special telephone number for disabled travellers.

BRITISH AIRWAYS
Head Office: Waterside, PO Box 365 Harmondsworth, Middlesex UB7 0GB
Tel: Admin/Reservations: (0345) 222111
web: www.british-airways.com
Minicom: (0345) 007706
UK routes: London Heathrow-Aberdeen, Belfast, Edinburgh, Glasgow, Islay, Jersey, Kirkwall, Manchester, Newcastle, Shetland (Sumburgh), Stornoway Wick.
London Gatwick-Aberdeen, Bristol, Edinburgh, Glasgow, Guernsey, Inverness, Jersey, Manchester, Newcastle, Newquay, Plymouth, Stornoway.
London City-Sheffield
Aberdeen-Belfast Int'l, Birmingham, Bristol, Cardiff, Glasgow, Leeds Bradford, Manchester, Newcastle, Newquay, Plymouth, Shetland (Sumburgh), Southampton, Stornoway.
Belfast City-Edinburgh, Glasgow, Guernsey, Jersey, Liverpool, Manchester, Sheffield, Southampton.
Belfast Int'l-Birmingham, Cardiff, Edinburgh, Glasgow, Manchester, Newcastle, Southampton.
Birmingham-Edinburgh, Glasgow, Inverness, Kirkwall, Newcastle, Shetland (Sumburgh), Stornoway, Wick.
Bristol-Edinburgh, Glasgow, Guernsey, Jersey, Manchester, Newcastle, Plymouth
Cardiff-Edinburgh, Glasgow.
Edinburgh-Glasgow, Guernsey, Inverness, Kirkwall, Manchester, Newquay, Plymouth, Southampton, Stornoway, Wick.
Glasgow-Inverness, Islay, Kirkwall, Manchester, Newquay, Plymouth, Southampton, Stornoway.
Guernsey-Manchester.
Inverness-Kirkwall, Shetland (Sumburgh), Stornoway.
Jersey-Manchester.
Kirkwall-Shetland (Sumburgh), Stornoway.

Leeds Bradford-Southampton.
Londonderry-Glasgow, Manchester.
Manchester-Newquay, Plymouth,
Southampton.
Newcastle-Newquay, Plymouth,
Southampton.
Shetland (Sumburgh)-Shetland
(Lerwick/Tingwall), Wick.
For all routes call reservations on the
number above for full clarification.
Specific literature for both disabled
passengers and staff. No medical form
required if stable disability. Airline offers
Special Services Desks and Meet & Greet
service, advise at least two days prior to
flight. Also includes special procedures on
check-in, lounge facilities, assistance
through the airport and boarding the
aircraft. Allow additional 30 minutes above
normal check-in time for special services
application. Wheelchairs are available on
request, both from check-in to aircraft,
and in-flight. Electric wheelchair
restrictions; passengers must transfer to a
ground wheelchair operated by the airline
at check-in. Taken through terminal in
this chair. Own wheelchair taken at check-
in and battery removed. Chair and battery
loaded into hold of aircraft and stored
separately for duration of flight. On arrival
chair is re-assembled and delivered to
baggage hall. Special seats are allocated at
time of booking, although on day of flight,
alterations to seating plan can be made.
These seats have moveable armrests and
seat belt extensions also are available. No
clinical air pumps or Stoma masks
available. No adapted WCs on domestic
services although most have emergency
cord and grab bars. Long-haul flight
aircraft have specially designed WC. No
aisle wheelchairs, except on long- haul.
Special meals provided, advance notice
required. The only special phone number
for disabled passengers is the minicom:
(0345) 007706.

BRITISH MIDLAND
Donington Hall, Castle Donington, Derby DE74
2SB
Tel: (01332) 854000   Fax: (01332) 854632
web: www.britishmidland.com
UK Routes: East Midlands-Aberdeen,

Belfast, Edinburgh, Glasgow, Jersey.
Aberdeen-Manchester. Belfast-Heathrow
(T1). Edinburgh-Heathrow (T1),
Manchester. Glasgow-Leeds Bradford,
Manchester. Teesside-Heathrow (T1).
No literature for disabled passengers.
Medical form usually not required.
Disabled passengers normally pre-boarded
and disembarked last. Normal check-in
time as per timetable, but if assistance
required do allow additional time for this.
Wheelchairs available for transfer from
check-in to aircraft. Non-spillable batteries
can be carried provided the battery is
disconnected and securely attached to the
wheelchair and terminals insulated to
prevent short circuit. Spillable batteries can
be carried provided the wheelchair can be
handled and secured in an upright position
and meets conditions for non-spillable
batteries. Dedicated rows on each aircraft.
Seats in these rows have moveable
armrests. No clinical air pumps or Stoma
masks. Assist handle provided in each WC.
No aisle wheelchairs available in cabin.
Special meals include diabetic, gluten-free,
low sodium/salt, low cholesterol and low
calorie that can be provided if pre-ordered
before 1600hrs on day prior to departure.
No special telephone/fax number for
disabled passengers. General customer
enquiries are able to assist.

JERSEY EUROPEAN AIRWAYS
Hangar 3, Exeter Airport, Exeter,
Devon EX5 2BD
Tel: (Reservations) (0990) 676676
Fax: (01392) 366151
web: www.jersey-european.co.uk
UK Routes: Guernsey-Belfast City,
Birmingham, Exeter, Jersey, Glasgow,
London Gatwick, London Luton,
Southampton, London City-
Leeds/Bradford, Jersey, Aberdeen.
No literature for disabled travellers.
Medical form not required. No special
procedures. Normal check-in. Dry cell
battery electric chairs acceptable with
advance notice. Special seat no: 00
allocated close to exit. Seat has moveable
armrests, leg rests, seat belt extension,
quadriplegic harness. No clinical air
pumps or Stoma masks. No specially

27

designed WC. No aisle wheelchairs. Special meals available for dietary and medical requirements. No special telephone/fax numbers.

KLM
ETS Ltd, Amsterdam Way, Norwich,
Norfolk NR6 6HA
Tel: (Reservations) (08705) 074074
Fax: (01603) 778111
web: www.klmuk.com
UK routes: No literature for disabled travellers. Medical form usually not required, although FREMEC form sometimes is needed when extreme circumstances apply. Normal check-in. Seats have moveable armrests, leg rests and seatbelt extensions, but no quadriplegic harnesses. Stoma masks not available, passengers should carry their own. No specially designed WC. No wheelchairs in cabin. Only dietary meals available. All agents trained to deal with special needs through usual booking numbers as above.

MANX AIRLINES
Isle of Man (Ronaldsway) Airport, Ballasalla,
Isle of Man IM29 2JE
Tel: (Reservations) (01624) 824313 or
(0345) 256256   Fax: (01624) 826031
UK routes: Isle of Man-Aberdeen, Birmingham, Cardiff, Edinburgh, Glasgow, Guernsey, Jersey, Leeds Bradford, Liverpool, London Heathrow, London Luton, London Stansted, Manchester, Southampton. Cardiff-Jersey No specific literature for disabled passengers, except safety Braille cards on aircraft. No medical form required unless passenger had to get medical clearance for travel. All disabled passengers are pre-boarded. Check-in no later than 45 minutes prior to departure. Wheelchairs have to be within size and with totally disconnected battery, dry cell only. Specific seating in rows 1/2 or nearest to exit, but not at emergency exits. Seats have seat belt extensions and on some aircraft moveable arm rests. No clinical air masks or Stoma pumps. No adapted WCs on aircraft. No aisle wheelchairs on board for use in cabin. Special meals are

available, that should be pre-booked when reserving seat: Tel: (01624) 826006 Fax: (01624) 826004.

RYANAIR
Dublin Airport, Co. Dublin, Eire
Tel: Reservations (0353) 1 6097800
Fax: (0353) 1 6097801
UK routes: London Stansted-Glasgow Prestwick.
No specific literature for disabled passengers. No medical form required. Full assistance to wheelchair-bound passengers travelling in their own wheelchairs. Advise when booking of any special needs. Check-in at least one hour prior to departure. No wheelchair transfer provided from check-in to aircraft. No restrictions regarding transport of personal electric chairs. Rows 2 and 3 on aircraft are prioritised for disabled passengers. Moveable arms rests and seat belt extensions available in these rows. No clinical air pumps or Stoma masks. No specially adapted WCs. No aisle wheelchairs for use in cabin. Airline does not offer meals. No special phone number for disabled passengers.

RAILWAYS
For all bookings, seat reservations, information about all stations,
tel: (018457) 413775.
web: www.railtrack.co.uk/travel/
Timetables on-line.
Crossing London: London Transport operates a Stationlink bus service between Paddington, Marylebone, Euston, St. Pancras, Kings Cross, Liverpool Street, Fenchurch Street, London Bridge, Waterloo and Victoria. The buses have adapted low floors and ramps. There are also Airbus services from Kings Cross, Victoria, Euston and Paddington stations to Heathrow Airport, serving all terminals, that are accessible. For information contact:
LONDON TRANSPORT UNIT FOR DISABLED PASSENGERS
172 Buckingham Palace Road,
London SW1 9TN
Tel: (020) 7 918 3312

TRAIN OPERATORS

ANGLIA RAILWAYS
Assistance: Tel: (01473) 693333
Minicom: (01603) 630748 or (0845) 6050600

CENTRAL TRAINS
Assistance: Tel: (08457) 056027
web: www.centraltrains.co.uk

CHILTERN RAILWAYS
Mobility Impaired: Tel: (01296) 332113/4
web: www.chilternRailways.co.uk

**CONNEX SOUTH CENTRAL/
CONNEX SOUTH EASTERN**
Customer Services: Tel: (08706) 030405
Fax: (08706) 030505
Minicom: (01233) 617621

FIRST GREAT EASTERN RAILWAY
Special Needs: Tel: (08459) 505050
Minicom: (08459) 606099

FIRST GREAT WESTERN TRAINS CO.
Special Needs: Tel: (0845) 7413775

GATWICK EXPRESS
Assistance: Tel/Minicom: (0990) 301530

GREAT NORTH EASTERN RAILWAY
Special Needs: Tel: (0145) 7225444

FIRST NORTH WESTERN TRAINS
Special Needs: Tel: (0845) 6040231
HEATHROW EXPRESS
Disabled Assistance: Tel: (020) 7 313 1041

LTS
Special Needs: Tel/Minicom: (01702) 357640

MERSEYRAIL
Special Needs: Tel: (0151) 7022071
(Minicom available)

MIDLAND MAINLINE
Special Needs: Tel: (0114) 2537654
Minicom: (0845) 7078051

NORTHERN SPIRIT
Special Needs: (0845) 6008008

SILVERLINK
Special Needs: Tel: (01923) 207818

Fax: (01923) 207023
Minicom: (01923) 256430

SOUTHWEST TRAINS
Special Needs: Tel: (0845) 6050440

STATIONLINK (LONDON)
Low floor bus linking all main stations
Tel/Minicom: (020) 7 918 3312

THAMES TRAINS
Special Needs: Tel: (0118) 9083607
web: www.thamestrains.co.uk

THAMESLINK
Special Needs: Tel: (020) 7 620 6333
Minicom: (020) 7 620 5561
Stationlink bus: Tel: (020) 7 918 3312

VALLEY LINES
Special Needs: (02920) 449944

VIRGIN TRAINS
Special Needs: (0845) 7443366
Minicom: (0845) 7443367

WALES & WEST
Special Needs: Tel: (0845) 3003005
Minicom: (0845) 7585469

WEST ANGLIA GREAT NORTHERN (WAGN)
Special Needs: (0345) 226688
Minicom: (0345) 125988

ROAD

NATIONAL EXPRESS COACH
Tel: (099) 010104 for nearest operator
web: www.nationalexpress.co.uk/
Network of long-distance buses and coaches. Site includes timetable, fares and booking on-line. NE cannot carry battery-operated wheelchairs, only folding types in the boot. Normally require seven days' notice. Coaches have some features to help disabled passengers; kneeling facility, reserved seats closest to entrance, guide and hearing dogs carried free. Details of journey are logged with driver to ensure awareness of special needs. Staff at manned stations on hand to help.

FERRIES

All companies stress the importance of stating one's needs when booking, sea travel is less uniform than air travel. Tides etc, particularly on smaller vessels, can make a difference as to which deck boarding for passengers with mobility difficulties is assigned. Therefore certain facilities may not be available during all voyages. All companies seem to be disabled-aware and all stress that their crew will be more than happy to help. Many companies also offer discounts for disabled passengers.

CALEDONIAN MACBRAYNE
The Ferry Terminal, Gourock, Renfrewshire
PA19 1QP
Tel: (Reservations) (0990) 650000
Fax: (01475) 635235
e-mail: reservations@calmac.co.uk
web: www.calmac.co.uk
UK routes: Firth of Clyde islands and peninsulas. Islay, Colonsay and Gigha. Mull and Inner Hebrides. Isles of Skye, Raasay and Small Isles. Outer Hebrides. No specific literature. No medical form required. Let car marshall know details of travel in advance. Lift from vehicle deck to passenger area that is on one level. Older ships have no accessible WC or restaurant. Each new ship is more accessible. Access from shore to vessel is via car deck.
The nature of the routes requires this service to be more than just a car ferry, cargo, coffins, etc also are carried.

CONDOR FERRIES LIMITED
Condor House, New Harbour Road South, Hamworthy, Poole, Dorset BH15 4AJ
Tel: (Reservations) (01305) 761551
Fax: (01305) 760776
UK routes: Weymouth and Poole-Guernsey and Jersey.
No specific literature, but brochure gives detailed information on vessels. No medical form required. Advance notice required. Lift from vehicle deck to main passenger area. Accessible WC with alarm. Restaurants on some vessels are accessible but if not, there is at-seat service. Discounts available through the DDA.

ISLE OF MAN STEAM PACKET CO. Owned by Sea Containers
Tel: (Reservations) (01624) 661661
Fax: (01624) 645697
e-mail: res@steam-packet.com
web: www.steam-packet.com
UK routes: Liverpool-Isle of Man, Heysham-Isle of Man, Heysham-Belfast. No specific literature. No medical form required. Advance notice required. Lift from vehicle deck to main deck that is on one level. 1 adapted WC, 2 adapted cabins. Accessible restaurant. Movement from ship to shore and vice versa is accessible.

ISLES OF SCILLY STEAMSHIP CO.
Quay Street, Penzance, Cornwall TR18 4BD
Tel: (01736) 362009
UK route: Penzance-St. Mary's.
No specific literature. No medical form needed. No special procedures for boarding. No lift. Main passenger area on one level except buffet, but staff are helpful. 1 adapted WC, smaller than regulation size but accessible by some wheelchairs. No special access from shore to vessel or vice versa.

NORSE IRISH FERRIES
Victoria Terminal 2, West Bank Road, Belfast BT3 9JN
Tel: Reservations: (02890) 779090
Fax: (012890) 775520
web: Norse-Irish-Ferries.co.uk
Liverpool Office: North Brocklebank Dock, Bootle, Merseyside L20 1BY
Tel: (Reservations) (0151) 944 1010
Fax: (0151) 922 0344
UK route: Liverpool-Belfast.
No specific literature. No medical form required. Notice recommended. Lift from vehicle deck to main passenger area that is on one level. 1 accessible WC and restaurant. Disabled friendly access from shore to vessel.

ORKNEY FERRIES LTD
Shore Street, Kirkwall, Orkney, Scotland KW15 1LG
Tel: (Reservations) (01856) 872044
Fax: (01856) 872921
UK routes: Mainland (Kirkwall)-all 10

islands. No specific literature. No medical form required. Notify in advance. No special boarding procedures. Lifts on some vessels. Some vehicles decks have some facilities on that level. No special access to shore from vessel and vice versa.

P & O IRISH FERRIES LTD
Cairnryan, Nr. Stranraer, Wigtownshire, Scotland DG9 8RG
Tel: (Reservations) (0870) 242666
Fax: (01581) 200282
UK route: Cairnryan-Larne (N. Ireland). No specific literature. No medical form required. May be boarded anytime during embarkation. Lifts from vehicle deck to main passenger area that is on one level. Accessible WCs and restaurant. Minibus available ship to shore.

P & O SCOTTISH FERRIES LTD
PO Box 5, Jamiesons Quay, Aberdeen AB11 5NP
Tel: (Reservations) (01224) 572615
Fax: (01224) 574411
UK routes: Aberdeen-Lerwick, Stromness and Scrabster-Stromness. No specific literature. No medical form required. Boarding depends on availability of lifts. Lifts connect vehicle deck and main passenger area that are on different levels. Accessible WC and restaurant. No minibus but short distance from quayside to vessel.

RED FUNNEL FERRIES
12 Bugle Street, Southampton SO14 2JY
Tel: (Reservations) (01703) 334010
Tel: (Special Needs) (01703) 333811
Fax: (01703) 639438
e-mail: sales@redfunnel.co.uk
web: www.redfunnel.co.uk
UK route: Southampton-Isle of Wight. Specific literature available. No medical form required. No special boarding procedures, but inform terminal staff of requirements. Lift sometimes available from vehicle deck to main passenger area that is on one level and accessible, except for upper deck area. Accessible WCs and restaurants/buffet. No special access from shore to vessel and vice versa.

SEA CAT Owned by Sea Containers, see Isle of Man Steam Packet Co.
General Booking Tel: (08705) 523523
UK Route: Isle of Man-Belfast.

SEA CAT SCOTLAND Owned by Sea Containers, see Isle of Man Steam Packet Co.
General Booking Tel: (08705) 523523
UK routes: Stranraer and Troom-Belfast.

STENA LINE
Charter House, Park Street, Ashford, Kent TN24 8EX
Tel: (Reservations) (08705) 707070
Fax: (01233) 202231
Minicom: (01233) 615678
web: www.stenaline.co.uk
UK routes: Stranraer-Belfast (HSS). No specific literature. No medical form required. Boarding depends on disability. Lifts from vehicle deck to main passenger area that is one level on new high-speed vessels. Accessible WCs and restaurants. Ramps from shore to vessel.

WIGHTLINK LTD
Wightlink House, 70 Broad Street, Portsmouth, Hants PO1 2LB
Tel: (0990) 827744
Tel: (01705) 812011 call in advance for assistance
Fax: (01705) 855257
web: www.wightlink.co.uk
UK routes: Portsmouth-Fishbourne. Portsmouth Harbour-Ryde Pier Head. Lymington-Yarmouth.
Information in general timetable. No medical form necessary. No special boarding procedures. Some vessels have lifts from vehicle deck to main passenger areas, some of which are on one level. Accessible WC on board and in terminals. Accessible restaurant. No special access from shore to vessel or vice versa. Passengers should contact road staff for assistance on arrival. Disabled persons travel card available with discounts for travel, and is well worth applying for.

BRITISH ARTS FESTIVAL VENUES

BRITISH ARTS FESTIVAL ASSOCIATION
The Library, 3rd Floor, 77 Whitechapel High Street, London E1 7QX
Tel: (020) 7 247 4667
Fax: (020) 7 247 5010
e-mail: bafa@netcomuk.co.uk
web: www.artsfestivals.co.uk

53rd ALDEBURGH FESTIVAL OF MUSIC AND THE ARTS
Aldeburgh Productions, High Street, Aldeburgh, Suffolk IP1 5AX
Admin: (01728) 452935
Box Office: (01728) 453543
Fax: (01728) 452715
e-mail: enquiries@aldeburghfestivals.org
web: www.aldeburgh.co.uk

ARUNDEL FESTIVAL
Arundel Festival, The Mary Gate, Arundel, West Sussex BN18 9AT
Tel: (01903) 883690   Fax: (01903) 884243
e-mail: arundel.festival@argonet.co.uk
web: www.argonet.co.uk/arundel.festival

BATH INTERNATIONAL MUSIC FESTIVAL
BATH LITERATURE FESTIVAL
Admin: 5 Broad Street, Bath, Somerset BA1 5LJ. Tel: (01225) 462231
Fax: (01225) 445551
Tel: (Box Office) (01225) 463362
Fax: (01225) 310377

VENUES:
Assembly Rooms,
Bennett Street,
Bath BA2 2QH
Tel: (01225) 477789 Fax: (01225) 477709

Bath Abbey: Abbey Office,
13 Kingston Buildings, Bath BA1 1LT
Tel: (Bookings) (01225) 422462
Fax: (01225) 429990
P-E [♿] on-street, free after 1800   RE [♿]
ED [♿] INT [♿] WC [♿] AUD [♿] 6
spaces, accessed across church to south aisle, seats at edge of nave.

Chew Magna: Not accessible.

Forum, 1a Forum Buildings, St. James' Parade, Bath BA1 1UG
Tel: (01225) 463556 Fax: (01225) 460651
CP-orange badge parking on both sides of Somerset St. where ramped entrance leads directly into auditorium.

Guildhall, High Street, Bath BA1 5AW
Tel: (01225) 477724 Fax: (01225) 477442
CP [♿] 2 outside Guildhall, 1 outside market
RE [♿] Market Gates entrance   ED [♿]   INT [♿]
WC [♿] on ground & first floors-RADAR key

Keynsham Methodist Church: Charlton Road, Keynsham BS31 2J
Tel: (0117) 9149408
CP Unknown
RE [♿] Permanent ramped access -gradient unknown.
WC [♿] Back of church.

Malmesbury Abbey, Paris Office,
Old Squash Court, Holloway,
Malmesbury, Wilts SN16 9BA
Tel: (01666) 826666
CP [♿] Ordinary spaces and some single yellow line parking outside church.   RE [♿]

Pavilion, North Parade, Bath BA2 4EU
Tel: 901225) 477235   Fax: (01225) 481306
CP [♿]   RE [♿] ramped to door at RHS of building
WC [♿] Main Foyer (Bar Area) RADAR key.

Pump Room, Stall Street, Bath
Tel: (01225) 477765   Fax: (01225) 477476
CP [♿] Designated outside Guildhall and single yellow lines in Cheap Street and York Street (rear of Pump Room)   WC [♿] Specific with level access

Royal Bath Literary and Scientific Institution:
NOT ACCESSIBLE

St. John's Church, South Parade, Bath
Tel: (01225) 464471
CP [♿] outside church (single yellow (line).

Wells Cathedral, West Cloister, Wells, Somerset BA5 2PA
Tel: 901749) 674483   Fax: (01749) 677360
CP [♿] Designated spaces by gap in wall on Cathedral Green with slope to NW Door   RE -ramped.
WC [♿] Outside W Front (through gate near SW door)

BELFAST FESTIVAL AT QUEEN'S
Festival House, 25 College Gardens,
Belfast BT9 6BS
Admin: (02890) 067687
Fax: (02890) 663733
Tel: (Booking-Box Office) (02890) 665577
e-mail: festival@qub.ac.uk
web: www.qub.ac.uk/festival

CANTERBURY FESTIVAL
Festival Office, Christ Church Gate,
The Precincts, Canterbury, Kent CT1 2EE
Tel: (01227) 452853 Fax: (01227) 781830

CHARD FESTIVAL OF WOMEN IN MUSIC
Admin: (01460) 66115   Fax: (01460) 66048
e-mail: chardfest@compuserve.com
Main traditional venue that is accessible
was closed in 1999 for major building
works and access is badly compromised for
2000, but much improved in future.
For full details of access to all venues
telephone above.

CHELMSFORD CATHEDRAL FESTIVAL
Guy Harlings, 53 New Street, Chelmsford,
Essex CM1 1AT
Tel: (Admin) (01245) 359890
Fax: (01245) 289456
Booking-Box Office: Civic Theatre Box office,
Fairfield Road, Chelmsford CM1 1JG
Tel: (01245) 606505

Chelmsford Cathedral
CP 🦽 (Designated in Waterloo Lane, or behind *Rat &
Parrot* pub opposite Cathedral main entrance)
RE- 🦽   ED 🦽
INT 🦽 (Box office at different location – see above).
WC 🦽 (not on site - disabled facilities in public WC in
Market Road)   AUD 🦽 (seats removed to
accommodate wheelchairs as requested)   B/R 🦽

CHELTENHAM INTERNATIONAL FESTIVAL OF MUSIC
Town Hall, Imperial Square, Cheltenham,
Glos. GL50 1QA
Admin: (01242) 521621
Box Office: (01242) 227979
Fax: (01242) 573902

e-mail: townhall@cheltenham,gov.uk
web: www.cheltenhamfestivals.co.uk/music

51st CHELTENHAM FESTIVAL OF LITERATURE
Booking as International Festival of Music.

CHESTER SUMMER MUSIC FESTIVAL
8 Abbey Square, Chester CH1 2HU
Tel: (01244) 320722 Fax: (01244) 341200
e-mail: csmf@dial.pipex.com

CHESTER CATHEDRAL
12 Abbey Square, Chester CH1 2HU
Tel: (01244) 324756   Fax: (01244) 341110
e-mail: office@chestercathedral.org.uk
see page 71 for full details

Chester Gateway Theatre
Hamilton Place, Chester CH1 2BH
Tel: (Admin) (01244) 344238
Fax: (01244) 344237
Booking-Box Office: (01244) 340392
Fax: (01244) 317217
SD 🦽 (designated bays in Hamilton Place)   CP no
RE 🦽 (passenger lift from street level, level access
from lift)   INT 🦽   L 🦽   WC 🦽
AUD 🦽 (max. 6 wheelchair spaces, with companion
space adjacent)   B/R 🦽 (bar in main entrance foyer)

CHESTER TOWN HALL
VERY LIMITED ACCESS.

CHICHESTER FESTIVITIES
Canon Gate House, South Street, Chichester,
West Sussex PO19 1PU
Tel: (Admin) (01243) 785718
Box office: (01243) 780192
Fax: (01243) 528356
e-mail: chi.fest@argonet.co.uk
web: www.argonet.co.uk/chifest

DARTINGTON INTERNATIONAL SUMMER SCHOOL
Dartington Hall, Totnes, Devon TQ29 6DE
Tel: (Admin) (01803) 867068
Booking-Box Office: (01803) 865988
Fax: (01803) 868108.
Booking with form by post.
Dartington Hall:
CP 🦽   RE 🦽   ED 🚶   INT 🦽
WC 🦽   AUD 🦽   B/R 🦽

33

Barn Theatre:

CP [♿] RE [♿] ED [♿] INT [♿]
WC [♿] AUD [♿] (4 designated wheelchair positions). Route is straight through foyer to wheelchair balcony at back of venue.
B/R [♿] (slight incline to door).

EDINBURGH INTERNATIONAL FESTIVAL
The Hub, Castlehill, Edinburgh EH1 2NE
Tel: (Admin) (0131) 473 2099
Fax: (0131) 4732002
e-mail:eif@eif.co.uk
web: www.go-edinburgh.co.uk
Booking-Box Office: (0131) 4732000
Fax: (0131) 4732003
Textphone: (0131) 4732098

Festival produces good leaflet on access to all venues. The Hub is fully accessible, with level access to ground floor facilities.
Edinburgh Festival Theatre: 13-29 Nicolson Street, Edinburgh EH8 9FT
CP [♿] Public in Crighton Street RE [♿] pavement ramp – level access at side. AUD [♿] designated spaces in centre stalls.
WC [♿] Designated on Levels 1,2 &3
R/B [♿] Café on ground floor. Others by lift.

VENUES
Edinburgh Playhouse: 18-22 Greenside Place, Edinburgh EH1 3AA
CP [♿] Public, 40m. away
RE [♿] Ramped access or 3 steps
INT [♿] level access AUD [♿] Designated spaces in middle of rear circle
WC [♿] off main Foyer R/B [♿] Circle level is accessible

King's Theatre: 2 Leven Street, Edinburgh EH3 9LQ
CP [♿] Orange badge parking on single yellow line nearby.
RE [♿] Ramped adjacent Box Office or 3 steps.
AUD [♿] 4 designated spaces in stalls.
WC [♿] Adapted on stalls level. R/B N/A.

Royal Lyceum Theatre: 30 Grindlay Street, Edinburgh EH3 0AX
CP [♿] 5 orange badge spaces on Grindlay Street, adjacent Usher Hall. RE [♿] Level access. ED [♿]
AUD [♿] Designated spaces in rear stalls, levelled and raised. Transfer available at row ends with removable armrests.

WC [♿] Adapted on ground floor.
B/R [♿] Level access. Removable seats.

The Queen's Hall: Clerk Street, Edinburgh EH8 9JG
CP [♿] Single yellow line in front of hall REC [♿]
Ramped to automatic double door AUD [♿]
Designated spaces on ground floor, at centre and sides.
WC [♿] Adapted on ground floor with level access, handrails
B/R [♿] Ground floor level access to double door. Self service. Removable seats.

Usher Hall: Lothian Road, Edinburgh EH1 2EA

CP [♿] 5 Orange badge spaces on Grindlay Street adjacent Usher Hall.

RE [♿] Ramped with handrails AUD [♿] 10 designated spaces in stalls. WC [♿] 2 adapted on ground floor either side of Hall.
B/R [♿] level access, on ground floor.

Lumiere Cinema: Reid Concert Hall: St. Cecilia's Hall and Ross Theatre
NOT ACCESSIBLE.

EXETER FESTIVAL
City Centre Marketing, Exeter City Council, Paris Street, Exeter, Devon EX1 1NN
Tel: (01392) 265118 Fax: (01392) 265695
e-mail: gerri.bennett@exeter.gov.uk
web: www.exeter.gov.uk

FISHGUARD MUSIC FESTIVAL
Festival Office, Fishguard, Pembrokeshire, Wales SA65 9BJ
Tel/Fax: (01348) 873612

HARROGATE INTERNATIONAL FESTIVAL
1 Victoria Avenue, Harrogate, North Yorks HG1 1EQ
Tel: (01423) 562303 Fax: (01423) 521264
e-mail: info@harrogate-festival.org.uk
web: www.harrogate-festival.org.uk

VENUES
Christchurch, Church Square, Harrogate HG1 4SW

Tel: (Admin and Box Office) (01423) 530750
Fax: (01423) 858343
CP [♿] (reservable designated in front of church)
RE [♿]   ED [♿]   INT [♿]   WC [♿]
AUD [♿] (10 designated spaces - space of companion)
R/B n/a

Harlow Carr Botanical Gardens,
Crag Lane, Harrogate HG3 1QB
Tel: (Admin and Box Office) (01423) 565418
Fax: (01423) 530663
CP [♿]   RE [♿]   ED [♿]   INT [♿]   WC [♿]
AUD-n/a   R/B [♿]

Harrogate International Centre,
Kings Road, Harrogate HG1 5LA
Tel: (Admin) (01423) 500500
Fax: (01423) 537210
Tel: (Box Office) (01423) 537230
Fax: (01423) 537202
CP [♿]   RE [♿]   ED [♿]   INT [♿]   L [♿]
WC [♿]   AUD [♿]   B/R [♿]

Harrogate Theatre
Oxford Street, Harrogate
Tel: (Admin) (01423) 502710
Fax: (01423) 563205
Booking Box office: (01423) 502116
Fax as above
SD [♿] (unrestricted road parking after 6.00pm)
CP [♿]   RE [♿]   ED [♿]   INT [♿]   L-n/a
WC [♿]   AUD [♿] (4 designated wheelchair spaces less
than 90cm w x 140cm d: no adjacent space for companions)
B/R [♿] (stalls bar behind auditorium through 2 sets of
doors)

Old Swan Hotel
Swan Road, Harrogate HG1 2SR
Tel: (Admin and Box Office) (01423) 500055
Fax: (01423) 501154
CP [♿]   RE [♿]   ED [♿]   INT [♿]   L [♿]
WC [♿]   AUD [♿]   B/R [♿]

St. Wilfred's Hall,
Duchy Road, Harrogate
Admin: (01423) 503259
Box office: 55 Mallinson Oval, Harrogate.
Tel: (01423) 879271 evenings only
CP [♿]   RE [♿]   ED [♿]   WC [♿]

HENLEY FESTIVAL OF MUSIC AND THE ARTS
14 Friday Street, Henley-on-Thames,
Oxon RG9 1AH

Tel: (Admin) (01491) 843400
Fax: (01491) 419482
Booking Box office: (01491) 843404
e-mail: info@henley-festival.co.uk
web: www.henley-festival.co.uk
Open air event, conditions of turf
dependent on weather.
CP [♿]   RE [♿]   ED [♿]   B/R [♿]
WC [♿] (located in centre of enclosure behind main
grandstand)   AUD [♿] (20 positions in open area in
front of grandstands, no spaces for companions)

HIGHLAND FESTIVAL
40 Huntly Street, Inverness, Inverness-shire,
Scotland IV3 5HR
Tel: (01463) 719000   Fax: (01463) 716777
e-mail: info@highlandfestival.demon.co.uk
More than 50 venues across Highlands
and Islands. For wheelchair access please
call Festival Information Line on (01463)
71112 where details are available of
Highland Artlink that assists people with
disabilities attending events in the
Inverness and Ross and Cromarty areas
through a network of volunteer driver
link-workers.

Eden Court, Bishops Road,
Inverness IV3 5SA
Admin: (01463) 239841
Fax: (01463) 713810
Booking Box Office: (01463) 234234
CP [♿]   RE [♿]   ED [♿]   INT [♿]
WC-3 (located at Box office)
AUD [♿] (11 positions, 3 in stalls, 8 in boxes, accessed
via box office, plus companion seating)
B/R [♿] (level front entrance and level reception hall
leading to facilities).

HUDDERSFIELD CONTEMPORARY
MUSIC FESTIVAL
Department of Music,
The University of Huddersfield,
Huddersfield, West Yorks HD1 3DH
Tel: (Admin) (01484) 425082/472103
Fax: (01484) 472957
e-mail: hcmf@hud.ac.uk
web: www.hud.ac.uk/events/hcmf/
welcome.html
Booking Box Office: (01484) 430528
Minicom: as above.

Fax: (01484) 425336
The festival produces a comprehensive access information leaflet.

VENUES

Canalside West Lecture Theatre
CP [♿] (University car park adjacent Canalside West by prior arrangement with Festival Office)
RE [🚶] (Firth St. entrance)   WC [🚶] (main foyer)
B/R n/a

Hudawi Cultural Centre
CP [🚶] (adjacent theatre)   RE/INT [🚶] ramp access
WC [🚶] (ground floor)   B/R n/a

Lawrence Batley Theatre,
Queen's Square, Queen Street, Huddersfield,
West Yorks HD1 2SP
Details as per booking office
CP [♿]   RE [♿]   ED [♿]   INT [♿]   L [♿]
WC [♿]   AUD [♿]   B/R [♿]

Recital Hall
CP [♿] (AS St. Paul's)   RE/INT [🚶] (2 steps into building, further 3 steps into auditorium. Steward assistance.
WC [🚶] (main foyer)
B/R [🚶] (common room, down 3 steps)

St. Paul's Hall
Access to ground floor only.
CP [♿] (spaces in University CP adjacent to Hall by prior arrangement with Festival Office)
RE [♿]   ED [♿]   WC [🚶]   B/R [♿] (Foyer)

St. Thomas's Church
CP [♿] (adjacent CP)   RE/INT [🚶] West Door entrance only (give prior notice)   WC -n/a
B/R [♿] (in foyer)

Town Hall
CP [🚶] (Princess Street)   RE [♿] (Ramp to entrance on Corporation Street, main entrance steps.)
ED [♿]   INT [🚶]   L [🚶]
WC [🚶] (Coronation St. entrance)
B/R [♿] (Access via lift to bar and Old Courtroom.)

UCI
CP [♿] (designated adjacent cinema)
RE [♿]   ED/INT [♿] (ramp/passenger lift)
WC [🚶] (on each floor)   B/R [🚶]

University Dance Studio
St. Peter's Building
Not Accessible.

ISLE OF MAN
26th MANANAN INTERNATIONAL FESTIVAL
Erin Arts Centre, Victoria Square, Port Erin,
Isle of Man IM9 6LD
Tel: (Admin and Booking) (01624) 832858
Fax: (01624) 836658
e-mail: erinartscentre@enterprise.net
web: www.manxman.co.im/music/mananan

Erin Arts Centre
CP [♿]   RE [♿]   ED [♿]   INT [♿]
WC [♿] (adjacent bar)   AUD [♿] (ramped access 1:12, 4 wheelchair positions, companion space nearby)
B/R [♿]

LAKE DISTRICT SUMMER MUSIC
Stricklandgate House, 92 Stricklandgate,
Kendal, Cumbria LA9 4PU
Tel: (01539) 733411 Fax: (01539) 724441
e-mail: info@ldlsm.org.uk
web: www.ldsm.org.uk

LEICESTER INTERNATIONAL MUSIC FESTIVAL
New Walk Museum, 53 New Walk,
Leicester LE1 7EA
Admin Tel/Fax: (0116) 2472043

VENUES:
New Walk Museum and Art Gallery
53 New Walk, Leicester LE1 7EA
Booking Box Office: (0116) 2554100
Fax: (0016) 2473005
CP [♿]   RE [♿]   ED [♿]   INT [♿]   L [♿]
WC [♿]   AUD [♿] (Variable no. of wheelchair positions, accessed from foyer down ramp (1:12) and up another ramp (1:12) into auditorium.
B/R [♿] (ground floor: tables moveable)

The Guildhall
Guildhall Lane, Leicester LE1 5FQ
Booking-Box Office: (0116) 2532569
Fax: (0116) 2539626
SD [♿]   CP [🚶]   RE [♿]   ED [♿]
INT [🚶]   WC [🚶]   AUD [♿]   B/R n/a

De Montfort Hall
Tel: (0116) 2333139

LLANGOLLEN INTERNATIONAL MUSICAL EISTEDDFOD
Eisteddfod Office, Abbey Road, Llangollen,
Denbighshire, North Wales LL20 8NG
Tel: (01978) 860236
Fax: (01978) 861300
e-mail: @lime.uk.com
Web: HYPERLINK http://www.lime.uk.com

Royal International Pavilion
Address as above
Tel: (Admin) (01978) 860236
Fax: (01978) 861300
Booking Box Office: (01978) 861501
CP 🔾 (plus courtesy car from car park to pavilion for
severely disabled visitors)   RE 🔾   ED 🔾
INT 🔾
WC 🔾 (numerous locations)
Aud 🔾 (14 positions in A and L stands, plus companion
seating)   B/R 🔾

LONDON
CITY OF LONDON FESTIVAL
June/July 2000
Bishopsgate Hall, 230 Bishopsgate,
London EC2M 4HW
Tel: (020) 7 377 9540
Fax: (020) 7 3771972
e-mail: fest@fircon.co.uk
web: www.city-of-london-festival.org.uk
A programme of world-class arts events in
the City's finest buildings. Prices and
venues vary depending on event. Access
information available with booking
brochure (published April 2000). To join
mailing list for access information in
brochure, contact the above.
Tickets: Barbican Box Office:
Tel: (020) 7 638 8891

BOC COVENT GARDEN FESTIVAL OF OPERA AND THEATRE MUSIC
47 The Market, Covent Garden Piazza,
London WC2E 8RF
Tel: (020) 7 379 0870
(for disabled access info.)
web: www.cgf.co.uk
Paul Gray, Marketing Manager, having
visited and checked the many venues
involved here, felt it impossible to
summarise every venue for access. The
above personal booking service number for

the Festival Office will allow direct
contact with him or a colleague and each
individual's needs will be assessed and in
majority of cases, facilitated. He confirms
a strong commitment to access for all.

GREENWICH AND DOCKLANDS INTERNATIONAL FESTIVAL
6 College Approach, Greenwich,
London SE10 9HY
Tel: (020) 8 305 1818   Fax: (01871) 305 1188
e-mail: greencok@globalnet.co.uk
web: www.festival.org

INTERNATIONAL FESTIVAL OF THEATRE
19/20 Great Sutton Street,
London EC1V 0DR
Admin: (020) 7 490 3964
Box Office: (020) 7 312 1995
Fax: (020) 7 490 3976
e-mail: info@liftfest
web: www.lift-info.co.uk
Biennial event bringing worldwide
innovative new theatre and performance
to London. Emphasis on connection
between London's diverse communities
and the diversity of the world. The
relationship with all the city's communities
especially those often excluded from the
arts, including disabled communities, is
very important to LIFT organisers.
Dates: early summer 2001. An access
guide is being produced that will include
volunteer companion, large print, audio-
brochures, signed performances, heavily
discounted tickets as well as access
details and facilities for each of the 10-15
venues. Contact above for a guide.

SOUTHWARK FESTIVAL
16 Winchester Walk, London SE1 9AQ
Admin/Fax: (020) 7 403 7474
Box Office: (020) 7 403 7400
e-mail: swkfest@aol.com

VENUES
SPITALFIELDS FESTIVAL
75 Brushfield Street, London E1 6AA
Tel: (Admin) (0207) 327 0287
Fax: (0207) 7 247 0494
Booking Box Office: (0207) 377 1362
Fax: as above
e-mail: spitfest@easynet.co.uk

Christ Church
Commercial Street, London E1
SD [♿] (front of church)
CP n/a (driver park in Whites Row Corporation of London CP opposite church)
RE [♿] (main entrance has steps, but accessible lift at side of church, from street level accesses entrance)
ED [♿]   INT [♿]   L [♿]   WC [♿]
AUD [♿] (ramped, unknown gradient, 4 wheelchair positions but flexible, companion seating adjacent. Accessed through main doors into front of church, down slight ramp to side aisles to seats.)
B/R [🚶] (accessed out of main entrance, lift to street level, path to marquee, down slight slope.)

NORFOLK AND NORWICH FESTIVAL
The Ticket Shop, Guildhall, Gaol Hill,
Norwich, Norfolk NR2 1NF
Tel: (01603) 764764 Fax: (01603) 766699
e-mail: info@nn.fest.eastern-arts.co.uk

NORTH WALES MUSIC FESTIVAL
High Street, St. Asaph, Clwyd,
Wales LL17 0RD
Tel: (01745) 584508 Fax: (01745) 710243

ROSS-ON-WYE INTERNATIONAL FESTIVAL
The Mews, Mitcheldean, Glos. GL17 0SL
Tel: (01594) 541070 Fax: (01594) 54446
e-mail: Ross_Festival@compuserve.com
web: www.rossfest.wynet.co.uk

SALISBURY FESTIVAL
Box Office: Salisbury Playhouse, Malthouse Lane, Salisbury, Wilts SP2 7RA
Tel: (01722) 320333
Festival Office: 75 New Street,
Salisbury SP1 2PH
Tel: (01722) 323888

THAXTED FESTIVAL
Clarence House, Thaxted, Essex CM6 2PJ
Admin and Booking Office:
Tel/Fax: (01371) 831421

VENUE
Thaxted Church
CP [♿]   RE [♿]   ED [♿]
WC [♿] (local authority disabled WC in St. Margaret Street)   AUD [♿] (4 reserved spaces plus companion space accessed from church door direct to wheelchair spaces at same level across church floor.)
B/R [♿]

THREE CHOIRS FESTIVAL at WORCESTER
Administrator, 5 Deansway,
Worcester WR1 2JG
Tel: (Box Office) (01905) 212600
Fax: (01905) 745661
e-mail: Lucasorg@compuserve.com
web: www.3choirs.org

WINDOW ON THE WORLD
INTERNATIONAL MUSIC FESTIVAL
40A Bell Street, Fish Quay, North Shields
Tel: (0191) 2005414 Fax: (0191) 2008910
e-mail: wowfest@connectfree.co.uk
web: www.wowfest.co.uk
Outdoor Event. Largest free music festival in Europe
CP [🚶] Accessible Park and Ride service from Unskill Centre, Unskill Terrace, North Shields.
E [♿] West End of Park and Ride to level site.
INT - Free Event   WC [🚶] Adapted WCs. At all toilet areas.
AUD - Seating only available in 1 marquee area, cabaret style seating at tables.   Wheelchairs available.

YORK EARLY MUSIC FESTIVAL
65 Rawcliffe Lane, York YO30 5SJ
Tel: (Admin) (01904) 645738
Fax: (01904) 612631
Booking Box Office: (01904) 658338
e-mail: HYPERLINK
mailto:yemf@netcomuk.co.uk

VENUES
Merchant Adventurer's Hall, Fossgate
SD [♿]   CP [♿]   RE [♿] (Use Undercroft entrance)
ED [♿] (Undercroft)   INT [♿]   WC [🚶]
AUD [♿] (ground level, flexible)   First Floor not accessible.

The National Centre for Early Music
St. Margaret's Church
Purpose built/adapted and accessible.

CP ⬚   RE ⬚   ED ⬚   INT ⬚
WC ⬚   (new annexe off church)   Aud ⬚
(ground level, flexible, accessed straight from doors to
seats).   B/R ⬚

St. Michael-le-Belfrey Church, Petergate
SD ⬚   CP ⬚   RE ⬚   ED ⬚
INT ⬚   WC n/a   AUD ⬚   (level access, 3-4
designated positions, access through main and interval
doors to pews)   B/R n/a

St. -Olave's Church, Marygate
SD ⬚   CP ⬚   RE ⬚   ED ⬚   INT
⬚
WC-n/a   AUD ⬚   (wheelchairs sit at side and back of
pews)   B/R n/a

York Minster
SD ⬚   CP ⬚   RE ⬚   ED ⬚
INT ⬚   WC ⬚   AUD ⬚   (ground level,
flexible)   B/R n/a

YORK MILLENNIUM MYSTERY PLAYS
PO Box 510, York YO30 5YT
Tel: (01904) 635444 Fax: (01904) 612631
e-mail: enquiry@mysteryplays2000.org

VALE OF GLAMORGAN FESTIVAL
St. Donats Arts Centre, St. Donats Castle,
Nr. Llantwit Major, Vale of Glamorgan,
Wales CF61 1WF
Admin: (01446) 792151
Box Office: (01446) 794848
Fax: (01446) 794711

MILLENNIUM PROJECTS

ENGLAND

BRISTOL
@BRISTOL.
Deanery Road, Harbourside, Bristol BS1 5DB
Tel: (0117) 9092000   Fax: (0177) 9099920
Minicom: (0117) 914 3475
web: www.at-bristol.org.uk
Located on Harbourside in the heart of
the city. Comprises two new attractions:
Wildscreen-at-Bristol that recreates the
extraordinary diversity of the natural
world, and Explore-at-Bristol that entices
visitors to delve into science stories that
seek to explain how the world works. Also
Open Spaces-at-Bristol, with public art,
including light features and sculptures,
tree-lined seating areas, plus shops, cafes
and restaurants.
Designated Car Parking available in large
underground car park close to lift access
to main square. Smooth path links all
facilities with clear route throughout
exhibitions. Centre of @Bristol in New
World Square. Pedestrian area and
pedestrian routes continue throughout
the site across 66 acres.

NATIONAL CYCLE NETWORK
Opening June 2000
Sustrans, 35 King Street, Bristol BS1 4DZ
Tel-Information: (0117) 9290888
Tel-Head Office: (0117) 9268893
Fax: (0117) 9294173
web: 222.sustrans.org.uk
The first phase of the National Cycle
Network will open in June 2000, with
5000 miles of continuous routes running
right through urban centres and reaching
all parts of the UK. This is part of a larger
Network of 9000 miles planned for
completion by 2005. The full network will
pass within two miles of half the population,
providing safe links to work, to schools,
to friends and family, to shops and stations.
As well as being a safe, attractive, high-
quality network for cyclists, the network
will be entirely traffic-free, built along old
railway lines, canal towpaths, forestry
tracks, riversides and urban spaces for
use by pedestrians, cyclists and, in places,

39

wheelchair users. The project is being co-ordinated by the charity, Sustrans, and involves over 400 local authorities, as well as businesses, land- owners, environmental bodies and others.

New tours are opening all the time and each one will be signed and mapped using an award-winning format. At present there are currently 15 maps available. The network will open with a nationwide celebration called Ride the Net in June 2000.

CORNWALL
THE EDEN PROJECT
Opening Spring 2001
Watering Lane Nursery, Pentewan,
St. Austell PL26 6BE
Tel: (01726) 222900   Fax: (01726) 222901
web: www.edenproject.com

Created to raise public awareness and understanding of, and responsibility for, the stewardship of nature, and to play a part in research and field-based projects. Eden will explain and interpret the work of many organisations engaged in sustainable approaches to agriculture, urban living, commerce and conservation both worldwide and locally. The home of this world-class visitor destination is a dramatic global garden the size of 50 football pitches, based in the natural theatre of a china clay pit overlooking St. Austell Bay. There will be thousands of important and beautiful plants from our own temperate zone, the humid tropics and the warm temperate zones, the latter two housed in giant conservatories.

We are advised that 90 per cent of the Eden Project will be accessible to visitors with mobility difficulties. For full clarification please contact Dominic Cole the Landscape Architect, on (020) 7 383 5784.

GREATER MANCHESTER
THE LOWRY
The Lowry Centre, West Pavilion, Harbour City, Manchester M5 2BH
Tel: (0161) 955 2032   Fax: (0161) 955 2021
e-mail: info@thelowry.org.uk
web: www.thelowery.org.uk

Waterfront complex in Salford Quays to include 1650 seat Lyric theatre, gallery to present works by L S Lowry, children's

hands-on gallery, national industrial centre for virtual reality. Project also will include new footbridge and public plaza.

HAMPSHIRE
THE RENAISSANCE OF PORTSMOUTH HARBOUR
Civic Offices, Guildhall Square,
Portsmouth PO1 2BG
Tel: (01705) 834176
Fax: (01705) 876414
web: www.millenium-city.co.uk

Development focusing on creation of international maritime leisure complex.

LEICESTERSHIRE
NATIONAL SPACE SCIENCE CENTRE
Opening February 2001
Leicester Promotions Ltd., 7-9 Every Street,
Town Hall Square, Leicester LE1 6AG
Tel: (0116) 2856734
Fax: (0166) 2555726
web:www.thisisleicestershire.co.uk/leicester promotions

Unique and exciting education and leisure facility based on space science. The scheme comprises four main elements; Exhibition Centre, Millennium Dome, Challenger Learning Centre, Research Centre.

SD ♿   CP ♿   E ♿   RF ♿   L ♿
C ♿   S ♿   WC ♿   RFE ♿   (Tower)

LONDON/GREATER LONDON
THE MILLENNIUM DOME
see London (Greater) attractions

THE MILLENNIUM SEED BANK,
Royal Botanic Gardens, Kew, Richmond,
Surrey TW9 3AB
Tel: (020) 8 332 5607
Fax: (020) 8 332 5610
web: www.rbgkew.org.uk/seedbank

Project to collect 25,000 species of UK and worldwide flora and freeze them for conservation. Also will provide world-class building of high architectural quality, access for public to view scientific process and opportunity to train new scientists.

BRITISH MUSEUM GREAT COURT
Opening September 2000
91 Great Russell Street, London WC1B 3PF
Tel: (020) 7 323 8988   Fax: (020) 7 580 3454
web: www.british-museum.ac.uk/court.htm
Renovation and roofing of Great Court will open up inner court for first time in 150 years, creating dramatic new public space.

MERSEYSIDE
THE NATIONAL DISCOVERY PARK, CHAVASSE PARK, LIVERPOOL
Opening December 2000
c/o Liverpool Cathedral, St. James Mount, Liverpool L1 7AZ
Tel: (0151) 709 6271   Fax: (0151) 709 1112
Concept built around rapid growth in IT, broadcasting and multi-media linked with public discovery, training, education and leisure. Discovery Centre will be glass-covered park with new bridge. Centre will house Space Time Machine and pedestrian footbridge will link project with Albert Dock development.

NORFOLK
NEW TECHNOPOLIS
Opening Early 2001
2nd Floor, Blackburn House,
1 Theatre Street, Norwich, Norfolk NR2 1RG
Tel: (01603) 610524   Fax: (01603) 610150
web: www.norfolk.gov.uk/announce.htm
Project linking three primary facilities, the Millennium Library, Business and Learning Centre, Heritage Attraction around new urban square, creating major new civic meeting place within the city centre. Complex also will include learning shop, multi-media auditorium, underground car park and range of bars and restaurants. We are advised that complex is being designed as fully accessible.

TYNE AND WEAR
INTERNATIONAL CENTRE FOR LIFE
Market Keepers House, Times Square, Scotswood Road,
Newcastle upon Tyne NE1 4EP
Tel: (0191) 261 6006
Fax: (0191) 261 4150
web: www.life-secret.co.uk

WEST MIDLANDS
MILLENNIUM POINT-BIRMINGHAM
Opening September 2001
Team Council House, Victoria Square, Birmingham B1 1BB
Tel: (0121) 303 2361
Fax: (0121) 303 4317
web: www.birmingham.gov.uk/millennium
Centre of technology and learning with four elements. Discovery centre, Technology Innovation Centre, University of the First Age and the Hub. Facilities include IMAX, shops and conference facilities.

YORKSHIRE – EAST
THE DEEP, KINGSTON-UPON-HULL
Opening April 2001
79 Ferensway, Hull, East Yorks HU2 8LE
Tel: (01482) 615789   Fax: (01482) 615645
web: www.hull.ac.uk/
World Ocean Discovery Centre based around an aquarium with supplementary buildings creating marine complex. Located at confluence of Rivers Hull and Humber. Built on four levels, it will include exhibits using IT and interactive displays to examine the sea life of the world's oceans from pre-historic times to present day.

SD ♿   CP ♿   E ♿   RF ♿   L ♿
C ♿   S ♿   WC ♿   RFE ♿

YORKSHIRE – SOUTH
THE EARTH CENTRE
Opened 1999
Doncaster Road, Denaby Main, Doncaster, South Yorks DN12 4EA
Tel: (01709) 512000   Fax: (01709) 512010
e-mail: info@earthcentre.org.uk
web: www.earthcentre.org.uk
Earth Centre's 26 acres of indoor and outdoor attractions, gardens, play areas, events, theatre, a restaurant and shop, all focus on sustainable living in an entertaining and thought-provoking way. The centre is a working example of sustainable living, built using environmentally sound materials and methods, on the regenerated sites of two former coal mines. The exhibitions and gardens are enthralling in their own right, but also are part of messages the centre wants to convey. Through the sound and light exhibition of Planet

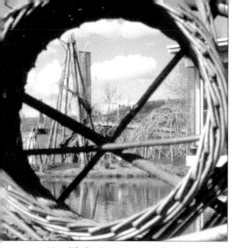

New life for Doncaster at The thought-provoking Earth Centre.

Earth Experience the message is that we are destroying the planet on which we live. Action for the Future exhibition delivers the message that we need not despair because people worldwide are taking action for a sustainable future. The centre brings hope for the future in a practical way showing we can take action at home, at work, and at school.

SHEFFIELD – REMAKING THE HEART OF THE CITY
Opening April 2001.
Press Office, Sheffield City Council, Town Hall, Sheffield, South Yorks S1 2HH
Tel: (0114) 2736604   Fax: (0114) 2734752
web: www.sheffieldcity.co.uk/heart/index.htm
The project comprises a Winter Garden, a temperate plant house, Millennium Art Gallery housing exhibitions from the V&A Museum collection, the Ruskin Gallery and the Hawley collection of Sheffield-made tools, and three public squares – the Peace Gardens, Town Hall Square and Hallam Square. All sites will be accessible.

MAGNA, ROTHERHAM
Soft opening Late 2000
Official opening Easter 2001
Sheffield Road, Templeborough, Rotherham S60 1DX
Tel: (01709) 720002   Fax: (01709) 820092
Conversion of existing, but redundant, Templeborough Steel Mill in Rotherham into an attraction focusing on British industry, combined with conference and

exhibition centre. Exhibits will include robotics demonstrations, interactive computers, live video links and virtual reality displays.

SD ♿ CP ♿ E ♿ RF ♿ L ♿
C 🚶 S ♿ WC ♿ RFE ♿

NORTHERN IRELAND – BELFAST
THE ODYSSEY PROJECT
Opening November 2000
2 Queen's Quay, Belfast BT3 9QQ
Tel: (028) 90 451055   Fax: (028) 90 451052
web: theodyssey.co.uk
First major development on the east side of the River Lagan and is seen as a catalyst for future regeneration. Buildings are located on the Queens Quay and Abercorn basin water frontages. From much designated parking, Sydenham Road entrance and all other main entrances are accessible via flat or gently sloping ramps or pathways, not exceeding 1:12. WC facilities throughout are designed for flexibility, including use by wheelchair users. Cinemas have integrated wheelchair spaces. Science Centre – three floors, accessed by lift, (passenger and 50-pax. lift) and wide doors: Arena – north entrance level access for public and disabled sports/events participants access. Disabled showers/unisex WCs. Six principal viewing areas, accommodation for 76 disabled persons.

SCOTLAND – GLASGOW
BRITISH WATERWAYS MILLENNIUM LINK
Opening April 2001
British Waterways, Canal House,
1 Applecross Street, Glasgow G4 9SP
Tel: (0141) 332 6936   Fax: (0141) 331 1688
web: www.britishwaterways.co.uk
This project is restoring navigation across the Forth and Clyde and Union Canals, from coast to coast and from Glasgow to Edinburgh. Design criteria for new bridges, facilities and path improvements takes access for people with disabilities into account, based on BT's *Countryside for All* guidelines and several local projects. The towpath is being widened to 1.8m wherever possible. Also in liaison with Countryside Access Forums. The Seagull Trust already provides free cruises for

groups of people with disabilities from bases at Ratho, Falkirk and Kirkintilloch, and many canalside pubs, for example the Bridge Inn at Ratho, are accessible. Many new facilities likely to be attracted to communities along the route of Millennium Link canals, probably operated by private business, not British Waterways. They may be able to advise on access details of pubs, boats, restaurants etc as they emerge.

GLASGOW SCIENCE CENTRE
Opening Easter 2001
4th Floor, The Eagle Building,
215 Bothwell Street, Glasgow G2 7EZ
Tel: (0141) 2044448   Fax: (0141) 2287100
New national science centre, located on five-acre site on south bank of River Clyde, that is part of Pacific Quay development of reclaimed docklands. Centre will enable visitors to explore science through inter-active exhibits and outreach activities. Development aimed at full access to centre.

WALES – CARDIFF
WALES MILLENNIUM CENTRE
Opening late 2001
Good Relations, Bay Chambers,
West Bute Street, Cardiff CF1 6YS
Tel: (01222) 344888
Providing a focus for Welsh culture, identity and talent, this will be an international showcase for musicals, opera, dance, museum displays and exhibitions.

CARMARTHENSHIRE
THE NATIONAL BOTANIC GARDEN OF WALES
Middleton Hall, Llanarthe,
Carmarthenshire SA32 8HG
Tel: (0155) 668768   Fax: (01558) 668933
web: www.gardenofwales.org.uk
Creating a Botanic Garden for Wales, dedicated to protection of threatened plant species. Universal access to buildings and features is being designed wherever possible with wheelchair accessibility. Working closely with relevant access groups, especially The Gateway Project enabling access to historic parks and gardens of Wales for under-represented groups. Access will be available at all levels of the Garden from the Great Glasshouse and Middleton Square to the Broadwalk and lakeside paths.

MAJOR UNITED KINGDOM ORGANISATIONS CONCERNED WITH DISABILITY

ARTHRITIS CARE
18 Stephenson Way, London NW1 2HD
Tel: (020) 7 916 1500   Fax: (020) 7 916 1505
Free Helpline: (0800) 8004050 12-4pm
e-mail: arthritis.care@virgin.net
web: www.arthritiscare.org.uk
Advice and practical help for people with arthritis.

ARTSLINE
54 Chalton Street, London NW1 1HS
Tel/Mincom: (020) 7 388 2227
Fax: (020) 7 3832653
e-mail: artsline@dircon.co.uk
London's major information and advice centre for disabled people on arts and entertainment. Produces excellent comprehensive series of guidebooks on theatres, cinemas, arts venues, museums etc. Also produces guide to access at Edinburgh cinemas. For access information to all of these contact Artsline.

ASSOCIATION FOR SPINA BIFIDA AND HYDROCEPHALUS (ASBAH)
Asbah House, 42 Park Road,
Peterborough PE1 2UQ
Tel: (01733) 555988   Fax: (01733) 555985
e-mail: postmaster@asbah.demon.co.uk
web: www.asbah.demon.co.uk/

BRITISH COUNCIL OF ORGANISATIONS OF DISABLED PEOPLE (BCODP)
Litchurch Plaza, Litchurch Lane,
Derby DE24 8AA
Tel: (01332) 295551
Fax: (01332) 295580
Minicom: (01332) 295581
e-mail: general@bcodp.org.uk
web: www.bcodp.org.uk
National umbrella organisations for groups controlled by disabled people.

BRITISH POLIO FELLOWSHIP
Eagle Office Centre, The Runway,
South Ruislip, Middlesex HA4 6SE
Tel: (020) 8 8421898
Fax: (020) 8 8420555
e-mail: british.polio@dial.pipex.com

43

Charity supporting people with polio, runs own holiday accommodation.

BRITISH RED CROSS SOCIETY
9 Grosvenor Crescent, London SW1X 7EJ
Tel: (020) 7 235 5454   Fax: (020) 7 235 3501
web: www.redcross.org.uk

CYSTIC FIBROSIS TRUST
11 London Road, Bromley, Kent BR1 1BY
Tel: (020) 8 464 7211   Fax: (020) 8 313 0472
web: www.cftrust.org.uk

DEPARTMENT OF TRANSPORT MOBILITY UNIT
1/11 Gt. Minster House, 76 Marsham Street, London SW1P 4DR Tel: (020) 7 893 3000
Deals with implementation of transport provisions of the DDA plus access to pedestrian environment.

DIAL UK
St. Catherine's Hospital, Tickhill Road, Balby, Doncaster, South Yorks DN4 8QN
Tel/Minicom: (01302) 310123
Fax: (01302) 310404
e-mail: dialuk@aol.com
web: members.aol.com/dialuk
Supports many local disability information and advises services.

DISABILITY DISCRIMINATION ACT HELPLINE
Tel: (0345) 622633
Minicom: (0345) 622644
e-mail: ddahelp@stra.sitel.co.uk
web: www.disability.gov.uk

DISABILITY INFORMATION TRUST
Mary Marlborough Lodge, Nuffield Orthopaedic Centre, Headington, Oxford OX3 7LD
Tel: (01865) 227600
Assessment and testing of disability equipment and publishing of in-depth information.

DISABLED DRIVERS ASSOCIATION
Ashwellthorpe, Norwich, Norfolk NR16 1EX
Tel: (01508) 489449   Fax: (01508) 488173
e-mail: DDAHQ@aol.com
web: www.disabled-drivers.org.uk
Fights to improve mobility and access for disabled people. Publishes excellent *Magic Carpet* magazine.

DISABLED DRIVERS MOTOR CLUB
Cottingham Way, Thrapston, Northants NN14 4PL
Tel: (01832) 734724   Fax: (01832) 733816
e-mail: ddmc@ukonline.co.uk
web: www.web.ukonline.co.uk/ddmc
Helps and encourages disabled people to gain mobility.

DISABLED LIVING FOUNDATION
380-384 Harrow Road, London W9 2HU
Tel: (020) 7 289 6111   Fax: (020) 7 266 2922
Minicom: (020) 7 432 8009
e-mail: dlfinfo@dlf.org.uk
web: www.dlf.org.uk
Aims to make everyday life easier for people with disabilities.

DISS
Harrowlands, Harrowlands Park, Dorking, Surrey TH4 2RA
Tel: (01306) 742130   Fax: (01306) 741740
Minicom: (01306) 742128
e-mail: diss@diss.org.uk
Disability information service that has developed the data base, DissBASE, an invaluable source of information.

ENGLISH HERITAGE
Customer Services, PO Box 570, Swindon, Wilts SN2 2YR
Tel: (020) 7 973 3434   Fax: (020) 7 973 3430
web: www.english-heritage.org.uk
Produces a comprehensive *Guide for Visitors with Disabilities* to all its properties.

HOLIDAY CARE
2nd Floor, Imperial Buildings, Victoria Road, Horley, Surrey RH6 7PZ
Tel: (01293) 774535   Fax: (01293) 784647
Minicom: (01293) 776943
Reservations: (01293) 773716
e-mail: holiday.care@virgin.net
web: freespace.virgin.net/hol.care
Central source of holiday and travel information for disabled and disadvantaged people. Offers details on accessible accommodation, attractions and transport and help with reservations.

HOTELIERS FORUM
(Part of Disability Partnership Initiative)
Nutmeg House, 60 Gainsford Street,

London SE1 2NY
Tel: (020) 7 403 9433   Fax: (020) 7 403 3957
e-mail: hoteliers@disabilitypartnership.co.uk
web: www.disabilitypartnership.co.uk
Aims to make the hospitality sector a leader in disability equality in the fields of service provision and employment.

LONDON TRANSPORT UNIT FOR DISABLED PASSENGERS
172 Buckingham Palace Road,
London SW1W 9TN
Tel/Minicom: (020) 7 918 3312
Fax: (020) 7 918 3876
e-mail: lt.udp@ltbuses.co.uk
web: www.londontransport.co.uk
Dedicated to securing better access to London's public transport system and providing information to mobility impaired passengers.

MOTABILITY
Goodman House, Station Approach, Harlow,
Essex CM20 2ET
Tel: (01279) 635666   Fax: (01279) 632035
web: www.motability.co.uk

MULTIPLE SCLEROSIS SOCIETY OF GT. BRITAIN and N. IRELAND
25 Effie Road, London SW6 1EE
Tel: (020) 7 610 7171   Fax: (020) 7 736 9861
Freephone Helpline: (0800) 8008000
e-mail: info@mssociety.org.uk
web: www.mssociety.org.uk
Provides information and support for people affected by MS.

MULTIPLE SCLEROSIS SOCIETY IN SCOTLAND
The Rural Centre, West Mains, Ingleston,
Newbridge, Edinburgh EH28 8NZ
Tel: (0131) 472 4106   Fax: (0131) 220 5188
45 branches throughout Scotland aiming to provide and promote welfare of people with MS and their families.

MUSCULAR DYSTROPHY GROUP
7-11 Prescott Place, London SW4 6BS
Tel: (020) 7 720 8055   Fax: (020) 7 498 0670
e-mail: info@muscular-dystrophy.org.uk
web: www.muscular-dystrophy.org.uk

NATIONAL CENTRE FOR INDEPENDENT LIVING
250 Kennington Lane, London SE11 5RD

Tel: (020) 7 587 1663   Fax: (020) 7 582 2469
Minicom: (020) 7 587 1177
e-mail: :ncil@ncil.demon.co.uk
web: www.bcodp.org.uk

NATIONAL INFORMATION FORUM
PP 10/101 BT Burne House, Bell Street,
London NW1 5BZ
Tel: (020) 7 402 6681   Fax: (020) 7 402 1259
e-mail: niforum@talk21.com
web: www.nif.org.uk
Works for improved provision of disability information.

NATIONAL TRUST DISABILITY UNIT
36 Queen Anne's Gate, London SW1H 9AS
Tel: (020) 7 222 9251   Fax: (020) 7 222 5097
e-mail: accessforall@nttrust.org.uk
web: www.nationaltrust.org.uk
Welcomes and provides for disabled visitors at a majority of its properties. Produces an excellent access guide.

QUEEN ELIZABETH'S FOUNDATION FOR DISABLED PEOPLE
Leatherhead Court, Woodlands Road,
Leatherhead, Surrey KT22 0BN
Tel: (01372) 841100   Fax: (01372) 844072

PHAB
Summit House, Wandle Road, Croydon,
Surrey CR0 1DF
Tel: (020) 8 667 9443   Fax: (020) 8 681 1399
e-mail: phab@ukonline.co.uk
web: www.phab.england.org.uk
Works for the integration of people with and without physical disabilities within the community through social clubs and activities and through holidays and courses.

ROYAL ASSOCIATION FOR DISABILITY AND REHABILITATION (RADAR)
12 City Forum, 250 City Road, London EC1V 8AF
Tel: (020) 7 250 3222   Fax: (020) 7 250 0212
Minicom: (020) 7 250 4119
e-mail: radar@radar.org.uk
web: www.radar.org.uk
National charity working for disabled people. Produces many publications relating to civil rights, mobility, employment and travel, with excellent UK and worldwide holiday guides and holiday fact packs.

SCOPE

6 Market Road, London N7 9PW
Tel: (020) 7619 7296   Fax: (020) 7619 7380
web: www.scope.org.uk
For people with cerebal palsy, scope offers a
wide range of projects and professional help.

SPINAL INJURIES ASSOCIATION

76 St. James Lane, London N10 3DF
Tel: (020) 8 444 2121   Fax: (020) 8 444 3761
Freephone Helpline: (0800) 980 0501
e-mail: sia@spinali.demon.co.uk
web: www.spinal.co.uk
This National Charity exists because life
does not stop when you become paralysed.
Offers advice on all aspects of disability.
Comprehensive web site with items such
as lists of disabled living centres.

TRIPSCOPE

Alexandra House, 241 High Street, Brentford,
Middlesex TW8 ONE.
Tel: (08457) 585641
e-mail: tripscope@cableinet.co.uk
and
The Vassall Centre, Gill Avenue
Bristol BS16 2QQ
Tel: as London
e-mail: tripscopesw@cableinet.co.uk
Provides a nationwide travel and transport
information service for disabled and
elderly people. Produces *Door to Door*, an
excellent transport guide.

TOURISM FOR ALL

11 Y Waen, Gwernaffield, Flintshire CH7 5DP
Tel: (01352) 740552   Fax: (01352) 740515
e-mail: jenny.murphy@virgin.net
web: www.disabilitynet.co.uk/groups/tourism
/index.html
Works to create and support mainstream
tourism, hospitality and leisure industries
that are accessible to all customers and
staff, irrespective of disability, age or income.

SPECIALIST TOUR/HOLIDAY ORGANISATIONS

ACCESS TRAVEL (LANCS) LTD

6 The Hillock, Astley, Lancs M29 7GW
Tel: (01942) 888844   Fax: (01942) 891811
e-mail: des@access-travel.co.uk
web: www.access-travel.co.uk
Arranges an extensive variety of holidays
to many destinations for disabled people.

A.T.S. TRAVEL LTD

1 Tank Lane, Purfleet, Essex RM19 1TA
Tel: (01708) 863198
Specialist agency arranging tailor-made
holidays throughout UK, Europe and
worldwide.

CAMPING FOR THE DISABLED

c/o National Mobility Centre,
Unit 2, Atcham Estate, Shrewsbury,
Shropshire SY4 4YG
Tel: (01743) 761889
e-mail: mis@nmcuk.freeserve.co.uk
Publish a list of adapted campsites.

CAN BE DONE LIMITED

7-11 Kensington High Street, London W8 5NP
Tel: (020) 8 907 2400   Fax: (020) 8 909 1854
e-mail: cbdtravel@aol.com
web: www.canbedone.co.uk
Individually tailored holidays and tours
designed to be accessible for wheelchair
users and for touring at a leisurely pace.

CHALFONT LINE HOLIDAYS

4 Medway Parade. Perivale,
Middlesex UB6 8HR
Tel: (020) 8 997 3799   Fax: (020) 8 991 2892
e-mail: holidays@chalfont-line.co.uk
web: www.chalfont.line.co.uk
Escorted holidays for disabled people in
UK and abroad. Specially adapted coach
with side lift, clamped wheelchair spaces.

LEONARD CHESHIRE FOUNDATION

30 Millbank, London SW1P 4QD
Tel: (020) 7 802 8200   Fax: (020) 7 802 8250
web: www.leonard-cheshire.org
Runs holiday properties for disabled persons.

DISABLED LIVING
Redbank House, 4 St. Chad's Street,
Cheetham, Manchester M8 8QA
Tel: (0161) 832 3678   Fax: (0161) 835 3591
e-mail: information@disabledliving.co.uk
Group holiday provision for disabled
people of all ages in both UK and abroad.

GROOMS HOLIDAYS
For Self-Catering and Boating Holidays
PO Box 36, Cowbridge,
Vale of Glamorgan CF71 7GB
Tel: (01446) 771311   Fax: (01446) 775060
e-mail: gmo@cwcom.net
web: www.johngrooms.org.uk/holidays

HOLIDAYS FOR YOU AND ME
Syn-y-don, Morawell Close, Croesgoch,
Haverfordwest, Pembrokeshire,
Wales SA62 5JS
Tel/Fax: (01348) 837833
e-mail: tycymru@lineone.net
web: www.jpmarketing.co.uk/holidays
Independently run small company
specialising in all types of accommodation
in the UK with disabled access. Very
comprehensive brochure.

CAR HIRE – LYNX HAND CONTROLS
Mansion House, St. Helens Road, Ormskirk,
Lancs. L39 4QJ
Tel: (01695) 573816   Fax: (01695) 581500
e-mail: info@lynxcontrols.com
web: www.lynxcontrols.com
Produces hand control equipment that
can be fitted to a hire car. Suitable only
for someone with a lower limb disability.
Also supplies push-pull systems if the
need arises. Lynx works with most of the
major car hire companies as well as many
smaller firms covering all the UK.

SPECIAL FAMILIES HOME SWAP REGISTER
Erme House, Station Road, Plympton,
Devon PL7 2AU
Tel: (01752) 347577   Fax: (01752) 344611
e-mail: med_serv@globalnet.co.uk
web: www.mywebpage.net/special-
families/index
Subscription based allowing swapping of
specially adapted homes UK wide. Short
breaks, full length holidays and visits.

WHEELCHAIR TRAVEL LTD
1 Johnston Green, Guildford, Surrey GU2 6XS
Tel: (01483) 233 640   Fax: (01483) 237 772
e-mail: info@wheelchair-travel.co.uk
web: www.wheelchair-travel.co.uk
Comprehensive private transport service
for wheelchair users including self-drive
rental accessible minibuses, Fiat Fiorino
cars and hand-controlled cars, accessible
luxury taxis, tour/airport transfers.

WINGED FELLOWSHIP TRUST
Angel House, 20-32 Pentonville Road
London N1 9XD
Tel: (020) 7 833 2594   Fax: (020) 7 278 0370
e-mail: admin@wft.org.uk
web: www.wft.org.uk
Operates five fully accessible holiday centres
at Netley (Hants), Redhill (Surrey), Chigwell
(Essex), Nottingham and Southport
(Merseyside). See under separate counties.

SPECIALIST SPORTS/ OUTDOOR ASSOCIATIONS
BRITISH DISABLED FLYING CLUB
Pantiles, The Street, Tendering,
Essex CO16 0BL
Tel/Fax: (01255) 830198
e-mail: deltaftrot@aol.com
web: www.englishinternet.com/deltafoxtrot/
contacts.htm

BRITISH DISABLED WATER SKI ASSOCIATION
The Tony Edge National Centre,
Heron Lake, Hythend, Wraysbury,
Middx. TW19 6HW
Tel: (01784) 483664   Fax: (01784) 482747
e-mail: heron.lake@ukonline.co.uk
web: www.bd.wsa.org.uk
Centres throughout the UK, open
between April and October. The aim is to
introduce newcomers to the sport who,
because of their disabilities, would not
have considered this challenge possible.
Accessible changing facilities and WCs,
wetsuits and lifejackets included.

BRITISH MOTORSPORTS ASSOCIATION FOR THE DISABLED
PO Box 120, Aldershot, Hants GU11 3TF
Tel: (01252) 319070

BRITISH SKI CLUB FOR THE DISABLED
Springmount, Berwick St. John, Shaftesbury,
Dorset SP7 0HO
Tel: (01747) 828515

**BRITISH WHEELCHAIR ATHLETICS
ASSOCIATION**
28 Congreve Way, Bardsey, Leeds,
West Yorks LS17 9DG
Tel: (01937) 572668

BRITISH WHEELCHAIR SPORTS FOUNDATION
Ludwig Guttman Sports Centre, Bernard
Crescent, Harvey Road, Aylesbury,
Bucks HP21 9PP
Tel: (01296) 484848 Fax: (01296) 24171

DISABILITY SPORTS ENGLAND
Mary Glen Haig Suite, Solecast House,
13-27 Brunswick Place, London N1 6DX
Tel: (020) 7 490 4919   Fax: (20) 7 490 4914

**GREAT BRITAIN WHEELCHAIR RUGBY
ASSOCIATION**
Firf Trellech, Monmouth, Wales NP5 4PQ
Tel: (01600) 860373

HANDICAPPED ANGLERS TRUST
Slivericks Oast, Ashburnham, Nr. Battle,
East Sussex TN33 9PE
Tel: (01435) 830891

HANDICAPPED SCUBA ASSOCIATION
6 Parkwood Grove, Charlton Kings,
Cheltenham, Glos. GL53 9JP
Tel: (01625) 586302

JUBILEE SAILING TRUST
Jubilee Yard, Hazel Road, Woolstone,
Southampton, Hants SO19 7GB
Tel: (01703) 449108   Fax: (01703) 449145

**NATIONAL ASSOCIATION OF SWIMMING
CLUBS FOR THE HANDICAPPED**
The Willows, Mayles Lane, Wickham,
Hants PO17 5ND
Tel: (01329) 833689

**NATIONAL HANDICAPPED SKIERS
ASSOCIATION**
c/o Harlow Ski School, Hammarskjold Road,
Harlow, Essex CM20 2JF
Tel: (01279) 444100   Fax: (01279) 413556

NATIONAL WHEELCHAIR TENNIS ASSOCIATION
c/o British Tennis Foundation,
The Queen's Club, West Kensington,
London W14 9EG
Tel: (020) 7 381 7051   Fax: (020) 7 381 6507

RIDING FOR THE DISABLED ASSOCIATION
Avenue R, National Agricultural Centre,
Kenilworth, Warwicks CV8 2LY
Tel: (01203) 696510 Fax: (01203) 696532
Aims to provide riding and driving
opportunities to disabled people.

RYA SAILABILITY
The Stables, Blind Burn Hall, Wark, Hexham,
Northumberland NE48 3HE
Tel: (01434) 230464 *or*
Romsey Road, Eastleigh, Hants SO50 9YA
Tel: (01703) 627400   Fax: (01703) 620545
In Hexham, RYA owns Sea Legs, a
catamaran adapted for disabled people.
Available for charter with qualified
skippers available on request. Sailability
also offers other water-based holidays.

UPHILL SKI CLUB
6 Market Road, London N7 9PW
Tel: (020) 7 619 7100
Winter sports holidays in Scotland.

THE STACKPOLE CENTRE
Home Farm, Pembroke, SA71 5DQ
Tel: (01646) 661425
Facilities include indoor pool and
activities include canoeing, abseiling,
horse riding, fishing. Self-catering
cottage or group house accommodation
and b&b full board.

CHURCHTOWN OUTDOOR ADVENTURE CENTRE
SCOPE Lanlivery, Bodmin,
Cornwall, PL30 5BT
Tel: (01208) 872148
All ability courses in sailing, canoeing,
orienteering, camping, rock climbing.

ENGLAND

Tower Bridge. Still one of the most impressive buildings on the London skyline.

MAJOR TOURIST BOARDS

BRITISH TOURIST AUTHORITY AND ENGLISH TOURISM COUNCIL
Thames Tower, Black's Road, London W6 9EL
Tel (020) 8563 3000   Fax: (020) 8563 0302
web: www.visitbritain.com
web: britannia.com/
web: www.englishtourism.org.uk

BTA/ETB also run immediate response query line called SCOOT. Tel: (0800) 192 192.

CUMBRIA TOURIST BOARD
(County of Cumbria, including Lake District)
Ashleigh, Holly Road, Windermere,
Cumbria LA23 2AQ
Tel: (01539) 444444   Fax: (01539) 444 041
e-mail: mail@cumbria tourist board.co.uk
web: www.golakes.co.uk

EAST OF ENGLAND TOURIST BOARD
(Counties of Beds., Cambs., Essex, Herts., Norfolk and Suffolk)
Toppesfield Hall, Hadleigh, Suffolk IP7 5DN
Tel: (01473) 822922   Fax: (01473) 823063
e-mail: englandtouristboard@compuserve.com
web: www.visitbritain.com/east-of-england

EAST MIDLANDS TOURIST BOARD
(Counties of Derby, Leics., Lincs., Northants and Notts.)
Exchequergate, Lincoln LN2 1PZ
Tel: (01522) 531 521   Fax: (01522) 532 501

HEART OF ENGLAND TOURIST BOARD
(Counties of Cherwell, Glos., Hereford and Worcs./Salop, Staffs., War., West Midlands and West Oxon.)
Woodside, Larkhill Road, Worcester WR5 2EF
Tel: (01905) 763436   Fax: (01905) 763450
e-mail: market@heart-eng_tourist-board.org.uk
web: www.visitbritain.com

LONDON TOURIST BOARD
(Greater London area)
26 Grosvenor Gardens, London SW1W 0DU
Tel: (020) 7932 2000
Fax: (020) 7932 0222
web: www.londontown.com

NORTH WEST TOURIST BOARD
(Counties of Cheshire, Gtr. Manchester, Lancs., Merseyside and High Peak District of Derbys.)
Swan House, Swan Meadow Road, Wigan Pier, Wigan, Lancs. WN3 5BB
Tel: (01942) 821222   Fax: (01942) 820002
e-mail: info@nwtb.u-net.com
web: www.visitbritain.com/north-west-england

NORTHUMBRIA TOURIST BOARD
(Counties of Cleveland, Durham, Northumberland and Tyne & Wear)
Aykley Heads, Durham DH1 5UX
Tel: (0191) 821222   Fax: (0191) 3860899
e-mail: marketing@ntb.org.uk
web: www.ntb.org.uk/

SOUTH EAST ENGLAND TOURIST BOARD
(Counties of east Sussex, Kent, Surrey and west Sussex).
The Old Brew House, Warwick Park, Tunbridge Wells, Kent TN2 5TU
Tel: (01892) 540766   Fax: (01892) 511008
e-mail: enquiries@seetb.org.uk
web: www.seetb.org.uk/

SOUTHERN TOURIST BOARD
(Counties of Berks., Bucks., east and north Dorset, Hants.. Oxon. and Isle of Wight)
40 Chamberlayne Road, Eastleigh,
Hants SO50 5JH
Tel: (01703) 620006   Fax: (01703) 620010
e-mail: 100651,.3040@compuserve.com
web: www.visitbritain.com

WEST COUNTRY TOURIST BOARD
(Counties of Cornwall, Devon, west Dorset, Somerset, Wilts. and Isles of Scilly)
60 St. Davids Hill, Exeter, Devon EX4 4SY
Tel:(01392) 425426   Fax: (01392) 420891
e-mail: post@wctb.co.uk

YORKSHIRE TOURIST BOARD
(Counties of north, south and west Yorks., and Humberside)
312 Tadcaster Road, York YO2 2HF
Tel: (01904) 707961   Fax: (01904) 701404
e-mail: e.n.c@dialpipex.com
web: www.ytb.org.uk

BEDFORDSHIRE

BEDFORD

County town with modern shopping centre and open market twice a week. Entertainment in Corn Exchange, whilst more leisurely pursuits include viewing the embankment gardens and the many historical buildings.

TOURIST INFORMATION CENTRE
10 St. Paul's Square, Bedford MK40 1SL
Tel: (01234) 215226

DISABILITY INFORMATION SERVICE (ABOVE SHOPMOBILITY)
First Floor, 1 The Howard Centre, Horne Lane, Bedford MK40 1HU
Tel/Fax: (01234) 349988
Mincom: (01582) 470968
e-mail: drc_beds@compuserve.com
Bedford CC publish booklet *Community Transport Handbook* with much relevant information, available from TIC or BCC (Transport) Tel: (01234) 228399/228337

BUSES – GENERAL INFORMATION
Tel: (01234) 228337

Arriva – The Shires, Marchwood House, 934-974 St. Albans Road, Garston, Watford, Herts WD2 6NN
Tel: (01923) 673121

BEDFORD SHOPMOBILITY
1 The Howard Centre, Horne Lane, Bedford MK40 1UH
Tel: (01234) 348000

TRAINS
Midland Main Line:
Special Needs: Tel: (0114) 2537654
Minicom: (0845) 7078051

Silverlink:
Special Needs: Tel: (01923) 207818
Fax: (01923) 207023
Minicom: (01923) 256430
Thameslink:
Special Needs: Tel: (0207) 6206333
Minicom: (0207) 6205561

Stationlink bus: Tel: (0207) 9183312

TAXIS:
AGS Cars. Tel: (01234) 218888
1 Metrocab with straps, no ramps.

Ampthill Taxis: Tel: (01525) 841841
1 Nissan Serena, no fittings.

Chands Taxis: Tel: (01589) 150293
1 FX4 with ramp, clamps and straps.

Rae's Taxis: Tel: (01973) 452002
1 Fairway with ramp, clamps and straps.

Sembhi's Taxis: Tel: (01589) 520439
1 FX4 with ramp, clamp and straps.

BEDFORD RED CROSS
99 Ashburnham Road, Bedford MK40 1EA
Tel: (01234) 349166

ATTRACTIONS
BEDFORD MUSEUM
Castle Lane, Bedford MK40 3XD
Tel: (01234) 353323   Fax: (01234) 273401
Housed in former brewery, the museum is within the grounds of Bedford Castle, beside the Great Ouse river embankment. Wide range of exhibits and collections tell human and natural history of north Bedfordshire, together with delightful rural room sets and Old School Museum. Located close to 2 town centre car parks.
SD 🦽   CP n/a   E 🦽   RF 🦽
L 🦽   S 🦽   WC 🚹

JOHN BUNYAN MUSEUM and LIBRARY
Mill Street, Bedford MK40 3EU
Tel/Fax: (01234) 213722
Contains most of known possessions of John Bunyan and many editions of his 60 recognised works including "The Pilgrim's Progress" in 168 foreign languages.
SD 🦽   CP 🦽   E 🦽   RF 🦽   L 🦽
C 🦽   S 🚹   RFE 🚹   WC n/a

BROMHAM MILL
Bridge Road, Bromham, Bedford MK43 8LP
Tel: (01234) 824330
By the river Great Ouse, this C17th restored water mill offers flour milling demonstrations, and has an art gallery

with exhibition programmes and craft displays. Upstairs gallery not accessible.

SD ♿   CP ♿   E ♿ via fire door.
RF ♿   C ♿   S ♿   WC 🚹

RIVERSIDE WALK

2 miles easy going, all hard paths suitable for wheelchairs. Starting from the north west bank at Town Bridge, the walk follows a route to the edge of town marked by County Bridge and returns along the Embankment Gardens. Follow the path from the Bridge (Charter Walk) past red brick Shire Hall designed by eminent Victorian architect Alfred Waterhouse, alongside being the market place. This path (Queen's Walk) takes you past the Star Club and walking towards County Bridge you pass the moorings at Queens Reach, before the path takes you up to the bridge past the river-front development of Sovereign Quay.

BIGGLESWADE

Known as a busy market-gardening area with many historical pubs from its days as a flourishing coach stop.

ATTRACTION
SWISS GARDEN
Biggleswade Road, Old Warden, Biggleswade
Tel: (01234) 228330
Fax: (01234) 228315

Go back to early C19th when interests in ornamental gardening and picturesque architecture were first combined. Within 10 acres wander among splendid shrubs and rare trees at the centre of which is the tiny romantic Swiss Cottage, although there are other exotic structures. There is also a fernery and grotto. A wheelchair route around the garden is available, together with loan of wheelchairs.

SD ♿   CP 🚹   E ♿
C 🚹   WC 🚹   RFE ♿

DUNSTABLE

The town was built at the junction of Watling Street and the prehistoric Icknield Way with the wonderful, windy Downs offering amazing views.

ATTRACTION
WHIPSNADE WILD ANIMAL PARK
Dunstable LU6 2LF
Tel: (0990) 200123   Fax: (01582) 872649

One of Europe's largest conservation centres with over 2,500 animals set in 600 acres of beautiful parkland. See the park by car and explore wherever you wish to stop, or on foot. Wheelchairs available.

SD ♿   CP ♿   E ♿   RF ♿
C 🚹   S 🚹   WC 🚹   RFE ♿

LEIGHTON BUZZARD

Large, pleasant market town with many buildings of interest.

ATTRACTIONS
LEIGHTON BUZZARD RAILWAY
Page's Park Station, Billington Road,
Leighton Buzzard LU7 8TN
Tel: (01525) 373888   Fax: (01525) 377814

5.5-mile train ride through mix of housing, industry and open countryside, following original authentic route created in 1919. Trip lasts for one hour.
One carriage capable of carrying up to four wheelchairs, operating on 11.15, 12.45, 14.15 and 15.45 departure trains.

SD ♿   CP 🚹   E 🚹   RF 🚹
C ♿   S ♿   WC 🚹   RFE ♿

MEAD OPEN FARM
Stanbridge Road, Billington, Nr. Leighton
Buzzard LU7 9HL
Tel: (01525) 852954

Working family farm with wide range of traditional animals and rare breeds. Pet's corner with lots of hands-on activities. Falconry displays, tractor trailer rides and children's play area. Surface in yard area is flat concrete with slight slope. Paddocks are flat with grass surface – accessible in dry weather – no steps at any point.

SD ♿   CP ♿   E ♿   RF ♿   WC ♿

LUTON

Largest town in the county with delightful parks.

HOTEL
THISTLE LUTON

Arndale Centre, Luton LU1 2TR
Tel: (01582) 734199   Fax: (01582) 402528
No. of Accessible Rooms: 1
Accessible Facilities: Lounge, Restaurant
(1st floor, via accessible lift). Large,
modern property located in central Luton,
next door to the Arndale Shopping Centre.

LUTON MUSEUM and ART GALLERY
Wardown Park, Luton LU2 7MA
Tel: (01582) 546722   Fax: (01582) 546763
e-mail: burgessl@luton.gov.uk
Victorian mansion in Wardown park with
exhibits on natural and cultural history of
the area, including development of hat
industry in C19th and C20th. NB: Entrance
via door to left of front entrance.
Wheelchairs available.

SD 🚾   CP 🚾   E 🚾   RF 🚾
C 🚾   S 🚾   WC 🚾

STOCKWOOD CRAFT MUSEUM and GARDENS
Stockwood Country Park, Farley Hill,
Luton LU1 4BH
Tel: (01582) 738714   Fax: (01582) 546763
e-mail: burgessl@luton.gov.uk
Exterior exhibits include sculpture, period
and winter gardens, plus interior
exhibition galleries. Wheelchairs available.

P 🚾   E 🚾   C 🚾   S 🚾
WC 🚾   RFE 🚾   WC 🚾 craft museum

WOODSIDE WILDFOWL PARK
Mancroft Road, Slip End Village,
Luton LU1 4DG
Tel: (01582) 841044
A vast farm shop, poultry centre, children's
farm and leisure complex with daily
handling, feeding and learning about
poultry. Wheelchairs available.

SD 🚾   CP 🚾   E 🚾   RF 🚾
C 🚾   S 🚾   WC 🚾

SANDY
Small, but growing town in pleasant
countryside. Home of the Royal Society for
the Preservation of Birds.

ATTRACTION
RSPB, THE LODGE NATURE RESERVE and
VISITOR CENTRE.
The Lodge, Sandy SG19 2DL

Tel: (01767) 680551   Fax: (01767) 683508
UK headquarters of the RSPB with
heathland, woodland and meadow, lakes
and formal gardens. Several exotic trees
including the Atlas cedar. Useful map of
areas of access available.

SD 🚾   CP 🚾   RF 🚾   S 🚾
WC 🚾   RFE 🚾

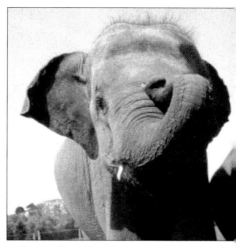

*Full access for all at Whipsnade Wild
Animal Park.*

WOBURN
Old village situated in picturesque
wooded countryside.

HOTEL
BEDFORD ARMS THISTLE   CAT   🚾
George Street, Woburn MK17 9PX
Tel: (01525) 290441   Fax: (01525) 290432
No. of Accessible Rooms: 20. Bath.
Accessible Facilities: Lounge, Dining
room. Originally an inn, now completely
modernised, located in town centre.

ATTRACTION
WOBURN SAFARI PARK
Woburn Park, Woburn MK17 9QN
Tel: (01525) 290407   Fax: (01525) 290489
e-mail: wobsafari@aol.com
Within Woburn Abbey, over 300 acres of
Safari Park with varied animal species
collection.

SD 🚾   CP 🚾   RF 🚾
C 🚾   SHOP 🚾   WC 🚾

BERKSHIRE

WEST BERKSHIRE TOURISM
e-mail: tourism@westberks.gov.uk
web: www.westberks.gov.uk

ASCOT

Famous for its racecourse, started by
Queen Anne in 1711. The Ascot Gold Cup
was first presented in 1807. Few of the
original buildings remain.

SPORTING VENUE
ASCOT RACECOURSE
Ascot, Berks. SL5 7JN
Admin: (01344) 878505
Booking-Box Office: (01344) 876456
Fax: (01344) 628299
NB. June meeting pre-booked, ticket only.
No pre-booking for other meetings.

CP ♿ RTE ♿ ED ♿
INT ♿ (assistance available) L ♿
WC ♿ (except no hinged support rail). Located in
Royal Enclosure, Grandstand and Silver Ring.
SS ♿ open – platform designated.
Route to Grandstand is tarmac, slight gradient to
grandstand, out onto lawned area
and platform. B/R ♿

BRACKNELL

Berkshire's only new town.

TOURIST INFORMATION CENTRE
The Look Out Discovery Park, Nine Mile Ride,
Bracknell RG12 7QW
Tel: (01344) 869896 Fax: (01344) 869343

HOTEL
COPPID BEECH HOTEL ♿
John Nike Wake, Binfield,
Nr. Bracknell RG12 8TF
Tel: (01344) 303333 Fax: (01344) 301200
No. of Accessible Rooms: 16. Shower
Accessible Facilities: Lounge, Restaurant,
Leisure Club with Pool, Sauna, Spa Alpine-
style hotel with extensive leisure facilities.

LEISURE FACILITY
CORAL REEF, BRACKNELL'S WATER WORLD

Nine Mile Ride, Bracknell RG12 7JQ
Tel: (01344) 862525 Fax: (01344) 869146
e-mail: coral.reef@bracknell-forest.gov.uk
Various pools for adults and children.

SD ♿ CP ♿ E ♿ RF ♿ L ♿
C ♿ S ♿ WC ♿ RFE ♿

MAIDENHEAD

Pleasant residential town popular for
boating on the Thames. Walks along the
towpath are rewarding.

TOURIST INFORMATION CENTRE
The Library, St. Ives Road,
Maidenhead SL6 1QU
Tel: (01628) 781110 Fax: (01628) 796408

ATTRACTION
COURAGE SHIRE HORSE CENTRE
Cherry Garden Lane, Maidenhead Thicket,
Maidenhead SL6 3QD
Tel: (01628) 824848
Free guided tours of prize-winning shire
horses, dray rides, farriers shop, harness
maker displays, small animal and bird area.

SD ♿ CP ♿ E ♿ C n/a
S ♿ WC ♿ RFE ♿

NEWBURY
TOURIST INFORMATION CENTRE
The Wharf, Newbury RG14 5AS
Tel: (01635) 30267 Fax: (01635) 51962

SPORTING VENUE
NEWBURY RACECOURSE
The Racecourse, Newbury RG14 7NZ
Admin and Booking-Box Office: (01635) 40015
Fax: (01635) 528358
e-mail: newbury.races@pop3.hiway.co.uk
web: www.sporting-life.com/racing/newbury

CP ♿ RE ♿ ED ♿ INT ♿
L ♿ WC ♿ SS ♿ B/R ♿

READING

County town with fine Georgian buildings.

TOURIST INFORMATION CENTRE
The Town Hall, Belgrave Street,
Reading RG1 1QH
Tel: (0118) 9566226 Fax: (0118) 9399885

READING BOROUGH COUNCIL
Town Hall, Blagrave Street,
Reading RG1 1QH
Tel: (0118) 9399873

ACCESS OFFICER
Civic Centre, Reading RG1 7TD
Tel: (0118) 9390900   Fax: (0118) 9589770
Minicom: (0118) 9390700

DIAL Berkshire
Tel: (0118) 9390900

DISABILITY INFORMATION NETWORK
Freepost (TG2750), Church Hill House,
Crowthorne Road, Bracknell RG12 7EP
Tel: (01344) 301572
Minicom: (01344) 427757
e-mail: ask@brin.demon.co.uk
web: www.azariah.org.uk/bdin
Maintains a comprehensive disability-
related library with wide range of
information, including holidays.

BUSES
Reading Buses, The Travel Shop, 9 Duke
Street, Reading
Tel: (0118) 9594000   Fax: (0118) 9575379
Minicom: (0118) 9027630
e-mail: info@reading-buses.co.uk
Some vehicles are fitted with kneeling
facility and some routes operated by Super
Low Floor vehicles.

TAXIS
Hackney Carriages: Tel: (0118) 9670670
30 FX4s.

YRB Ltd: Tel: (0118) 9599030
2 minibuses with lift, clamp and straps.

Checkers Cars: Tel: (0118) 9595959
1 FX4 with ramp, clamps and straps.

TRAINS
First Great Western – Special Needs:
Tel: (0845) 7413775
Thames Trains – Special Needs:
Tel: (0118) 9083607
web: www.thamestrains.co.uk
Virgin Trains – Special Needs:
Tel: (0845) 7443366
Minicom: (0845) 7443367

Wales & West – Special Needs:
Tel: (0845) 3003005
Minicom: (0845) 7585469

CAR PARKS
6-hour free Orange badge parking in Broad
Street Mall.
Tel: (0118) 9390900
Minicom: (0118) 9390700

SHOPMOBILITY
Readibus, 2nd Floor, Broad Street Mall,
Reading RH2 0JX
Tel: (0118) 9310000   Fax: (0118) 9753070
Minicom: (0118) 9310000

HOTEL
COURTYARD BY MARRIOTT
Bath Road, Padworth, Reading RG7 5HT
Tel: (0118) 971 4411
Fax: (0118) 971 4442
No. of Accessible Rooms: 2. Bath
Accessible Facilities: Lounge, Restaurant.

READING HOLIDAY INN
Caversham Bridge, Richfield Avenue,
Reading RG1 8BD
Tel: (0118) 9259988   Fax: (0118) 9391665
No. of Accessible Rooms: 1.
Accessible Facilities: Ramped access to
Lounge and Restaurant. Purpose-built
hotel located next to Caversham Bridge,
overlooking River Thames.

RENAISSANCE READING HOTEL
Oxford Road, Reading RG1 7RH
Tel: (0118) 9586222   Fax: (0118) 9597842
web: www.renaissancehotels.com
No. of Accessible Rooms: 1. Bath.
Accessible Facilities: Lounge, Restaurant
Deluxe hotel in town centre close to
pedestrianised shopping and
entertainment.

WINDSOR
Famous for its castle, home of British
monarchs for almost 900 years. Recently
restored after 1992 fire. Largest inhabited
castle in the world. Known also for Eton,
England's famous public school. An
attractive town with Georgian and Victorian
buildings, many interesting walks.

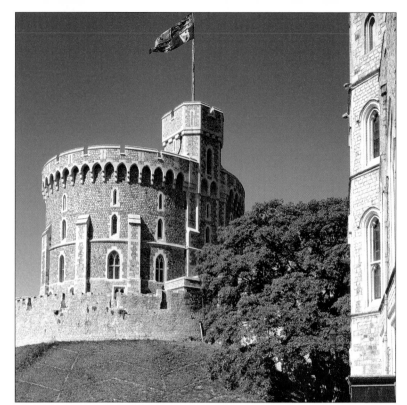

The flag now flies cheerily over the newly restored Windsor Castle.

TOURIST INFORMATION CENTRE
24 High Street, Windsor SL4 1LH
Tel: (01753) 743900   Fax: (01753) 743904

HOTEL
OAKLEY COURT HOTEL 🚶
Windsor Road, Water Oakley,
Windsor SL4 5UR
Tel: (01753) 609988   Fax: (01628) 637011
e-mail:oakleyct@atlas.co.uk
No. of Accessible Rooms: 2
Accessible Facilities: Lounge, Restaurant
(both via ramps). Victorian Gothic
mansion set in 35 acres overlooking River
Thames. Used in the 60s as location for
Hammer Horror films.

ATTRACTIONS
LEGOLAND WINDSOR
Winkfield Road, Windsor SL4 4AY
Tel: (0990) 040404   Fax: (01753) 626300
web: www.legoland.co.uk
Set in 1,500 acres of Windsor Great Park
with many hands-on activities, rides,
themes, playscapes and millions of Lego

bricks. Also peaceful areas with
restaurants and facilities.
SD ♿ CP ♿ E ♿ RF ♿ C ♿
S ♿ WC ♿ RFE ♿

WINDSOR CASTLE
Windsor SL4 1NJ
Tel: (01753) 868286   Fax: (01753) 832290
Originally built for William the
Conqueror 900 years ago to guard western
approach to London. State apartments
contain fine works of art, armour,
pictures and interiors. Damaged by fire in
1992, now completely restored.
NOTE: NO PARKING FACILITIES.
All areas within precincts of Castle
accessible, except Queen Mary's Dolls
House and some semi state rooms within
State Apartments open only in winter.
Principal restored areas that form year-
round visitor route are accessible. Lift
available to State Apartments.
SD n/a CP n/a E ♿ RF ♿
L ♿ WC ♿

BRISTOL

Thriving ancient city-port developed originally for wool export and C18th slave trading, with resultant fine terraces and grand buildings built on the ensuing riches. Clifton, once a village on the steep cliffs above the port, is the most attractive part, and location of the university. Brunel's famous suspension bridge is located here.

TOURIST INFORMATION CENTRE
St. Nicholas Church, St. Nicholas Church Street, Bristol BS1 1UE
Tel: (0117) 9260767   Fax: (0117) 9297703
e-mail: bristol@tourism. gov.uk
web: www.tourism.bristol.gov.uk

BUSES
Easyrider: Tel: (0117) 9778759
General Bus/Park & Ride Information:
Tel: (0117) 9555111

TAXIS
Bristol Hackney Cabs: Tel: (0117) 9538638
15 adapted vehicles.
Peter's Taxis: Tel: (0117) 9714141
2 adapted vehicles.
Streamline Taxis: Tel: (0117) 9264001

TRAINS
First Great Western – Special Needs:
Tel: (0845) 7413775
Virgin Trains – Special Needs: (0845) 7443366
Minicom: (0845) 7443367
Wales & West: (0845) 3003005
Minicom: (0845) 7585469

CAR PARKS
Some free unlimited Orange badge parking.
Tel: (0117) 9223006

SHOPMOBILITY
Unit 26, Castle Gallery, Upper Mall,
The Galleries Shopping Centre, Broadmead,
Bristol BS1 3XE
Tel: (0117) 9226342

HOTELS
SWALLOW ROYAL
College Green, Bristol BS1 5TA
Tel: (0117) 9255100   Fax: (0117) 9251515
No. of Accessible Rooms: 2

Accessible Facilities: All public areas, except pool. Quality city centre hotel next to the cathedral restored to former Victorian glory with contemporary luxury.

CROWNE PLAZA BRISTOL
Victoria Street, Bristol BS1 6HY
Tel: (0117) 9769988   Fax: (0117) 9255040
No. of Accessible Rooms: 2
Accessible Facilities: Lounge, Restaurant
Modern hotel in city centre close to Temple Meads Railway station.

THISTLE BRISTOL
Broad Street, Bristol BS1 2EL
Tel: (0117) 9291645   Fax: (0117) 9227619
No. of Accessible Rooms: 6. Bath
Accessible Facilities: Restaurant.
Quality hotel in the centre of the city.

ACCESSIBLE ATTRACTIONS
BRISTOL INDUSTRIAL MUSEUM
Princes Wharf, City Docks, Bristol BS1 4RN
Tel: (0117) 9251470   Fax: (0117) 9297318
Displays of motor and horse-drawn vehicles, plus locally built aircraft. Railway exhibits include an industrial locomotive. Local port displays also.

SD CP E RF
C n/a S WC

All ship shape and Bristol fashion at the Industrial Museum.

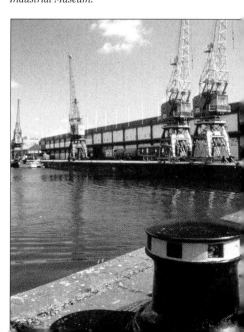

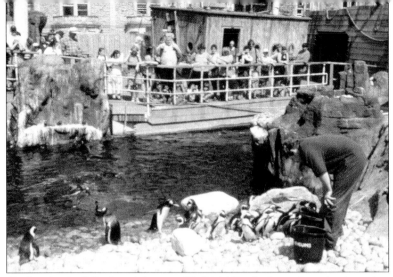

Feeding time is all the time at the accessible Bristol Zoo Gardens cafes and restaurants.

BRISTOL ZOO GARDENS
Clifton, Bristol BS8 3HA
Tel: (0117) 9738951   Fax: (0117) 9736814
e-mail: information@bristolzoo.org.uk
web: www.bristolzoo.org.uk

Over 300 species of wildlife in delightful gardens, notable for gorilla exhibit, walk-through aviary. Also aquarium reptile house, bug and twilight worlds.

SD	♿	CP	🚶	E	♿	RF	♿
C	🚶	S	🚶	WC	🚶	RFE	🚶

SS GREAT BRITAIN
Great Western Dock, Gas Ferry Road,
Bristol BS1 6TY
Tel: (0117) 9260680   Fax: (0117) 9255788

The first ocean-going, propeller-driven, iron ship in history, designed by Brunel and built and launched in Bristol in 1843. Now being restored to original appearance.

SD	♿	CP	♿	E	♿	RF	♿	C	♿
S	♿	WC	🚶	RFE	♿		

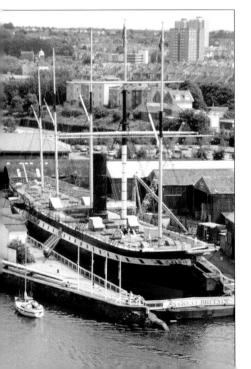

THEATRE
BRISTOL OLD VIC
King Street, Bristol BS1 4ED
Admin: (0117) 9493993
Booking-Box Office: (0117) 9877877
Minicom: (0117) 9264388
Fax: (0117) 9493996
e-mail: bristol.old.vic@cablenet.co.uk

Complies Part M, Building Regulations.

SD ♿   CP 🚶 Nearest Public CP – Queen Charlotte Street, Orange badge spaces.   No Taxi Rank
RE ♿   ED ♿   INT ♿
L ♿ (wheelchair lift)   WC ♿ (Adapted, unisex, on ground floor)   AUD ♿   B/R ♿

Additional Notes: Concessionary prices for you and companion. Level entrance to steps (lift), level to wheelchair spaces.

SS Great Britain – not quite rustproof.

BUCKINGHAMSHIRE

BUCKS DISABILITY INFORMATION
Tel: (01908) 231344

CHILTERN MULTIPLE SCLEROSIS CENTRE
Scarlett Avenue, Halton, Aylesbury HP22 5PG
Tel: (01296) 696133

BEACONSFIELD

Old town with historical buildings separated from the new town by over 0.25 miles of wooded country.

ATTRACTION
BEKONSCOT MODEL VILLAGE
Warwick Road, Beaconsfield HP9 2PL
Tel: (01494) 672919
Fax: (01494) 675284
e-mail: bekonscot@dial.pipex.com
web: www.bekonscot.org.uk
Oldest model village in the world founded in 1929. It portrays rural England in the 1930s with six villages each with their miniature population going about their daily routines. Many moving models including a gauge-1 model railway that runs throughout the

They say rural England is shrinking, but really!

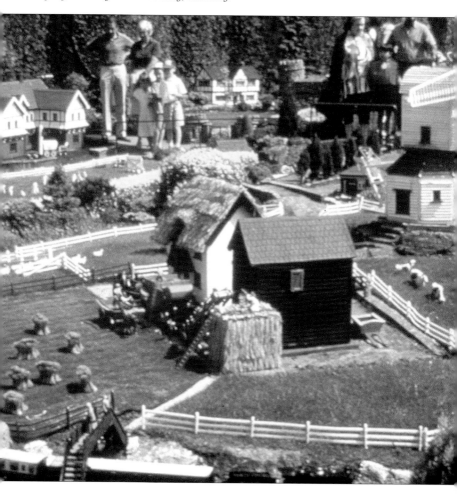

1.5-acre site. Width of some of the paths is a little narrow.

SD  CP   E   C
S n/a WC 👤 RFE 👤

BURNHAM

Fairly large residential village known for its forest of Burnham Beeches, one of the country's finest beauty spots.

HOTEL

THE GROVEFIELD HOTEL
Taplow Common Road, Burnham SL1 8LP
Tel: (01628) 603131   Fax: (01628) 668078
web: macdonaldhotels.co.uk/grovefield-hotel
No. of Accessible Rooms: 1. Bath Accessible Facilities: Lounge, Restaurant, Bar. Elegant property set in seven acres of lawns surrounded by woodland. Originally the country retreat of John Fuller, of brewing fame and still retains many original architectural features.

HIGH WYCOMBE

Large town of importance since Roman times. Now a modern town surrounded by many areas of natural beauty.

ATTRACTION

HUGHENDEN MANOR ESTATE (NT)
High Wycombe HP14 4LA
Tel: (01494) 755573
Home of Benjamin Disraeli, Victorian Prime Minister from 1848 until his death in 1881. House contains many personal items: lovely walks in surrounding park and colourful gardens.

SD n/a CP   E 👤 FR 👤
C 👤 S 👤 WC 👤 RFE 👤

MILTON KEYNES

New town built in 1960s, arranged on grid/roundabout system, surrounded by pleasant countryside.

TOURIST INFORMATION CENTRE

The Food Centre, 411 Secklow Gate East, Central Milton Keynes MK9 3NE

Tel: (01908) 232525   Fax: (01908) 235050

BRITISH RED CROSS
Westfield Road, Bletchley, Milton Keynes MK2 2RA
Tel: (01908) 370996
They also operate a wheelchair short-term loan service Tel: (01908) 678768

BUSES

No easy access/low-floor buses at present, but planned. Information on services:
Community Information Centre, Central Library, 555 Silbury Boulevard, Milton Keynes MK9 3HL
Tel: (01908) 254055   Fax: (01908) 254086

TAXIS

Hackney Carriages: Tel: (0802) 847503
12 London-style cabs.
No private hire cars available.

TRAINS

Connex: Customer Services:
Tel: (0870) 6030405
Fax: (0870) 6030505
Minicom: (01233) 617621
Silverlink – Special Needs:
Tel: (01923) 207818
Fax: (01923) 207023
Minicom: (01923) 256430
Virgin Trains – Special Needs:
Tel: (0845) 7443366
Minicom: (0845) 7443367

CAR PARKS

Free unlimited orange-badge parking.

SHOPMOBILITY

Shopping information Centre, CMK Shopping Building, Midsummer Arcade, Milton Keynes
Tel: (01908) 670231

HOTEL

HILTON NATIONAL 👤
Timbold Drive, Kents Hill Park, Milton Keynes MK7 6HL
Tel: (01908) 694433   Fax: (01908) 695533
No. of Accessible Rooms: 2. Bath Accessible Facilities: Lounge, Restaurant Bright, modern hotel close to the M1.

CAMBRIDGESHIRE

CAMBRIDGESHIRE TOURISM
The Old Library, Wheeler Street
Cambridge CB2 3QB
Tel: (01223) 322640   Fax: (01223) 457588
Comprehensive *Guide to Cambridge for Disabled People* covering most of what one needs to know.

BRITISH RED CROSS
2 Shaftesbury Road, Cambridge CB2 2DW
Tel: (01223) 354434

CAMBRIDGE PASSENGER TRANSPORT INFORMATION LINE
Tel: (01223) 717740

DIRECTIONS PLUS
Affiliated to DIAL. Disabled persons information project with factsheet with much information covering whole country.
Tel: (01223) 569600
Textphone: (01223) 569601
Fax: (01223) 506470
e-mail: directions.plus@dial.pipex.com
web: www.direction-plus.org

BUSES
Stagecoach Cambus. Tel: (01223) 423578
Whippet Coaches: Tel: (01480) 463792
Park & Ride Buses: Tel: (01223) 717755

HICOM
Histon and Impington Community Minibus may be available for hire:
Neil Davis, 3 Somerset Road, Histon, Cambridge CB4 4JS
Tel: (01223) 232514/233349
All these companies operate some low floor buses on some routes.

TAXIS
Camtax: Tel: (01223) 313131
2 FX4s with ramps, 1 minibus with ramps, clamps and straps.
Intercity: Tel: (01223) 301301
1 FX1.
Regency: Tel: (01223) 311311
1 Nissan Cargo.
Cabco: Tel: (0800) 123444

TRAINS
Anglia Railways: Assistance:
Tel: (01473) 693333
Minicom: (01603) 630748 or (0845) 6050600
Central Trains: Assistance:
Tel: (0845) 7056027
web: www.centraltrains.co.uk
West Anglia Great Northern: Special Needs –
Tel: (0345) 226688
Minicom: (0345) 125988
General Advice: (0345) 81819

SHOPMOBILITY
5th Floor, Lion Yard Car Park
Tel: (01223) 457452
Grafton Centre East
Tel: (01223) 461858
Textphone: (01223) 463219

CAMBRIDGE MOBILITY
Wheelchair Hire
Tel: (01223) 844666

CAMBRIDGE
Ancient university town with row of colleges lining the River Cam and overlooking the Backs on the other side of the river. This area of lawns and trees is delightful. Modern shopping in historical surroundings adds to the unique atmosphere created by the university, river and gardens.

HOTELS
HOLIDAY INN
Downing Street, Cambridge CB2 3DT
Tel: (01223) 464466   Fax: (01223) 464440
No. of Accessible Rooms: 2. Bath
Accessible Facilities: Lounge, Restaurant
Modern city centre hotel with reserved parking.

CAMBRIDGE GARDEN HOUSE MOAT HOUSE
Granta Place, Mill Lane, Cambridge CB2 1RT
Tel: (01223) 259988   Fax: (01223) 316605
No. of Accessible Rooms: 1
Accessible Facilities: Lounge, Restaurant

Purpose-built hotel in peaceful setting with grounds overlooking River Cam.

SORRENTO HOTEL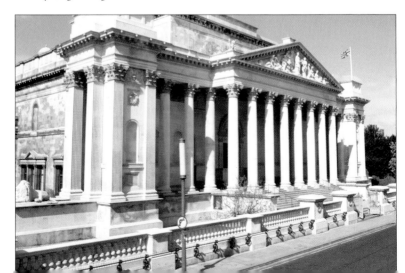
196 Cherry Hinton Road, Cambridge CB1 7AN
Tel: (01223) 243533   Fax: (01223) 213463
No. of Accessible Rooms: 1. Bath Accessible Facilities: Lounge, Restaurant (ramped at 1:11), Outdoor patio/eating area. Medium-sized private and family-run hotel 1.5 miles from city centre. Progressive staff.

ATTRACTIONS
ANGLESEY ABBEY GARDENS and LODE MILL (NT)
Lode CB5 9EJ
Tel/Fax: (01223) 811200
Gardens and ground floor of Mill accessible, Abbey not so. Founded in 1135 as a religious house, becoming a secular property by C16th. Purchased by the first Lord Fairhaven in 1926. He created a superb landscaped garden with great statuary and trees for all seasons and a working water mill.

SD 🚻   CP 🚹   RF 🚹   C 🚹
S 🚹   WC 🚹   RFE 🚻

CAMBRIDGE UNIVERSITY BOTANIC GARDEN
Cory Lodge, Bateman Street,
Cambridge CB2 1JE
Tel: (01223) 336265   Fax: (01223) 336278
e-mail: gardens@hermes.cam.ac.uk
web: www.plantsci.cam.ac.uk/WWW/botgdn
Founded in 1762, in its present site since 1846, there are 40 acres including nine national collections. Also a Winter Garden, Chronological Bed, Scented Garden and a collection of native British plants. Glasshouses contain sub-tropical and tropical plants.

SD 🚻   CP 🚹   E 🚻   RF 🚻   L n/a
C 🚹   S 🚹   WC 🚹

CHILFORD HALL VINEYARD
Linton, Cambridge CB1 6LE
Tel: (01223) 892641   Fax: (01223) 894056
18-acre vineyard for tasting and buying, plus winery tour to learn how English wine is produced.

SD 🚻   CP 🚹   E 🚻   RF 🚹   C 🚹
S 🚹   WC 🚹

THE FITZWILLIAM MUSEUM
Trumpington Street, Cambridge CB2 1RB
Tel: (01223) 332900   Fax: (01223) 332923
Small, personal museum with permanent collections of antiquities, applied arts, coins, manuscripts and paintings, together with ever-changing exhibitions. Admittance at rear of building where set down is available. From Trumpington Street, approach by lane opposite Brown's Restaurant.

SD 🚻   CP n/a   E 🚻   RF 🚻   L 🚻
C 🚻 (access dependent on staff available to accompany visitors in wheelchairs in lift and through non-public area)   S 🚹   WC 🚹

The imposing frontage of The Fitzwilliam Museum.

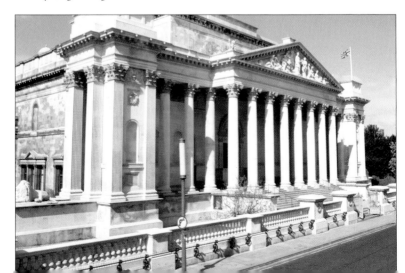

IMPERIAL WAR MUSEUM
Duxford Airfield, Duxford,
Nr. Cambridge CB2 4QR
Tel: (01223) 835000   Fax: (01223) 837267
Former Battle of Britain fighter station
and home to Europe's largest collection of
historic aircraft. Experience the American
Air Museum and Land Warfare exhibitions.

SD 🦽   CP 🚶♿   E 🦽   RF 🦽   L n/a
C ♿   S 🦽   WC 🦽   RFE 🦽

ELY
Famous for its great cathedral, there are
also pleasant walks and beautiful views.

TOURIST INFORMATION CENTRE
Oliver Cromwell's House,
29 St. Mary's Street, Ely CB7 4HF
Tel: (01353) 662062

HOTEL
TRAVELODGE   🚶
Witchford Road, Ely CB6 3NN
Tel/Fax: (01353) 668499
No. of Accessible Rooms: 2. Bath
Accessible Facilities: Restaurant.
Spacious accommodation in modern building
located at roundabout of A10 and A142.

ATTRACTION
ELY CATHEDRAL
Chapter House, The College, Ely CB7 4DL
Tel: (01353) 667735   Fax: (01353) 665658
Magnificent Norman cathedral set amidst
medieval monastic buildings.

SD 🦽   CP 🚶   E 🦽   (South door)
RF 🦽   (except Refectory door that is ramped at 1:6)
C 🦽   S 🦽   WC 🚶   RFE 🦽

HUNTINGDON
Attractive county town with narrow main
street, stretches of Georgian buildings,

TOURIST INFORMATION CENTRE
Princes Street, Huntingdon PE18 6PH
Tel: (01480) 388588   Fax: (01480) 388591

SPORTING VENUE
HUNTINGDON STEEPLECHASES LTD
The Racecourse, Brampton,
Huntingdon PE18 8NN

Booking-Box Office: (01480) 453373
Fax: (01480) 455275

CP 🦽   RE 🦽   ED 🦽♿
WC 🚶   (Members Enclosure)
SS 🚶   Wheelchair platform designated. Route via Paddock
Enclosure Grandstand near main entrance.   B/R 🦽

PETERBOROUGH
Known as a market town with a fine cathedral,
historic buildings and good shops.

HOTELS
SWALLOW HOTEL   🦽♿
Lynch Wood, Peterborough Business Park,
Peterborough PE2 6GBA
Tel: (01733) 371111   Fax: (01733) 236725
No. of Accessible Rooms: 2
Accessible Facilities: Lounge, Restaurant.
Modern hotel located opposite East of
England Showground.

PETERBOROUGH MOAT HOUSE   🚶
Thorpe Wood, Peterborough PE3 6SG
Tel: (01733) 289988   Fax: (01733) 262737
No. of Accessible Rooms: 1
Accessible Facilities: Lounge, Restaurant
Modern hotel on outskirts of town,
overlooking 500-acre country park.

ATTRACTION
NENE VALLEY RAILWAY
Wansford Station, Stibbington,
Peterborough PE8 6LR
Tel: (01780) 784444   Fax: (01780) 784440
The golden age of steam – 7.5 mile track
following River Nene meandering from HQ
at Wansford Station to Peterborough
passing through the 500-acre ferry
Meadows Country Park.

SD 🦽   CP 🚶♿   E 🦽   RF 🦽   L n/a
C 🦽   S 🦽   WC 🦽   RFE 🦽

PEAKIRK WATERFOWL GARDENS TRUST
Deeping Road, Peakirk,
Peterborough PE6 7NP
Tel: (01733) 252271
20 acres of woodland, water and formal
gardens with many species of duck, goose,
swan ands flamingo, located seven miles
north of Peterborough.

SD 🦽   CP 🚶♿   E 🦽   RF 🦽   C 🚶
S 🦽   WC 🚶   RFE 🦽

CHANNEL ISLANDS

JERSEY

Largest and most southerly of the islands, set in the Bay of St. Malo, 14 miles from the French coast. Originally part of Normandy, coming under English rule when William the Conqueror invaded England. Loyal to the British Crown but has its own government and is not part of the European Community. Landscape of rugged north coast, central country lanes and southern bays.

JERSEY TOURISM
Liberation Square, St. Helier,
Jersey JE1 1BB
Tel: (01534) 500700
Fax: (01534) 500 808
e-mail: :jtourism@itl.net
web: www.jtourism.com

BUSES/COACHES
Pioneer Coaches: Tel: (01534) 725100
One 37-seater vehicle with lift, one 42-seater vehicle with proper disabled lift, one 17-seater vehicle taking folding wheelchairs.

Jersey Bus: Tel: (01534) 21201
No low-floor buses yet.

TAXIS
Flying Dragon/Clarendon:
Tel: (01534) 888333
3 adapted vehicles.
Luxicabs: Tel: (01534) 887000
4 adapted vehicles.
Andy Tague: Tel: (01534) 758476
1 adapted vehicle.

On Jersey there are height and width restrictions on small country roads that render large vehicles impractical. It is the states that refuse licences, rather than transport companies not wanting to become disabled friendly.

FERRIES see Introduction

AIRLINES see Introduction

CAR PARKS
Free 4- or 2-hour orange badge parking.

WHEELCHAIR HIRE
Available from:
Guardian Medical Supplies:
Tel: (01534) 732335   Fax: (01534) 759465
Travelsmith: Tel: (01534) 737317

GROUVILLE
Located in the south-east, joining with St. Clements to form many miles of sweeping bays. Grouville Bay is the finest on the island, reaching from Gorey harbour to La Roque Point. Many Martello towers and forts built during Napoleonic wars.

HOTEL
BEAUSITE HOTEL
Grouville Bay, Grouville JE3 4DJ
Tel: (01534) 857577   Fax: (01534) 857211
No. of Accessible Rooms: 3
Accessible Facilities: Lounge, Restaurant, Pool. The hotel's original granite farm buildings date back to 1636 and public rooms retain a traditional style. The remainder is modern. The property looks out onto the Royal Jersey Golf Course and the Bay of Grouville.

ATTRACTION
THE JERSEY POTTERY
Gorey Village, Grouville JE3 9EP
Tel: (01534) 851119   Fax: (01534) 856403
e-mail: jsypot@itl.net
See complex manufacturing process of hand-painted ceramics in the 600 unique lines of this commercial pottery with beautiful gardens and restaurant.

SD n/a   CP 🚹♿   E ♿   RF ♿   C ♿
S ♿   WC 🚹

ST. BRELADE
Parish makes up the south-western tip of island, seaside resorts in sheltered bays.

JERSEY LAVENDER
Rue Du Pont Marquet, St. Brelade JE3 8DS
Tel: (01534) 42933 Fax: (01534) 45613
The first lavender was planted in 1983 and now extends to approximately nine acres. The farm exhibits the processes involved in extracting the oil and in creating exclusive Jersey lavender products on this working farm. The owners took advice from the local disabled access group when designing the layout, but because this is a working farm, access to some areas without a robust pusher is a little difficult.

SD   CP  E   RI C

S WC G Wheelchairs available.

ST. CLEMENT
Situated just east of St. Helier with lovely arable countryside and long stretches of sandy beaches. This is Jersey's smallest parish with granite outcrop of Rocqueberg and 3m menhir testifying to probable neolithic origin.

ATTRACTION
SAMARES MANOR GARDENS
Inner Road, St.Clement JE2 6QW
Tel: (01534) 870551 Fax: (01534) 768949
14 acres of lovely gardens, including a Japanese garden and one of Britain's largest herbal gardens. Also a craft centre and farm animals.

SD   CP   E   C S WC

ST. HELIER
Capital of the island with paved shopping streets and lanes, combined with night spots, restaurants and entertainment.

HOTELS
GRAND HOTEL
Esplanade, St. Helier JE4 8WD
Tel: (01534) 22301 Fax: (01534) 737815
No. of Accessible Rooms: 1. Bath Accessible Facilities: Lounge, Restaurant.

ATTRACTIONS
JERSEY MUSEUM
The Weighbridge, St. Helier JE2 3NF
Tel: (01534) 633300 Fax: (01534) 633301
e-mail: jersmus@itl.net

Award-winning museum telling the Story of Jersey that brings together the island's collections in a very striking exhibition. The art gallery offers paintings, etchings and sculpture and a new theatre presents a picture of Jersey's unique place in history.

SD CP E C S WC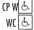

MARITIME MUSEUM
New North Quay, St. Helier
Tel: (01534) 633340 Fax: (01534) 633301
Hands-on exhibits, historic objects and new art and sculpture celebrate the relationship of the islanders and the sea. Feel the force of gale, float your own ships, and experience pitch and roll of life at sea.

SD CP W E RF L   S   WC

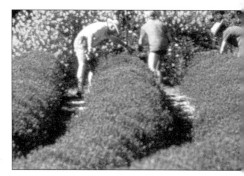

Can't you just smell the Lavender.

ST. LAWRENCE
ATTRACTION
FLYING FLOWERS
Jersey Flower Centre, St. Lawrence JE3 1GX
Tel: (01534) 865665 Fax: (01534) 866000
Home of the largest mail-order floral company in the world. Giant glasshouses, Flamingo Lake, Wildfowl Sanctuary, Koi Carp reserve, exotic birds and wildflower meadowland.

SD CP E RF C S WC   RFE

GERMAN UNDERGROUND HOSPITAL
Les Charrieres Malorey, St. Lawrence JE3 1FU
Tel: (01534) 863442 Fax: (01534) 865970
Remarkable engineering feat of the German Occupation and an evocative reminder of events that began in July 1940.

Vast complex dug deep into a hillside. Continuous video presentation with memorabilia bring life of islanders at war to life.

SD n/a   CP ♿   E ♿   RF ♿   L ♿
C ♿   S ♿   WC 🚶

ST. OUEN
HOTEL
MAISON DES LANDES HOTEL   ♿
St. Ouen JE3 2AA
Tel: (01534) 481683 Fax: (01534) 485327
No. of Accessible Rooms: All Accessible
Facilities: Lounge, Dining room, Indoor
Pool. Purpose-built hotel for disabled
guests and their families and fully
accessible to wheelchair users. Hoists,
wheelchairs and other equipment
available, but personal care not provided.

TRINITY
Largest parish, but one of the least
populated, a rural area with fine granite
farmhouses and picturesque small lanes.
Boulay Bay, on the north coast, is a
tranquil cove with cliff paths through
wonderful heather. Holy Trinity Parish
Church dates back to the 12th century.

PALLOT HERITAGE STEAM MUSEUM
Rue de Bechet, Trinity JE3 5BE
Tel: (01534) 865307 Fax: (01534) 865506
Collection of displays on mechanical and
farming heritage. Host to Liberation Day
Steam Fayre early May and Steam
Threshing Fayre in autumn.

SD ♿ CP ♿ E ♿ RF ♿ C 🚶 WC 🚶

GUERNSEY
30 miles from France and 80 from the
English coast. Covering about 25 square
miles there are 20 bays and beaches, wooded
valleys, spectacular cliffs, marshland and
rolling countryside. The islands remain
part of the Duchy of Normandy and are
self-governing with their own parliament.

DEPARTMENT OF TOURISM
PO Box 23, St. Peter Port GY1 3AN
Tel: (01481) 723552 Fax: (01481) 721256
e-mail: enquiries@tourism.guernsey.net

web: www.guernseytourism.gov.gg

STATES TRAFFIC COMMITTEE:
Tel: (01481) 243400
Publishes leaflet entitled "Transport and the
Disabled in Guernsey".

GUERNSEY ASSOCIATION OF PEOPLE WITH DISABILITIES
Tel: (01481) 724102/722435

BUSES
No low-floor buses on island.

TAXIS
Ace Taxis: Tel: (01481) 121180
One adapted vehicle.

WHEELCHAIR HIRE
St. John Ambulance: Tel: (01481) 729268

CASTEL
ATTRACTION
FORT HOMMET GUN CASEMATE
Fort Hommet, Castel.
Correspondence, c/o Occupation Museum,
Forest GY8 0BG
Tel: (01481) 238205
Fully restored German bunker with
original 10.5cm gun, located on Fort
Hommet headland in Vazon Bay.

SD ♿ CP ♿ E ♿ C n/a S 🚶
WC n/a

FERMAIN BAY
Close to St. Peter Port, reached by steep
valley road, one of Guernsey's prettiest bays.

HOTEL
LA FAVORITA   🚶
Fermain Bay GY4 6SD
Tel: (01481) 235666
Fax: (01481) 235413
web: www.favorita.com
No. of Accessible Rooms: 11
Accessible Facilities: Lounge, Bar,
Restaurant (1st floor, via accessible lift).
Originally a country house that retains
its character. Set in a wooded valley
leading down to Fermain Bay with fine
views over the sea towards Jersey.

FOREST

Bordered by beautiful cliffs and the Bays of Petit Bot and Portlet, much of the cliff area is inaccessible to wheelchairs, but at the parish centre is the ancient church of St. Marguerite de la Foret, the patron saint of dentists, that is accessible.

ATTRACTION
GERMAN OCCUPATION MUSEUM
Forest GY8 0BG
Tel: (01481) 230205

The Channel Islands was the only British territory to be occupied by the Germans during WWII. The museum tells the story from 1940/45 through a large collection of authentic occupation items and tableaux of bunker rooms and a street. The military, occupation and civilian rooms and the prison are accessible .

SD   CP   E   RF   C
S ⌂   WC ⌂   RFE ⌂

ST. MARTINS
HOTEL
LA VILLETTE HOTEL ⌂
St. Martins GY4 6QG
Tel: (01481) 235292   Fax: (01481) 237699
e-mail: reservations@lavillettehotel.co.uk
web: www.lavillettehotel.co.uk
No. of Accessible Rooms: 1. Bath
Accessible Facilities: Lounge, Restaurant
Attractive property surrounded by trees and lawns.

ST. PETER PORT

Capital of Guernsey, a town that has grown uphill with many of its attractive narrow streets meandering upwards. Much of the town is pedestrianised but the main High Street is cobbled.

HOTEL
ST. PIERRE PARK HOTEL ⌂
Rohais, St. Peter Port GY1 1FD
Tel: (01481) 728282   Fax: (01481) 712041
e-mail:stppark@itl.net
No. of Accessible Rooms: 2. Bath
Accessible Facilities: Open plan
Lounge/Bar, Restaurants (2), 1 on ground floor, one lower ground via accessible lift.

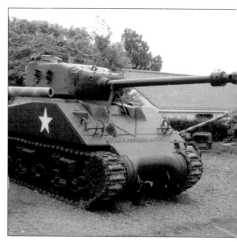

Forbidding example of the amazing display at the German Occupation Museum.

Set amidst 45 acres of quiet mature parkland, this 5-star hotel is superb.

ATTRACTION
GUERNSEY MUSEUM and ART GALLERY
Candie Gardens, St. Peter Port GY1 1UG
Tel: (01481) 726518   Fax: (01481) 715177
e-mail: admin@museum.guernsey.net
Purpose-built to relate the history of the island, with audio visual theatre and both permanent art gallery and special exhibitions all year round.

SD ⌂   CP n/a   E ⌂   RF ⌂   C ⌂
S ⌂   WC

VALE

An area of lovely sandy bays, particularly Pembroke, offering good access from smooth shallow slipway at eastern end and car park adjoining bay. Chouet Bay has a slipway to hard sand as does Ladies Bay, but Port Soif Bay is difficult to access.

HOTEL
PENINSULA HOTEL ⌂
Les Dicqs, Vale GY6 8JP
Tel: (01481) 48400   Fax: (01481) 48706
No. of Accessible Rooms: 2. Bath
Accessible Facilities: Lounge, Restaurant, Gardens. Surrounded by five acres of gardens, located on tranquil grassy peninsula leading to a sandy bay.

CHESHIRE

CHESHIRE DISABILITIES FEDERATION
Vale Royal Disability Access and
Information Service
Council House, Church Road,
Northwich CW9 5PD
Tel: (01606) 350611
Produce excellent *Cheshire Welcome
Guide* with attractions and
accommodation inspected by members of
the Federation and Holiday Care Service.

HALTON DISABILITY SERVICE
Castlefields Avenue, North Runcorn
Tel: (01928) 590361

ALTRINCHAM
Industrial and residential centre
surrounded by picturesque villages,
ancient churches and broad stretches of
placid water.

ATTRACTION
DUNHAM MASSEY HALL (NT)
Altrincham WA14 4SJ
Tel: (0161) 9411025   Fax: (0161) 9297508
The house, park and garden owe their
design and character mostly to the 2nd
Earl of Warrington (1675-1758). Over 30
house rooms are open and the garden
contains remnants from past layouts
including the moat, Elizabethan mount
and C18th. orangery. Ancient trees
outline the avenues of the park with a
1610 water mill, now a sawmill, with
working machinery. Much of the hall is
difficult because of staircases, but there
are plans to obtain a motorised stair-
climber in near future. Park and gardens
have level easy paths, but there is a
cobbled area around the stable block
that houses a restaurant and a shop. Two
manual wheelchairs and two battery-
powered wheelchairs are available free of
charge. NB. Entrance has three steps.

SD 🚶 CP 🚶 E 🚶 RF 🚶 L ♿
C   S   WC   G

CHESTER
Known as the black-and-white city, and
famous for its half-timbered buildings,
Chester's foundations are Roman as are
the original forts that still surround it.
There is plenty of shopping here, an
historic feel, plus entertainment.

CHESTER TOURISM
Chester City Council, The Forum,
Chester CH1 2HS
Tel: (01244) 402150   Fax: (01244) 315789
web: www.chestercc.gov.uk

TOURIST INFORMATION CENTRES
Town Hall, Northgate Street, Chester
Tel: (01244) 402111   Fax: (01244) 400420
e-mail: tis@chestercc.gov.uk

Vicars Lane, Chester, CH1 1QX
Tel: (01244) 351609   Fax: (01244) 403188

Chester Railway Station, Station Road,
Chester CH1 3NT
Tel: (01244) 322220   Fax: (01244) 322211

CHESHIRE C.C. TRANSPORT CO. ORDINATION
Rivacre Business Centre, Mill Lane,
Ellesmere Port L66 3TL
Tel: (01244) 603041 (for Chester area)
Publish "Getting There", a guide to public
transport for people with mobility problems.

BUSES
Cheshire Buslines: Tel: (01244) 602666
Arriva: Tel: (01244) 661195
First Crosville: Tel: (01244) 381515
Fax: (01244) 373849
All operate some low-floor buses.
Also operate Women's Safe Transport
Tel: (01244) 372535
Park & Ride: Tel: (01244) 602666
City-Rail link: Tel: (01244) 602666

TAXIS
Taxi Rank at Bus Station
Chester Radio Taxis: Tel: (01244) 372372
26 wheelchair-accessible vehicles.
John Morris Taxis: Tel: (01244) 851032
1 taxi with all fittings.

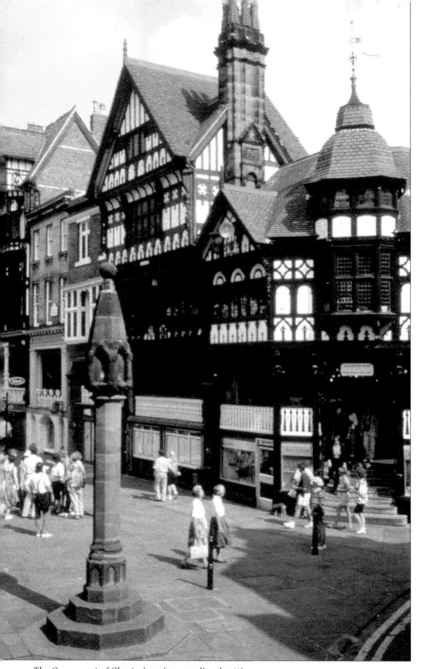

The Cross, part of Chester's unique medieval setting.

TRAINS

Central Trains: Assistance:
Tel: (0845) 7056027
web: www.centraltrains.co.uk
First North Western: Special Needs –
Tel: (0845) 6040231
Merseyrail: Special Needs –
Tel: (0151) 7022071 (minicom available)
Virgin Trains: Special Needs –
(0845) 7443366
Minicom: (0845) 7443367
Wales & West: Special Needs –
Tel: (0845) 3003005
Minicom: (0845) 7585469

CAR PARKS
Some free Orange badge parking.
Tel: (01244) 343503

SHOPMOBILITY
Kale Yards, Frodsham Street Car Park,
Chester CH1 3JH
Tel: (01244) 312626

CHESTER ACCESS OFFICER
Chester City Council
Tel: (01244) 402442
Minicom: (01244) 320915
DIAL House-Chester
Tel/Minicom: (01244) 345655

CHESTER ACCESS GROUP
Tel: (01244) 378276

HOTELS
CHESTER MOAT HOUSE
Trinity Street, Chester CH1 2BD
Tel: (01244) 899988 Fax: (01244) 316118
No. of Accessible Rooms: Unknown
Accessible Facilities: Restaurant
Quality hotel with superb views over the
racecourse and the Welsh hills.

ABBEY COURT HOTEL
Liverpool Road, Chester CH2 1AG
Tel: (01244) 374100 Fax: (01244) 379240
web: www.macdonaldhotels.co.uk/abbey-
court-hotel/
No. of Accessible Rooms: Several on the
ground floor. Accessible Facilities:
Lounge, Restaurant, Bars (some steps).
Elegant porticoed hotel close to the medieval
city centre and 3 miles from the M53.

THE CHESTER GROSVENOR
Eastgate, Chester CH1 1LT
Tel: (01244) 324024 Fax: (01244) 313246
e-mail: reservations@chestergrosvenor.co.uk
web: www.chestergrosvenor.co.uk
No. of Accessible Rooms: 1. Bath
Accessible Facilities: Drawing Room,
Restaurants (2). Luxurious 5-star hotel,
owned by the 6th Duke of Westminster
under the Grosvenor Estates, located in the
city centre, adjacent to the Eastgate Clock.

DENE HOTEL
95 Hoole Road, Chester CH2 3ND

Tel: (01244) 321165 Fax: (01244) 350277
No. of Accessible Rooms: 12. Bath
Accessible Facilities: Lounge, Restaurant
Set in its own grounds, adjacent to
Alexandra Park. 1 mile from Chester.

GREEN BOUGH HOTEL
60 Hoole Road, Chester CH2 3NL
Tel: (01244) 326241 Fax: (01244) 326265
e-mail: greenboughhotel@cwcom.net
web: SmoothHound.co.uk/hotels/
greenbo.html
No. of Accessible Rooms: 2
Accessible Facilities: Lounge, Dining room.
Elegant family-run hotel with homely
atmosphere in Victorian surroundings.
NB. Two steps into main entrance.

HOOLE HALL
Warrington Road, Hoole, Chester CH1 3PD
Tel: (01244) 350011 Fax: (01244) 320251
No. of Accessible Rooms: 1. Roll-in
Shower. Accessible Facilities: Lounge,
Restaurant. Converted C18th manor
house set in five acres of grounds, two
miles from Chester.

ROWTON HALL HOTEL
Whitchurch Road, Rowton, Chester CH3 6AD
Tel: (01244) 335262 Fax: (01244) 335464
No. of Accessible Rooms: 7
Accessible Facilities: Lounge,
Restaurant, Pool, Sauna, Spa. 1779 manor
house set in eight acres of parklands and
gardens, two miles from Chester.

ATTRACTIONS
CHESTER CATHEDRAL
12 Abbey Square, Chester CH1 2HU
Tel: (01244) 324756 Fax: (01244) 341110
e-mail: office@chestercathedral.org.uk
Well-preserved example of a medieval
monastic complex with all main periods of
Gothic architecture to be seen. Fine
medieval woodwork in quire stalls of 1380.

SD ⬜ CP n/a E ⬜ RF ⬜ C ⬜
S ⬜ WC ⬜ RFE ⬜

CHESTER VISITOR and CRAFT CENTRE
Vicars Lane, Chester CH1 1QX
Tel: (01244) 351609 Fax: (01244) 403188
e-mail: g.tattum@chestercc.gov.uk
Video presentation introducing history,

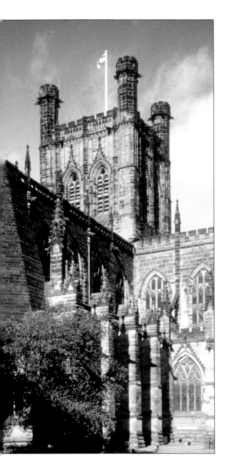

Gothic as built, Chester's beautiful cathedral.

main features and place of interest. Stroll through typical Chester street in Victorian times with sights, sounds and smells. Also working craft shops.

SD ♿ CP 🚶 E ♿🚶 RF ♿
C ♿ S ♿ WC ♿

MOULDSWORTH MOTOR MUSEUM
Smithy Lane, Mouldsworth CH3 8AR
Tel: (01928) 731781

Located six miles east of Chester and housed in a 1937 art deco building, this is a collection of vintage, post vintage, classic cars, motorcycles and early bicycles.

SD ♿ CP 🚶 E ♿ WC 🚶

ZOOLOGICAL GARDENS
Upton-by-Chester, Chester CH2 1LH
Tel: (01244) 380280   Fax: (01244) 371274

e-mail: marketing@chesterzoo.co.uk
web: www.demon.co.uk/chesterzoo

The largest zoo in the UK, notable for breeding rare and endangered species, and an enormous variety of animals. There is an excellent guide and map. With the exception of waterbuses and Oakfield WC, the zoo is accessible with long level sections and gentle slopes. The ramps are steep at orang utans, penguins, Europe of the Edge Aviary, and at the Tropical Realm and Exotic Birds sections. The overhead railway is accessible, compartments will take a wheelchair. A small, free fleet of four-wheel drive electric scooters is housed at the staff and pedestrian entrance at Caughall Road, *not the main entrance*. There are three reserved parking spaces close by, but book in advance. Adult wheelchairs are available for hire at low cost at the first-aid centre by the main entrance.

SD ♿ CP ♿ E ♿ RF ♿
C 🚶 S ♿ WC ♿

CONGLETON
Known for its cattle market. There are a few half-timbered houses remaining.

TOURIST INFORMATION CENTRE
Town Hall, High Street, Congleton CW12 1BN
Tel: (01260) 271095   Fax: (01260) 298243

BED & BREAKFAST
SANDHOLE FARM   🚶
Hulme Walfield, Congleton CW12 2JH
Tel: (01260) 224419   Fax: (01260) 224766
No. of Accessible Rooms: 2
Accessible Facilities: Lounge, Dining room.
Country farmhouse where an original L-shaped stable block has been converted .

ATTRACTION
LITTLE MORETON HALL (NT)
Congleton CW12 4SD
Tel: (01260) 272018

The most famous and probably the finest timber-framed moated manor house in the UK. Fine wall paintings and knot garden of particular note.

SD ♿ CP 🚶 E ♿ RF 🚶
C 🚶 S 🚶 WC ♿ RFE ♿🚶

CREWE

Large industrial town, famous as a railway junction. Modern town centre.

HOTEL
OLD VICARAGE HOTEL
Knutsford Road, Cranage, Holmes Chapel, Crewe CW4 8FS
Tel: (01477) 532041 Fax: (01477) 535728
No. of Accessible Rooms: 1
Accessible Facilities: Lounge, Restaurant. C17th, A Grade II listed building on the banks of the river Dane in the village of Cranage, Holmes Chapel. Located a mile from the M6 (J.18).

HUNTERS LODGE HOTEL
Sydney Road, Crewe CW1 1LU
Tel: (01270) 583440
No. of Accessible Rooms: 1. Bath
Accessible Facilities: Lounge, Restaurant. A rural family-run hotel, a mile from the city centre.

MACCLESFIELD

Once a leading silk manufacturing town with good C18th and C19th mills remaining that contribute to the town's character. The Georgian Town Hall and the market cross, now situated in the West Park, are worth viewing. Also in the park are old iron stocks and a 30-ton boulder brought from Cumberland by ice-age glaciers. Macclesfield Forest, 5 miles east, is a tiny village on the edge of a wide stretch of wild country with crags and narrow valleys.

TOURIST INFORMATION CENTRE
Town Hall, Macclesfield SK10 1DX
Tel: (01625) 504114 Fax: (01625) 504116

SELF-CATERING
LOWER HOUSE COTTAGE
Wildboarclough, Nr. Macclesfield SK11 0BL
Tel: (01260) 227229
No. of Accessible Units: 1. Roll-in-Shower
No. of Beds per Unit: 1.
Accessible Facilities. Secluded cottage on the edge of the Peak District. River nearby. Fishing included.

THE OLD BYRE
Pye Ash Farm, Leek Road, Bosley, Macclesfield SK11 0PN
Tel: (01260) 273650
No. of Accessible Units: 1. Roll-in shower.
No. of Beds per Unit: 5. Traditional working farm on the edge of the Peak District.

STRAWBERRY DUCK HOLIDAYS
Bryher Cottage, Bullgate Lane, Bosley, Macclesfield SK11 0PP
Tel: (01260) 223591
No. of Accessible Units: 1. Roll-in Shower
No. of Beds per Unit: 4.
Accessible Facilities: Lounge, Kitchen, Patio. Award-winning converted cottage close to the Peak District National Park overlooking Cheshire plain in the tiny village of Bosley. Nearby there are pubs and restaurants with wheelchair access.

ATTRACTION
JODRELL BANK SCIENCE CENTRE, PLANETARIUM and ARBORETUM
Lower Withington,
Nr. Macclesfield SK11 9DL
Tel: (01477) 571331 Fax: (01477 571695
e-mail: sc@jb.man.ac.uk
Focus of the centre is the Lovell telescope receiving radio waves from deep space. At the Science Centre explore the science of Earth, energy and space and also enjoy the Nature Experience. Divided into three distinct categories – Exhibition Spaces, Planetarium and Arboretum. Very interactive and hands on.

SD | CP | E | RF | C n/a
S n/a | WC | RFE

NANTWICH

Old market town on the River Weaver, surrounded by rich agricultural area producing the famous Cheshire cheese. A fire in 1583 destroyed many original buildings, but rebuilding gave the town a wealth of Elizabethan structures still standing.

TOURIST INFORMATION CENTRE
Church House, Church Walk,
Nantwich CW5 5RG
Tel: (01270) 610983 Fax: (01270) 610880

HOTELS

ROOKERY HALL [♿]
Worleston, Nantwich CW5 6DQ
Tel: (01270) 610016   Fax: (01270) 626027
No. of Accessible Rooms: 30. Bath
Accessible Facilities: Lounge, Restaurant.
Luxury award winning hotel set in 200
acres of countryside.

THE PEACOCK [♿]
221 Crewe Road, Nantwich CW5 6NE
Tel: (01270) 624069   Fax: (01270) 610113
No. of Accessible Rooms: 2. Bath
Accessible Facilities: Restaurant
Located two miles from Nantwich, good
location for Wales and the Potteries.

ATTRACTION

STAPELEY WATER GARDENS and PALMS TROPICAL OASIS
London Road, Stapeley,
Nantwich CW5 7JL
Tel: (01270) 623868   Fax: (01270) 624919
Glass pavilion of the Palm Tropical oasis is
home to exotic flowers, fish and birds, plus
two-acre Water Garden centre housing,
among other things, the national collection
of water-lilies.

CP    E [♿]   C [♿]   S [♿]   WC [♿]

NORTHWICH
Old town recently modernised. Shopping
centre. Black and white houses also are
modern but give the town an historic feel.

TOURIST INFORMATION CENTRE
Chester Way, Northwich
Tel: (01606) 353500

HOTEL
QUALITY FRIENDLY FLOATEL [♿]
London Road, Northwich CW9 5HD
Tel: (01606) 44443
No. of Accessible Rooms: 2
Accessible Facilities: Lounge (ground fl.)
Restaurant, Bar (1st floor, via lift)
Unique floating hotel on River Weaver

ACCESSIBLE ATTRACTIONS
ARLEY HALL AND GARDENS
Nr. Northwich CW9 6NA
Tel: (01565) 777353   Fax: (01565) 777465

The Hall, replacing a Tudor version, is
Jacobean in style with fine ceilings, oak
panelling and a splendid library. The gardens,
that have evolved since Tudor times, are
notable for a double herbaceous border laid
in 1846. Ninety per cent accessible with
only rootery and sundial garden inaccessible.

SD [♿]   CP [♿]   E [♿]   RF [♿]
C [♿]   S [♿]   WC [♿]   RFE (gardens) [♿]

BLAKEMERE CRAFT CENTRE
Chester Road, Sandiway,
Northwich CW8 2EB
Tel/Fax: (01606) 883261
Restored Edwardian stable block housing
18 craft shops.

SD [♿]   CP [♿]   E [♿]   RF [♿]   L [♿]
C [♿]   S [♿]   WC [♿]   RFE [♿]

NORTON PRIORY MUSEUM and GARDENS
Tudor Road, Manor Park, Runcorn WA7 18X
Tel: (01928) 569895
In this C12th home of Augustinian canons,
stone masons and tile makers were
commissioned to decorate the priory church.
The museum displays examples of their
work, plus a model of the priory. 16 acres of
lovely woodland gardens with contemporary
sculpture trail. The mid C18th walled garden
has themed areas including old roses and
herbaceous borders. A truly tranquil place.

SD [♿]   CP [♿]   RF [♿]   C [♿]   S [♿]
E [♿] (ramped at gradient of 1:11)
WC [♿]   RFE [♿]

SANDBACH
Small historic town with winding streets,
cobbled market place and timbered houses.

HOTEL
SAXON CROSS HOTEL [♿]
Holmes Chapel Road, Sandbach CW11 9SE
Tel: (01270) 763281   Fax: (01270) 768723
No. of Accessible Rooms: 34. Bath
Accessible Facilities: Lounge, Restaurant
Modern ground-storey building situated
close to the M6 motorway

BED AND BREAKFAST
CANAL CENTRE
Hassall Green, Sandbach CW11 4YB
Tel/Fax: (01270) 762266

No. of Accessible Rooms: 1. Roll-in shower. Accessible Facilities: Lounge, Dining room, Canal Lockside and Garden C18th family-run guest house by the lockside of the Trent and Mersey Canal. Near the M6 (J17).

STYAL

Picturesque little village with white cottages and an old mill that stands where the River Bollen flows swiftly through a deep wooded glen.

ATTRACTION
STYAL COUNTRY PARK and QUARRY (NT)
Styal SK9 4LA
Tel: (01625) 527468   Fax: (01625) 539267
e-mail: quarrybankmill@rmplc.co.uk
web: www.rmplc.co.uk/orgs/quarrybankmill
The Greg family gave the Styal Estate that includes the mill and mill workers' village, plus surrounding woods and farmland, to the NT in 1939, and little has changed since. In the deep valley and woodlands are fields, ponds, flowers and birds. Discover how cotton is made into cloth. Use the mill entrance and the mill kitchen for access to catering. WC is in the inner yard opposite the mill kitchen. The route for wheelchair-bound visitors includes a step-lift and runs through the heart of the mill on one level. The mini-tour is quite arduous, but ramps and seats are provided wherever possible throughout the museum. Outdoor Attractions: Via Twinnies Bridge Car Park (0.25 mile from the main entrance), leading to a special wheelchair route through willow Ground Wood to the mill pool. There is no access through to the mill yard.

SD   CP    E   RF   L
C [人]   S n/a   WC [人]   RFE [人]

TARPORLEY

Regular winner of Best Kept Village in Cheshire competition.

HOTELS
THE SWAN   [人]
50 High Street, Tarporley CW6 0AG
Tel: (01829) 733838   Fax: (01829) 732932

No. of Accessible Rooms: 3
Accessible Facilities: Lounge, Restaurant
C16th coaching inn in the centre of a charming Georgian village. The hotel has been home to England's oldest Hunt Club since the late 18th century.

WILD BOAR HOTEL   [人]
Whitchurch Road, Beeston,
Tarporley CW6 9NW
Tel: (01829) 260309   Fax: (01829) 261081
No. of Accessible Rooms: 10
Accessible Facilities: Lounge, Restaurant, Bar, Grounds

WARRINGTON

An industrial town with the locks of the Manchester Ship Canal.

TOURIST INFORMATION CENTRE
21 Rylands Street, Warrington WA1 1EJ
Tel: (01925) 442180   Fax: (01925) 442149

HOLIDAY INN GARDEN COURT   [人]
Woolston Grange Avenue, Woolston,
Warrington WA1 4PX
Tel: (01925) 838779   Fax: (01925) 838859
No. of Accessible Rooms: 1. Bath
Accessible Facilities: Lounge, Restaurant.
Modern comfortable hotel.

PARK ROYAL INTERNATIONAL HOTEL   [人]
Stretton Road, Stretton, Warrington WA4 4NS
Tel: (01925) 730706   Fax: (01925) 730740
No. of Accessible Rooms: 1. Bath
Accessible Facilities: Lounge, Restaurant.
Once the site of an old vicarage and adjacent to C19th church, set in 40 acres of grounds and situated two minutes from the M56 (J10) in a picturesque village.

BED AND BREAKFAST
TALL TREES LODGE   [人]
Tarporley Road, Lower Whitley,
Warrington WA4 4EZ
Tel: (01928) 790824   Fax: (01928) 791330
No. of Accessible Rooms: 1.
Accessible Facilities: Breakfast Room.
Family-run lodge in Cheshire's heartland on the A49, south of M56 (J.10) and 10 minutes from Warrington.

ATTRACTIONS
GULLIVER'S WORLD
Warrington WA5 5YZ
Tel: (01925) 230088   Fax: (01925) 637354
Family theme park aimed at children
between three and 14 with over 40 exciting
rides, All rides have at least one step.

SD 🦽   CP 🚶   E 🚶   RF 🦽
C 🦽   S 🦽   WC 🚶

WALTON HALL GARDENS
Walton Lea Road, Higher Walton,
Warrington WA4 6SN
Tel: (01925) 261957   Fax: (01925) 861868
e-mail: waltonhall@warrington.gov.uk
Located in the heart of the Mersey Forest,
with mature parkland and ornamental
gardens with trees and shrubs from all
over the world, plus spacious lawns, picnic
areas, children's zoo, heritage centre. The
hall is not open to the public, but the
gardens are.

SD 🦽   CP 🦽   E 🦽   RF 🦽   C 🦽   S 🦽
WC 🦽   RFE (heritage centre, children's zoo) 🦽

WIDNES
Located between Runcorn and Liverpool.

TOURIST INFORMATION CENTRE
Tel: (0151) 4242061

HOTEL
EVERGLADES PARK HOTEL   🦽
Derby Road, Widnes WA8 0UJ
Tel: (0151) 4952040   Fax: (0151) 4246536
No. of Accessible Rooms: 4. Bath
Accessible Facilities: Lounge, Restaurant
Modern, private hotel in the country, a few
minutes from the M62 (J7) and close to
the town centre.

ATTRACTION
**CATALYST. THE MUSEUM OF THE CHEMICAL
INDUSTRY**
Gossage Building, Mersey Road,
Widnes WA8 0DF
Tel: (0151) 4201121   Fax: (0151) 4952030
e-mail: info@catalyst.org.uk
Previous winner of the Northwest Tourism
Visitor Attraction of the Year. Science and
technology come alive here through a host
of interactive exhibits and hands-on
displays that you can tug, tease and test.
Explore the impact of chemicals on
everyday life through scenes from the past
and multi-media programmes. There are
anoramic views across the River Mersey
from the roof-top observatory. The route
from the car park, that has designated
spaces, is along a sloping path of about
100m, with a gradient of 1:29 to the
entrance. There are handrails both sides of
the path. There is also close street parking
available at the side of the museum. There
are two wheelchairs on site, and level
access to the first-floor gallery and
observatory is via a glass lift.

SD 🦽   CP 🦽   E 🦽   RF 🦽
L 🦽   (non-motorised chairs)   C 🦽
S 🦽   WC 🦽

SPIKE ISLAND
Mersey Road, Widnes
Tel: (0151) 4203707
Just below the Catalyst Museum with
shared car parking, Spike Island was the
birthplace of the British chemical industry.
In late C19th it was dominated by huge
factories, and a maze of railway lines
crossed the Sankey Canal. By the early
C20th more efficient processes made the
old factories obsolete. In 1975 the land was
reclaimed and Spike Island was
transformed into acres of grassland,
woodland and watersides. There is a
ramped visitor centre alongside the Sankey
Canal with exhibitions that bring to life the
extraordinary history of the island. This is a
lovely quiet area for watching wildlife or to
sit and let the world go by.

WILMSLOW
Small town, outwardly a modern shopping
centre, in the deep valley of the Bollin river.

HOTEL
DEAN BANK HOTEL   🦽
Adlington Road, Wilmslow SK9 2BT
Tel: (01625) 524268
No. of Accessible Rooms: 3. Roll-in shower.
Accessible Facilities: Restaurant
Family-run hotel in a countryside location,
ten minutes from Manchester Airport.

CORNWALL

CORNWALL TOURIST BOARD
Pydar House, Pydar Street, Truro TR1 1EA
Tel: (01872) 274057   Fax: (01872) 240423
e-mail: tourism@visit.cornwall.gov.uk

DIAN (DISABILITY INFORMATION AND ADVICE NETWORK)
Marie Therese House, Hayle TR27 4HW
Tel: (01736) 751300
ALLDIS publish "Discover" at Marie Therese House. Tel: (01736) 759113.

AGE CONCERN
Tel: (01872) 223388
Provide minibuses with lifts, clamp and ramps in Bodmin, Falmouth, Launceston, Liskeard, Newquay, Penzance, St. Austell and Truro.

CORNWALL FRIENDS MOBILITY CENTRE
Tel: (01872) 254920   Fax: (01872) 254921
e-mail: mobility@rcht.swest.nhs.ik
Offers breakdown service for wheelchairs, scooters etc.

SPECIAL NEEDS SERVICES
Tel: (01326) 376011
Based in Falmouth, working with Tripscope. Will do anything, go anywhere, including nursing home transfer.

BUSES
Western National: West Cornwall
Tel: (01209) 719988
SE Cornwall Tel: (01742) 222666
Mid and North Cornwall Tel: (01208) 79898
(includes North Devon Red Bus and Truronian)
Truronian have one route (T1), Perranporth to The Lizard, that has raised kerbs for access by motorised wheelchairs at principal stops. This and other routes operate Easy Access buses that kneel at ordinary stops enabling wheelchairs to be pushed on board.

TRAINS
Great Western Trains: Tel: (01793) 499458
South West Trains: (020) 7620 5620
Virgin Trains: (0870) 7891234

FERRIES
All local ferry operators are willing to assist passengers with difficulties, but many embarkation points are inaccessible because of steep steps, rocks, beaches etc. Helford Passage-Helford Village: steep steps.
St Maws-Place: inaccessible. Falmouth-Flushing: steep steps. Feock-Philleigh: steep slope at low water, easier at high tide, but only from a car. Fowey-Polruan: steep steps. Fowey-Bodinnick: Car ferry. Plymouth-Mt. Edgcumbe: possible except at very low tide. Plymouth-Torpoint: car ferry. Padstow-Rock: inaccessible.

SPECIALIST OUTDOOR ACTIVITIES
CHURCHTOWN
Lanlivery, Bodmin PL30 5BT
Tel: (01208) 872148   Fax: (01208) 873377
This is Scope's accessible Adventure and outdoor education centre. Accessible residential courses for disabled persons with activities options including sailing, canoeing, orienteering, rock climbing, swimming, hands on farming.

BOSCASTLE
This is a classic beauty spot with a charming small harbour and old stone cottages. The main area of the village is in steep woods behind the harbour. It has very old houses and an unusual long, broad street that climbs straight and steeply up the hill.
A car is essential.

TOURIST INFORMATION CENTRE
Cobweb Car Park, Boscastle PL35 0HE
Tel/Fax: (01840) 250010

HOTEL
THE OLD COACH HOUSE   🚶
Tintagel Road, Boscastle PL35 0AS
Tel: (01840) 250398
Fax: (01840) 250346
e-mail: parsons@old-coach.demon.co.uk
No. of Accessible Rooms: 2. Roll-in shower. Accessible Facilities: Lounge. Set in a beautiful former coach house of the early 1700s, that has been now been restored and fully modernised.

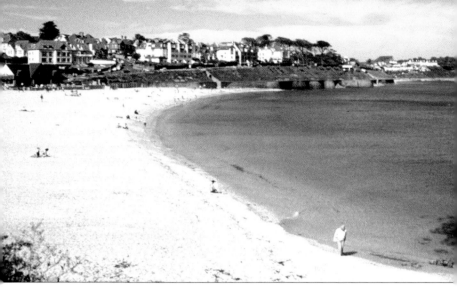

Falmouth, a beach of perfect childhood memories.

NB: No dining room, breakfast is served in the conservatory.

FALMOUTH

In a beautiful setting with a large natural harbour and the most temperate climate of any British resort, Falmouth has beaches, public gardens, scattered hotels and villas lying on the south side, while in the north there are harbours and docks backed by a shopping centre and charming narrow streets.

TOURIST INFORMATION CENTRE
28 Killigrew Street, Falmouth TR11 3PN
Tel: (01326) 312300   Fax: (01326) 313457

BUSES
Truronian: Tel: (01872) 273453
Some easy-access buses.

TAXIS
Special Needs Services
(see under country heading)
Abacus Cabs: Tel: (01326) 212141
1 Eurocab with ramps and clamps.
Acorn Mobility: Tel: (01326) 373890
1 Minibus adapted for three wheelchairs with ramps, lifts, clamps and belts.
Falmouth and Penryn Radio Taxis:
Tel: (01326) 315194/312404
3 TXIs with ramps.

Kendall, DR: Tel: (01326) 316610
1 TXI.

TRAINS
Wales & West: Special Needs –
Tel: (0845) 3003005
Minicom: (0845) 7585469
Both Falmouth stations have ramps.

HOTEL
BROADMEAD HOTEL
Kimberely Park Road, Falmouth TR11 2DD
Tel: (01326) 315704   Fax: (01326) 311048
No. of Accessible Rooms: 2. Bath.
Accessible Facilities: Lounge, Restaurant.
Hotel near town centre.

HELSTON

Delightful town, its most interesting streets being the main one, Coinagehall and Cross Streets, boasting lovely shops and a pleasant stroll.

HELSTON, LIZARD PENINSULA and TIN MINING COUNTRY TOURIST INFORMATION CENTRE
79 Meneage Street, Helston TR13 8RS
Tel: (01326) 565431   Fax: (01326) 572803

ATTRACTION
FLAMBARDS VILLAGE THEME PARK
Culdrose Manor, Helston TR13 0QA
Tel: (01326) 573404   Fax: (01326) 573344

e-mail: flambards@connexions.co.uk

Three themed attraction areas, Flambards Victorian village, Britain in the Blitz and Cornwall Aero park together with many rides.

SD ♿ CP ♿ E ♿ RF ♿ S ♿
WC ♿ RFE ♿

LAUNCESTON

The town stands on a hill crowned by the ruins of its castle. The present town is an agricultural centre with a weekly market. It is an extremely attractive town with narrow streets and interesting buildings. Outstanding among these is the St. Mary Magdalene Church, unique except for its C14th tower. Its outside walls are entirely covered with carvings.

TOURIST INFORMATION CENTRE
Market House Arcade, Market Street
Launceston PL15 8EP
Tel: (01566) 772321   Fax: (01566) 772322

SELF-CATERING
ROUNDHOUSE COTTAGE 🚶
Trenannick Cottages, Trenannick, Warbstow,
Launceston PL15 8RP
Tel/Fax: (01566) 781443
No. of Accessible Units: 1
No. of Beds per Unit: 2 + sofa bed
Accessible Facilities: Roll-in Shower, Lounge, Kitchen/Diner, Gardens. Situated

Rush hour at Looe harbour.

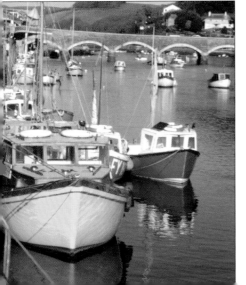

at the end of a private drive in a south facing hollow, the cottages are converted from C18th farm buildings in three acres of grounds. Roundhouse Cottage was once the building that ground corn and was operated by a horse walking in a circle – hence the name. At the rear is the main building with its own drive and garden and a huge oak beam running through its centre. Space is limited in the bedroom and bathroom, otherwise probably would be Category 2.

LISKEARD

Progressive small town, lively in atmosphere with some pleasant Georgian and Victorian architecture. Hosts the busiest livestock market in East Cornwall.

HOTEL
WHEALTOR HOTEL ♿
Caradon Hill, Pensilia, Liskeard PL14 5PJ
Tel: (01579) 362281
No. of Accessible Rooms: 7.
Accessible Facilities: Lounge, Bar, Restaurant. Purpose built, small moorland hotel. Minibus available.

SELF-CATERING
ROSECRADDOC LODGE ♿
Liskeard PL14 5BU
Tel/Fax: (01579) 346768
No. of Accessible Units: 2. 1 with Roll-in Shower: 1 with Bath. No. of Beds per Unit: 4
1 unit has bath, 1 has wheel-in shower.
Accessible Facilities: Kitchen-living room, Dining room, level lawn and patio. Rosecraddoc, an area of rolling farmland, is two miles northeast of Liskeard. The modern, traditionally built bungalows are situated in gardens and woodland, once part of Rosecraddoc Manor grounds.

LOOE

This tourist-orientated fishing port and seaside resort becomes very overcrowded in summer, but is a delightful spot.

TOURIST INFORMATION CENTRE
The Guildhall, Fore Street, East Looe
Tel: (01503) 262072
Fax: (01503) 265426 – Seasonal

SELF-CATERING
PENVITH BARN COTTAGES
St. Martins by Looe, Looe PL13 1NZ
Tel/Fax: (01503) 240772
e-mail: anne@penvith.demon.co.uk
web: www.pilgrims.com/penvith-barns
No. of Accessible Units: 2
No. of Beds per Unit: 5
Accessible Facilities: Open plan Kitchen,
Lounge, Patio. Swallow and barn owl.
Cottages have been converted from a part
C16th. stone barn. Facing south, they
overlook open paddocks, a small copse and a
field and are set in lovely unspoilt
countryside. Three miles' drive from Looe.

GRANITE HENGE BUNGALOWS
Trelawne Cross, Looe PL13 2BT
Tel: (01503) 272772   Fax: (01503) 272060
No. of Accessible Units: 10. Shower
No. of Beds per Unit: 9 x 3 beds: 1 x 6 beds.
Accessible Facilities: Lounge, Dining room,
Pool. Situated on the edge of National Trust
countryside, 5 minutes from Looe and
Polperro. Small, privately owned holiday
complex of 10 cottage style bungalows with
heated pool and peaceful gardens.

KATIE'S COTTAGE
Bocaddon Farm, Lanreath, Looe PL13 2PG
Tel/Fax: (01503) 220245
e-mail: alimaik@aol.com
No. of Accessible Units: 1. Roll-in Shower.
No. of Beds per Unit: 4
Accessible Facilities: Kitchen/Living Area.
Stone barn conversion on 350-acre dairy
farm, seven miles from Looe. Lanreath
village is a quiet backwater with tea rooms,
farm and country museum and shop.

ATTRACTION
LANREATH FOLK and FARM MUSEUM
Nr. Looe PL13 2NX
Tel: (01503) 220321
Hands-on exhibits reflect Cornwall's history.
Facilities are limited, there is no catering,
shop or WC, but this is worth a visit.

SD 🚹   CP 🚹   E 🚹

NEWQUAY
The county's most popular seaside resort.
Wonderful beaches, renowned for surfing.

TOURIST INFORMATION CENTRE
Municipal Offices, Marcus Hill,
Newquay TR7 1BD
Tel: (01637) 854020   Fax: (01637) 854030
e-mail: info@newquay.co.uk

BUSES
Western Greyhound. Tel: (01637) 871871

TAXIS
Ace Taxis: Tel: (01637) 852121
2 Fairways and 1 Minibus
Summercourt Travel: Tel: (01726) 861108

TRAINS
Virgin Trains (summer Saturdays only):
Special Needs – Tel: (0845) 7443366
Minicom: (0845) 7443367
Wales & West – Special Needs:
Tel: (0845) 3003005
Minicom: (0845) 7585469
Newquay station has a ramp.

HOTEL
CHYNOWETH LODGE HOTEL
1 Eliot Gardens, Newquay TR7 2QE
Tel: (01637) 876684
No. of Accessible Rooms: 1. Bath.
Accessible Facilities: Lounge, Pool, Sauna,
Spa. Small, family-owned hotel of 9 rooms
in flat, residential area near Tolcarne beach.

ATTRACTION
NEWQUAY ZOO
Trenance Park, Newquay TR7 2LZ
Tel: (01637) 873342   Fax: (01637) 851318
Preservation is a major issue here where
attractions include penguin pool, monkey,
lion and tropical houses, together with a
maze, assault course and oriental garden.

SD 🚹   CP 🚹   E 🚹   RF 🚹
C 🚹   S 🚹   WC 🚹   RFE 🚹

TRERICE (NT)
Kestle Mill, Newquay TR8 4PG
Tel: (01637) 875404   Fax: (01637) 879300
Three miles from Newquay, tucked away
among narrow lanes, is this Elizabethan
manor house built in 1571 with Dutch-
style gabled façade, elaborate plaster
ceilings, fine C17th and C18th oak and
walnut furniture and oriental and English
porcelain to view. In the garden there is a

picnic area and a lawnmower museum. Two wheelchairs are available along with a useful map/leaflet on access.

SD ♿ | CP ♿ | E ♿ | RF ♿
C ♿ | S ♿ | WC 🚹

PADSTOW
North coast fishing town with unspoiled narrow streets converging on its harbour.

TOURIST INFORMATION CENTRE
Red Brick Building, North Quay, Padstow
Tel: (01841) 533449   Fax: (01841) 532356
e-mail: padstowtic@visit.org.uk

SELF-CATERING
TREGINEGAR HOLIDAY BUNGALOWS   ♿
St. Merryn, Nr. Padstow PL28 8PT
Tel/Fax: (01841) 521042
No. of Accessible Units: 4
No. of Beds per Unit: 4. Roll-in Shower
Accessible Facilities: Lounge, Kitchen.
Attached to the Treginegar Guest House, situated off the beaten track in rural surroundings, four miles from Padstow, 12 from Newquay. Within a two-mile radius are seven superb bays with clean sandy beaches.

TREVORRICK FARM   🚹
St. Issey, Nr. Padstow PL27 7QH
Tel/Fax: (01841) 540574
No. of Accessible Units: 1. Bath
No. of Beds per Unit: 4/5
Accessible Facilities: Lounge/Diner, Kitchen. Serendipity Cottage is a bow-windowed cottage, one of six stone cottages converted from old farm buildings and arranged around a central garden alongside an C18th farmhouse. Situated near Camel Estuary overlooking Petherick Creek, a haven for wildlife. Padstow and great beaches close by.

REDRUTH
Known for its copper mining, there are traces of a major iron-age fort, hut circles and a semi-ruined castle.

ATTRACTION
CORNISH MINES AND ENGINES (NT)

Agar Road, Pool, Redruth TR15 3EB
Tel/Fax: (01209) 315027
Enormous beam engines used in tin mining industry for pumping water and lifting men and ore from workings below ground.

SD ♿ | CP ♿ | E ♿ | RF ♿ | L 🚹
C 🚹 | S ♿ | WC 🚹 | RFE 🚹

ST. AUSTELL
China and clay capital with pedestrian precinct of overhead walkways and plenty of modern buildings. Close to Porthpean and Kopehaven seaside spots.

TOURIST INFORMATION CENTRE
14 Church Street, Mevagissey PL26 6SP or By-Pass Service Station, Southbourne Road, St. Austell PL25 4RS
Tel/Fax: (01726) 76333

ATTRACTION
THE LOST GARDENS OF HELIGAN
Pentewan, St. Austell PL26 6EN
Tel: (01726) 845100   Fax: (01726) 845101
e-mail: info@heligan.com
Over 80 acres of beautiful gardens and grounds including walled gardens with exotic fruit houses, kitchen, grotto, Italian and sundial gardens. Also a 22-acre sub-tropical jungle garden and 30-acre lost valley – a natural woodland. Large areas of the gardens are accessible and not to be missed. Wheelchairs available for loan.

SD ♿ | CP 🚹 | E ♿ | RF ♿ | C 🚹
S 🚹 | WC 🚹 | RFE-Gardens ♿

ST. IVES
The shape and situation of this town is magnificent and remains mostly unspoilt. Streets are narrow and steep leading to excellent shops and museums.

TOURIST INFORMATION CENTRE
The Guildhall, Street-an-Pol, St. Ives TR26 2DS
Tel: (01736) 796297   Fax: (01736) 798309

HOTEL
CHY-an-DOUR HOTEL   ♿
Trelyon Avenue TR26 2AD
Tel: (01736) 796436   Fax: (01736) 795772
No. of Accessible Rooms: 1. Roll-in

Shower. Accessible Facilities: Lounge, Restaurant. C19th former sea captain's house extended to form an attractive hotel with panoramic views of St. Ives Bay, Porthminster beach and harbour. NB: town centre and beaches are downhill.

ATTRACTION
TATE GALLERY ST. IVES
Porthmeor Beach, St. Ives TR26 1TG
Tel: (01736) 796543   Fax: (01736) 794480
web: www.tate.org.uk

The gallery, opened in June 1993, presents modern art created in or associated with Cornwall. It is a striking building, full of light and intriguing perspectives. There are no permanent collections, displays are based on selected works from the Tate Gallery's national collection that also includes loans from other public or private collections. The gallery also presents works by contemporary artists.
Facilities are accessible by the lift.

SD ♿   CP n/a   e ♿   RF ♿   I ♿
C ♿   S ♿   WC ♿

TRURO
Commercial and administrative centre of the county with a three-spired cathedral completed in 1910. Georgian townhouses, pedestrianised shopping and Victoria Gardens add to the town's ambience.

TOURIST INFORMATION CENTRE
Tel: (01872) 274555

BUSES
Truronian City Service (T5):
Tel: (01872) 273453
Regular easy access buses.

TAXIS
City Taxis: Tel: (0800) 318708
1 metrocab with ramp.

TRAINS
Virgin Trains: Special Needs –
Tel: (0845) 7443366
Minicom: (0845) 7443367
Wales & West: Special Needs –
Tel: (0845) 3003005
Minicom: (0845) 7585469

ATTRACTION
ROYAL CORNWALL MUSEUM
River Street, Truro TR1 2SJ
Tel: (01872) 272205   Fax: (01872) 240514

Fine displays covering Cornish history particularly mining, and including the well-known mineral collection; and also the New Gallery on local natural history and costumes.

CP n/a   E ♿   RF ♿
L ♿   C ♿   S ♿   WC ♿

TRLISSICK GARDEN
Feock, Truro TR3 6QL
Tel: (01872) 862090   Fax: (01872) 865808

A garden within a 500-acre estate of park and farmland, particularly famous for its large collection of hydrangeas and rhododendrons and exotic plants, plus a Cornish apple orchard.

CP ♿   E ♿   RF ♿   C ♿
S ♿   WC ♿   RFE (garden) ♿

TREWITHEN GARDENS
Grampound Road, Truro TR2 4DD
Tel: (01726) 883647   Fax: (01726) 882301

Renowned 30-acre landscaped garden with many rare trees and shrubs.

SD ♿   CP ♿   E ♿   RF ♿
C ♿   S ♿   WC ♿   RFE ♿

81

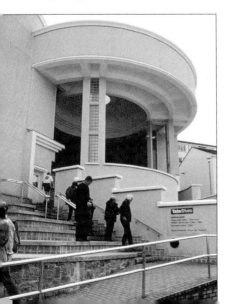

London-on-Sea, the Tate Gallery at St. Ives.

COUNTY DURHAM

An area of 861 square miles, Co. Durham is recognised as an area of outstanding natural beauty.

CO. DURHAM TOURISM
County Hall, Durham DH1 5UF
Tel: (0191) 3833698   Fax: (0191) 3833657
e-mail: cdpd@durhamcc.octacon.co.uk

NORTHUMBRIA TOURISM
web: www.ntb.org.uk

ACCESS DIRECTORY
Much information on transport services throughout County Durham available from Miss Chris Graham, The Public Transport Group, Durham City Council.
Tel: (0191) 3833337.

BARNARD CASTLE
Picturesque town, an excellent base for discovering the delights of Teesdale. Lovely riverside walks here, especially to Egglestone Abbey on the Yorkshire side.

TOURIST INFORMATION CENTRE
Woodleigh, Flats Road,
Barnard Castle DL12 8AA
Tel: (01833) 690909/630272

SELF-CATERING
EAST BRISCOE FARM COTTAGES
Baldersdale, Barnard Castle DL12 9UL
Tel: (01833) 650087
e-mail: pejowi@aol.com
No. of Accessible Units: 2. Bath.
Low Barn Cottage
Studio Cottage
Situated in beautiful Teesdale, on a 14-acre Riverside estate, this 1713 farmhouse and its adjoining barns were converted in the early 90s to charming cottages. In 1998 they received the Northumbrian TB Self-Catering of the Year special award. Each cottage has access to a patio area, a shared conservatory and lawned garden. Explore the estate's fields and woods where you can. Cotherstone, two miles away, has pubs and a shop: four miles farther on is Barnard Castle, a popular market town.

ATTRACTION
THE BOWES MUSEUM
Barnard Castle DL12 8NP
Tel: (01833) 690606   Fax: (01833) 637163
French chateau-style mansion built in 1869, housing a fine collection of paintings by El Greco, Goya, Canaletto and others, plus porcelain and silver, furniture, ceramics and tapestries.

| SD n/a | CP 🚶 | E ♿ | RF ♿ | L 🚶 |
| C 🚶 | S ♿ | WC 🚶 | RFE ♿ | |

BISHOP AUCKLAND
Country home of bishops of Durham since C12th with Auckland Castle, their official residence, surrounded by 800-acre Bishops' Park.

TOURIST INFORMATION CENTRE
Town Hall, Market Place,
Bishop Auckland DL14 7NP
Tel: (01388) 604922

HOTEL
REDWORTH HALL HOTEL
Redworth, Newton Aycliffe,
Nr. Bishops Auckland DL5 6NL
Tel: (01388) 772442   Fax: (01388) 775112
No. of Accessible Rooms: 5. Accessible Facilities: Restaurants (2), Bar, Health Club (disabled chair lift into pool). Imposing and impressive Elizabethan-style manor built around a 300-year-old great hall in 25 acres of woodland. Located a few miles south of Bishop Auckland on A6072.

CHESTER-LE-STREET
Old historic town with stone beach, a market place for surrounding areas.

HOTEL
THE OAK TREE INN
Tantobie, Nr. Chester-le-Street,
Stanley DH9 9RF
Tel: (01207) 235445
No. of Accessible Rooms: 1
Accessible Facilities: Lounge, Restaurant
Once a manor house dating from 1700,

now carefully restored and furnished with antiques. 10 minutes' drive from Beamish and 20 minutes from Durham.

ATTRACTION
BEAMISH, NORTH OF ENGLAND OPEN AIR MUSEUM
Beamish, Nr. Chester-le-Street DH9 0RG
Tel: (01207) 231811   Fax: (01207) 290933
e-mail: beamish@ neoam.demon.co.uk
web: www.merlins.demon.co.uk/beamish
Award-winning museum set in 300 acres recreating northern life in early C19th and C20th. Six main areas; The Town, Colliery Village, Home Farm, Pockerly Manor, Railway Station and 1825 Railway, a replica of Stephenson's Locomotion No 1, the world's first passenger train. Linked by footpaths, a bus and circular tram track. Very large open-air site with some steep gradients, not ideal for wheelchairs, but the museum provides a good leaflet for visitors with mobility problems and it is worth the effort to see it. The town is cobbled, and co-op shops are accessible from the street. Sweet shop/factory is accessible from an alley on the RHS of the shop. The garage is accessible from street. The dentist (two houses) and The Sun Inn pub (no food) are accessible on the ground floor.
Colliery Village – The pit yard surface is crushed stone. The chapel/school is accessible from the rear. The pit cottages have steps, so look in the windows.
Colliery – The surface is crushed stone, the engine shed and drift mine are accessible.
Home Farm – Not accessible, there is a steep slope of 60m from the tram stop.
Pockerly Manor – Rest stops on steep slope of 100m. Gardens and ground floor are accessible, railway station and Old House aren't. Stephenson Locomotion 1 carriage is accessible by slope to the platform. There is no suspension so the track is bumpy.

DURHAM
One of the most visually exciting university cities in the UK, this was once a secure fortress against the Scots and Danes. Towering above a loop in the river Wear, Durham Cathedral, with the castle close by, gives a fine sense of Norman splendour.

TOURIST INFORMATION CENTRE
Market Place, Durham DH1 3NJ
Tel: (0191) 3843720

BUSES
General Information: Tel: (0191) 3833337
Arriva: Tel: (0345) 124125
Super low-floor services
Stagecoach: Tel: (0191) 2761411
Super low-floor services
Go Northern: Tel: (0845) 6060260

TAXIS
Nova Travel: Tel: (01207) 270327
2 Renault Master vehicles.

Crossroad Coaches: Tel: (0191) 3710291
5 minibuses in varying sizes with all fittings.
Greencroft Minicoaches: Tel: (01207) 235079
4 minibuses with all fittings.
Nightingale Coaches: Tel: (01207) 529729
11 vehicles with all fittings, various sizes.

TRAINS
Great North Eastern Railway: Special Needs –
Tel: (0845) 225444
Minicom: (0191) 2330173
Virgin Trains: Special Needs –

Full up on top!

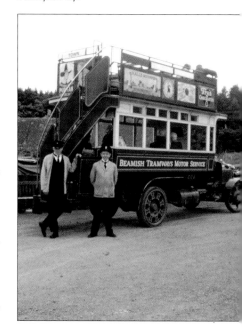

Tel: (0845) 7443366
Minicom: (0845) 7443367

CAR PARKS

Free orange badge parking in all council car parks.

HOTEL ACCOMMODATION
ROYAL COUNTY HOTEL ♿
Old Elvet, Durham DH1 3JN
Tel: (0191) 386 6821
No. of Accessible Rooms: 1. Bath
Accessible Facilities: Lounge, Restaurant
Elegant city-centre hotel overlooking
River Wear, rich with antiques and
paintings.

CROSSWAYS HOTEL and RESTAURANT ♿
Dunelm Road, Thornley,
Nr. Durham DH6 3HT
Tel: (01429) 821248   Fax: (01429) 820034
No. of Accessible Rooms: 1. Bath.
Accessible Facilities: Lounge, Restaurant
Family-owned and managed country hotel
five miles east of Durham, originally one
of 21 public houses existing during the
hay-days of the mining industry. A dog
track existed alongside the pub and
greyhound racing remains very popular.

RAMSIDE HALL HOTEL and GOLF CLUB 🚶
Carrville, Durham DH1 1TD
Tel: (0191) 3865282   Fax: (0191) 3860399
e-mail: ramsidehall@easynet.co.uk
web: www.ramsidehall.co.uk
No. of Accessible Rooms: 2. Bath
Accessible Facilities: Lounge (three steps
or portable ramp): Restaurants (three
steps, portable ramp for upper and lower
levels). Charming private hotel with
lovely gardens leading down to the river.

BED AND BREAKFAST
THE BRACKEN GUEST HOUSE 🚶
Bank Foot, Shincliffe, Durham DH1 2PB
Tel: (0191) 3862966
Fax: (0191) 384 5423
No. of Accessible Rooms: 1. Accessible
Facilities: Restaurant.
Set in two acres of private grounds, in a
rural location, a mile from Durham city
centre.

WATERSIDE GUEST HOUSE 🚶
Elvet Waterside, Durham DH1 3BW
Tel: (0191) 3846660   Fax: (0191) 3846996
No. of Accessible Rooms: 2. Shower
Accessible Facilities: Lounge, Dining room
This is a charming small property, opened
since August 1997 and situated on the
banks of the River Wear just a short
distance from the city centre. Evening
meals may be available.

ATTRACTION
DURHAM ART GALLERY and LIGHT INFANTRY MUSEUM
Aykley Heads, Durham DH1 5TU
Tel: (0191) 384 2214   Fax: (0191) 386 1770
e-mail: durham.gallery@durham.gov.uk
The museum has continually changing
exhibitions in the gallery and tells the
Light Infantry regimental history through
its collection of artefacts.
SD ♿ CP 🚶 E ♿ RF ♿ L ♿
C 🚶 S 🚶 WC 🚶 RFE 🚶

WOLSINGHAM

Entrance to some of the finest Weardale
scenery, Wolsingham is built mostly of
stone and boasts a beautiful parish
church.

SELF-CATERING
BRADLEY BURN HOLIDAY COTTAGES 🚶
Bradley Burn Farm, Wolsingham,
Weardale DL13 3JH
Tel/Fax: (01388) 527 285
e-mail:
SelfCatering@bradleyburn.demon.co.uk
web: bradleyburn.demon.co.uk
No. of Accessible Units: 2.
No. of Beds per Unit: 2-4
Accessible Facilities: Stable Cottages –
Lounge, Kitchen. Harvest Cottage – Open
Plan Living Area. Two of the five
renovated cottages overlook the pretty
stream with fields and woods beyond on
this family-run farm of 360 acres on the
eastern edge of the north Pennines.
Bradley Burn was part of a C12th
settlement where prince bishops hunted
deer each autumn. Part of the original
hunting lodge at Bradley Hall still exists.

CUMBRIA

CUMBRIA TOURIST BOARD
Ashleigh, Holly Road,
Windermere LA23 2AQ
Tel: (015394) 44444   Fax: (015394) 44041
Web: www.golakes.co.uk

CYMBRIA COUNTY COUNCIL
Public Transport Team, Citadel Chambers,
Carlisle CA3 8SG
Tel: (01228) 606000
web: www.cumbria.gov.uk
Produces "Getting Around Cumbria",
information on buses and trains.

ALSTON
The highest market town in England is
now a holiday centre offering a wonderful
choice of drives around sweeping moorland
scenery.

TOURIST INFORMATION CENTRE
Alston Railway Station, Alston CA9 3JB
Tel: (01434) 381696 (Seasonal)

SELF-CATERING
GREY CROFT   [⚐]
Crossgill Farm, Garrigill, The Raise,
Alston CA9 3HE
Tel: (01434) 381383
No. of Accessible Units: 1. Bath
No. of Beds per Unit: 6
Accessible Facilities: Lounge, Dining room,
Kitchen. Spacious bungalow on the fringe
of Raise hamlet with open views to the
south, one mile from Alston.

ATTRACTION
SOUTH TYNEDALE RAILWAY
The Railway Station, Alston CA9 3JB
Tel: (01434) 381696
Narrow-gauge railway between Alston and
Kirkhaugh along South Tyne valley.

SD [♿] CP [⚐] E [♿] (wheelchair space in carriage)
RF [⚐] C [⚐] (No provision at Alston: refreshment
vehicle at Northern Terminus Platform).
S [⚐]   WC n/a   RFE [♿]

AMBLESIDE
Busy tourist centre, protected from north
and east winds by mountains, and open to
warmer air from the south.

TOURIST INFORMATION CENTRE
Borrans Road, Ambleside LA2 0EN
Tel: (01539) 432582

SELF-CATERING
NATIONWIDE
Borrans Close, Ambleside
Book through Grooms Holidays
No. of Accessible Units: 1. Roll-in Shower
No. of Beds per Unit: 6
Accessible Facilities: Garden. Spacious
bungalow close to Lake Windermere.

HAWKSHEAD HOLIDAY HOMES   [⚐]
Rogerground House, Hawkshead, Ambleside
Booking through I.G.Mackie, 2 Rowanside,
Prestbury, Macclesfield, Cheshire SK10 4BE
Tel: (01625) 828624
No. of Accessible Units: 1. Bath
No. of Beds per Unit: 4
Accessible Facilities: Open plan Lounge/
Dining/Kitchen (kitchen not adapted). The
Monk's Barn is one of six holiday homes
within walled grounds with lawns and
flowering shrubs, 0.5 mile from
Hawkshead. Laundry room and sheltered
open air pool.

BARROW-IN-FURNESS
Barrow developed from a tiny C19th hamlet
into the biggest iron and steel centre in
the world and then to a major British
shipbuilding force, all within 40 years.

TOURIST INFORMATION CENTRE
Forum 28, Duke Street, Barrow LA14 1HU
Tel: (01229) 894 784

ACCESSIBLE ATTRACTIONS
THE DOCK MUSEUM
North Road, Barrow-in-Furness LA14 2PW
Tel: (01229) 870871   Fax: (01229) 811361
Straddling a Victorian graving dock, this
museum offers exhibition gallery, film
show and landscaped dock site.

SD [♿]   CP [♿]   E [♿]   RF [♿]
L [♿]   C [⚐]   S [♿]   WC [⚐]

BOWNESS-ON-WINDERMERE

On the shore of Lake Windermere, there is much activity centred on the lake and a winding main street with attractive shops.

TOURIST INFORMATION CENTRE

Glebe Road, Bowness Bay, Bowness on Windermere LA23 3HJ
Tel: (015394) 42895 (Seasonal)

HOTEL
THE BURNSIDE HOTEL

Bowness on Windermere LA23 3EP
Tel: (015394) 42211   Fax: (015394) 43824
No. of Accessible Rooms: 15. Roll-in Shower. Facilities: Lounge, Restaurant, Pool, Sauna, Spa. Set in mature gardens overlooking Lake Windermere and 300 metres from the Steamer Pier and village.

BURN HOW GARDEN HOUSE HOTEL

Belfield Road,
Bowness-on-Windermere LA23 3HH
Tel: (015394) 46226   Fax: (015394) 47000
e-mail: burnhowhotel@btinternet.com
web: www.burnhow.co.uk
No. of Accessible Rooms: 4.
Accessible Facilities: Lounge, Restaurant. Charming hotel with delightful furnishings. Two minutes from Lake Windermere. Rooms for disabled guests have direct access to a rose garden and patio.

SELF-CATERING
BIRCH COTTAGE

Deloraine Holiday Homes
Helm Road,
Bowness-on-Windermere LA23 2HS
Tel: (015394) 45557   Fax: (015394) 43221
e-mail: gordon@deloraine.demon.co.uk
web: www.deloraine.demon.co.uk
No. of Accessible Units: 2
No. of Beds per Unit: 6. Roll-in shower
Accessible Facilities: Open plan living/dining/kitchenette. Adjoining sun room. Terrace path round house with garden views. Converted and enlarged from traditional stone and slate structure, retaining timber features. Located within the grounds of an Edwardian mansion 300m above Lake Windermere in 1.5 acres of landscape.

ATTRACTIONS
WINDERMERE LAKE CRUISES

Bowness Bay Boating Division,
Bowness-on-Windermere LA23 3HQ
Tel: (015394) 43360   Fax: (015394) 43468
Cruise between Lakeside, Bowness and Ambleside on large steamers, Swan and Teal and the smaller Tern. A number of different trips are offered of about 1.5 hours' duration, including a champagne evening cruise. We checked the pier facilities at Bowness only, but understand that adaptive WCs are available at Lakeside and Ambleside also. Car parking is available at both these sites next to the piers.

SD 🚿   CP n/a (200m away)   E ♿ (to pier)
RF ♿ (ramped boarding onto steamers, dependent on water height, summer when water is lower, a little steep, but manageable and staff are very helpful)
C ♿ (on board),
♿ Boatman's Café in Bowness coach/car park.
WC 🚽 (on pier, on board facility not accessible)

WORLD OF BEATRIX POTTER ATTRACTION

Crag Brow,
Bowness-on-Windermere LA23 3BX
Tel/Fax: (015394) 88444
e-mail: beatrixpotter@hop-skip-jum.com
web: www.hop-skip-jump.com
Multi-award-winning attraction in which to discover a magical indoor recreation of Peter Rabbit and Jemima. Where else can you call on Mrs. Tiggy-Winkle? Three-dimensional displays on Hill Top, Beatrix Potter's home and inspiration for many of the tales. A must!
The approach to the entrance is steep, but all staff have completed the Welcome All course and want to help.

SD 🚿   CP n/a   E 🚶   RF ♿
C 🚿   S 🚿   WC 🚶

BROUGH

Located midway between Penrith and Barnard Castle, the closest town is Appleby-in-Westmoreland.

ATTRACTION
LANCERCOST PRIORY (EH)

Brampton, Nr. Brough CA8 2HQ
Tel: (016977) 73030

Augustinian priory founded in 1166. The nave of the church has survived and is still used as the local parish church, although the chancel and priory buildings are in ruins.

SD 👤   CP 👤   E 👤   RF 👤
S 👤   WC 👤   RFE 👤

CALDBECK

Most famous village in Northern Lakes, an area of dramatic fells. Birth and burial place of John Peel.

SELF-CATERING
MONKHOUSE HILL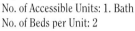
Sebergham, Caldbeck CA5 YHW
Tel/Fax: (016974) 76254
No. of Accessible Units: 1. Bath
No. of Beds per Unit: 2
Accessible Facilities: Open-plan Lounge/
Diner/Kitchen. Lovely views across paddock
from sitting area and bedroom. Mickle Rigg
Cottage is one of seven delightful stone,
oak-beamed cottages with panoramic views
set around a courtyard of this 300-year-old
farm in foothills of North Lakeland fells.

CARLISLE

Just north of Hadrian's Wall, with a small cathedral and vast amounts of Roman history. The city centre is compact, pedestrianised and accessible.

CARLISLE TOURISM AND MARKETING
Civic Centre, Rickergate, Carlisle CA3 8QG
Tel: (01228) 817150 Fax: (01228) 511370

CARLISLE TOURIST
INFORMATION CENTRE
Old Town Hall, Greenmarket, Carlisle CA3 8JH
Tel: (01228) 512444 Fax: (01228) 511758
web: www.historic-carlisle.org.uk

BUSES
Stagecoach Cumberland: Tel: (01228) 597222
Some low-floor, easy access routes.

TAXIS
A Newton: Tel: (01228) 520568
1 FX4 with all fittings.
Border Cabs: Tel: (01228) 534440
17 vehicles of varying sizes.

Staceys Minicoaches: Tel: (01228) 511127
Mercedes with all fittings.

TRAINS
First North Western: Special Needs –
Tel: (0845) 6040231

CAR PARKS
Free orange badge parking in all council-run car parks, some limited parking on-street.

SHOPMOBILITY
Level 2, The Lanes Car Park, East Tower Street, Carlisle CA3 8NX
Tel: (01228) 625950

ACCESSIBLE RESTROOMS
Many accessed by RADAR key, available for sale at TIC and Civic Centre, 7th floor. Bus Station (Lowther Street), Carlisle Cathedral (separate building at rear of the grounds), Civic Centre, Market Hall, Old Town Hall, Railway Station, St. Nicholas Toilets (Butchergate), Sands Centre, Tullie House Museum.

BED AND BREAKFAST ACCOMMODATION
7 Hether Drive 👤
Lowry Hill, Carlisle CA3 0ED
Tel: (01228) 527242
No. of Accessible Rooms: 1. Roll-in Shower.
Accessible Facilities: Lounge, Dining room
Detached bungalow in quiet location and easy access to the M6 (J44).

SELF-CATERING
ARCH VIEW 👤
Midtodhills Farm, Roadhead, Carlisle CA6 6PF
Tel/Fax (016977) 48213
No. of Accessible Units: 1. Shower
No. of Beds per Unit: 2/8
Accessible Facilities: Lounge, Kitchen/Diner.
Barn conversion and two cottages with lovely views on 320-acre working farm set in lovely Lyne valley near Scottish border.

GREEN VIEW LODGES 👤
Welton, Nr. Dalston, Carlisle CA5 7ES
Tel: (016974) 76230 Fax: (016974) 76523
No. of Accessible Units: 2
No. of Beds per Unit: 6
Accessible Facilities: Open plan Lounge/
Kitchen/Diner, Garden.

The site comprises traditional cottages, a converted chapel and pine lodges, of which two lodges are accessible. All properties overlook meadows. The tiny hamlet of Weldon nestles in the foothills of the northern fells, three miles from the National Park with Lake Ullswater and Keswick within 30 minutes' drive.

WILDSIDE 🚶
Mealsgate, Carlisle
Tel: (01694) 371420
No. of Accessible Units: 1. Bath
No. of Beds per Unit: 6
Accessible Facilities: Lounge, Dining room. Comfortable bungalow between market towns of Wigton and Cockermouth and four miles from the Lake District National Park boundary.

LAKESHORE LODGES 🚶
Thurstonfield, Carlisle VA5 6HBA
Tel: (01228) 576661   Fax: (01228) 576662
No. of Accessible Units: 1. Roll-in shower.
No. of Beds per Unit: 3
Accessible facilities: Lounge, Kitchen, Wheelchair accessible boat for fly fishing/ leisure. One mile pathway around lake and use of accessible bird hide. Chalets are on the lake shore. Tranquil surroundings with lots of nature, otters, red squirrels etc.

ATTRACTIONS
CARLISLE CATHEDRAL
Castle Street, Carlisle
(Office: 7 The Abbey, Carlisle CA3 8TZ)
Tel/Fax: (01228) 548151
Originally a Norman priory, built in 1122. Notable for its superbly decorated chancel roof and east window.

SD n/a   CP 🚶   E ♿   RF 🚶   C n/a
S ♿   WC 🚶   RFE ♿

SPORTING VENUE
CARLISLE RACECOURSE
Durdar Road, Carlisle CA2 4TS
Booking-Box Office: (01228) 522973
Fax: (01228) 591827
CP ♿ Free across road from club entrance and turnstiles. Trackside CP/picnic area on terraces £3.
RE ♿   ED ♿ (except Manual Door)
INT ♿   WC 🚶 (by paddock and by trackside CP)
SS ♿ Route through Club Entrance foyer: through

Paddock Entrance side gate at turnstiles: Trackside CP with adjacent WC. £3 (£5, Evenings, Sats. Bank Holidays).
B/R ♿

THEATRE
THE SANDS CENTRE
The Sands, Carlisle CA1 1SQ
Admin: (01228) 625208
Fax: (01228) 625666
Booking-Box Office: (01228) 625222
CP ♿   RE ♿   ED ♿   INT ♿
WC ♿ (ground floor opposite reception desk)
AUD ♿ Standing concerts – ramp erected against far wall for wheelchairs.
Bar/Restaurant ♿ (R. ground floor).
Note: Wheelchair spaces through main doors, on flat.

COCKERMOUTH
Home of William Wordsworth, this bustling market town is a perfect base for visiting the West Lakes and Fells. Nearest train station is Workington, 8 miles away.

TOURIST INFORMATION CENTRE
The Town Hall, Market Street,
Cockermouth CA13 9NP
Tel: (01900) 822634

WEST CUMBRIA TOURISM INITIATIVE
Unit 5, Lakeland Business Park,
Cockermouth CA13 0QT
Tel: (01900) 829990   Fax: (01900) 828049

HOTEL
SHEPHERDS HOTEL ♿
Egremont Road, Cockermouth CA13 0QX
Tel/Fax: (01900) 822673
No. of Accessible Rooms: 1
Accessible Facilities: Restaurant, Bar, Lift (Cat.1) to Shop, Exhibition and Sheep Show. Adjacent Lakeland Sheep and Wool centre.

PHEASANT INN 🚶
Bassenthwaite Lake, Cockermouth CA13 9YE
Tel: (01768) 776234   Fax: (01768) 776002
No. of Accessible Rooms: 3 Accessible Facilities: Lounges (3), Dining room. Bar. Charming old coaching inn, a traditional Cumbrian hostelry, set in lovely gardens and woodland.

SELF-CATERING
SIMONSCALES MILL ♿
Simonscales Lane,
Cockermouth CA13 9TG
Tel: (01900) 822594
No. of Accessible Units: 1. Bath.
No. of Beds per Unit: 4
Accessible Facilities: Lounge, Dining room. Fishing is from a flat river bank 30 metres from the front door. Originally a flax and bobbin mill, this property lies on the banks of the River Cocker, with a private patio overlooking the river. Just over a mile from Cockermouth.

IRTON HOUSE FARM ♿
Book through Holidays for You & Me.
Isel, Bassenthwaite, Cockermouth CA13 9ST
Tel: (01768) 776380
No. of Accessible Units: 1. Roll-in Shower.
No. of Beds per Unit: 2, T. The Granary is a self-contained cottage situated in the 240 acres of pasture and woodland that surrounds Irton House. The farm is a working sheep farm. Easy driving distance to many lakes favourites.

ATTRACTION
LAKELAND SHEEP AND WOOL CENTRE
Cumwest Visitor Centre, Egremont Road,
Cockermouth CA13 0QX
Tel/Fax: (01900) 822673
A visual show and different exhibits introduce the life of the countryside. A comprehensive indoor presentation includes a face-to-face with 19 different breeds of live sheep and surprising facts about each breed. There is a display of sheep dogs in the 300-seater arena.

SD ♿ CP ♿ E ♿ L ♿ C ♿
S ♿ WC ♿ RFE ♿

GRANGE-OVER-SANDS
Seaside resort backed by wooded fells, overlooking Morecambe Bay. Its parks are noted for flowering shrubs, alpines, rock and herbaceous plants.

TOURIST INFORMATION CENTRE
Victoria Hall, Main Street,
Grange-over-Sands LA11 6PT
Tel: (015395) 34026

HOTEL
NETHERWOOD HOTEL ♿
Lindale Road, Grange-over-Sands LA11 6ET
Tel: (015395) 32552   Fax: (015395) 34121
No. of Accessible Rooms: 1. Bath.
Accessible Facilities: Lounge, Restaurant, Pool. C19th country residence set in 11 acres of gardens overlooking Morecambe Bay.

GRASMERE
Famous as Wordsworth's home from 1799, the area around the village and lake has superb scenery.

TOURIST INFORMATION CENTRE
Red Bank Road, Grasmere LA22 9SW
Tel: (015394) 35245

ATTRACTION
DOVE COTTAGE and THE WORDSWORTH MUSEUM
The Wordsworth Trust, Dove Cottage,
Grasmere LA22 9SH
Tel: (015394) 35544   Fax: (015394) 35748
e-mail: enquiries@wordsworth.org.uk
web: www.wordsworth.org.uk
This award-winning museum displays the trust's unique collection of manuscripts, books and paintings, interpreting the great poet's life and work. Dove Cottage was Wordsworth's home from 1799-1808. There are guided tours of the cottage and its artefacts, all wonderfully preserved in enchanting surroundings. The trust has been incredibly helpful to our researchers. NB: The cottage is accessible, although the kitchen has narrow door, so retreat through Dorothy's bedroom! Museum entrance is ramped at 1:5 and not easily accessible.

SD ♿ CP ♿ E-COTTAGE ♿ MUSEUM n/a
C ♿ S ♿ WC ♿

KENDAL
This ancient town is just outside the Lakes, surrounded by attractive Westmoreland fells on three sides with many parks and open spaces.

TOURIST INFORMATION CENTRE
Town Hall, Highgate, Kendal LA9 4DL
Tel: (015395) 725758

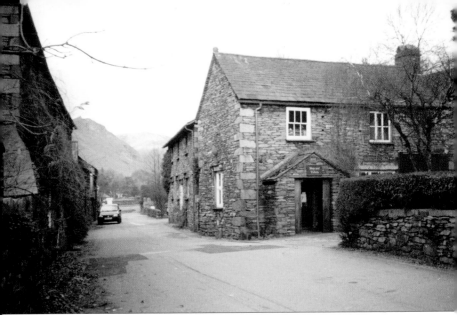

The award-winning Dove's Cottage.

SOUTH LAKELAND DISTRICT COUNCIL LEISURE SERVICES DEPT.
South Lakeland House, Lowther Street, Kendal
Tel: (015397) 33333 Fax: (015397) 40300

BED AND BREAKFAST
MITCHELLAND FARM BUNGALOW
Crook, Nr. Kendal LA8 8LL
Tel: (015394) 47421

No. of Accessible Rooms: 1. Bath
Accessible Facilities: Lounge, Garden. Family home shared with owners' who are dedicated to wheelchair access (retired nurse with holiday-care experience). Situated on a delightful working farm between Kendal and Bowness. There are plans to extend the accessible accommodation with a second purpose-built bathroom and a self-catering unit. Category 1 apart from two slightly narrow doorways. Unwilling to join NAS because there are many full and independent wheelchair users who might be deterred by Category 2 grading.

SELF-CATERING
BARKINBECK COTTAGE
Barkin House, Gatebeck, Kendal LA8 0HX
Tel: (015395) 67277/67122

No. of Accessible Units: 1. Roll-in Shower.
No. of Beds per Unit: 1 double/2 single
Accessible Facilities: Lounge, Dining room.
Converted barn on small working farm

between Kendal and Kirby Lonsdale in peaceful, unspoilt, open countryside.

GREENBANK
Crosthwaite, Kendal LA8 8TD
Tel/Fax: (015395) 68598

No. of Accessible Units: 1. Shower
No. of Beds per Unit: 2
Accessible Facilities: Lounge.
Delightful old farmhouse located in Winster valley with access to central lakes, local limestone scars and quiet Kendal area fells.

ATTRACTION
LEVENS HALL ESTATE GARDENS
Levens Hall, Kendal LA8 0PD
Tel: (015395) 60582   Fax: (015395) 60669
e-mail: levens.hall@farmline.com

House not accessible, but the Gardens are. Famous award-winning gardens were laid out around 1694. The topiary, beech hedges and colourful seasonal bedding create an amazing impact.

SD ♿	CP ♿	E-(Garden) ♿	RF ♿
C ♿	S ♿	WC ♿	RFE (Garden) ♿

KESWICK
Major Lakeland town popular with poets, artists and visitors. Keswick has narrow streets and buildings of old grey stone.

TOURIST INFORMATION CENTRE
Moot Hall, Market Square, Keswick CA12 5HR
Tel: (01768) 772645
e-mail: information@moothall.u-net.com
web: www.keswick.org

KESWICK TOURISM ASSOCIATION
50 Main Street, Keswick CA12 5JR
Tel: (01768) 773607   Fax: (01768) 775738

BUSES
Stagecoach Cumberland:
Tel: (01228) 597222
Some low-floor, easy-access routes.

TRAINS
Virgin
Scotrail
First Northwestern
Cumbrian Coastal Railway

HOTELS
WOODLAND COUNTRY HOUSE
Ireby, Nr. Keswick CA5 1EX
Tel: (016973) 71791   Fax: (016973) 71482
No. of Accessible Rooms: 3. Bath
Accessible Facilities: Lounge, Dining
room, Bar. Privately owned and managed
guest house set within delightful gardens.

DERWENTWATER HOTEL
Portinscale, Keswick CA12 5RE
Tel: (017687) 72538   Fax: (017687) 71002
e-mail: derwentwater.hotel@dial.pipex.com
No. of Accessible Rooms: 6. Bath.
Accessible Facilities: Lounge, Dining room.
Wonderful lakeshore location in 16 acres of
conservation grounds with panoramic views.

SELF-CATERING
CALVERT TRUST
Little Crosthwaite, Keswick
Book through Grooms Holidays or Calvert
Trust. No. of Accessible Units: 3
No. of Beds per Unit: 6, 6 and 16.
South Barn is set in two acres of
panoramic grounds at the foot of Skiddaw
peak, four miles from Keswick. Grooms
Cottage and the Coach House form part of
a listed building where William
Wordsworth once lived, located on
northern outskirts of Keswick, at the foot
of Latrigg.

ATTRACTION
MIREHOUSE HISTORIC HOUSE and GARDENS
Mirehouse, Keswick CA12 4QE
Tel/Fax: (017687) 72287
Grand C17th house with much original
furniture and portraits and works of
Francis Bacon, Carlyle and Tennyson.
Walled garden picnic area and lake where
Tennyson wrote much of Morte d'Arthur.
Four woodland adventure playgrounds for
children. Those parts of the house open to
the public are accessible to wheelchairs.
The main drive and the Bee Garden are
accessible. The garden behind the house is
reached by wheeling on the grass close to
the house. Directions for rose garden access
is given on the useful leaflet provided.
SD   CP   E (House)
C   WC

KIRKBY STEPHEN
Old picturesque market town situated on
the moors with an Anglo Saxon church.

TOURIST INFORMATION CENTRE
Market Square, Kirkby Stephen CA17 4QN
Tel: (017683) 71199

HOTEL
FAT LAMB HOTEL
Crossbank, Ravenstonedale,
Kirkby Stephen CA17 4LL
Tel: (015396) 23242   Fax: (015396) 23285
No. of Accessible Rooms: 2. Bath.
Accessible Facilities: Lounge, Restaurant,
Garden, Viewing point overlooking nature
reserve. Lovely property dating back to the
mid-1600s located midway between the Lake
District and Yorkshire Dales National Parks.

BLACK SWAN HOTEL
Ravenstonedale, Kirkby Stephen CA17 4NG
Tel: (015396) 23204   Fax: (015396) 23604
No. of Accessible Rooms: 1. Bath
Accessible Facilities: Lounges, Restaurant,
Bar. This is a true country hotel built of
lakeland stone in 1899 with comfortable
public rooms, books and magazines and
log fires. Ravenstone is a sleepy, unspoilt
village with Kendal and Penrith half an
hour to the west and Kirkby Stephen very
close by.

SELF-CATERING
COLDBECK HOUSE
Ravenstonedale, Kirkby Stephen
Tel/Fax: (015396) 23230
No. of Accessible Units: 1. Roll-in Shower
No. of Beds per Unit: 4 single/1 double/cot
Accessible Facilities: Lounge, Dining
room, garden,family pub opposite.
Recently renovated self-contained wing
built in 1881 attached to the owner's
farmhouse that was built in early C19th.
Ravenstonedale is a small unspoilt village
set at the foot of the Howgills that lie
between the Lakes and the Yorkshire
Dales.

NEWBY BRIDGE
Charming village on the River Leven with
unusual stone bridge with arches of
unequal size.

ATTRACTION
AQUARIUM OF THE LAKES
Lakeside, Newby Bridge LA12 8AS
Tel/Fax: (015395) 30153
Follow the life story of a Lakeland River
from mountain top to Morecambe Bay.

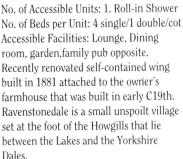

PENRITH
Ancient and historic town, a touring
centre for the Eden Valley. Connections
with Wordsworth and his family.

TOURIST INFORMATION CENTRES
Penrith Museum, Middlegate,
Penrith CA11 7PT
Tel: (01768) 867466

HOTEL
MOSEDALE HOUSE
Mosedale, Mungrisdale, Penrith CA11 0XQ
Tel: (017687) 79371
No. of Accessible Rooms: 1. Roll-in
Shower. Accessible Facilities: Lounge,
Restaurant, Gardens, Path through small
wood, Horse Riding, Wheelchair. Small
and homely family guest house with lovely
views across the Caldew valley to Bowscale
fell from the lounge. From the enclosed

yard there is direct access for wheelchair
users to relatively quiet lanes and the
riverside. Age Concern Eden Shopmobility
Service base a powered scooter here that
guests can book.

SHAP WELLS HOTEL
Shap, Penrith CA10 3QU
Tel: (01931) 716628   Fax: (01931) 716377
web: www.shapwells.com
No. of Accessible Rooms: 2. Roll-in
Shower
Facilities: All public rooms, except Games
room. Large family owned traditional and
comfortable Victorian hotel set in 30 acres
of woodland and gardens high in the Shap
Fells. NB: the area around the hotel is
hilly.

SELF-CATERING
HOWSCALES
Kirkoswald, Penrith CA10 1JG
Tel: (01768) 898666   Fax: (01768) 898710
web: www.oas.co.uk/howscales
No. of Accessible Units: 1. Bath.
No. of Beds per Unit: 2
Accessible Facilities: Lounge, Dining
room
300-year-old farm with barns and byres
converted into cottages surrounding a
central courtyard. Set in secluded open
countryside with views to the lakes and
the Pennines.

MOORFOOT
Clifton, Penrith CA10 2EP
Tel: (01768) 892596
No. of Accessible Units: 1. Roll-in Shower
No. of Beds per Unit: 4-6
Accessible Facilities: Lounge, Dining
room, Kitchen. One of three barns, Lilac
Barn is built in lovely Cumbrian stone, in
this small village three miles south of
Penrith.

PATTERDALE HALL ESTATE
Glenridding, Penrith CA11 0PJ
Tel/Fax: (01768) 482308
e-mail: patterdaleestate@phel.demon.co.uk
web: www.phel.demon.co.uk
No. of Accessible Units: 3.
No. of Beds per Unit: 6
Accessible Facilities: Lounge/Diner,

Kitchen. Three pine lodges of 16 self-catering properties of various types located on a working hill farm at the southern end of Ullswater. The estate has wooded grounds reaching from the shores of the lake to the lower slopes of the Helvellyn range. Patterdale is a good base for touring the Lakes.

ATTRACTION
RHEGED DISCOVERY CENTRE
Redhills, Penrith CA11 0DQ
Tel: (01768) 868000   Fax: (01768) 868002
e-mail: enquiries@rheged.com
web: www.rheged.com

In the Dark Ages, Rheged was a kingdom of magic, myth and mystery. This new attraction, housed in the largest earth-covered building in the UK, celebrates the history and mystery of Cumbria and the Lake District with the first all-British large format film taking viewers back in time through centuries. There is also the huge glass atrium of Mountain Hall with special Cumbrian shops, plus restaurant and coffee shops. Interior features include babbling brooks and massive limestone crags to ensure the visitor feels as if in the very heart of Cumbria. Opened Easter 1999 as a millennium attraction. Full wheelchair access to all seven levels, via three lifts. Located close to the M6 (J40, towards Keswick). Not to be missed!

| SD ♿ | CP ♿ | E ♿ | RF ♿ | L ♿ |
| C ♿ | S ♿ | WC ♿ | RFE ♿ | |

WETHERIGGS COUNTRY POTTERY
Clifton Dykes, Penrith CA10 2DH
Tel: (01768) 892733   Fax: (01768) 892722
e-mail: info@wetheriggs-pottery.co.uk
web: www.wetheriggs-pottery.co.uk

Working pottery since 1855, the only steam powered country pottery in the UK. The museum offers a history of the pottery and an opportunity to throw a pot.All this combines with garden and patio terracotta to produce a fascinating day out.

| SD ♿ | CP ♿ | E ♿ | RF ♿ |
| C ♿ | S ♿ | WC ♿ | RFE ♿ |

RAVENGLASS
Known to have one of the best preserved Roman sites in the north.

ATTRACTION
MUNCASTER CASTLE, GARDENS AND OWL CENTRE
Muncaster Castle, Ravenglass CA18 1RQ
Tel: (01229) 717614   Fax: (01229) 717010

Winner of 1999 Tourism for All Award, every effort is being made to develop the castle into a fully accessible site. Attractions include stunning gardens in 77 acres of woodland, cultivated and wild areas: the castle, family home of the Penningtons since early C13th, and the Owl Centre, HQ of the World Owl Trust with over 180 birds.

Gardens – paths paved or shale in some places, tricky with some steep slopes. Wonderful terrace views accessible from disabled parking, via old St. Michael Church and down a grass slope toward the castle.

Castle – three exterior and one interior step to the accessible ground floor. A ramp is planned. Access from disabled parking is quite steep but surfaced. Wonderful views of Scarfell Pike, the highest in England.

Owl Centre – 90% of aviaries are accessible via ramps and pathways. Shop, WC and catering are within the Stable Courtyard and are very accessible. An interactive Vole Maze is new, encouraging habitat awareness.

| CP ♿ | E ♿ | RF ♿ | C ♿ |
| S ♿ | WC ♿ | | |

SEDBERGH
A hill town and busy market town, set below the slate Howgill fells, more like the Lake district than the Yorkshire dales.

TOURIST INFORMATION CENTRE
72 Main Street, Sedbergh LA10 5AD
Tel: (015396) 20125

SELF-CATERING
BAINBRIDGE COURT   ♿
Castleshaw Farm, Bainbridge Road,
Sedbergh LA10 5BA
Tel: (015396) 21000   Fax: (015396) 21710
e-mail: nigel.close@virgin.net

No. of Accessible Units: 1. Bath. No. of Beds per Unit: 4. Accessible Facilities: Lounge, Dining room.

WINDERMERE

The largest lake in England with thickly wooded shores. Very popular tourist town, noted for its watersports and Yacht Club.

TOURIST INFORMATION CENTRE
Victoria Street, Windermere LA23 1AD
Tel: (01539) 446499

HOTEL ACCOMMODATION
HAWKSMOOR 🚶
Lake Road, Windermere LA23 2EQ
Tel: (015394) 42110
No. of Accessible Rooms: 3. Bath. Accessible Facilities: Lounge, Dining room. NB. Dinner is not available during August or on Bank Holidays. Surrounded by gardens with woodland to the rear this charming guest house is situated between Windermere and Bowness-on-Windermere.

LINTHWAITE HOUSE HOTEL 🚶
Crook Road, Windermere LA33 3JA
Tel: (015394) 88600   Fax: (015394) 88601
e-mail: handmade@linhotel.u-net.com
No. of Accessible Rooms: 1 (one in progress).
Accessible Facilities: Lounge, Restaurant
This privately owned, country house hotel won Hotel of the Year 1994. Set in 14 acres of gardens overlooking Lake Windermere. Great views, and reputedly fine food.

ATTRACTION
WINDERMERE STEAMBOAT MUSEUM
Rayrigg Road, Windermere LA23 1BN
Tel: (015394) 45565   Fax: (015394) 48769
e-mail: steam@insites.co.uk
Web: www.steamboat.co.uk
Historic collection of steam and motor boats in peaceful lakeside setting. Also cruises on original Edwardian steamboats with embarkation assistance from staff.

SDn/a	CP 🚶	E ♿	RF 🚶
C ♿	S ♿	WC 🚶	RFE 🚶

There are many trips available on Windermere.

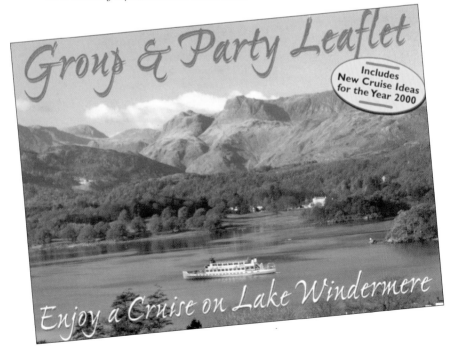

DERBYSHIRE

DERBYSHIRE COALITION OF DISABLED PEOPLE

Victoria Buildings, 117 High Street,
Clay Cross, Chesterfield S45 9DZ
Tel: (01246) 865305
A campaigning pressure group working for
and on behalf of disabled people.

DERBYSHIRE ASSOCIATION FOR THE DISABLED

Amber Vale Resources Centre,
Long Close, Cemetery Lane,
Ripley Tel: (01773) 512076

DERBYSHIRE CENTRE FOR INTEGRATED LIVING

Long Close, Cemetery Lane, Ripley.
Tel: (01773) 740246

ASHBOURNE

Gateway to the Izaak Walton country of
Dovedale, this is a small market town
where little has changed since 1645.

SELF-CATERING
THE COTTAGE BY THE POND
Beechenhill Farm, Ilam, Ashbourne DE6 2BD
Tel/Fax: (01335) 310274
e-mail: beechenhill@btinternet.com
web:www.cressbrook.co.uk/ashborn/beechen/
No. of Accessible Units: 1. Roll-in Shower.
No. of Beds per Unit: 6
Accessible Facilities: Lounge, Dining room
92-acre working dairy farm located in Ilam
between Dovedale and the Manifold Valley
in the Peak District National Park. The
cottage looks south over fields and animals.

LAKE VIEW
Yew Tree Lane, Bradley, Ashbourne DE6 1PG
Tel: (01335) 370577   Fax: (01335) 342707
No. of Accessible Units: 1. Roll-in Shower
No. of Beds per Unit: 6
Accessible Facilities: Lounge, Dining room,
Kitchen, Hydrotherapy Pool part of complex.

*Beauty and dignity at Chatsworth,
the most noble of stately houses.*

BAKEWELL

Small market town built almost entirely in
warm, brownish stone. It lies in a sheltered
valley of the Derbyshire Wye with rolling
wooded hills.

ATTRACTION
CHATSWORTH
Bakewell DE45 1PP
Tel: (01246) 582204   Fax: (01246) 583536
Palatial home of the Duke and Duchess of
Devonshire since 1549 with a fine art
collection in 26 richly furnished rooms. The
garden is one of the finest in England, laid out
by Capability Brown, and is famous for the
work of the head gardener, Joseph Paxton in
C19th. Notable for Cascade and Emperor
Fountain and Angel Conner water sculpture.
THE HOUSE IS NOT ACCESSIBLE.
The garden, farmyard, shops and restaurant
are accessible to a greater or lesser degree as
below. A useful leaflet is given out that
indicates routes and their terrain. Three
electric scooters and four manual wheelchairs
are available free for use in the garden.

SD 🦽   CP 🦽   C 🚶   S 🚶   WC 🚶

PEAK DISTRICT NATIONAL PARK AUTHORITY

Aldern House, Baslow Road,
Bakewell DE45 1AE
Tel: (01629) 816200   Fax: (01629) 816310
The park can be divided into two parts, the
Dark and White Peak. To the north and down
each side lies high, desolate moor lands,
named the Dark Peak for vegetation, peat
and weathering of gritstone. The southern
and middle, separated from the moors by
shale valleys is the White Peak area.

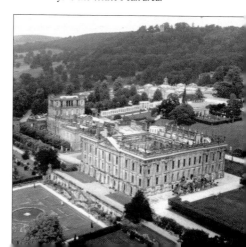

Farming, delightful villages, drystone walls, green fields and woods. The hills impose some difficulties, but worth the effort.

PLACES IN THE PARK WITH ACCESS

Bakewell (Granby Road). Large car park, level tarmac path along river, level kerbed pathway to information centre with ramped entrance. Adaptive restroom.

Curbar Gap. Popular beauty spot with small car park and paths constructed to provide reasonably level access for wheelchair users to viewpoints close to Curbar Edge and right up to Baslow Edge with dramatic views across Derwent Valley.

Derwent. Car Park. Fairly level tarmac paths to views of Derwent Dam and Ladybower Reservoir. Adaptive restroom.

Dovedale. Car Park with fairly level road leading beside river for 0.5 mile to Stepping Stones. This road is closed to traffic at weekends and rarely used at other times. Adaptive restroom.

Dove Stone Reservoir. Circular path around entire reservoir offers moorland scenery. Large car park with tarmac gradient to level track overlooking the reservoir.

Edale. Large car park. Narrow road with slight gradient leads through village. Adaptive restroom.

Goyt Valley - Goyt's Lane. Wheelchair route along a one-mile section of former Cromford and High Peak Railway. Route winds through open moorland. Reserved car parking opposite entrance to route. Adaptive restroom.

Ernwood Reservoir. Reserved car parking near west end of dam. Ramp link to a level road alongside reservoir. Adaptive restroom.

Hathersage. No car park adjacent to street but the main village street is wide enough for parking. Adaptive restroom.

Ladybower. Reserved spaces at Heather Dene car park, plus wheelchair-accessible route. Platform for use of wheelchair anglers opposite fishery office and specially adapted boat with electric outboard.

Redmires Reservoir. Nr. Sheffield. Accessible footpath and new car park.

Tideswell Dale. Car park, firm level track 0.25 miles long to picnic site, continuing to Litton Mill where path through Water-cum-Jolly Dale can be joined. Adaptive restroom.

Tissington and High Peak Trails. Level tracks from Ashbourne and Hopton Top meeting at Parsley Hay and continuing north. Surface variable, but reasonably firm. Gradients where bridges have been removed. Bridle gates not fitted with special catches.

Water-cum-Jolly Dale. Access to level concession path through fine limestone dale. Path sometimes used by anglers with cars.

PEAK CYCLE HIRE

All centres have some or all of a range of cycles suitable for use by people with disabilities. This range includes tandems, trikes, and duet wheelchair cycles.

Mapleton Lane, Ashbourne, Derbys. DE6 2AA. Tel and Fax: (01335) 343156
Just north of town centre on Tissington Trail: a disused railway line of scenic beauty, traffic free and 13.5 miles long.

Fairholmes, Derwent, Sheffield. S30 2AQ. Tel and Fax: (01433) 651261
Off the A57 in Derwent Valley. Cycle beside historic Derwent and Ladybower reservoirs through beautiful woodland.

Parsley Hay, Buxton, Derby. SK17 0DG. Tel and Fax: (01298) 84493
At the junction of Tissington and High Peak Trails. Over 30 miles of traffic-free cycling through amazing limestone scenery.

Old Station Car Park, Waterhouses, Staffs. ST10 3EG. Tel and Fax: (0153) 308609
Located behind Crown Hotel. A 9-mile route through two super river valleys along the Manifold Track converted railway line.

Visitor Centre, Middleton-by-Wirksworth, Derbys. DE4 4LS. Tel: (01629) 823204 Fax: (01629) 825336
On the High Peak Trail near Middleton. 17.5 miles of traffic-free route with link to Tissington Trail.

Information Centre, Station Road, Hayfield, Stockport. SK12 5ES. Tel: (01663) 746222 Fax: (01663) 741581
In Hayfield Village, 2.5 mile trail with plenty of access to surrounding hills via bridleways.

BUXTON

Small but rather grand town having once been a fashionable spa. There is a Regency crescent, restored Edwardian theatre, museums, pump room and pavilion with antique fairs.

HIGH PEAK TOURIST INFORMATION CENTRE
The Crescent, Buxton SK17 6BQ
Tel: (01298) 25106   Fax: (01298) 73153
e-mail: tourism@high peak.gov.uk
web: www.highpeak.gov.uk

SELF-CATERING
CRESSBROOK HALL COTTAGES 🧑‍🦽
Cressbrook Hall, Cressbrook,
Nr. Buxton SK17 8SY
Tel: (01298) 871289   Fax: (01298) 871845
e-mail: Len-Hull@cressbrook-
hall.swinternet.co.uk
No. of Accessible Units: 3. Roll-in Shower.
No. of Beds per unit: 2-8
Accessible Facilities: Lounge, Dining
room, Sauna. Charming cottages within
Cressbrook Village in the Peak District,
within grounds of Cressbrook Hall.

CASTLE DONINGTON
The site of the first Norman castle, built by
Henry de Lacy, Earl of Lincoln, the town
has some lovely houses and cottages
incorporating the original stone. Also a
surprisingly attractive power station.

HOTEL
THISTLE EAST MIDLANDS AIRPORT 🚶
Castle Donington DE74 2SH
Tel: (01332) 850700   Fax: (01332) 850823
No. of Accessible Rooms: 3. Bath
Accessible Facilities: Lounge, Restaurant,
Sauna. Very close to the airport, this
modern hotel is set in its own large
grounds, and has antique furnishings.

CHESTERFIELD
Known for the church's crooked spire and
its strong links with George Stephenson,
who spent his last years at Tapton House.

HOTEL
ABBEYDALE HOTEL 🚶
Cross Street, Chesterfield S40 4TD
Tel: (01246) 277849   Fax: (01246) 558223
No. of Accessible Rooms: 1. Shower
Accessible Facilities: Lounge, Dining
room. Situated in quiet, residential area of
town, this is a family-run hotel.

SELF-CATERING
CHESTNUT and WILLOW COTTAGES 🚶
Priestfield Grane, Old Brampton, Chesterfield
S42 7JH
Tel: (01246) 566159
No. of Accessible Units: 2
No. of Beds per Unit: CH-3: WI-2
Accessible Facilities: CH-Lounge,
Kitchen/Diner, Patio
WI – Lounge/Diner, Kitchen, Patio and
Lawn. Secluded cottages on a farm with
surrounding grassland leading to Linacre
Reservoir and Nature Trails, close to Peak
Park, Bakewell and Chesterfield.

ATTRACTIONS
CHESTERFIELD MUSEUM AND ART GALLERY
St. Mary's Gate, Chesterfield S41 7TY
Tel: (01246) 345727   Fax: (01246) 345720
Rich town heritage explored in different
aspects of Chesterfield's history.

SD 🧑‍🦽	CP n/a	E 🧑‍🦽	RF ♿
C n/a	S ♿	WC ♿	RFE ♿

EYAM HALL GARDENS
Eyam, Hope Valley S32 5QW
Tel: (01433) 631976   Fax: (01433) 731603
e-mail: hicwvi@globalnet.co.uk
Family owned house for over 320 years
with a beautiful walled garden where
outdoor plays and concerts are performed.
Setting down point outside house is gravel
mixture, some loose. Located in the centre
of Eyam village, just off the A623, 20
minutes from Chesterfield, Bakewell and
Sheffield.

SD 🧑‍🦽	CP 🧑‍🦽	E ♿	RF 🧑‍🦽
C ♿	S 🚶	WC 🚶	RFE ♿

HARDWICK HALL (NT)
Doe Lea, Chesterfield DE S44 5QJ
Tel: (01246) 850430   Fax: (01246) 854200
In 1597, Bess of Hardwick, the most
powerful woman after the queen in Tudor
England, moved into this, one of the
greatest of all Elizabethan houses. Superb
collections, a glorious park, and a Tudor
herb garden.

SD ♿	CP 🚶	E ♿	RF ♿
C 🚶	S 🚶	WC 🚶	
RFE - Hall and Garden ♿			

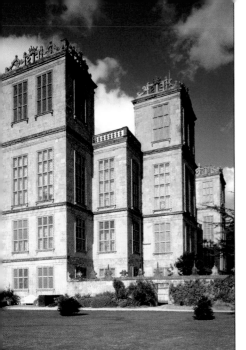

Towering Hardwick Hall.

DERBY

Blessed with open spaces and interesting old houses. The most striking building is the cathedral that retains much from its past. Home of Sir Henry Royce, Rolls-Royce has been associated with Derby since 1908.

DERBY TOURISM

Assembly Rooms, Market Place, Derby DE1 3AH
Tel: (01332) 256201   Fax: (01332) 256137

DERBY CITY COUNCIL

Roman House, Friargate, Derby DE1 1XB
Tel: (01332) 255925   Fax: (01332) 255989
Minicom: (01332) 256666
e-mail: mick.watts@derby.gov.uk
Produces *Derby Access Guide for Disabled People.*

DISABILITY DIRECT

Tel: (01332) 299449

BUSES

Derby Busline: Tel: (01332) 292200
Arriva: Tel: (01332) 572707
Trent: Tel: (01773) 712265

TAXIS

Hackney Carriages: Tel: (01332) 757575
10 TX1s with all fittings.

TRAINS

Midland Mainline: Special Needs —
Tel: (0114) 2537654
Minicom: (0145) 7078051
Virgin Trains: Special Needs:
Tel: (0845) 7443366
Minicom: (0845) 7443367

CAR PARKS

Free three-hour orange badge parking in all council-owned car parks and some off-street.

SHOPMOBILITY

The Coach Park, Derby Bus Station,
The Moreledge, Derby DE1 2AY
Tel: (01332) 200329

HOTEL

BEST WESTERN MIDLAND HOTEL   [♿]
Midland Road, Derby DE1 2SQ
Tel: (01332) 345894   Fax: (01332) 293522
e-mail: sales@midland-derby.co.uk
web: www.midland-derby.co.uk
No. of Accessible Rooms: 88, via accessible lift. Accessible Facilities: Lounge, Restaurant. Quality hotel situated near the city centre, close to the M1 (J25).

ATTRACTIONS

DERBY INDUSTRIAL MUSEUM
Silk Mill Lane, off Full Street, Derby DE1 3AR
Tel: (01332) 255308   Fax: (01332) 716670
Located in C18th silk and flour mills with exhibits on local industries.
SD [♿]   CP [♿]   E [♿]   RF [♿]   L [♿]
S [♿]   WC [♿]   RFE [♿]

DERBY MUSEUM AND ART GALLERY
The Strand, Derby DE1 1BS
Tel: (01332) 293111   Fax: (01332) 716670
Fine display of Derby porcelain and mid-C18th painting by Joseph Wright of Derby plus many changing exhibitions.
SD [♿]   CP n/a   E [♿]   RF [♿]   L [♿]
C n/a   S [♿]   WC [♿]   RFE [♿]

DENBY POTTERY VISITORS CENTRE
Denby, Nr. Derby DE5 8NX
Tel: (01773) 740799   Fax: (01773) 740749

Modern complex with wide open spaces between the Visitor Centre that houses several shops, museum and seconds shop, ramped at gradient of 1:19, and a cookery demonstration area with several wheelchair spaces. The craftsman's workshop tour is limited to two wheelchairs per tour. The Guided Pottery Tour is not accessible.

SD ♿ CP ♿ E ♿ RF ♿
L ♿ Craftsman's tour on first floor.
C 🚶 S ♿ WC 🚶

THE AMERICAN ADVENTURE THEME PARK
Pit Lane, Ilkeston, Nr. Derby DE7 5SX
Tel: (01773) 531521   Fax: (01773) 530238
web: www.adventureworld.co.uk

Theme park based on pioneers from the western to space in an epic story. Small family rides allow all users to have fun so long as restraint criteria are met. There are also restraint consideration on Skycoaster, Runaway Train, Niagara Rapids, Missile and Motion Master. There is an evacuation consideration on the Log Flume, but a High Loading Platform for the Twin Looper.

SD ♿ CP ♿ E ♿ RF ♿
C ♿ S ♿ WC 🚶

SPORTING VENUE
DERBY COUNTY FOOTBALL CLUB
Pride Park Stadium, Derby DE24 8XL
Admininistration and Booking-Box Office:
(01332) 667531

Complies with Part M, Building Regulations.

CP ♿ RE ♿ ED ♿ IN ♿ L 🚶
WC 🚶 SS ♿ B/R ♿

THEATRE
DERBY PLAYHOUSE
Eagle Centre, Derby DE1 2NF
Administration: (01332) 363271
Fax: (01332) 294412
Booking-Box Office: (01332) 363275

CP ♿ RE ♿ ED ♿ INT ♿
L ♿ WC ♿ AUD ♿ B/R ♿

MATLOCK
Riber Castle is the most famous landmark in the Matlocks. The famous wishing stone in Lumsdale is nearby. Many terrific views here.

SELF-CATERING
DARWIN FOREST COUNTRY PARK
Two Dales, Matlock

Book through Grooms Holidays
No. of Accessible Units: 2
No. of Beds per Unit: 4 and 6
Accessible Facilities: Open plan lounge, diner/kitchen.

All aboard for Derby's industrial museum.

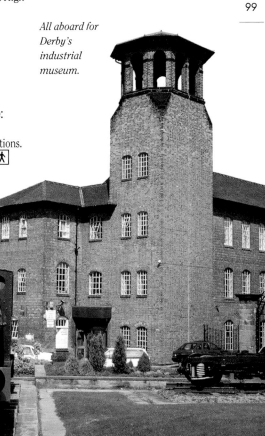

Adapted lodges in 44 acres of woodland and lush parkland.

MIDDLEHILLS FARM
Grange Mill, Matlock DE4 4HY
Tel/Fax: (01629) 650368
e-mail: l.lomas@btinternet.com
No. of Accessible Units: 1
No. of Beds per Unit : 2-4. Roll-in Shower
Accessible Facilities: Open plan Lounge/
kitchen/diner.
NB: Lateral transfer space to WC is 20cm
short. Clematis Cottage is one of three facing
each other on a tarmac-surfaced area on a
small working farm five miles from Matlock in
the Peak National Park. It is close to many
interesting attractions.

ATTRACTIONS
THE NATIONAL TRAMWAY MUSEUM
Crich, Matlock DE4 5DP
Tel: (01773) 852526 Fax: (01773) 852326
A vast array of indoor diversions and rides
through history on vintage trams. The access
Tram is a 1969 model from Berlin and is
specially adapted. An extra-wide door and
hydraulic lift is fitted for easy access. It carries
4 people in their wheelchairs and runs on
demand, so pre-book.

SD 🦽   CP 🦽   E 🦽   RF 🦽
L 🦽   C 🦽   S 🦽   WC 🚶

Mole and Badger check out accessibility.

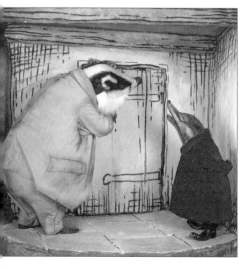

RIDGEWAY
Rural heart of the Moss Valley, south-east
of Sheffield.

ACCESSIBLE ATTRACTION
RIDGEWAY CRAFT CENTRE
Main Road, Ridgeway S12 3XR
Set in restored and converted C17th
farmhouse, visitors can watched skilled
crafts people at work on modern and
traditional crafts.
The Smithy: Paul Mossman Pottery:
Tel: (0114) 251158.
West Byre: Silver and Gold Jewellery:
Tel: (0114) 2477028
Garden Room: Tiffany Land Stained Glass:
Tel: (0114) 2477104
East Byre: Chocolatier:
Tel: (0114) 2478626
Farmhouse Kitchen: Kent House Country
Kitchen. Tel: (0114) 2473739
CP 🦽   WC 🦽

ROWSLEY
Located on the A6 between Bakewell and
Matlock in the new Peak Village retail centre.

ATTRACTIONS
PARK VILLAGE ESTATES
Chatsworth Road, Rowsley DE4 2JE
Tel: (01629) 735326 Fax: (01629) 735128
e-mail: infor@peakvillage
Outlet shopping and leisure centre.
SD 🦽   CP 🦽   E 🦽   RF 🦽
C 🦽   S 🦽   WC 🚶

WIND IN THE WILLOWS
Peak Village, Rowsley DE4 2NP
Tel: (01629) 733433 Fax: (01629) 734850
e-mail: toad@hop-skip-jump.com
Every scene from this delightful adventure
story is brought to life in a recreation of
the English countryside undercover.
Lighting, sound and AV techniques, and
innovative and exciting displays present an
animal's eye view of woods, meadow and
riverbank. 4 wheelchairs available for loan.
SD 🦽   CP 🦽   E 🦽   RF 🦽
C 🦽   S 🦽   WC 🦽   RFE 🦽

DEVONSHIRE

TOURIST OFFICE
web: www.devon-cc.gov.uk/tourism

DISABILITY INFORMATION SERVICE
Tel/Minicom: (01803) 552175
Fax: (01803) 556060

BARNSTAPLE
One of the oldest boroughs in Britain, the town has a fine estuary setting with a C16th arch bridge.

TOURIST INFORMATION CENTRE
36 Boutport Street, Barnstaple EX31 1RX
Tel: (01271) 375000   Fax: (01271) 374037

HOTEL
BRACKEN HOUSE
Bratton Fleming, Barnstaple EX31 4TG
Tel: (01598) 710320
No. of Accessible Rooms: 1. Bath.
Accessible Facilities: Lounge, Restaurant.
Originally an 1840 rectory, the house is now a small and intimate eight-bedroom hotel. Situated on the western edge of Exmoor and standing in eight acres of garden, woodland and paddock, including a small lake.

SELF-CATERING
CALVERT TRUST EXMOOR
Wistlandpound, Kentisbury,
Barnstaple EX31 4SJ
Tel: (01598) 763560   Fax: (01598) 763400
e-mail: Calvert.Exmoor@btinternet.com
No. of Accessible Units: 3. Roll-in Shower
No. of Beds per Unit: 4-7.
Accessible Facilities: Dining room, TV Lounge, bar, heated indoor pool with spa and steam room. Opened in 1996 providing holidays with adventure for disabled people, their families and friends. Accommodation is in a converted farm complex. Accessible to all, set around an inner courtyard garden. Fully catering accommodation in mainly twin-bedded rooms, all with en-suite shower and wc and accessible for wheelchair users.

COUNTRY WAYS
Little Knowle Farm, High Bickerton,
Umberleigh, Nr. Barnstaple EX37 9BJ
Tel/Fax: (01769) 560503
No. of Accessible Units: 1.
No. of Beds per Unit: 2-6
Converted barns hidden away on a small farm with delightful gardens and many superb views.

BRADWORTHY
Bradworthy is the northern apex of the triangle of Bradworthy, Bude and Holsworthy. Located two miles from Tamar Lakes, with National Trust Coastline and Bude's sandy beach 10 miles away.

SELF-CATERING
KIMWORTHY COTTAGES
Bradworthy EX33 7RP
No. of Accessible Units: 3
No. of Beds per Unit: Little Kimworthy 2: Wren and Jay Cottages 4 + cot.
Accessible Facilities: Open plan Lounge/Kitchen/Diner. Three lovely pine and brick cottages sharing a three-acre garden with a lawned play area, an outdoor pool and partially landscaped gardens full of shrubs and flowers.

BUDLEIGH SALTERTON
Red cliffs, large-pebbled beach leading to the mouth of the River Otter.

TOURIST INFORMATION CENTRE
Fore Street, Budleigh Salterton EX9 6NG
Tel: (01395) 445275

SELF-CATERING
LEMPRICE FARM
Yettington, Budleigh Salterton EX9 7BW
Tel: (01395) 567037 Fax: (01395) 567585
No. of Accessible Units: 1. Roll-in Shower.
No. of Beds per Unit: 4/6/4
Accessible Facilities: Lounge, Dining room. Yettington is small hamlet adjacent to Woodbury Common, a mile west of East Budleigh. The adjoining farm was the birthplace of Sir Walter Raleigh. The cottages are set in a very peaceful location with a lake and open countryside all around.

101

COLYTON

A neat, busy small town supplying a rich farm vale. Its church is remarkable for its octagonal lantern top.

SELF-CATERING
SMALLICOMBE FARM
Northleigh, Colyton EX13 6BU
Tel: (01404) 831310   Fax: (01404) 831431
Winner of Best Self-Catering Accommodation in England from Holiday Care Service in 1996.
No. of Accessible Units: 2. Roll-in Showers
No. of Beds per Unit: 1 double and 1 twin or 1 bunk-bed.
Accessible facilities: Lounge, Dining room, Games room with snooker, table tennis, skittles, darts, level concrete farmyard. Smallicombe means narrow valley in which the farm nestles in this unspoilt part of Devon. Home of the prize winning Smallicombe Herd of rare breed pigs. Close to Honiton and the coast from Lyme Regis to Sidmouth.

CULLOMPTON

Hemyock is situated in Blackdown Hills, a good centre for touring Exmoor and Dartmoor.

SELF-CATERING
HEMYOCK CASTLE
Hemyock, Cullompton EX15 3RJ
Tel: (01823) 680745
No. of Accessible Units: 1. Shower
No. of Beds per Unit: 6. Lounge has bed settee downstairs, other bedrooms upstairs.
Accessible Facilities: Lounge, Kitchen, Private sitting area overlooking level grassed area. Shared gardens mostly level. Mow Barton is one of four holiday cottages converted in 1993 from an open linhay and stable block. Located in the grounds of a medieval castle built in 1380 that surround the even older fortified manor house.

DREWSTEIGNTON

Standing above Fingle Gorge in the north-east of Dartmoor National Park. Thatched cobhouses surrounded the central square.

SELF-CATERING
CLIFFORD LODGE BARN
Clifford Bridge, Drewsteignton EX6 6QE
Tel: (01647) 24445
No. of Accessible Units: 1. Roll-in Shower
No. of Beds per Unit: 4
Accessible Facilities: Kitchen/Diner. Lift to lounge upstairs. Garden, patio.
Barn conversion situated deep in the heart of Upper Teign Gorge, within Dartmoor National Park, ideal base for exploring South Devon.

EXETER

Cathedral city dating back to Roman times with a wealth of historical interest and displays, combined with a lively shopping centre and the leisurely bank of the River Exe.

BUSES
Dartline Coaches: Tel: (01392) 444343
Various vehicles with all fittings.

Stagecoach Devon: Tel: (01392) 494001

TAXIS
Hookways Greenslades Coaches:
Tel: (01392) 469210
One 40-seater coach with lift and clamps, available countrywide.

Exeter Hackney Carriages:
Tel: (01392) 277770
1 Metrocab with all fittings.

Ross Cabs: Tel: (07971) 169620
Seven-seater Mercedes with all fittings.

Connect 49: Tel: (01392) 491010
One Minibus with lift and ramp.

Freedom Wheels: Tel: (01392) 464206
Serving Exeter and surrounding area. Could be residents only, but worth a call.

TRAINS
First Great Western: Special Needs –
Tel: (0845) 7413775

Virgin Trains: Special Needs –
(0845) 7443366
Minicom: (0845) 7443367

Wales & West: Special Needs —
Tel: (0845) 3003005
Minicom: (0845) 7585469

Exeter St. Davids station is suitable for wheelchairs using ramp access.

SHOPMOBILITY
Deck F, King William Street Car Park,
King William Street, Exeter EX4 6PD
Tel: (01392) 494001

HOTEL
ST. ANDREWS HOTEL 🚶
28 Alphington Road, Exeter EX2 8HN
Tel: (01392) 276784   Fax: (01392) 250249
No. of Accessible Rooms: 1. Bath.
Accessible Facilities: Lounge, Restaurant.
Converted from a large Victorian house, this long-established family-run hotel is bright and spacious and located near the city centre.

ATTRACTION
KILLERON HOUSE AND GARDEN (NT)
Broadclyst, Nr. Exeter EX5 3LE
Tel: (01392) 881345   Fax: (01392) 883112
Rebuilt in 1778 as a comfortable family house, home to Paulise de Bush costume collection. Exhibition in stable courtyard, plus hillside garden. Volunteer-driven motorised buggies available. Wheelchairs also available.

SD ♿   CP ♿   E ♿   RF 🚶
L ♿ Stairclimber   C 🚶
S ♿ wheelchair lift to upper level   WC 🚶
G 🚶

THEATRE
NORTHCOTT THEATRE
Stocker Road, Exeter EX4 6QX
Admin: (01392) 2562182.
Booking-Box Office: (01392) 493493
Fax: (01392) 499641
CP ♿   RE ♿ (Queen's Drive, not Main Entrance)
ED ♿   INT ♿   WC ♿ (sited in upper foyer, next to Queen's Drive entrance)
AUD ♿ (Wheelchair lift, 2 spaces)
B/R ♿ (Queen's Drive entrance)

GREAT TORRINGTON
Home to Dartington Crystal. Great Torrington has an interesting parish church and good views across the river Torridge towards Dartmoor from Castle Hill. The castle is no longer standing.

Royal Horticulturial Society's beautiful Rosemoor Garden.

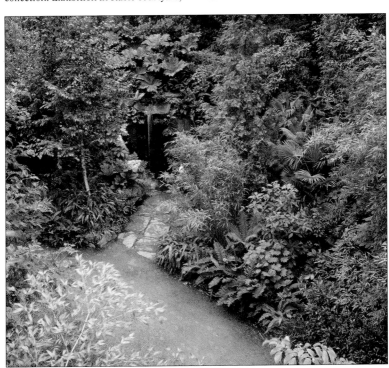

103

ATTRACTION

DARTINGTON CRYSTAL LTD
Linden Close, Torrington EX38 7AN
Tel: (01805) 626262   Fax: (01805) 626263
e-mail: enquiries@dartington.co.uk
web: www.dartington.co.uk
Home to the famous glass, the factory is viewed from inaccessible overhead galleries, but the Visitor Centre has an exhibition on the story of glass, demonstrations of engraving lampwork and studio glass-making.

ROYAL HORTICULTURAL SOCIETY ROSEMOOR GARDEN

Great Torrington EX38 8PH
Tel: (01805) 624067   Fax: (01805) 624717
40-acre site with mature planting in Lady Anne Berry's Garden and arboretum and a recent formal garden by a winding rock gorge planted with ferns and bamboos, together with herb, cottage, foliage, winter and fruit and vegetable gardens.

ILFRACOMBE

Holiday and retirement resort, with many public gardens.

TOURIST INFORMATION CENTRE

The Landmark Sea Front,
Ilfracombe EX34 9BX
Tel: (01271) 863001   Fax: (01271) 862586

BED AND BREAKFAST

SUNNYMEADE COUNTRY HOTEL
Dean Cross, West Down, Ilfracombe EX34 8NT
Tel: (01271) 863668
e-mail: Sunnymeade@btinternet.com
No. of Accessible Rooms: 2. Shower.
Accessible Facilities: Lounge, Dining room.
Charming small hotel surrounded by rolling green hills, in a fine location among North Devon's lovely scenery and wildlife.

IVYBRIDGE

Gateway to Dartmoor and good for exploring Erme Valley and Erme Plym trail to Plymouth.

TOURIST INFORMATION CENTRE

Leonards Road, Ivybridge PL21 0SL
e-mail: ivybridge@south-hams-dc.gov.uk

SELF-CATERING

VENN FARM
Ugborough, Ivybridge PL21 0PE
Tel: (01364) 73240
Total No. of Accessible Units: 2. Roll-in Shower. No. of Beds per Unit: 8 + 4.
Facilities: Lounge in one unit, Dining room. The Granary and Hams barns are built of lovely yellowstone and overlook unspoilt countryside.

NEWTON ABBOT

Purposeful, busy and unpretentious town surrounded by beautiful villages.

BED AND BREAKFAST

NEW COTT FARM
Poundsgate, Newton Abbot TQ13 7PD
Tel/Fax: (01364) 631421
No. of Accessible Rooms: 4. Bath
Accessible Facilities: Conservatory, Dining room. 130-acre sheep farm set in Dartmoor National Park with lovely views and a good base for exploring the Devon countryside. The farm bungalow with accessible rooms is situated in a large garden just away from the farmyard. Dinner is also available.

SELF-CATERING

WOODER MANOR
Widecombe-in-the-Moor,
Newton Abbot TQ13 7TR
Tel/Fax: (01364) 621391
No. of Accessible Units: 2
No. of Beds per Unit: 2-4. Chinkwell-bath: Hameldown roll-in shower.
Accessible Facilities: Lounge/kitchen/diner. Large shared garden. Lower Chinkwell and Lower Hameldown are two of six cottages on working family farm of 150 acres in a picturesque valley in Dartmoor National Park. Surrounded by unspoilt woodland, moors and granite tors. Widecombe village

is 0.5miles along a quiet, level country lane. The famous Widecombe Fair, dating back to about 1850, still takes place annually on the second Tuesday in September.

ATTRACTION
HEDGEHOG HOSPITAL AND FARM
Prickly Ball Farm, Denbury Road,
Newton Abbot TQ12 6BZ
Tel/Fax: (01626) 362319
e-mail: hedgehog@hedgehog.org.uk

A busy hands-on farm that also has a hedgehog hospital, treating and returning them to the wild. See, touch and learn about them. This is a small farm with undercover areas, but grassed areas are inevitably bumpy. Advice from local Access Team implemented. Wheelchair for hire.

SD	♿	CP	♿	E	♿	RF	🚹
C	♿	S	🚹	WC	🚹	RFE	🚹

SPORTING VENUE
NEWTON ABBOT RACECOURSE
Newton Abbot TQ12 3AF
Admin and Booking-Box Office:
(01626) 353235   Fax: (01626) 336972

CP	♿	RE	♿	ED	♿ (except Manual Door)
INT	🚹	L	♿	WC	🚹	SS	♿
B/R	♿ (Lift access)				

OKEHAMPTON
Market town on northern boundary of Dartmoor that prospered during the wool period of the 18th and 19th centuries.

BED AND BREAKFAST
WEEK FARM 🚹
Bridestowe, Okehampton EX20 4HZ
Tel: (01837) 861221

No. of Accessible Rooms: 1
Accessible Facilities: Lounge, Dining room. C17th farmhouse surrounded by wonderful scenery, where three generations of the same family have welcomed guests. Close to several local events and attractions.

SELF-CATERING
ANGLERS UTOPIA PARADISE HOLIDAYS ♿
The Gables, Winsford, Halwill Junction,
Beaworthy EX21 5XT
Tel/Fax: (01409) 221559

No. of Accessible Units: 3. Bath.

No. of Beds per Unit: 3.
Anglers Big Wheel – 4-bedroomed villa.
Anglers Access – 2-bedroomed villa.
Anglers Freedom – 2-bedroomed villa
Accessible Facilities: Fishing. Family run venture of 12 lakes on a 70-acre estate. Pagoda shelters available on most lakes and purpose-built pathways to most lakes. Suitable for non-anglers also, with the peace and quiet of the countryside.

BLAGDON FARM COUNTRY HOLIDAYS ♿
Ashwater, Beaworthy, Nr.
Okehampton EX21 5DR
Tel: (01409) 211509   Fax: (01409) 211510
e-mail: Blagfarm@netcom.co.uk

No. of Accessible Units: 8. Roll-in Showers. No. of Beds per Unit: 6 sleep up to 6, 2 sleep up to 4.
Accessible Facilities: Open plan lounge/diner/kitchen, balcony with patio doors. Indoor heated pool with hoist, Hard surfaced nature trails. Delightful small development of quality bungalows built in 1995, designed to be wheelchair-friendly. Situated on the shore of a 2.5-acre game fishing lake in a superb rural setting, close to the ancient port town of Holsworthy and 10 miles from Launceston and the beaches of Bude and Widemouth.

PAIGNTON
The town's fine features include the red sandstone St. John's Church, Oldway Mansion and an outstanding zoo.

ATTRACTION
PAIGNTON ZOO ENVIRONMENTAL PARK
Totnes Road, Paignton TQ4 7EU
Tel: (01803) 697500   Fax: (01803) 523457

One of the country's largest zoos set in 75 acres of gardens where many endangered species are nurtured, including African lions and Sumatran tigers.
NB. BECAUSE OF THE NATURE OF THE ZOO, ONE NURSE/ATTENDANT PER FIVE DISABLED VISITORS IS REQUIRED.
It does require a fair bit of effort to wheel around, but so long as you bear this in mind, the facilities provide a good day out. There is a variety of bird, lions and pandas and of monkeys including orang-utans,

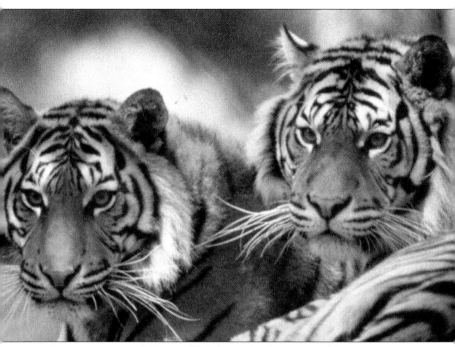

Seen any tasty mortals? Inscrutable Paignton Zoo tigers eye up visitors.

macaques and gorillas, in natural habitats.

SD 🦽   CP 🦽   E 🦽   C 🦽
S 🦽   L 🦽   WC 🚶

Features: Access indoors to monkey and rhino houses, the Ark, restaurant and bar. Orang-utan and nocturnal houses have steps to negotiate. Wheelchairs are available free.

THE PAIGNTON AND DARTMOUTH STEAM RAILWAY
Queens Park Station, Torbay Road, Paignton TQ4 6AF
Tel: (01803) 555872   Fax: (01803) 664313
Steam trains run along the Torbay coast to Churston and on through the Dart estuary to Kingswear. Wonderful scenery throughout.

SD 🦽   CP n/a (Brit. Rail next door)
E 🦽 (special ramp to take wheelchairs onto the train)
RF 🦽   S 🚶   WC 🚶   RFE 🚶

PLYMOUTH
A city of distinct parts: it is well worth while wandering through the modern central area and the Barbican, both offer excellent views, and Plymouth Hoe offers one of the country's great harbour views.

HOTELS
COPTHORNE HOTEL   🦽
Armada Way, Plymouth PL1 1AR
Tel: (01752) 224161   Fax: (01752) 670688
No. of Accessible Rooms: 1. Bath
Accessible Facilities: Lounge, Restaurant.
Located in the city centre.

NEW CONTINENTAL HOTEL   🚶
Millbay Road, Plymouth PL1 3LD
Tel: (01752) 220782   Fax: (01752) 227013
No. of Accessible Rooms: 4
Accessible Facilities: Lounge, Restaurant.
NB: The side door entrance is ramped through the main corridor.
Privately owned Victorian hotel adjacent to the Pavilion Conference and Leisure Centre and the city centre.

NOVOTEL PLYMOUTH   🚶
Marsh Mills, Plymouth PL6 8NH
Tel: (01752) 221422   Fax: (01752) 223922
No. of Accessible Rooms: 2. Bath
Accessible Facilities: Lounge, Restaurant, Pool. Modern hotel situated on the outskirts of the town.

PLYMOUTH MOAT HOUSE
Armada Way, Plymouth PL1 2HJ
Tel: (01752) 639988   Fax: (01752) 673816
No. of Accessible Rooms: 2
Accessible Facilities: All public areas, via a lift. A modern high-rise hotel in a superb location overlooking the Hoe.

BED AND BREAKFAST
OSMOND GUEST HOUSE
42 Pier Street, West Hoe, Plymouth PL1 3BT
Tel: (01752) 229705   Fax: (01752) 269655
No. of Accessible Rooms: 2. Shower
Accessible Facilities: Dining room
three-storey converted Edwardian house situated on Plymouth Hoe close to the sea front and main points of interest.

ATTRACTIONS
PLYMOUTH DOME
The Hoe, Plymouth PL1 2NZ
Tel: (01752) 603300   Fax: (01752) 256361
Hi-tec centre where visitors can explore an Elizabethan street, sail an epic voyage, stroll on an ocean liner, witness the Blitz.

SD 🦽   CP 🦽   E 🚹   RF 🦽   L 🦽
C 🦽   S 🦽   WC 🚹   RFE 🚹

THEATRE
THEATRE ROYAL
Royal Parade, Plymouth PL1 2TR
Admin: Tel: (01752) 668282
Fax: (01752) 262633
Booking-Box Office: (01752) 267222
Minicom: (01752) 600290
Fax: (01752) 252546
Complies with Part M, Building Regulations.

SD 🦽   CP Nearest Public – Civic Centre
Taxi Rank: Royal Parade, outside theatre.
RE 🦽   ED 🦽   IN 🦽   L 🦽
WC 🦽   Drum Foyer   AUD 🚹   B/R 🦽

Route to wheelchair spaces via Door 1, wheelchair lift to stalls foyer and access via Doors 2 and 3 to stalls.

SOUTH MOLTON
Pleasant and lively small town with an attractive, mainly Georgian, square.

TOURIST INFORMATION CENTRE
1 East Street, South Molton EX36 3BU
Tel/Fax: (01769) 574122

SELF-CATERING
HAZEL COTTAGE
Bournebridge House, Meshaw,
Nr. South Molton EX36 4NL
Tel/Fax: (01884) 860134
No. of Accessible Units: 1. Bath.
No. of Beds per Unit: 4
Accessible Facilities: Lounge, Dining room. Formerly a pig sty! Now a pretty cottage, one of three located at the head of a quiet valley in 6.5 acres amid rolling countryside.

TEIGNMOUTH
The promenade and sandy beaches border the town with family entertainment on the sea front and pier. Teignmouth has a busy working port and fishing quay.

HOTEL
CLIFFDEN
Dawlish Road, Teignmouth TQ14 8TE
Tel: (01626) 770052   Fax: (01626) 770594
No. of Accessible Rooms: 4. Bath
Accessible Facilities: Lounge, Restaurant, Pool. This hotel is owned by the Guide Dogs for the Blind Association. It is a listed Victorian building set in formal grounds of over six acres overlooking a small valley forming lovely gardens. These give direct access to East Cliff Beach.

SELF-CATERING
TREVIMIDER
12 Hermosa Road, Teignmouth TQ14 9JZ
Tel: (01626) 775623
No. of Accessible Units: 1
No. of Beds per Unit: 1. Roll-in Shower
Accessible Facilities: Lounge, Kitchenette, south-facing garden. Part of large house, but self-contained and comfortable ground floor flatlet. Located close to the town centre and beaches.

TIVERTON
Prosperous industrial and agricultural town on the River Exe.

TOURIST INFORMATION CENTRE
Phoenix Lane, Tiverton TA1 3PF
Tel: (01884) 255827   Fax: (01884) 257594

HOTEL
TIVERTON HOTEL ♿
Blundells Road, Tiverton EX16 4DB
Tel: (01884) 256120 Fax: (01884) 258101
No. of Accessible Rooms: 2. Bath
Accessible Facilities: Lounge, Restaurant
This is a modern hotel on the edge of
the town.

SELF-CATERING
THE BARN ♿
Huntsham, Tiverton EX16 7NQ
Tel: (01398) 361519
No. of Accessible Units: 1. Bath
No. of Beds per Unit: 5-6 + cot.
Accessible Facilities: Lounge, Dining
room, South facing courtyard with
barbecue. Offers Internet short breaks,
learning to discover the Net. Huntsham is
a conservation hamlet: the barn is a
converted stone barn.

ATTRACTIONS
KNIGHTSHAYES COURT AND GARDENS (NT)
Knightshayes, Tiverton EX16 7RQ
Tel: (01884) 254665 Fax: (01884) 243050
Begun in 1869, the rich interior
combines medieval romanticism with
Victorian dècor, giving rare insight into
elegant countryhouse life. The gardens
are notable for their water lily pool, rare
shrubs and topiary.The ground floor is
very spacious, ideal for wheelchairs. Two
chairs are available on loan, one at the
house and one at reception.

SD ♿ CP 🚶 E 🚶 RF 🚶 L 🚶
C 🚶 S 🚶 WC 🚶 RFE 🚶

TIVERTON CASTLE
Tiverton EX16 6RP
Tel: (01884) 253200 Fax: (01884) 254200
Built in 1106 and dominating the River
Exe, only one original circular Norman
tower remains. Grade 1 listed. Access to
the building's interiors is very limited,
but the inner baillie with walled garden,
that is in the process of rehabilitation, is
well worth a visit.

SD ♿ CPn/a E 🚶 RF 🚶
S 🚶 WC 🚶

TORQUAY
The most glamorous, grandly sited and
well- planned of all west country resorts
with fine beaches and ambitious modern
buildings.

THE ENGLISH RIVIERA TOURIST BOARD
Vaughan Parade, Torquay TQ2 5JG
Tel: (01803) 297428   Fax: (01803) 214885
email: tourist.board@torbay.gov.uk
web: www.torbay.gov.uk/tourism/contents.htm
Produces Information for Disabled People.

BUSES
Stagecoach Devon: Tel: (01803) 613226

TAXIS
Brian Ling: Tel: (01803) 324028
One London cab with all fittings.

Torbay Cab Co: Tel: (01803) 213521
Three vehicles, all with all fittings.
Tel: (01803) 616969
One TX1 with all fittings.

TRAINS
Wales and West: Special Needs –
Tel: (0845) 3003005
Minicom: (0345) 585469

Torquay station is on the flat and taxis
can take wheelchairs right inside the
station.

CAR PARKS
Corporate Services Dept., Civic Offices,
Torquay TQ1 3DS
Tel: (01803) 201201
Free parking for visitors with mobility
allowance (at the higher rate). Major
council car parks have reserved spaces: the
Orange badge is recognised for on-street
parking.

WHEELCHAIR HIRE
Torex Hire Ltd,
95 Newton Road,
Torquay TQ2 7AR
Tel: (01803) 613031

HOTELS
FAIRMOUNT HOUSE HOTEL 🚶
Herbert Road, Chelston, Torquay TQ2 6RW

Tel/Fax: (01803) 605446

No. of Accessible Rooms: 2. Bath
Accessible Facilities: Lounge, Restaurant,
Conservatory Bar. Charming small hotel,
set above Cockington Valley on south
facing hillside. Built in 1900 as a large
family home, there are mature gardens
and patios. Accessible garden level rooms
open out directly onto a paved area above
the main lawn. Accessed by a slightly
circuitous, ramped route through the side
garden. Located close to Cockington
Country Park.

FROGNEL HALL HOTEL

Higher Woodfield Road, Torquay TQ1 2LD
Tel: (01803) 298339   Fax: (01803) 215115

No. of Accessible Rooms: 2. Bath
Facilities: Lounge, Restaurant, Sauna,
Garden. Lovely adapted Victorian mansion
in two acres of peaceful private gardens
with fine views. In a quiet corner of
Torquay, but close to the harbour, sea and
town centre.

SELF-CATERING
THE CORBYN SUITES

Torbay Road, Torquay TQ2 6RH
Tel: (01803) 215595

No. of Accessible Units: 2 (Forbes C.3 and
Wallace C.2)
No. of Beds per Unit: Forbes-2S: Wallace-
1D, 2S
Accessible Facilities: Both have
lounge/diner, kitchen. Quality suites with
classical Georgian proportions situated
within 50m of the beach and a mile from
local shops. Nearby is Torre Abbey
Mansion and Meadows. Close to the
railway station.

1 PARK ROAD

St. Marychurch, Babbacombe, Torquay
Book through Grooms Holidays
No. of Accessible Units: 1. Shower
No. of Beds per Unit: 6
Accessible Facilities: Lounge, Kitchen
This apartment is a short walk from the
pedestrianised shopping area in the
delightful seaside town of Babbacombe,
tucked into a little sandy bay.

WOOLACOMBE

Enjoy a wonderful sand and surf beach,
with the town enclosed by steep moorland
slopes rather than cliffs.

HOTEL
THE CLEEVE HOUSE HOTEL

Mortenhoe, Wollacombe EX34 7ED
Tel/Fax: (01271) 870719

No. of Accessible Rooms: 1. Roll-in Shower.
Accessible Facilities: Lounge, Restaurant.
Mortenhoe is situated in an area of
outstanding natural beauty. This small
privately owned and managed hotel has
most attractive gardens and is two miles
from the beach and 100m from the village.

YELVERTON

This old settlement has ponies wandering
all over its flat common, and the best
inland golf course in Devon.

BED AND BREAKFAST
HEADLAND WARREN FARM

Postbridge, Yelverton PL20 6TB
Tel: (01822) 880206

No. of Accessible Rooms: 2
Accessible Facilities: Kitchen. Lounge/
Diner (on first floor, accessed by stairlift).
One of the few remaining longhouses.
These 600-year-old plus farm buildings
now consist of an original farmhouse, a
converted barn for those with disabilities,
an attached cottage and stables. Remote
but easily located 30 minutes from Exeter
off the B3212. Headland Warren is in its
own 600 acres of National Park moorland
in the middle of the Two Moors Way.

SELF-CATERING
MIDWAY

Book through Leigh Farm, Roborough,
Plymouth PL6 7BS. Tel: (01752) 733221

No. of Accessible Units: 1. Bath
No. of Beds per Unit: 6
Accessible Facilities: Lounge, kitchen,
dining room, conservatory, garden. Large
detached house, recently converted into
two self-contained holiday apartments with
a lovely garden. Situated in quiet crescent
in sleepy village of Crapstone, a mile from
Yelverton and nine from Plymouth.

DORSET

DORCHESTER COALITION OF DISABLED PEOPLE.
Room 1, Poole Advice Centre,
54 Lagland Street, Poole BH15 1QG
Tel: (01202) 668593
Provides information throughout Dorset.

DORSET COUNTY COUNCIL
Colliton Park, Dorset
Tel: (01305) 251000
Minicom: (01305) 267933

WHEELCHAIR HIRE
One-to-One Care, 37 Haven Road,
Canford Cliffs, Poole BH13 7LE
Tel: (01202) 709121
County-wide, but makes relevant charge for delivery.

BEAMINSTER
Set in beautiful countryside of steep hills dividing deep cups of farmland, this is one of the most appealing towns of its size.

SELF-CATERING
RIVERSIDE
Bakers Hill Farm, Mosterton, Beaminster
Bookings through Mrs. Young,
61 Clifton Road, Southampton SO40 7GA
Tel: (01703) 771729
No. of Accessible Units: 1. Shower.
No. of Beds per Unit: 6
Accessible Facilities: Open plan lounge/ kitchen. Bungalow on farm.

BLANDFORD FORUM
Home of sculptor and painter Alfred Stevens, this is the hub of a rich farming area and has a very handsome and uniform Georgian red-brick and stone town centre.

SELF-CATERING
LUCCOMBE
Milton Abbas, Blandford Forum DT11 0BE
Tel: (01258) 880558   Fax: (01258) 881384
No. of Accessible Units: 1.Shower.
No. of Beds per Unit: 4

Accessible Facilities: Lounge, Dining room. Pound Cottage Equestrian Centre specialising in riding for the disabled 0.5 miles from Luccombe. 650-acre dairy/arable working farm close to historic thatched village of Milton Abbas. The converted 150-year-old brick and flint-built barns and stables house a variety of cottage-style units, of which Old Sty has accessible grading 3. The Cakehouse, not graded, is considered accessible also and has two bedrooms.

ATTRACTION
CAVALCADE OF COSTUME MUSEUM
Lime Tree House, The Plocks,
Blandford Forum DT11 7AA
Tel: (01258) 453006   Fax: (01258) 454084
Unique collection of over 500 items exhibiting clothes and accessories from the 1730s to the 1950s. Immediate access to four rooms, one with a ramp 1:5, to access three other rooms. Steward assistance guaranteed, visitors are taken down backwards. Off these three rooms are four steps to another large area, stewards carry wheelchairs.

SD   CP   E   RF
C   S   WC

BOURNEMOUTH
Wide streets, a pier, a pavilion and a theatre. Many parks and gardens scattered close to the town centre. Spectacular views of the Isle of Wight can be seen from the cliffs.

BOURNEMOUTH TOURISM AND TOURIST INFORMATION CENTRE
Westover Road,
Bournemouth, BH1 2BU
Tel: (01202) 451702   Fax: (01202) 451743
TIC: Tel: (01202) 451700

BOURNEMOUTH BOROUGH COUNCIL
Central Office, 9 Madeira Road,
Bournemouth BH1 1QN
Tel: (01202) 458000
Publishers of *Bournemouth Disabled Visitors' Guide*.

BOURNEMOUTH HELPING SERVICES
29A Alma Road, Winton
Bournemouth BH9 1AB
Tel: (01202) 536336

BRITISH RED CROSS (Bournemouth)
52 Portchester Road, Bournemouth BH8 8JY
Tel: (01202) 553433

BUSES
Wilts and Dorset
27 The Triangle, Bournemouth
Tel: (01202) 291288
Some low-floor buses, some raised kerbs.

TAXIS
Central Taxis: Tel: (01202) 394455
One vehicle with all fittings.
United Taxis: Tel: (01202) 556677
Three vehicles with all fittings.
Warren Cars: Tel: (01202) 555511
One minibus with all fittings.

TRAINS
Connex: Customer Services:
Tel: (0870) 6030405
Fax: (0870) 6030505
Minicom: (01233) 617621
South West Trains: Special Needs –
Tel: (0845) 6050440
Minicom: (0845) 6050441
Virgin Trains: Special Needs –
(0845) 7443366
Minicom: (0845) 7443367

Bournemouth Station has a flat entry to both sides, three orange badge spaces (platform 2 entrance), manual entry to ticket office (90cm wide), flexible seating, level access to platforms and sloped subway. Unisex WCs and buffet on platform 2 with flexible seating. Saloon cars and cabs available from the rank by platform 3, card/payphones on each platform (149cm high), no lifts, wheelchair ramps plus three wheelchairs.

CAR PARKS
Orange badge scheme operates in borough council car parks and some others.
Tel: (01202) 451365/451200

SHOPMOBILITY
Sovereign Centre Car Park, Boscombe, Bournemouth
Tel: (01202) 399700

HOTEL
CARRINGTON HOUSE HOTEL ♿
Knyveton Road, Bournemouth BH1 3QQ
Tel: (01202) 369988 Fax: (01202) 292221
No. of Accessible Rooms: 1
Accessible Facilities: Restaurant (lift access), lounge.
Set in quiet residential area with good children's facilities.

THE CONNAUGHT HOTEL ♿
West Hill Road, Bournemouth BH2 5PH
Tel: (01202) 298020 Fax: (01202) 298028
No. of Accessible Rooms: 4. Roll-in Shower.
Accessible Facilities: Lounge, Restaurant, Conservatory Bar, Pool, Sauna, Whirlpool, Gymnasium, Snooker Room.
Delightful hotel with a wide variety of leisure facilities located 200 metres from the town centre and the beach.

ATTRACTIONS
RUSSELL-COTES ART GALLERY AND MUSEUM
East Cliff, Bournemouth, BH1 3AA
Tel: (01202) 451800 Fax: (01202) 451851
Noted for its collection of Victorian and Edwardian paintings, plus sculpture, decorative art and furniture and modern art, all housed in East Cliff Hall, built in 1897. Catering and Shop accessed through Garden entrance.

SD ♿ CP ♿ E ♿ C ♿ S ♿
WC ♿ L ♿

BRIDPORT
Georgian houses and a handsome arcaded town hall are of interest here.

SELF-CATERING
SHEPHERDS COTTAGE ♿
Rudge Farm, Chilcombe, Bridport DT6 4NF
Tel: (01308) 482630 Fax: (01308) 482635
e-mail: sue@rudge-farm.co.uk
No. of Accessible Units: 1. Bath
No. of Beds per Unit: 4
Accessible Facilities: Lounge/Diner, Kitchen. Converted old farm buildings, retaining many original features ranged round a flower decked, cobbled yard overlooking the lakes in the paddock below. The village is about five miles from

Bridport. A good base for exploring West
Dorset, and designated as an Area of
Outstanding Natural Beauty.

CONWAY HOUSE
Bettiscombe, Bridport DT6 5NT
Tel/Fax: (01308) 868313
e-mail: conway@wdi.co.uk
No. of Accessible Units: 1. Roll-in Shower
No. of Beds per Unit: 4-6
Accessible Facilities: Lounge/Dining room
combined. Bungalow with lovely views.

CHARMOUTH
Jane Austen found Charmouth a nice place
for "sitting in unwearied contemplation".
Its hillside street is still lined with thatched
houses and some Regency bow windows.
The town is in one of the few gaps in the
hills that break into the cliffs overlooking
the sweep of Lyme Bay. Beautiful beach.

SELF-CATERING
THE POPLARS
Woodfarm Caravan Park, Axminster Road,
Charmouth DT6 6BT
Tel/Fax: (01297) 560697
e-mail: 1.pointing@zetnet.co.uk
No. of Accessible Units: 1. Roll-in Shower
No. of Beds per Unit: 4 + cot
Accessible Facilities: Lounge, kitchen/diner.
Self-catering flat within camping and
caravan park nestling in Char Valley with
views over Lyme Bay. Close to the Heritage
Coast and lovely villages.

DORCHESTER
Made famous by the novels of Thomas
Hardy, today Dorchester is a livestock
marketing and farmers' shopping centre with
a large brewery and other light industries.

TOURIST INFORMATION CENTRE
Unit 11, Antelope Walk, Dorchester DT1 1BE
Tel: (01305) 267992   Fax: (01305) 266079.
Publishes "West Dorset for visitors with
special needs". Includes Bridport, West Bay,
Beaminster, Lyme Regis and Sherborne.

DORCHESTER TOWN COUNCIL
North Square, Dorchester. Tel: (01305) 266861

BUSES
First Southern National: Tel: (01305) 783645
Some low-floor, easy-access buses.
Wilts and Dorset: Tel: (01202) 673555
Some low-floor, easy-access buses.

TAXIS
Access Taxis: Tel: (01305) 768190
Two vehicles with all fittings.
Coach House Travel: Tel: (01305) 267644
Four 57-seater vehicles with all fittings.
Transport Business Unit: Tel: (01305) 224899
67 vehicles of various sizes with all fittings.

TRAINS
South West Trains: Special Needs –
Tel: (0845) 6050440
Minicom: (0845) 6050441
Wales and West: Special Needs –
Tel: (0845) 3003005
Minicom: (0845) 7585469
Dorchester South Station. Tel: (01305) 264423.
Two orange badge spaces, ramp from street
to ticket office, wide manual door, ramp to
up platform, level to down platform. Disabled
ladies WC, saloon cars available at rank, card/
pay telephone, 149cm high, ramp available.
Dorchester West. Unmanned. Level access
to platform 1, to platform 2 via footbridge.
Alternative access from Damers Road via
wide steps and partly unmade path. No WCs.

CAR PARKING
Orange badge spaces available free for first
three hours. Car parks located in Dorchester
Town Information Leaflet from TIC.

SELF-CATERING
THE BARN AT BAGLAKE FARM
Litton Cheney, Dorchester DT2 9AD
Tel: (01308) 482222   Fax: (01308) 482226
No. of Accessible Units: 1. Bath.
No. of Beds per Unit: 3
Accessible Facilities: Lounge, dining room.
Little Cheney is along the Bride Valley, eight
miles from Dorchester and within three of the
sea and Chesil Beach. The Barn is one third
of a thatched barn converted into a cottage.

LOWER BURTON FARMHOUSE
Dorchester, Dorset DT2 7RZ
Tel/Fax: (01305) 250685
No. of Accessible Units: 1. Shower.

No. of Beds per Unit: 5. Accessible Facilities: Large living room, kitchen, garden. Ground floor wing of family farmhouse deep in Hardy country with large garden.

ATTRACTIONS
ATHELHAMPTON HOUSE AND GARDENS
Dorchester DT2 7LG
Tel: (01305) 858363   Fax: (01305) 848135
15th century house with many finely furnished rooms. Gardens contain the famous topiary pyramids, fountains, the River Piddle and fine flowering collections. Six ground floor rooms are accessible.

| SD ♿ | CP ♿ | E ♿ | RF ♿ | C ♿ |
| S ♿ | WC ♿ | RFE ♿ | | |

THE KEEP MILITARY MUSEUM
The Keep, Bridport Road, Dorchester DT1 1RN
Tel: (01305) 264060   Fax: (01305) 250373
The Keep is a Grade 11 listed building, gateway to the former barracks of the Dorsetshire Regiment in the 1870s. Many original features, including the cells, are retained. The regiment's story is told using touchscreen computers and a variety of creative displays from 1685 to the present.

| SD ♿ | CP ♿ | E ♿ | RF ♿ |
| L ♿ | S ♿ | WC ♿ | RFE ♿ |

GILLINGHAM
Set in the Blackmore Vale close by the River Stour.

SELF-CATERING
TOP STALL   ♿
Factory Farm, Fifehead Magdalen, Gillingham SP8 5RS
Tel/Fax: (01258) 820022
No. of Accessible Units: 1. Roll-in Shower
No. of Beds per Unit: 5
Accessible Facilities: Lounge, Dining room, Fishing from River Stour. Single storey cow stall conversion adjoining the farmhouse, a listed C18th former woollen and stocking factory, hence the name. Situated off the road with a garden enclosed by a stone wall, the village shops and inns of Marnhull are a mile away and

Shaftesbury six.

POOLE
Tremendous natural harbour with much of its shoreline still undeveloped. Famous for its Poole Pottery.

TOURIST INFORMATION CENTRE
The Quay, Poole BH15 1HE
Tel: (01202) 253253   Fax: (01202) 684531

HOTEL
THISTLE POOLE   ♿
The Quay, Poole BH15 1HD
Tel: (01202) 666800   Fax: (01202) 684470
No. of Accessible Rooms: 1.
Accessible Facilities: Lounge, restaurant (1st floor). Modern hotel close to Old Poole town overlooking the lovely natural harbour.

SELF-CATERING
ROCKLEY PARK
Poole.
Book through Grooms Holidays
No. of Accessible Units: 1. Roll-in Shower
No. of Beds per Unit: 6
Wooden forest-style chalet with views of Poole's natural harbour close by.

SANDFORD PARK
Holton Heath, Poole
Book through Grooms Holidays
No. of Accessible Units: 1
No. of Beds per Unit: 6
Luxury pinelog cabin set among woodland in Sandford Park.

ATTRACTION
COMPTON ACRES GARDENS
Canford Cliffs, Poole, Dorset BH13 7ES
Tel: (01202) 700778   Fax: (01202) 707537
e-mail: info@comptonacres.co.uk
Gardens of 9.5 acres with Japanese, Roman, Italian, water, rock and heather gardens, plus superb bronze and marble statuary.

| SD ♿ | CP ♿ | E ♿ | RF ♿ | C- ♿ |
| S ♿ | (ramped at 1:11) | WC ♿ | RFE-Garden ♿ | |

FARMER PALMER'S FARM PARK LTD
Organford, Poole

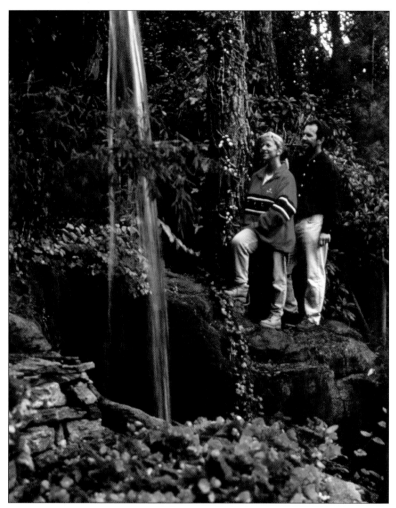

Lost in the beauty of Compton Acres gardens.

Tel: (01202) 622022 Fax: (01202) 632111
e-mail: farmerpalmers@bigfoot.co.uk
web:
www.dorsetweb.co.uk/leisure/farmerpalmers
The farm park operates alongside a 200-acre
working dairy farm. The park overlooks
lovely open grass fields and forest with a
wide woodland walk by the river. Trained
staff demonstrate handling and feeding of a
wide range of animals including goats,
pigs, lambs. Whatever the weather there
are undercover barns full of activities and
milk demonstration.

SD   CP   E   RF   C
S   WC   RFE

WATERFRONT MUSEUM
4 High Street, Poole BH15 1BW
Tel: (01202) 683138 Fax: (01202) 660896
e-mail: c.fisher@poole.gov.uk
2,000 years of history displayed in C18th
warehouse and adjoining medieval town
cellars (latter not accessible). Original
artefacts and reconstructions.

SD   CP n/a   E   RF   L
WC   RFE

SHAFTESBURY
Dorset's only hill-top town, to which King
Alfred gave a nunnery C880 and an Anglo-
Saxon town grew around it. The ancient,

wide, curved and cobbled Gold Hill is probably the most photographed street in Dorset, although the cobbles sadly prevent comfortable access to those in wheelchairs.

TOURIST INFORMATION CENTRE
8 Bell Street, Shaftesbury SP7 8AE
Tel: (01747) 853514   Fax: (01747) 850593
e-mail: tourism@ruraldorset.com
web: www.ruraldorset.com

HOTEL
THE COPPLERIDGE INN   [人]
Motcombe, Shaftesbury SP7 9HW
Tel: (01747) 851980   Fax: (01747) 851858
e-mail: thecoppleridgeinn@btinternet.com
No. of Accessible Bedrooms: All (10). Bath
Accessible Facilities: Lounge, Restaurant.
Converted C18th farmhouse set in 15 acres of meadow, woodland and gardens overlooking Blackmore Vale. The courtyard farm buildings have been converted into 10 bedrooms. Motcombe is two miles from Shaftesbury.

SELF-CATERING
HARTGROVE FARM COTTAGES   [&] [&] [人]
Hartgrove, Shaftesbury SP7 0JY
Tel: (01747) 811830
No. of Accessible Units: 3. Bath
No. of Beds per Unit: Each cottage sleeps 4, plus cot.
Bulbarrow Cottage   [&]
(Daily Mail Top 20 Holiday Cottages)
Melbury Cottage   [&]
(winner of Holiday Care Award)
Duncliffe Cottage   [人]
Accessible Facilities: All three have wood-burning stove and small private gardens. Arrangements with nearby leisure centre for swimming, hoist access. Much of the farmyard can be accessed in a wheelchair. Outstanding family dairy farm straddling a small hill between Cranborne Chase and Blackmore Vales 1.5 miles from thatched village of Fontwell Magna. Farm buildings now converted into character cottages.

ATTRACTION
SHAFTESBURY ABBEY
Park Walk, Shaftesbury SP7 8JR
Tel: (01747) 852910

Founded by King Alfred, the abbey became a centre of pilgrimage in medieval times as King Edward the Martyr was buried here in 981AD. He kept good company – King Canute died in the abbey. It survived until the dissolution of the monasteries and the excavated remains, open during the summer, are the subject of interesting museum and garden audio-tours.

SD [&]   CP [&]   E [&]   RF [人]
S [&]   WC [人]

SHERBORNE
Yellowstone town with a wealth of medieval buildings and fine Abbey Church of 705.

TOURIST INFORMATION CENTRE
3 Tilton Court, Diby Road, Sherborne DT9 3NL
Tel: (01935) 815341

ATTRACTION
WORLDLIFE and LULLINGSTONE SILK FARM
Compton House, Sherborne, Dorset DT9 4QN
Tel: (01935) 410706   Fax: (01935) 429957
Elizabethan manor house, accessible except for Silk Farm on first floor. Worldlife has evolved from Worldwide Butterflies, with displays on wildlife and environment. Butterflies fly free in a reconstruction of their natural habitat, including jungle and tropical palmhouse. Collection built up over 30 years with active breeding and hatching areas on view.

SD [&]   CP n/a   E [&]   RF [&]   C [&]
S [&]   WC [人]

SWANAGE
Cosy resort on a marvellous bay of yellow sands and white cliffs, flanked by downs grand for both walking and great views.

TOURIST INFORMATION CENTRE
The White House, Shore Road,
Swanage BH19 1LB
Tel: (01929) 422885   Fax: (01929) 423423

ATTRACTION
PUTLAKE ADVENTURE FARM
Langton Matravers, Swanage BH19 3EU
Tel: (01929) 422917
Over 50 breeds of cows, horses, pigs, goats,

etc that can be touched and a farm implement collection. A delightful attraction.

SD ♿ CP ♿ E ♿ RF 🚶 C ♿
S ♿ WC 🚶

WAREHAM

Attractive small town situated on a low ridge between the rivers Frome and Piddle. A shopping centre with friendly pubs and some light industry.

TOURIST INFORMATION CENTRE
Trinity Church, South Street,
Wareham BH20 4LU
Tel: (01929) 552740   Fax: (01929) 554491

HOTEL
KEMPS COUNTRY HOTEL   🚶
East Stoke, Nr. Wareham BH20 6AL
Tel: (01929) 462563   Fax: (01929) 405287
No. of Accessible Rooms: 6. Bath.
Accessible Facilities: Lounge, Restaurant.
Victorian rectory in its own grounds facing the Purbeck Hills.

BED AND BREAKFAST
THE OLD GRANARY   🚶
West Holme Farm, Wareham BH20 6AQ
Tel: (01929) 552972   Fax: (01929) 551616
web: www.rural-dorset.org.uk
No. of Accessible Rooms: 1. Roll-in Shower.
Facilities: Lounge, Dining room. Charming, recently converted old granary with PYO fruit, plant nursery and farm shop adjacent.

ATTRACTIONS
THE BLUE POOL
Furzebrook, Nr. Wareham BH20 5AT
Tel: (01929 551408)
Features include a designated wheelchair route, the surface varies in both width and surface with some gentle inclines and declines. Allow 45 minutes to get around, but there are numerous vantage points to view the pool without having to complete whole route.
The pool is surrounded by 25 acres of heather, gorse and pine trees, interlaced with sandy paths climbing to views of the Purbeck Hills. Originally a clay pit, in warmer weather the clay particles settle, resulting in the pool showing more green

shades: in cold weather the particles rise to the surface, making the pool look more blue than green. The museum traces the Furzebrook Estate industry from making tobacco pipes to pottery.

SD ♿ CP 🚶 E ♿ RF ♿ C ♿
S 🚶 WC ♿

THE HERITAGE CENTRE
West Lulworth, Wareham BH20 5RQ
Tel/Fax: (01929) 400587
Video and displays on Lulworth's history from prehistoric times to the present day.
SD n/a   CP 🚶 E 🚶 RF ♿ S ♿
WC 🚶 RFE 🚶

WEYMOUTH

Pleasant sea-front, with long, tall, late Georgian terraces backing the wide esplanade and sandy beach.

TOURIST INFORMATION CENTRE
The King's Statue, The Esplanade,
Weymouth DT4 7AN
Tel: (01305) 785747
e-mail: tourism@weymouth.gov.uk
web: www.weymouth.gov.uk

HOTEL
HOTEL CENTRAL   🚶
15-17 Maiden Street, Weymouth DT4 8BB
Tel: (01305) 760700   Fax: (01305) 760300
No. of Accessible Rooms: 3. Bath.
Accessible Facilities: Lounge, Restaurant, Lift. Located in town centre, very close to the beach with ferry terminal and Pavilion Theatre nearby.

ATTRACTIONS
ABBOTSBURY SWANNERY
New Barn Road, Abbotsbury,
Weymouth DY3 4SG
Tel: (01308)871858   Fax: (01308) 871092
Voted best family attraction in Dorset 1999. For over 600 years this colony of friendly mute swans has made its home here, Sheltered by Chesil Beach, this ancient site provides protection for many nesting swans and their broods. From the end of May you can wander around the nests safely to see the fluffy cygnets. An AV show about the

Swannery runs hourly. A must!

SD ♿ CP ♿ E ♿ RF ♿ C ♿ S ♿
WC ♿ (3 WCs. All Cat.1 -main toilet block between main car park and ticket-office/shop: Restaurant: inside Swannery).

DEEP SEA ADVENTURE
9 Custom House Quay, Old Harbour,
Weymouth DT4 8BG
Tel/Fax: (01305) 760690

Experience the Titanic Exhibition and encounter underwater exploration and maritime exploits both past and present.

SD ♿ CP 🚶 E 🚶 RF 🚶 L ♿
C ♿ S 🚶 WC 🚶 RFE ♿

WEYMOUTH SEA LIFE PARK
Lodmoor Country Park, Lodmoor,
Weymouth DT4 7SX
Tel: (01305) 761070   Fax: (01305) 760165

Spectacular marine displays, plus tropical jungle, blue whale splashpool and 3-D shark academy.

CP- council owned E ♿ RF ♿ C ♿
S ♿ WC 🚶 RFE ♿

WIMBORNE MINSTER
Centred on its distinctive church, dating from 1043, this small town is almost like a miniature cathedral city.

Time out at Knoll Gardens and nursery.

TOURIST INFORMATION CENTRE
29 High Street,
Wimborne Minster BN21 1HR
Tel: (01202) 886116   Fax: (01202) 841025

ATTRACTIONS
DORSET HEAVY HORSE CENTRE
Brambles Farm, Gottam Edmondsham,
Wimborne BH21 5RJ
Tel: (01202) 824040   Fax: (01202) 821402
e-mail: dhhc@btinternet.co.uk

Many different breeds of heavy horse and miniature and Shetland ponies are on show here. There is an interesting information centre and a good display of farm implements.

SD ♿ CP 🚶 E ♿ RF ♿ C 🚶
S 🚶 WC 🚶 RFE ♿

KNOLL GARDENS AND NURSERY
Hampreston,
Nr. Wimborne BH21 7ND
Tel: (01202) 873931   Fax: (01202) 870842

Six acres of compact and mostly level gardens with herbaceous borders and water gardens. The nursery has a concrete floor with raised beds and is mostly accessible. The garden is flat and partly inclined, care is required because surfaces, widths and gradients do vary.

SD ♿ CP 🚶 E 🚶 RF ♿ C 🚶
S ♿ WC 🚶 RFE 🚶

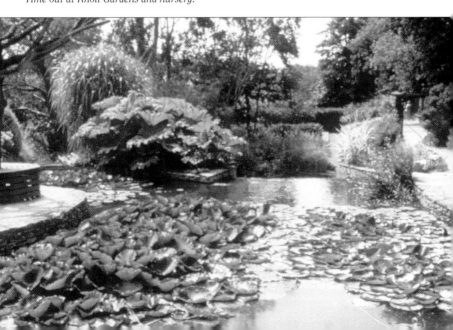

ESSEX

ESSEX TOURISM
Essex County Council, County Hall,
Chelmsford CM1 1LX
Tel: (01245) 437547   Fax: (01245) 355032
e-mail: tourism@essexcc.gov.uk
web: www.essexxx.gov.uk/tourism

ESSEX DISABLED PEOPLE'S ASSOCIATION
90 Broomfield Road, Chelmsford CM1 1SS
Tel: (01245) 253400   Fax: (01245) 346730
Minicom: (01245) 287177
e-mail: edpa@adpass.org
web: www.edpass.org   www.edpass.org

ESSEX COUNTRY TRANSPORT ENQUIRIES
Tel: (01245) 437707

BILLERICAY

Here in Mayflower Hall, some of the
Pilgrim Fathers met before setting sail for
America in 1620. The town also has its
place in history as the scene where
remaining participants in the Peasants
Revolt took refuge in Norsey Wood in
1381.

ATTRACTION
BARLEYLANDS FARM
Barleylands Road, Billericay CM11 2UD
Tel: (01268) 532253   Fax: (01268) 532032
e-mail: barleyfarm@aol.com
Farm museum depicting rural life in the past
with an animal centre, a glass-blowing studio
with a viewing gallery, and craft studios.

SD 🦽   CP 🦽   E 🦽   RF 🦽   C 🦽
S 🦽   WC 🦽

BRAINTREE

Pleasant town with several historical
buildings, shops and entertainment.

TOURIST INFORMATION CENTRE
Braintree Town Hall Centre, Market Place,
Braintree CM7 3YG
Tel: (01376) 557766

ATTRACTIONS

CRESSING TEMPLE
Witham Road, Cressing, Nr. Braintree
Tel: (01376) 584903 Fax: (01376) 584864
An ancient moated farmstead with two fine
mediaeval timbered barns built for the
Knights Templar, and a C16th walled garden.

SD 🦽   CP 🦽   E 🦽   RF 🦽   C 🦽
S 🦽   WC 🚶   RFE 🦽

THE WORKING SILK MUSEUM
New Mills, South Street, Braintree CM7 3GB
Tel: (01376) 553393   Fax: (01376) 330642
Web:www.humphriesweaving.co.uk
Fabric is woven on 150-year-old handlooms
for the National Trust, royal palaces, etc.
This is the last company of handloom silk
weavers. See the process from raw silk to
woven fabric.

SD 🦽   CP 🦽   E 🦽   RF 🚶   S 🦽
WC 🚶   RFE 🚶

CASTLE HEDINGHAM

Built on a hill overlooking the River Colne
is the great castle that has given the village
its name. Constructed by the de Vere
family c1140.

ATTRACTION
COLNE VALLEY RAILWAY
Yeldham Road, Castle Hedingham CO9 3DZ
Tel: (01718) 461174
Award-winning station for a pleasant ride
on a section of the railway of the former
Colne Valley line. Incorporating a large
collection of heritage railway rolling stock,
steam and diesel locomotives.

SD 🦽   CP 🦽   E 🦽   RF 🦽   C-n/a
S 🚶   WC 🚶   RFE 🦽

CHELMSFORD

The county town of Essex is large and well-
developed with a shopping complex and
fine sporting facilities.

TOURIST INFORMATION CENTRE
County Hall, Market Road,
Chelmsford CM1 1GG
Tel: (01245) 283400   Fax: (01245) 430705

ATTRACTION
CHELMSFORD AND ESSEX MUSEUM

Oaklands Park, Moulsham Street,
Chelmsford CM2 9AQ
Tel: (01245) 353066   Fax: (01245) 280642
Wide range of artefacts of the town's
history plus geological displays.

SD [♿]   CP [♿]   E [♿]   RF [🚶]   S [🚶]
WC [♿]   RFE [♿]

MOULSHAM MILL
Parkway, Chelmsford CM2 7PX
Tel: (01245) 608200   Fax: (01245) 608310
This a charming mill house the ground
floor of which has been converted into a
place for crafts of all kinds including lace
making, and sales of pottery, wooden
crafts etc. It is managed by Interact, the
charity that helps those with learning
difficulties back into the workplace.

SD [♿]   CP [♿] (slight incline down to entrance,
spaces should be symbolised in near future)
E [♿]   C [🚶]   S [♿]
WC [🚶] (fully accessible projected).

CHIGWELL
HOTEL
JUBILEE LODGE (Winged Fellowship)
Grange Farm, High Road,
Chigwell IG7 6DP
Tel: (020) 8501 2331
On the edge of Epping Forest with lawns
and gardens galore. All rooms have en
suite facilities and hoist tracking, with
variable height beds. 24-hour nursing.
Bar, conservatory, shop, and coffee lounge.
Adaptive transport.

CHINGFORD
ATTRACTION
QUEEN ELIZABETH'S HUNTING LODGE
Ranger's Road, Epping Forest, Chingford
London E4 7QH
Tel: (020) 8529 6681
Timber-framed hunting grandstand built
for Henry V111. Exceptional carpentry set
in Epping Forest with ancient oaks and
fine views. Wide and shallow staircase with
a stair walker. One staff member has been
trained in its use so call ahead.

SD [♿]   CP [♿]   E [♿]   RF [♿]   C [♿]
S [♿]   WC [🚶]   RFE [♿]

CLACTON-ON-SEA
A popular holiday resort with a pier, every
possible holiday amenity and form of
entertainment, and a giant scenic railway a
striking feature.

TOURIST INFORMATION CENTRE
23 Pier Avenue, Clacton-on-Sea CO15 1QD
Tel: (01255) 423400   Fax: (01255) 430906

HOTEL
HERTFORD HOUSE HOTEL   [♿]
11 Park Way, Clacton-on-Sea CO15 1BJ
Tel/Fax: (01255) 475994
No. of Accessible Rooms: All (13)
Accessible Facilities: Lounge, bining room,
bar, beach hut on sea front. Purpose-built
hotel for those with disabilities.

SELF-CATERING
GROOMSHILL
8 Holland Road, Clacton on Sea
Book through Grooms Holidays
No. of Accessible Units: 1. Roll-in Shower
No. of Beds per Unit: 7 Accessible
Facilities:
Comfortable bungalow tucked away on a
peaceful residential street with a secluded
garden. Close to local shops.

COLCHESTER
Britain's oldest recorded town was the first
capital of Roman Britain. A familiar sight
is undoubtedly Bourne Mill, built in 1591
and made famous in a number of paintings
by John Constable.

TOURIST INFORMATION CENTRE
1 Queen Street, Colchester CO1 2PG
Tel: (01206) 282920

BUSES
Some low-floor buses.
Tel: (01206) 769778

TAXIS
A1 Taxis: Tel: (01206) 544744
One adapted vehicle.

Colchester Airport Services:
Tel: (01206) 729927
One adapted vehicle for airport services.

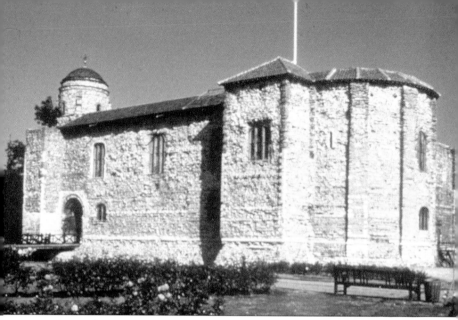

Norman doesn't come any bigger than this keep at Colchester Castle.

Five One Taxis: Tel: (01206) 515151
Five adapted vehicles.

TRAINS

Anglia Railways: Assistance:
Tel: (01473) 693333
Minicom: (01603) 630748 or
(0845) 6050600
Central Trains: Assistance:
Tel: (0845) 7056027
web: www.centraltrains.co.uk
First Great Eastern: Special Needs —
Tel: (0845) 9505050
Mincom: (0845) 9606099
Colchester station is manned most of time,
although there is not 24-hour cover.

CAR PARKS

Three-hour free orange badge spaces in
council-run car parks, some off-street parking.
Tel: (01206) 282222

SHOPMOBILITY

15 Queen Street,
Colchester CO1 2PH
Tel: (01206) 505256   Fax: (01206) 572570

HOTEL

FORTE POSTHOUSE COLCHESTER
Abbotts Lane, Eight Ash Green,

Colchester CO6 3QL
Tel: (01206) 767740   Fax: (01206) 766577
No. of Accessible Rooms: 1
Accessible Facilities: Lounge, restaurant
Located three miles from Colchester.

ATTRACTIONS

ABBERTON RESERVOIR NATURE RESERVE
Church Road, Layer-de-la-Haye, Colchester
Tel: (01206) 738172   Fax: (01206) 738292
Essex Wildlife Trust run this conservation
centre for wild duck, swans and other
water birds.

SD 🚹 | CP 🚹 | E 🚹 | RF 🚹 | S 🚹
WC 🚹 | RFE 🚹

BRIDGE COTTAGE (NT)
Flatford, East Bergholt, Colchester CO7 6OL
Tel: (01206) 298260   Fax: (01206) 299193
C16th cottage near Flatford Mill with John
Constable exhibition, famous for paintings of
this property and surrounding area. Flatford
Mill is not accessible to the general public.

SD 🚹 | CP 🚹 | E 🚹 | RF 🚹 | C 🚹
S 🚹 | WC 🚹 | RFE 🚹

CASTLE MUSEUM
Castle Park, Colchester CO1 1JJ
Tel: (01206) 282931   Fax: (01206) 282925
This is the largest surviving Norman keep
in Europe. It includes Roman displays,

hands-on activities and medieval and prison displays. Discover why Colchester was chosen to be the first capital of Roman Britain.

SD ♿ | CP n/a | E ♿ | RF ♿ | L- ♿
C 🚶 | S ♿ | WC 🚶 | RFE ♿

COLCHESTER LEISURE WORLD
Cowdray Avenue, Colchester CO1 1YH
Tel: (01206) 282000   Fax: (01206) 282024

Contains leisure, fitness and teaching pools, the latter two reached via a lift to the upper floor. The fitness pool has a hoist and a shower chair. In the leisure pool a carry chair is used to access the main area of the pool, apart from the flume area that is not accessible.
DISABILITY SPORT CO-ORDINATOR

CP ♿ | E ♿ | RF ♿ | L ♿ | C ♿ | WC ♿

COLCHESTER ZOO
Maldon Road, Stanway, Colchester CO3 5SL
Tel: (01206) 331292   Fax: (01206) 331392
e-mail: colchester.zoo@btinternet.com

Irregular levels add to the charm but detract from accessibility. The zoo produces a good Easy Route for wheelchair users, avoiding some steeper areas, but the terrain is varied. The wide variety of animals divide in five areas – the Beginning, Aquatic Zone, Lake Lands, The Slopes and The Heights. There is some undercover viewing and outside exhibits. A good day out. Spotless WCs and good quality food.

CP ♿ | E ♿ | RF ♿ 🚶 | C ♿
SC ♿ | WC 🚶 | RFE ♿

LAYER MARNEY TOWER
Nr. Colchester CO5 9US
Tel/Fax: (01206) 330784
e-mail: nicholas@layermarney.demon.co.uk

A fine example of Tudor architecture incorporating the tallest Tudor gatehouse in Britain. There is a long gallery, church, formal garden and farm. The farmyard is concrete. The farm walk is over earth and grass, requiring assistance. The upper garden is accessible with wide gravel paths, the lower garden is accessed by a steep ramp. The church has three high steps and there is no wheelchair access to the Tower.

SD ♿ | CP 🚶 | E ♿ | RF 🚶
C ♿ | S 🚶 | WC 🚶 | RFE 🚶

MANNINGTREE

Standing on the estuary of the River Stour. The village centre contains several Georgian and Victorian buildings of character.

ATTRACTION
ESSEX SECRET BUNKER
Crown Building, Shrublands Road, Misley, Manningtree CO11 1HS
Tel: (01206) 392271   Fax: (01206) 353847
e-mail: Bunker9248@aol.com

Nuclear War HQ that would have

121

Tudor magnificence reaching skyward at Layer Marney Tower.

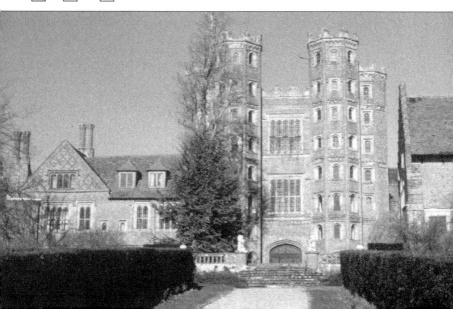

controlled the county in the event of a nuclear attack. Built in 1951, the two-level bunker remained operational until 1993. Fully restored and historically accurate, from the moment you enter the maze of passages and rooms you are in another world. Archive film and announcements emphasise the power of nuclear weapons.

SD 🚹 CP 🚹 E 🚹 RF 🚹 S 🚹 WC 🚹

SAFFRON WALDEN

Delightful historic town with a long history. Remains of an iron age fort at King Hill, evidence of Roman occupation and remains of a C12th castle. The town also hosts one of the few surviving town mazes.

TOURIST INFORMATION CENTRE
1 Market Place, Saffron Walden CB10 1HR

Tel: (01799) 510444

SELF-CATERING
WOODMORE COTTAGE 🚶
Whitensmere Farm Cottages, Ashdown, Saffron Walden CB10 2JQ
Tel/Fax: (01799) 584244
e-mail: GFORD@lineme.net
No. of Accessible Units: 1
No. of Beds per Unit: 5-8
Accessible Facilities: Lounge, dining room. Well converted C18th farm buildings cluster around south-facing garden. Woodmore Cottage features exposed beams and log-burning stove with its own private patio with garden furniture and barbecue.

ATTRACTION
MOLE HALL WILDLIFE PARK
Widdington, Newport,

Fine example of plaster work in historic Saffron Walden.

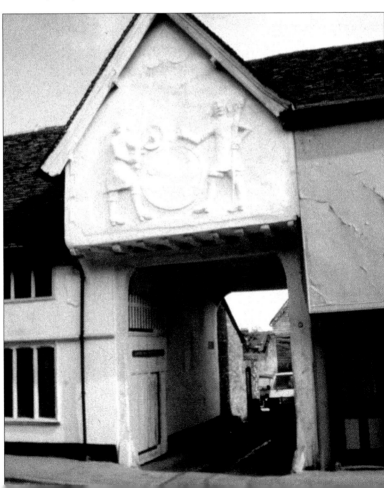

Nr. Saffron Walden CB11 3SS
Tel/Fax: (01799) 540400
e-mail: Molehall@aol.com

20 acres developed by a single family with a wide variety of animals including otters, chimpanzees, arctic foxes and flamingos, in delightful natural surroundings. A dominant feature is the fully moated private manor house, dating back to 1280.
The deer walk and butterfly pavilion are not suitable for wheelchairs because of high stiles and gravel respectively.

SD [♿]   CP [🚶] (shingle/grass)   E [♿]   RF [🚶]
C [🚶]   S [🚶]   WC [♿]

SOUTH OCKENDON
THURROCK ENVIRONMENTAL AND OUTDOOR EDUCATION CENTRE
Buckles Lane, South Ockendon RM15 6RS
Tel/Fax: (01708) 855228

Small attractive country park with 26-acre lake with activities year-round.

SD [♿]   CP [🚶]   E [🚶]   C [♿]   S [♿]
WC [🚶]   RFE-(Jetty) [🚶]

STANSTEAD
Known principally for its airport designed by Sir Norman Foster, now growing rapidly with excellent links to and from London.

TRAINS
Central Trains: Assistance:
Tel: (0845) 7056027
Web: centraltrains.co.uk
West Anglia Great Northern:
Special Needs – Tel: (0345) 226688
Minicom: (0345) 125988

HOTEL
HILTON STANSTEAD   [🚶]
Round Coppice Road,
Stansted Airport CM24 8SE
Tel: (01279) 680800   Fax: (01279) 680890
No. of Accessible Rooms: 6. Bath
Accessible Facilities: Lounge, restaurant
Quality airport hotel.

SOUTHEND-ON-SEA
Known as the holiday resort for Londoners, it has the longest pier in the world, stretching for 1.5 miles. Two funfairs offer amusement for all age groups and a wealth of day and night-time entertainment.

SOUTHEND TOURISM
Borough Council Marketing Division, Civic Centre, Victoria Avenue, Southend SS2 6ER
Tel: (01702) 215118   Fax: (01702) 215465
e-mail: marketing@southend.gov.uk

ATTRACTIONS
FOCAL POINT GALLERY
Southend Central Library, Victoria Avenue, Southend-on-Sea SS2 6EX
Tel: (01702) 612621 ext. 207
Fax: (01702) 469241
e-mail: admin@focalpoint.org.uk

Photographic gallery with exhibitions of a regional, national and international nature.

SD [♿]   CP [♿]   E [♿]   RF- [♿]   L [♿]
C [♿]   S n/a   WC [🚶]   RFE [♿]

SOUTHEND CENTRAL MUSEUM
Victoria Avenue, Southend-on-Sea SS2 6EW
Tel: (01702) 21513   Fax: (01702) 215631

Displays of archaeology, natural, social and local history and temporary exhibitions.
Use side entrance that is ramped at 1:16.

SD [♿]   CP [♿]   E [♿]   RF [♿]
C n/a   S [♿]   WC n/a

WESTCLIFFE-ON-SEA
A quiet resort notable for its Edwardian bandstand.

HOTEL
LULWORTH COURT   [♿]
Chalkwell Esplanade,
Westcliff-on-Sea SS00 8JQ
Tel: (01702) 347818
No. of Accessible Rooms: 10
Accessible Facilities: All
Holiday home owned by Queen Elizabeth's Foundation for Disabled People. Located on the seafront. 24-hour nursing care is provided with a full programme of outings and activities. There are two vehicles with tailgate lifts. This hotel offers nursing care and a holiday atmosphere where those with a disability and their carers can enjoy a real holiday.

GLOUCESTERSHIRE

GLOUCESTER TOURISM
Herbert Warehouse, The Docks,
Gloucester GL1 2EQ
Tel: (01452) 396620 Fax: (01452) 396622

PASSENGER TRANSPORT TEAM
Gloucestershire County Council, Shire Hall,
Bearland, Gloucester GL1 2TH
Tel: (01452) 425609 Fax: (01452) 425543
Timetable information.

BOURTON-ON-THE-WATER
This is the Venice of the Cotswolds. There
are cow-arched bridges and lovely
Cotswold stone houses.

HOTEL
CHESTER HOUSE HOTEL 🚶
Victoria Street, Bourton-on-the Water
GL54 2BG
Tel: (01451) 820266 Fax: (01451) 820471
e-mail: juliand@chesterhouse.u-net.com
web: www.bizarre.demon.co.uk/chester
No. of accessible Rooms: 5
Accessible Facilities: Lounge, restaurant.
Small, family-run hotel built of delightful
Cotswold stone with gardens.

ATTRACTIONS
BIRDLAND PARK LTD
Bourton-on-the-Water GL54 2BN
Tel: (01451) 820480 Fax: (01451) 822398
e-mail: sb.birdland@virgin.net
Set in seven acres of woodland, river ponds
and gardens, the setting is inhabited by
over 500 birds. Flamingos, pelicans, storks,
penguins, cranes, and waterfowl can be
seen, aviaries of parrots, falcons and toucans
plus tropical house and temperate houses.
SD ♿ CP n/a E ♿ RF 🚶 C 🚶
S ♿ WC 🚶 RFE ♿

COTSWOLD MOTOR MUSEUM AND TOY
COLLECTION
The Old Mill, Bourton-on-the-Water GL54 2BY
Tel: (01451) 821255
Located on River Windrush in a watermill.
SD ♿ CP ♿ E ♿ S ♿
WC 🚶 (village WC 80m from entrance)

CHELTENHAM
Set on a sheltered ridge between the high
Cotswolds and the Severn Vale, the town
enjoys an equable climate and is one of the
finest spa towns in Europe. There are many
fine examples of Regency architecture.
Cheltenham is notable also for its important
annual music festival and its racecourse.

TOURIST INFORMATION CENTRE
77 The Promenade, Cheltenham GL50 1PP
Tel: (01242) 522878

CHELTENHAM DISABILITY ADVICE CENTRE
St. Vincents Centre, Central Cross Drive,
Cheltenham GL50 4LA
Tel: (01242) 243030
Information about disability and support
services.

DISABILITY ACTION CHELTENHAM
PO Box 8, Cheltenham GL50 1YU
Tel: (01242) 237292
Run by people with disabilities for people
with disabilities, offering support, advice
and representation.

BUSES
Stagecoach: Tel: (01242) 224853
One low-floor route with raised kerbs.

TAXIS
Starline (evenings only):
Tel: (01242) 250250
One London cab with all fittings.

Station Taxis: Tel: (01242) 573355
One FX4 with all fittings.

TRAINS
Virgin Trains: Special Needs –
Tel: (0845) 7443366
Minicom: (0845) 7443367
Wales and West: Special Needs –
Tel: (0845) 3003005
Minicom: (0845) 7585469

Cheltenham Spa station is suitable for
wheelchairs using ramp access.

HOTEL
THE PRESTBURY HOUSE HOTEL
The Burgage, Prestbury, Cheltenham GL52 3DN
Tel: (01242) 529533   Fax: (01242) 227076
No. of Accessible Rooms: 1. Roll-in shower
Accessible Facilities: Bar, reception area, restaurants (two out of three), gardens. Country manor house hotel, main house dating back to early 1600s, typical late William and Mary design with Georgian wing added later. Standing in four acres of secluded grounds, the hotel is situated in the Burgage, an original road steeped in English history, particularly the Civil War. Now a quiet backwater, Prestbury is reputed to be the most haunted village in England.

ATTRACTIONS
CHELTENHAM ART GALLERY AND MUSEUM
Clarence Street, Cheltenham GL50 3JT
Tel: (01242) 237431   Fax: (01242) 262334
e-mail: ArtGallery@cheltenham.gov.uk
Museum houses a fine collection relating to William Morris' Arts and Crafts Movement. The gallery contains Dutch and British art from C17th onward. Oriental Gallery has Ming dynasty pottery and costumes, and a depiction of the true story of local hero Edward Wilson who joined Captain Scott on his tragic 1911 Antarctic Expedition.

SD 🚽   CP ♿   E 🚽   RF 🚽
L ♿   C 🚽   S 🚽   WC ♿
RFE ♿

COTSWOLD HERITAGE CENTRE
Northleach, Nr. Cheltenham GL54 3JH
Tel: (01451) 860715   Fax: (01451) 860091
Museum of rural life at a time when most people worked on the land. Hand and craft tool displays are housed in an C18th prison. The agricultural collection is displayed in a purpose-built gallery recalling Cotswold farm buildings. The Cotswold Land and People gallery and the Victorian kitchen in the cellar are not accessible.

SD n/a   CP ♿   E 🚽   RF 🚽
C ♿   S ♿   WC ♿

KEITH HARDINGíS WORLD OF MECHANICAL MUSIC
High Street, Northleach, Nr. Cheltenham GL54 3ET
Tel: (01451) 860181
Fax: (01451) 861133
Living museum of the various kinds of self-playing musical instruments, together with unique clocks in a workshop environment where items are still created and clocks repaired. Set in the joined buildings of the Oak house, parts of which are over 300 years old and Westwoods Grammar School that closed in 1902.

SD 🚽   CP ♿   E- ♿   S ♿   WC ♿

CIRENCESTER
There is an elegant parish church of St. John the Baptist, appreciated at a distance when the pinnacles and embattlements, that distinguish the Cirencester skyline, can be seen.

TOURIST INFORMATION CENTRE
Market Place, Cirencester GL7 2NW
Tel: (01285) 654180
Fax: (01285) 641182

SELF-CATERING
THE COTSWOLD HOBURNE
South Cerney, Nr. Cirencester
Book through Grooms Holidays
No. of Accessible Units: 3
No. of Beds per Unit: 4
Accessible Facilities:
Situated beside the lake in the Cotswold Water park holiday centre, close to the lovely village of Bibury.

ATTRACTION
BARNSLEY HOUSE GARDEN
Barnsley House,
Barnsley, Nr. Cirencester GL7 5EE
Tel: (01285) 740561
Fax: (01285) 740628
e-mail: cverey@barnsley
Noted for a vegetable garden planted as a French *potager orne* – a chequerboard of paths around fruit trees as pyramids and decorative kitchen plants. Laburnum and Lime walks and C18th

125

summerhouses.

SD ♿ CP ⧍ E ⧍ RF ⧍ S ⧍
WC ⧍ G ⧍

FOREST OF DEAN

Bordered to the west by the River Wye, and to the east by the Severn, the Royal Forest of Dean is one of England's foremost primeval forests, comprising over 23,000 acres and around 20 million trees. Once famous for its huge oaks, used for almost all British Navy ships at the time of the Armada, it now boasts breathtaking scenery and many walks.

BED AND BREAKFAST
THE FOUNTAIN INN ⧍
Fountain Way, Parkend, Nr. Lydney GL15 4JD
Tel: (01594) 562189   Fax: (01594) 564438
No. of Accessible Rooms: 1
Accessible Facilities: Dining room.
Built 200 years ago for the local mining population, now a charming pub with a garden in a delightful small village in the Royal Forest of Dean within the boundaries of the Cannop Valley Nature Reserve.

SELF-CATERING
BIG BARN COTTAGE ♿
Cinderhill House, St. Briavels,
Lydney GL15 6RH
Tel: (01594) 530393   Fax: (01594) 530098
e-mail: cinderhill.house@virgin.net
No. of Accessible Units: 1
No. of Beds per Unit: 2-6
Big Barn Cottage is one of three cottages set in the grounds of Cinderhill House. Each is stone built with fine views over the countryside to the Sugar Loaf Mountains and Brecon Beacons. St. Briavels is a good touring base with Cheltenham, Bath, Cardiff and Hereford within 45 minutes.

DRYSLADE FARM ⧍
English Bicknor, Coleford,
Forest of Dean GL16 7PA
Tel/Fax: (01594) 860259
No. of Accessible Units: 1
No. of Beds per Unit: 2D + 2S
Accessible Facilities: Lounge. Forest Enterprise with woodland paths.
184-acre farm with 20 acres of woodland in

a small village close to Monmouth. Accommodation consists of the ground floor flat of a late C18 farmhouse.

ATTRACTIONS
CLEARWELL CAVES
Nr. Coleford, Royal Forest of Dean GL16 8JR
Tel: (01594) 832535
These are ancient iron mines, you need to be adventurous because the story of iron is told in displays throughout the caves. Iron has been mined here since the Iron Age, 2,500 years ago, and continues today.

SD ♿ CP ♿ E ♿ RF ⧍ C ⧍
S ♿ WC- ⧍ RFE ⧍

DEAN FOREST RAILWAY
Norchard Railway Centre, Forest Road,
Lydney GL15 4ET
Tel/Fax: (01594) 845840
e-mail: fredb@globalnet.co.uk
Dean Forest Railway traces its history back to 1809, the Severn and Wye Railway preserving the last remnant of a once extensive forest railway. Steam-hauled passenger trains run from Norchard to Lydney Jcn (15 mins) but may extend northwards toward Parkend.

SD ♿ CP ⧍ at Norchard Centre only.
E- ♿ level to ramp for shop/museum, then level to station platform ramp. RF ⧍ C ⧍ S ⧍
Museum ♿ (through Shop with double doors).
WC ⧍ at Norchard Centre only.
TRAIN- ramp to adapted coach, taking 4 wheelchairs and 4 assistants. Wheelchair clamps and window views.

GLOUCESTER

The city has long been an inland port. A delightful city with some priceless C10th manuscripts, a Norman church and a fine cathedral, one of the centres of the Three Choirs Festival.

TOURIST INFORMATION CENTRE
28 Southgate Street,
Gloucester GL1 2DP
Tel: (01452) 421188

BUSES
Stagecoach: Tel: (01452) 523928
Gloucester City Bus – one low-floor route.

TAXIS
Andy Cars: Tel: (01452) 523000
One FX1 with all fittings.

EB Taxis: Tel: (01452) 305888
Two minibuses with all fittings.

Intacab: Tel: (01452) 527272
Two minibuses with all fittings.

TRAINS
Virgin Trains: Special Needs –
Tel: (0845) 7443366
Minicom: (0845) 7443367
Wales and West: Special Needs –
Tel: (0845) 3003005
Minicom: (0845) 7585469
Gloucester station is suitable for
wheelchairs using ramp access.

SHOPMOBILITY
Hampden Way, Gloucester
Tel: (01452) 302871   Fax: (01452) 396899

HOTEL
CHELTENHAM/GLOUCESTER MOAT HOUSE
Shurdington Road, Brockworth,
Gloucester G13 4PB
Tel: (01452) 519988   Fax: (01452) 519977
No. of Accessible Rooms: 2
Accessible Facilities: Lounge, restaurant,
pool, sauna, spa.
Modern hotel set in landscaped gardens
located just SW of the Forest of Dean
towards the Monmouth border.

MORETON-IN-MARSH
A very pleasant, prosperous-looking town
with a wide grass-verged main street, and
many C17th and C18th houses. An old
curfew bell still hangs in its tower that
overlooks the Fosse Way.

TOURIST INFORMATION CENTRE
Cotswold District Council Office,
Moreton-in-Marsh GL56 0AZ
Tel: (01608) 650881

HOTEL
TREETOPS
London Road, Moreton-in-Marsh GL56 0HE

Tel/Fax: (01608) 651036
No. of Accessible Rooms: 2. Shower
Accessible Facilities: Lounge, restaurant.
Family-run guest house in 0.75 acres of
secluded garden, a short distance from the
town centre.

NAILSWORTH
Located in softly wooded South Cotswold
Hills with a mix of architecture. C16th
cottages cling to the hillside while large
C17th wool merchants' houses present
imposing facades. Attractive Georgian
houses also can be seen.

BED AND BREAKFAST
APPLE ORCHARD HOUSE
Springhill, Nailsworth GL6 0LX
Tel: (01453) 832503   Fax: (01453) 836213
No. of Accessible Rooms: 1
Accessible Facilities: Lounge, dining
room, patio. Modern, elegant detached
house in an acre of garden with lovely
views of the Cotswold hills.

STOW-ON-THE-WOLD
The highest town in the Cotswolds,
situated where eight roads meet.

TOURIST INFORMATION CENTRE
Hollis House, The Square,
Stow-on-the-Wold GL54 1AF
Tel: (01451) 831082   Fax: (01451) 870083

ATTRACTION
COTSWOLD FARM PARK
Guiting Power,
Nr. Stow-on-the-Wold GL54 5UG
Tel: (01451) 850307   Fax: (01451) 850423
Premier UK rare breed survival centre and
a leading live animal exhibition with
demonstrations, tractor and trailer rides,
Barn houses educational interactive displays.

| SD | CP | E | RF |
| C | S | WC | RFE |

TETBURY
A quiet small market town, developed
during the mid C17th, situated almost on
the border with Wiltshire.

127

TOURIST INFORMATION CENTRE
33 Church Street, Tetbury GL8 8JG
Tel: (01666) 503552

HOTEL
HUNTERS HALL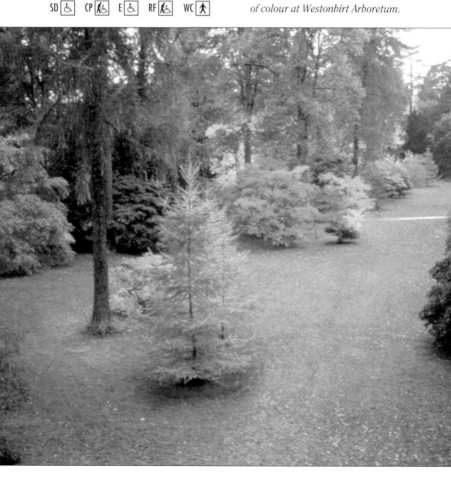
Kingscote, Nr. Tetbury GL8 8XZ
Tel: (01453) 860393   Fax: (01453) 860707
No. of Accessible Rooms: 2. Roll-in shower
Accessible Facilities: Lounge, restaurant.
Country hotel.

ATTRACTIONS
CHAVENAGE HOUSE
Chavenage, Nr. Tetbury GL8 8XP
Tel: (01666) 502329   Fax: (01666) 836778
Historic Elizabethan house of 1576, owned
by Colonel Nathaniel Stephens, MP for
Gloucestershire, during the Civil War
(1641-49). Contains fine tapestries, stained
glass windows and furniture.
SD CP E RF WC

WESTONBIRT ARBORETUM
Tetbury GL8 8QS
Tel: (01666) 880220   Fax: (01666) 880559
web: www.forestry.gov.uk
Over 18,000 trees from all over the world
have been planted here from 1829 to the
present day, producing 600 acres of
landscaped Cotswold countryside. There
are 17 miles of waymarked trails where
you will be accompanied by birds, badgers
and deer. Particularly notable for
rhododendrons, azaleas, magnolias and
the wild flowers of Silk Wood that can be
seen from March to June, and for the
autumn colour spectacular from late
September to early November.
SD CP E RF
C S WC RFE

*New England in the fall? No, just a blaze
of colour at Westonbirt Arboretum.*

HAMPSHIRE

HAMPSHIRE CENTRE FOR INDEPENDENT LIVING
4 Plantation Way, Whitehill,
Borden GO35 9HD
Tel: (01420) 474261

BASINGSTOKE

Although not a beautiful town, the modern development here is very interesting.

TOURIST INFORMATION CENTRE
Willis Museum, Old Town Hall, Market Place, Basingstoke RG21 7QD
Tel: (01256) 817681   Fax: (01256) 356231

HOTEL
AUDLEYS WOOD THISTLE HOTEL
Alton Road, Basingstoke RG25 2JT
Tel: (01256) 817555   Fax: (01256) 817500
e-mail: audleys.wood@thistle.co.uk
No. of Accessible Rooms: 1
Accessible Facilities: Lounge, restaurant C19th. mansion with preserved original features, set in seven acres of landscaped gardens and lightly wooded grounds on the edge of the Hampshire Downs. Located on the A339. Two miles from M3 (J6).

BASINGSTOKE COUNTRY HOTEL
Scures Hill, Nately Scures, Hook RG27 9JS
Tel: (01256) 764161   Fax: (01256) 768341
No. of Accessible Rooms: 6
Accessible Facilities: Lounge, restaurants (2), cocktail bar. Originally a private country residence, now an elegant country retreat located on the main A30 London road, but set well back. Set in 4.5 acres and surrounded by mature woodland.

FORDINGBRIDGE

A medieval bridge, much restored and widened, crosses the Avon here, giving the town its name. Set NW of the New Forest, the views are spectacular with outdoor pursuits popular.

SELF CATERING
SANDY BALLS HOLIDAY CENTRE
Godshill, Fordingbridge SP6 2JZ

Tel: (01425) 653042   Fax: (01425) 653067
web: www.sandy-balls.co.uk
No. of Accessible Lodges: 3
No. of beds per Lodge: 5
Accessible Facilities: Open plan lounge/kitchen. One lodge has wheel-in shower, others have bath. Site facilities accessed by level tarmac, including indoor pool with hoist, and gently ramped outdoor pool. Adaptive changing room, pizza restaurant and pub, and shop. A number of adapted WCs with RADAR key available from reception. Winner of England for Excellence 1998 Caravan Holiday Park of the Year and David Bellamy Gold Award. Bordered by the Avon and set in 120 acres of woods and parkland in the New Forest area.

ATTRACTION
ROCKBOURNE ROMAN VILLA
Rockbourne, Fordingbridge SP6 3PG
Tel: (01725) 518841
On the site of the remains of a 40-room Roman village, this on-site museum displays many artefacts found during its excavation.

SD 👤 CP 🧍 E 🧍 RF 👤 S 🧍
WC 🧍 RFE 👤

GOSPORT

Famous for its yacht and boat building, many of the buildings were destroyed in a C19th fire, but those remaining are still pretty.

BED AND BREAKFAST
WEST WIND GUEST HOUSE
197 Portsmouth Road, Lee on the Solent, Gosport PO13 9AA
Tel: (01705) 552550   Fax: (01705) 554657
e-mail: maggie@west-wind.co.uk
web: www.west-wind.co.uk
No. of Accessible Rooms: 1
Accessible Facilities: Dining room, beach access by ramped slipway (gradient 1:20). 50m from the beach. A one-mile promenade is fully accessible to wheelchair users.

LIPHOOK

Beautifully situated in the shadow of the downs, this is a charming village with a pond, pretty cottages and a famous late C17th posting inn.

ATTRACTION
HOLLYCOMBE STEAM COLLECTION
Iron Hill, Liphook GU30 7LP
Tel: (01428) 724900   Fax: (01428) 723682
Relive the days of the traditional fairground. The main attractions are fairground rides and railways. Wheelchair passengers can be accommodated on some, but not all, of these. Gardens are accessible but paths can be steep.

SD CP E RF C
S WC RFE

LYMINGTON
Pleasant town on the edge of the New Forest. Bright cottages and attractive Georgian and C19th houses in a broad high street.

TOURIST INFORMATION CENTRE
St. Barb Museum, New Street,
Lymington SO41 9BH
Tel/Fax: (01590) 672422

BED AND BREAKFAST
OUR BENCH
Lodge Road, Pennington,
Lymington SO41 8HH
Tel/Fax: (01590) 673141
e-mail: ourbench@newforest.demon.co.uk
No. of Accessible Rooms: 1
Accessible Facilities: Lounge, dining room, pool, sauna, Jacuzzi. Holders of ETB England for Excellence award in Tourism for All Categories, 1997. Large bungalow in 0.3 of an acre of garden in quiet village two miles from the New Forest. Evening meals are an optional extra.

ATTRACTION
BRAXTON GARDENS
Braxton Courtyard, Lynmore Lane,
Milford on Sea, Lymington SO41 0TX
Tel: (01590) 642008
Lovely walled garden and courtyard designed around red brick barns of an original Victorian farmyard. Fine selection of unusual herbs, alpines and shrubs.

SD CP E RF C
S WC n/a

NEW MILTON
Small town, close to New Forest. Lowland heath and mixed forestation.

BED AND BREAKFAST
ST. URSULA
30 Hobart Road, New Milton BH25 6EG
Tel: (01425) 613515
No. of Accessible Rooms: 1
Accessible Facilities: Lounge, dining room. Located two miles from the New Forest.

SELF-CATERING
NAISH HOLIDAY VILLAGE
New Milton
Book through Grooms Holidays
No. of Accessible Units: 3
No. of Beds per Unit: 4
Accessible Facilities: Paved patio. Timbered chalets in the New Forest with fine views across the Solent to the Needles and the Isle of Wight.

PETERSFIELD
Set in a wide valley, there are many elegant Georgian buildings in this market and agricultural town.

ATTRACTION
UPPARK (NT)
South Harting, Petersfield GU31 5QR
Tel: (01730) 825415   Fax: (01730) 825873
e-mail: supgen@smtp.ntrust.org.uk
Elegant late C17th house high on the South Downs with fine views. The mid C18th interior has been fully restored after a disastrous fire in 1989. The house contains a collection of grand tour paintings, fine ceramics and furniture. Evocative servants' rooms where H G Wells spent part of his youth. NB: Entrance ramp gradient 1:11.

SD CP E RF C
S WC Wheelchair available.

PORTSMOUTH
In naval terms the history of Portsmouth has long been important. Home to Charles Dickens and to Jones Hanway, inventor of the umbrella, Portsmouth as a town grew by itself, rather than to plan.

Many modern buildings and plenty of entertainment.

HAMPSHIRE

TOURIST INFORMATION CENTRE
Civic Offices, Portsmouth PO1 2BG
Tel: (023) 92 834086   Fax: (023) 92 834975
E-mail:pzhms310@hantsnet.hants.go.uk

PORTSMOUTH HARBOUR TOURISM
102 Commercial Road, Portsmouth PO1 1EJ
Tel: (023) 92 838382   Fax: (023) 92 730116
web: www.portsmouthharbour.co.uk

HOTEL
HILTON NATIONAL PORTSMOUTH
Eastern Road, Farlington, Portsmouth PO6 1UN
Tel: (023) 92 219111   Fax: (023) 92 210762
No. of Accessible Rooms: 2. Bath Accessible Facilities: Lounge (split level area with steps to raised section), restaurant (split level ramped to lower section), pool, sauna and steam room (accessible with assistance).Modern hotel situated on the A2020 at the junction of the A27(M) and 1.5 miles from the A3(M) from London. 4.5 miles from city centre.

ATTRACTIONS
FLAGSHIP PORTSMOUTH
Building 1/7 College Road, HM Naval Base, Portsmouth PO1 3LJ
Tel: (023) 92 870999   Fax: (023) 92 29525
e-mail: rob@flgship.org.uk
This is a working naval base so visitors with restricted mobility should be accompanied. After setting down, car parking is at the Victory Gate 600/800m from the visitor centre. There is orange badge parking in 4/5 spaces outside the centre. Wheelchairs are available from the visitor centre, Mary Rose, HMS Warrior 1860 and Royal Naval Museum. We recommend the special access route map.

HMS Victory
Tel: (023) 92 722351
Lord Nelson's famous flagship at Trafalgar, and the world's most outstanding example of maritime restoration. The tour involves fairly steep steps. A video tour is provided on the lower gundeck.

SD   CP n/a   E    RF
C   S   WC

HMS Warrior 1860
Tel: (023) 92 291379
World's first iron-hulled armoured warship that spanned the periods of wood, iron, sail and steam. Four decks are connected by steep steps but there is alternative access to two decks. A ramp gives access to the upper deck although tides may make the gradient steeper. A stairlift from the upper to the main gun deck requires a transfer from wheelchair to lift with staff assistance.

SD   CPn/a   E   RF   L
C   S   WC

Mary Rose Museum
Tel: (023) 92 812931
Amazingly preserved in the Solent for 437 years, the Mary Rose, Henry VIII's warship, was raised in 1982. A short audio-visual presentation is followed by a themed display on the many artefacts recovered, including weapons, clothing and pewterware. An absolute must! Fully accessible.

SD   CP n/a   E   RF
C   S-   WC

Royal Naval Museum
Tel: (023) 92 727562
Devoted to the Navy's history. Relics of Lord Nelson, artefacts, model ships and a wide range of displays. Ramps in all buildings. Little inaccessible to wheelchair users.

SD   CP n/a   E   RF   L
C   S   WC

SOUTHSEA MODEL VILLAGE
Lumps Fort, Eastney, Esplanade, Southsea, Portsmouth PO4 9RU
Tel: (023) 92 294706
1/12th scale models of over 40 buildings plus G scale miniature garden railway, toy museum and gardens watercourse.

SD   CP   E   RF
C   WC n/a

RINGWOOD
Situated by the River Avon, just outside the New Forest, but with heath and woodland close at hand. Houses here date from all periods, many with lovely thatched roofs.

131

TOURIST INFORMATION CENTRE
The Furlong, Ringwood BH24 1AZ
Tel/Fax: (01425) 470896

ATTRACTION
MOORS VALLEY COUNTRY PARK
Horton Road, Ashley Heath,
Nr. Ringwood BH24 2ET
Tel: (01425) 470721   Fax: (01425) 471656
Trails and a lake, with fishing from west
bank with a platform for wheelchair users.
A comprehensive map of trails is available,
only the Tree-Top Trail appears inaccessible,
but a companion is advised for all trails.

| SD | ♿ | CP | ♿ | E | ♿ | RF | ♿ |
| C | ♿ | S | ♿ | WC | 🚶 | RFE | ♿ |

For visitors in a wheelchair or those that have difficulty
walking, a battery-operated Easirider or pedal-powered
Tandem chair is available.

SOUTHAMPTON
Situated on a peninsula with the River Test
to the south and west of the city. Heavy
devastation during WWII has led to many
new buildings, although some fascinating
houses have remained.

TOURIST INFORMATION CENTRE
9 Civic Centre Road, Southampton SO14 7JP
Tel: (023) 80 221106   Fax: (023) 80 832082

SOUTHAMPTON TOURISM
Southampton City Council, 4th Floor Frobisher
House, Nelson Gate, Southampton SO4 1GX
Tel: (023) 80 832846   Fax: (023) 80 832929

SOUTHAMPTON DIAL
Tel: (023) 80 335473

BUSES
First Southampton: Tel: (023) 80 224854
Some low-floor routes
Solent Blue Line: Tel: (023) 80 223224
Stagecoach: Tel: (01256) 464501

Passenger Transport Group:
Tel: (01962) 845614
Publishers of *Connections*, bus and train
timetables.

TAXIS
A2B: Tel: (023) 80 223450

One adapted vehicle.
Cabmobility: Tel: (023) 80 899291
Three adapted vehicles.
Martax: Tel: (023) 80 616265
Four adapted vehicles.
Radio Taxis: Tel: (023) 80 339988
Four adapted vehicles.
Streamline Taxis: Tel: (023) 80 223355
One adapted vehicle.

TRAINS
Connex: Customer Services:
Tel: (0870) 6030405
Fax: (0870) 6030505
Minicom: (01233) 617621
Southwest Trains: Special Needs –
Tel: (0845) 6050440
Minicom: (0845) 6050441
web: www.swtrains.co.uk
Virgin Trains: Special Needs – (0845)
7443366
Minicom: (0845) 7443367
Wales and West: Special Needs –
(0845) 3003005
Minicom: (0845) 7585469
Southampton Parkway (airport) station.
Level access, but ensure you arrive at the
correct side of the station for direction of
travel. Six orange badge spaces; level access
via automatic door to ticket office; adapted
WC in station building; accessible taxis can
be ordered on request; standard height
pay/card phones; ramp; two wheelchairs
available.

Southampton Central Station. Level access
both sides; no orange badge spaces in long-
term car park; accessible automatic doors to
ticket office; lift to all platforms; unisex
adapted WCs on platforms 1 and 4; standard
height pay/card phones; ramps; wheelchairs
on each platform.

CAR PARKS
Contact local services:
Tel: (023) 80 832539

SHOPMOBILITY
7 Castle Way, Southampton SO14 2BX
Tel/Fax: (023) 80 631263
Minicom: (023) 80 228291

HOTELS
NETLEY WATERSIDE HOUSE
(Winged Fellowship)
Abbey Hill, Netley Abbey,
Southampton SO31 5FA
Tel: (023) 80 453 686

On the shores of Southampton Water, minutes away from local shops. Well placed for visits to Portsmouth Dockyard, Stonehenge etc. Large number of nurses and care assistants. Lounge, bar, shop, craft area. Garden sun house. Garden viewing platform over the water. Adaptive transport.

HILTON SOUTHAMPTON
Bracken Place, Chilworth,
Southampton SO16 3RB
Tel: (023) 80 702700   Fax: (023) 80 767233

No. of Accessible Rooms: 1. Bath. Accessible Facilities: Lounge, restaurant, pool, sauna. Bright and modern hotel north of the city at the junction of the M3/A33.

ATTRACTION
EXBURY GARDENS
Exbury, Nr. Southampton SO45 1AZ
Tel: (023) 80 891203   Fax: (023) 80 899940

200 acres of landscaped woodland with fine flowering shrub collections, ponds, rock gardens. The summer garden of 53 acres is ideal for picnics.

SD   CP   E   RF   C
S   WC   RFE

SOUTHAMPTON FOOTBALL CLUB
The Dell, Milton Road, Southampton SO15 2XH
Admin: (023) 80 220505

For details on the disabled enclosure contact **Mr. and Mrs. Frank Mortimer, 24 The Croft, Calmore, Southampton SO40 2GN. Tel: (023) 80 667547.**

The disabled enclosure is situated by the corner flag/players' entrance, at the Milton Road end. Experienced, designated stewards are stationed in enclosure.

CP – NO PARKING AVAILABLE but Orange badge holders are usually allowed to park on the road close to the disabled enclosure.

RE (steep slope)

WC (near entrance to disabled supporters' area)

B/R (steward available to obtain for you)

WINCHESTER
Important in Roman times, this became England's capital under the Anglo-Saxons: William the Conqueror kept Winchester as the capital and as late as the C17th, Charles II planned to build a palace here. The focal points are the C19th High Street and Guildhall, and there are many small alleyways with houses of all centuries.

TOURIST INFORMATION CENTRE
Guildhall, The Broadway, Winchester SO23 9LJ
Tel: (01962) 840500   Fax: (01962) 850348
e-mail: tourism@winchester.gov.uk
web: www.winchester.gov.uk

WINCHESTER GROUP FOR DISABLED PEOPLE
Tel: (01962) 840600

Publishers of *Access Guide to Winchester*.

PASSENGER TRANSPORT GROUP
Tel: (01962) 845614

BUSES
Stagecoach Hampshire Bus:
Tel: (01256) 464501

TAXIS
Wessex Cars: Tel: (01962) 877749
Five adapted vehicles.
Wintax: Tel: (01962) 866208
Two adapted vehicles.
Hackney Carriages: Ranks at The Broadway, Silver Hill and the station.
20 adapted vehicles.

TRAINS
South West Trains. Special Needs –
Tel: (0845) 6050440
Minicom: (0845) 6050441
web: www.swtrains.co.uk

Winchester Station: Tel: (01962) 213660
Some orange badge spaces; level entry to ticket office via automatic door; stairmate in operation, disabled WC on platform 2, taxi rank; standard height pay/card phones; wheelchair ramp.

CAR PARK
Free parking for orange badge holders in

all city car parks and use of residents' parking.
Tel: (01962) 848346

SHOPMOBILITY
Upper Parking Level, Brooks Car Park,
Winchester SP23 8QY
Tel: (01962) 842626

HOTEL
WINCHESTER MOAT HOUSE
Worthy Lane, Winchester SO23 7AB
Tel: (01962) 709988   Fax: (01962) 840862
No. of Accessible Rooms: 1
Accessible Facilities: Lounge, bar,
restaurant. Located on the edge of the city
in a quiet residential area.

MARWELL HOTEL
Thompsons Lane, Colden Common,
Nr. Winchester SO21 1JY
Tel: (01962) 777681   Fax: (01962) 777625
No. of Accessible Rooms: 4
Accessible Facilities: Lounge/bar, restaurant.
Delightful safari and colonial-style hotel,
with airy glass and timber walkways, set in
wooded grounds. Located six miles from
Winchester and adjacent to Marwell
Zoological Park.

BED AND BREAKFAST
SHAWLANDS
46 Kilham Lane, Winchester SO22 5QD
Tel/Fax: (01962) 861166
No. of Accessible Rooms: 1

Accessible Facilities: Lounge, dining room.
Guest house located in a quiet lane
overlooking fields, 1.5 miles from
Winchester city centre. Near the M3 (J11).

ATTRACTIONS
MARWELL ZOOLOGICAL PARK,
Colden Common, Marwell SO21 1JH
Tel: (01962) 777407   Fax: (01962) 777511
e-mail: marwell@marwell.org.uk
Over 150 species from Siberian tigers to
tamarins, from rhino to meerkat. Highlights
include penguin world with underwater
viewing, Encounter Village for pet and farm
animals, Tropical World for a rainforest
experience and aviaries for rare owls.

CP [♿]   E [♿]   RF [♿]   C [♿]
S [♿]   WC [♿]   RFE [♿]

WINCHESTER CATHEDRAL
The Close, Winchester SO23 9LS
Tel: (01962) 853137   Fax: (01962) 841519
Founded in 1079, this is the longest
medieval church in England. It is rightly
world-famous famous for its 12th-century
illuminated Winchester Bible and its black
marble font. Many kings lie here as do Jane
Austen and Izaak Walton. An absolute must.

SD [♿]   CP n/a   E [♿]   RF [♿]
C [♿]   S [♿]   WC [♿]   RFE [♿]

Winchester Cathedral.

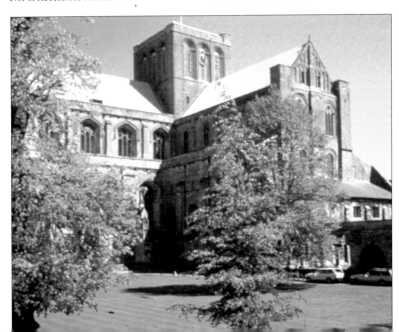

HEREFORD AND WORCESTERSHIRE

HEREFORDSHIRE TOURISM
Education Centre, Blackfriars Street,
Hereford HR4 9HS
Tel: (01432) 277286   Fax: (01432) 266156

WORCESTERSHIRE TOURISM
web: www.valenet.com

OUTDOOR ACTIVITIES
THE BRUCE WAKE CHARITY
Ayston, Oakham LE15 9AE
Tel: (01572) 822183
Berthed at Upton Marina on the River Severn,
10 miles south of Worcester, the narrow boat
Charlotte is designed for a wheelchair user
and an accompanying family of up to eight
passengers. Includes hydraulic lifts, ceiling
hoist, shower wheelchair, wide access ramp,
fingertip control panel. One and two-week
cruises available on River Severn, River Avon
and Staffs. & Worcs. canal.

GLOUCESTERSHIRE DISABLED AFLOAT RIVERS TRUST (DART)
Diocesan Office, 4 College Green, GL1 2LR
Tel: (01452) 410022
Specially built river boat designed to
provide residential facilities for disabled
persons. Moored at Upton-on-Severn, the
Dart cruises the rivers Severn and Avon
and the Gloucester/Sharpness canal
passing through beautiful countryside and
the historic towns of Tewkesbury,
Gloucester, Worcester, Evesham and
Stratford-on-Avon. Accommodation for 12
persons including five wheelchairs. Fully
accessible with lift and adapted WCs,
shower and galley.

ABBERLEY
Thriving village with good shops, pub and
hotel. Eleven miles from Worcester.

SELF-CATERING
OLD YATES COTTAGES   [icon]
Old Yates Farm, Abberley WR6 6AT
Tel: (01299) 896500   Fax: (01299) 896065
e-mail: rmgoodma@aol.com

No. of Accessible Units: 1. Bath
No. of Beds per Unit: 2
Beagle and Bassett Cottages can be linked
together and have commanding views
towards the Teme Valley. On a farm
growing grass and cereal crops built 100
years ago to house the squire's hounds. Now
converted, you'll certainly not feel in the
dog-house!

BROMSGROVE
Situated in the Lickey Hills, surrounded by
lush orchard country, Bromsgrove is an
ancient and sizeable market town. The
church, surrounded by yew trees planted
in 1790, has fascinating early C18th
tombstones.

HOTEL
STAKIS BROMSGROVE   [icon]
Birmingham Road, Bromsgrove B61 0JB
Tel: (0121) 4477888   Fax: (0121) 4477273
No. of Accessible Rooms: 2. Bath
Accessible Facilities: Lounge, bar,
restaurant, health club (pool, sauna, spa).
Quality hotel with extremely spacious
reception area and extra large rooms.
Located close to the M5 and M42 and
several attractions.

BROMYARD
Surrounded by orchards and hop fields.

ATTRACTION
LOWER BROCKHAMPTON/BROCKHAMPTON
ESTATE (NT)
Bringsty, Nr. Bromyard WR6 5UH
Tel: (01885) 488099
e-mail:vbkluc@smtp.ntrust.org.uk
Late C14th medieval moated manor house.
The hall, screens, parlour and garden are
accessible. Along the *Access for All* trail in
the Brockhampton woodlands majestic
oaks, ash trees and conifers abound as do all
types of wildlife. The trail passes Lawn
Pool, a glade with benches and picnic
tables and there is a series of sculptures

depicting the history of the estate and the area. An excellent leaflet is available about the trail.

SD 🚶 CP ♿ E 🚶 RF ♿ WC 🚶 RFE 🚶

EVESHAM

This is an important market town and the centre of the fruit-growing area of the Vale of Evesham. There are tree-lined walks and lawns along the banks of the Avon, many quality houses and old inns including the late C15th restored Booth Hall with fine timberwork. Part of the town's original medieval wall stands in Bridge Street.

HOTEL
NORTHWICK ARMS HOTEL   ♿
Waterside, Evesham WR11 6BT
Tel: (01386) 40322
No. of Accessible Rooms: 1. Bath
Accessible Facilities: Restaurant
Privately owned, attractive hotel, close to the town centre.

HAY-ON-WYE

At the northern end of the Brecon Beacons, this sleepy town is synonymous with books and bookshops as the site of the best-known literary festival in England. Held in the last week of May, the atmosphere is incredible.

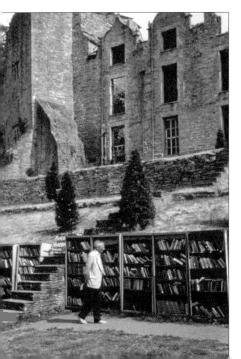

TOURIST INFORMATION CENTRE
Oxford Road, Haye-on-Wye HR3 5DG
Tel: (01497) 820144   Fax: (01497) 820015

HOTEL
THE HAVEN COUNTRY GUEST HOUSE
Hardwicke, Hay-on-Wye HR3 5TA
Tel/Fax: (01497) 831254
No. of Accessible Rooms: 1. Roll-in Shower
Accessible Facilities: Lounge, dining room, garden, tarmac around the house, garden grass may be tricky in damp weather.
NB. WC seat is 2.5cm lower than the criteria but otherwise everything is suitable. The wardrobe is cut down to size and the mirror and hanging rails are at accessible heights. This lovely early Victorian vicarage, built in 1850, is at the head of the Golden Valley close to Hay-on-Wye. It is owned by a charming family for whom nothing is too much trouble. Delightful atmosphere.

HEREFORD

Situated on a level plain bounded in the distance by low-lying hills. The Wye runs through the southern part of the town, under a medieval bridge. This is a cathedral city and an important agricultural centre. Many interesting buildings date from C4th.

TOURIST INFORMATION CENTRE
1 King Street, Hereford HR4 7BW
Tel: (01432) 268430   Fax: (01432) 342662

HEREFORD PUBLIC TRANSPORT
Tel: (01432) 260948

BUSES
Sargent Brothers: Tel: (01544) 230481
Operates access bus in city centre.
County Busline: Tel: (0345) 125436
Timetables and phone numbers of all local operators available.
Stagecoach Red & White: Tel: (01633) 485118

TAXIS
Ace Taxis: Tel: (01432) 343399
Four adapted vehicles.
Blue Line Taxis: Tel: (01432) 263000

Hay-on-Wye, a bibliophile's delight.

Two adapted vehicle.
Hereford Taxis: Tel: (01432) 343343
Two adapted vehicles.

TRAINS
Wales and West: Special Needs –
Tel: (0845) 3003005
Minicom: (0845) 7585469
Hereford station is suitable for
wheelchairs using ramp access.

CAR PARK
Contact Herefordshire DIAL.
15 St. Owen Street, Hereford
Tel: (01432) 277770

SHOPMOBILITY
Maylord Orchards, Hereford
Tel: (01432) 342166

HOTEL
STARTING GATE TRAVEL INN
Holmer Road, Holmer, Hereford HR4 9RS
Tel: (01432) 274853   Fax: (01432) 343003
Take the A49 Leominster road, the inn is
0.5 miles past the Hereford Leisure
Centre.

ATTRACTION
CHURCHILL HOUSE MUSEUM AND HATTON
GALLERY
Venus Lane, Aylestone Hill, Hereford HR1 1DE
Tel: (01432) 260693
Laid out in Regency house style with
superb grounds. C18th and C19th rooms,
costume displays and a gallery of works by
local artist Brian Hatton.
SD 🖐   CP 🚶   E 🖐
RF-(Shop). Gradient is 1:6-NA   WC 🚶

HEREFORD CIDER MUSEUM TRUST
21 Ryelands Street, Hereford HR4 0LW
Tel: (01432) 354207
Explore the story of traditional cider-
making with reconstructed cider
farmhouse and Champagne Cider cellars
and sample! Applying for funding for
wheelchair lifts and accessible WC
facilities.
SD 🖐   CP 🖐   E 🖐   RF 🖐
S 🖐   WC 🚶   RFE 🖐

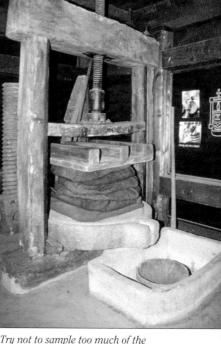

*Try not to sample too much of the
produce at the Cider Museum.*

KIDDERMINSTER
Lying on the Stour, the town is known for
its carpet manufacturing. There is
pleasant wooded countryside to the NW of
the town and in the centre there is a late
medieval red sandstone church.

HOTEL
THE GRANARY HOTEL and RESTAURANT 🚶
Heath Lane, Shenstone,
Kidderminster DY10 4BS
Tel: (01562) 777535   Fax: (01562) 777722
No. of Accessible Rooms: 1. Bath
Accessible Facilities: Lounge, restaurant.
Small, family-run hotel with views across
fields to Great Witley and Abberley Hills.

ATTRACTION
WORCESTERSHIRE COUNTY MUSEUM
Hartlebury Castle, Hartlebury,
Nr. Kidderminster DY11 7XZ
Tel: (01299) 250416   Fax: (01299) 251890
e-mail: museum@worcestershire.gov.uk
Hartlebury Castle was home to the Bishops
of Worcester for over 1000 years. In the
former servants' quarters in the north wing,
there are permanent exhibitions showing

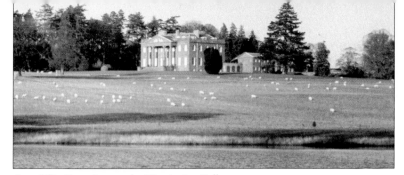

Caperbility Brown's grounds at Berrington Hall.

past lives of the county's inhabitants from Roman times to the present day.

SD ⬚   CP ⬚   E ⬚   RF ⬚
C ⬚   S ⬚   WC ⬚   RFE ⬚

LEOMINSTER

Set among pastureland, hop fields and orchards in countryside watered by three streams, Leominster has many medieval, Tudor and Georgian houses and is also rich in early English domestic architecture.

TOURIST INFORMATION CENTRE
1 Corn Square, Leominster HR6 8LR
Tel: (01568) 616460   Fax: (01568) 615546

ATTRACTION
BERRINGTON HALL (NT)
Leominster HR6 0DW
Tel: (01568) 615721   Fax: (01568) 613263
e-mail: vbeosb@smtp.ntrust.org.uk
An C18th Henry Holland-built house set in parkland designed by Capability Brown.

SD ⬚   CP ⬚   E ⬚   WC ⬚   RFE ⬚

MALVERN

The town has a continental flavour, being terraced on its hillside site. There are many interesting buildings and artefacts in the church dating mostly from the C15th.

MALVERN HILLS TOURISM and LEISURE SERVICES
Rockliffe House, 40 Church Street,
Gt. Malvern WR14 2AZ
Tel: (01684) 862 411   Fax: (01684) 862 441
Publishes a useful guide to disabled access to places of interest and beauty.

MALVERN TOURIST INFORMATION CENTRE
21 Church Street, Malvern WR14 2AA
Tel: (01684) 892 289   Fax: (01684) 892 872

SELF-CATERING
CIDAR MILL COTTAGE ⬚
Mutlows Farm Cottages, Drake Street, Welland,
Nr. Malvern WR13 6LP
Tel/Fax: (01684) 310878
No. of Accessible Units: 1. Bath
No. of Beds per Unit: 3
Accessible Facilities: Lounge/diner, kitchen. Private courtyard patio with raised flower/herb garden and furniture.
An old cow byre and a cider store have been converted into a spacious single-storey detached cottage. At the foot of the Malvern Hills three miles from Upton, the farm has acres of ancient orchards with wild flowers.

ATTRACTION
GREAT MALVERN PRIORY
6 Church Street,
Malvern WR14 2AY
Tel/Fax: (01684) 561020
Norman priory church, built 22 years after the Conquest and famous for its stained glass, of which original jewelled fragments remain in the east window, also for hundreds of detailed wall tiles made between 1453/6. Two rows of original dark oak monastic choir stalls, dating from C15th, also survived the Dissolution.

SD ⬚   CP ⬚   E ⬚   RF ⬚
S ⬚   WC ⬚   RFE ⬚

ROSS-ON-WYE

Modest market town set on a red sandstone cliff above a lovely sweep of the Wye.

TOURIST INFORMATION CENTRE
Edde Cross Street, Ross-on-Wye HR9 7BZ
Tel: (01989) 562768   Fax: (01989) 565057

HOTEL
MERTON HOUSE HOTEL   ♿
Eddie Cross Street, Ross-on-Wye HR9 7BZ
Tel/Fax: (01989) 563252
No. of Accessible Rooms: 13. Roll-in shower.
Accessible Facilities: Lounge, dining room.
Located on the edge of town, this beautiful
Georgian house has been adapted as a
holiday hotel for disabled people. Glorious
views across to the Welsh mountains.

WORCESTER
Built on both sides of the Severn, today the
principal part of the city is on the eastern
bank. Famous for its superb cathedral,
Royal Worcester porcelain and the Guildhall.

TOURIST INFORMATION CENTRE
The Guildhall, High Street,
Worcester WR5 1BA
Tel: (01905) 726311   Fax: (01905) 722481

CITY OF WORCESTER LEISURE SERVICES
Orchard House, Worcester WR1 3BW
TEL: (01905) 722306   Fax: (01905) 722350
e-mail: wcclies@netcomuk.co.uk
web: www.cityof worcester.gov.uk

MOBILITY HIRE
13 Droitwich Road, Worcester WR3 7LG
Tel: (0800) 592436
Wide range of wheelchairs and scooters for
hire, nationwide.

BUSES
First Midland Red: Tel: (01905) 763888
County Bus Line: Tel: (0345) 125436

DIAL Worcester
54 Friary Walk, Crowngate Centre,
Worcester WR1 3LE
Tel: (01905) 27790   Fax: (01905) 612692
Minicom: (01905) 22191

TAXIS
Associated Blue Star Taxis:
Tel: (01905) 610022
Two adapted vehicles.

Central Taxis: Tel: (01905) 22292
15 adapted vehicles.
Crown Radio Taxis: Tel: (01905) 357788
Two adapted vehicles.
Knights Radio Taxis: Tel: (01905) 617171
Two adapted vehicles.

TRAINS
Wales and West: Special Needs –
Tel: (0345) 125625
Minicom: (0345) 585469
Worcester Foregate and Shrub Hill are
suitable for wheelchairs using ramp access.

CAR PARKS
Free three-hour orange badge parking in
some council-owned car parks, some on-
street parking. A map is available from DIAL.

SHOPMOBILITY
Crowngate Shopping Centre, Worcester
Tel: (01905) 610523

HOTEL
FOWNES HOTEL   🚶
City Walls Road, Worcester WR1 2AP
Tel: (01905) 613151   Fax: (01905) 23742
No. of Accessible Rooms: 1
Accessible Facilities: Lounge, restaurant
Former Victorian glove factory converted
into an interesting-looking, modern hotel
in the city centre.

SELF-CATERING
HIDELOW LODGE   ♿
Hidelow House, Acton Green,
Acton Beauchamp, Worcester WR6 5AH
Tel: (01886) 884547   Fax: (01886) 884060
e-mail: hidelow@aol.com
web: www.cadenza.org/hidelow
No. of Accessible Units: 1. Shower.
Accessible Facilities: Lounge,
kitchen,private garden.
Newly refurbished detached stone building,
set in grounds of small secluded country
house with lovely views.

ATTRACTIONS
THE COMMANDERY CIVIL WAR CENTRE
Sidburgh,
Worcester WR1 2HU
Tel: (01905) 355071
NB. We have included this museum

because it is unique, but beyond the entrance and the shop, there is a heavily cobbled path to the museum. This was the Royalist headquarters at the Battle of Worcester in 1651. The museum tells the turbulent story of the English Civil War with scenes, models and interactive displays. Originally a monastic hospital, it was bought privately by the wealthy Wylde family after the Dissolution. From 1900-1975 the building housed a printing factory until purchased by the local council and restored. This is the only museum in England dedicated to the Civil War and, if the cobblestones can be managed, it is well worth a visit. At weekends activities such as re-enactments, historical crafts, etc. take place in the charming garden.

SD ♿ CP ♿ E ♿ RF- Cobblestones
C ♿ S ♿ WC ♿

THE MUSEUM OF WORCESTER PORCELAIN
Severn Street, Worcester WR1 2NE
Tel: (01905) 23221   Fax: (01905) 617807

The first Worcester porcelain, manufactured here in 1751, specialised in tableware and ornamental vases in distinctive vivid colours. The museum has a Georgian Gallery including vignettes of dining scenes, and shop fronts that show the collections in an historical context. The Victorian Gallery offers a contrast to the C18th displays as design and the social history of the Victorian era unfolds. There is an extensive shop and factory seconds shop, plus demonstrations. Much to see, do – and buy!

SD ♿ CP ♿ E ♿ RF ♿ L ♿
C ♿ S ♿ WC ♿

WORCESTER CATHEDRAL
The Dean and Chapter, 10A College Green, Worcester WR1 2LH
Tel: (01905) 21004 Fax: (01905) 611139

Dominated by a fine C14th. tower, much of the cathedral belongs to this period, although the See was founded in 650 and there have been previous buildings on this site. Among notable things to see are the monumental effigy of King John; the C16th. Prince Arthur's chantry, built by Henry VII for his son who died at Ludlow in 1502; fine misericords and works by famous sculptors.

There are superb glass windows and a modern altar hanging, in the colours of the liturgical year, representing the cathedral's pinnacles as reflected in the river Severn. Although the quire is on a higher level than the nave, it can be entered using a different entrance door. A ramped access (gradient:1:19) to the cloisters is clearly marked. The crypt, lady chapel, library and tower are not accessible.

SD ♿ CP n/a E- ♿ RF ♿ C ♿
S ♿ WC ♿

SPETCHLEY PARK GARDEN
Spetchley Park, Worcester WR5 1RS
Tel: (01905) 345213

Located three miles east of the city, this 100-acre deer park and 30-acre garden contains a large collection of trees and shrubs, many rare or unusual.

SD ♿ CP ♿ E ♿ RF- ♿
C ♿ RFE ♿

SPORTING VENUE
WORCESTER RACECOURSE
Pitchcroft, Worcester WR1 3EJ
Admin & Booking-Box Office: (01905) 25364
Fax: (01905) 617563

Complies with Part M, Building Regulations.

CP ♿ RE ♿ ED ♿ (except manual door)
INT ♿ L ♿ (attended)
WC ♿ (Gents, ground floor, Ladies, first floor)
SS ♿ (Lift access) Designated viewing platform by track at the winning post route through the grandstand main entrance and by lift to the first floor   B/R ♿

THEATRE
WORCESTER SWAN THEATRE
The Moors, Worcester WR1 3EP
Admin: (01905) 726969
Fax: (01905) 723738
Booking-Box Office: (01905) 27322

SD ♿   CP ♿ Public CP – Pitchcroft car park, rear of theatre, access via sloping road.
Taxi rank – city centre, payphone on the premises.
RE ♿ ED ♿ INT ♿
WC ♿ (access via double doors adjacent to auditorium
AUD ♿ B/R ♿
Add. Notes: Route to wheelchair spaces position 'A' on level through Aud. doors to Row A: position 'B' as above and across front of seating in Row A to far end of Row A. Transfer seating into wide seat at either end of Row A.

HERTFORDSHIRE

HERTFORDSHIRE ASSOCIATION FOR THE DISABLED
The Woodside Centre, The Commons,
Welwyn Garden City AL7 4DD
Tel: 01707 324581   Fax: 01707 371297
e-mail: herts_action@dial.pipex.com
The association runs an Easier Living
Exhibition of useful equipment with help
and advice, together with general
information and counselling services. They
offer a wheelchair-accessible taxi service,
holiday fact sheets and a purpose-built
hotel in Clacton.

HERTS and DISTRICT ADD/ADHD SUPPORT GROUP
23 Foxglove Bank, Royston SG8 9TH
Tel: (01763) 242782   Fax: (01762) 245892

HERTFORDSHIRE ACTION ON DISABILITY
Tel: (01707) 324581
Transport Service: Tel: (01707) 375159
Fax: (01707) 371297
e-mail: herts_action@dial.pipex.com

HERTFORDSHIRE TRAVEL LINE
Tel: (0345) 244344

BROXBOURNE
PARADISE WILDLIFE PARK
White Stubbs Lane, Broxbourne EN10 7QA
Tel: (01992) 470490   Fax: (01992) 440525

Touch and feed the paddock animals
including zebras and camels and meet lion
and tiger cubs in this family-run leisure park
Parking and approach   E   C
S   WC

HATFIELD
Divided into the old and the new, the
latter an industrialised area, the former
retaining its historic character with half-
timbered C16th houses and Georgian
properties.

ATTRACTION
HATFIELD HOUSE and GARDEN
Hatfield AL9 5NQ
Tel: (01707) 262823   Fax: (01707) 275719
Jacobean house built by Robert Cecil, the
1st Earl of Salisbury in 1611. This is where
Elizabeth I spent much of her childhood.
The state rooms are rich in world-famous
paintings, the old kitchen offers cooking
implements from long ago, and there are
superb examples of Jacobean craftsman-
ship throughout. NB. A special entrance
for wheelchair users is via a long even
pathway and electronic doors. The code is
given at the front entrance. The end of
the path is rather cobbled and bumpy.
SD   CP   E RF   L
C   S   WC   G

HEMEL HEMPSTEAD
Developed market town with attractive
stretches along the river Gade.

Diner is served. The state rooms at Hatfield House.

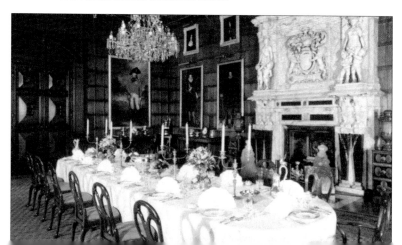

REACH OUT PROJECTS CANAL BOATS
Diocesan Education Centre, Hall Grove,
Welwyn Garden City AL7 4PJ.
Tel: (01707) 335968   Fax: (01707) 373089
e-mail: stalbansdys@enterprise.net
Reach out projects include Enable holidays
for a weekend or a few days that provide
resource for young people of all abilities.
Narrow and wide-beam boats are moored
on the Grand Union Canal and are
available for self-steer hire or skippered.

ST. ALBANS
This beautiful and ancient city was one of
the most important Roman towns. It has
an historic city centre with narrow, twisting
and hilly streets and several coaching inns
and houses of medieval construction.

TOURIST INFORMATION CENTRE
Town Hall, Market Place, St. Albans
Tel: (01727) 864511
Fax: (01727) 863533
web: www.stalbans.gov.uk

ST. ALBANS CITY and DISTRICT COUNCIL
St. Peter's Street, St. Albans AL1 3JE
Tel: (01727) 866100
Fax: (01727) 845658

BUSES
Arriva: (Helpline) Tel: (0345) 788788
Sovereign: Tel: (01727) 854732

TAXIS
Goldline Taxis: Tel: (01727) 840000
Four adapted vehicles.
Arena Taxis: Tel: 901727) 844844
One adapted vehicle.

TRAINS
Thameslink: Special Needs –
Tel: (0207) 6206333
Minicom: (0207) 6205561
Stationlink bus: Tel: (0207) 9183312

HOTEL
HERTFORDSHIRE MOAT HOUSE
London Road, Markyate,
Nr. St. Albans AL3 8HH
Tel: (01582) 449988 Fax: (01582) 842282
No. of Accessible Rooms: 140

Accessible Facilities: Restaurant, lounge
Re-opened in January 2000, convenient for
the M1 but with pleasant rural outlook.

ATTRACTION
THE GARDENS OF THE ROSE
Chiswell Green Lane, St. Albans AL2 3NR
Tel: (01727) 850461   Fax: (01727) 850362
e-mail: mail@rnrs. org.uk
Gardens of the Royal National Rose Society
with over 30,000 plants in 1,650 different
varieties, including old-fashioned and
modern roses and roses of the future. This
is the International Trial Ground for new
roses.

ROMAN THEATRE
Gorhambury Drive, St. Michaels,
St. Albans AL3 6AH
Tel: (01727) 835035
Built about AD160 and excavated in 1935,
this semi-circular theatre is unique.
about 60m across it held 1,600
spectators.

VERULAMIUM MUSEUM
St. Michaels Street, St. Albans AL3 4SW
Tel: (01727) 819339 Fax: (01727) 859919
A museum of everyday life in Roman
Britain, it stands on the site of
Verulamium, one of the most important
cities in Roman Britain. Excavated
objects range from mosaics to everyday
pottery and metalwork.

BOWMANS OPEN FARM
Coursers Road, London Colney,
St. Albans AL2 1BB
Tel: (01727) 822106 Fax: (01727) 826406
Farm trail past paddocks of pigs, cattle
and sheep and a working farmyard. Pets
Corner; tractor rides in an Adventure
Playground; watch cows being milked;
see hawks and falcons in the falconry
area; the wildlife on the lake and visit an
Indoor touching Barn.

De HAVILLAND HERITAGE and MOSQUITO AIRCRAFT MUSEUM

PO Box 107, Salisbury Hall, London Colney, St. Albans AL2 1EX
Tel: (01727) 822051

This is the oldest aviation museum in Britain. It opened in 1959 on uneven, but accessible land with 20 types of de Havilland aircraft with hands-on experience and working displays. The Mosquito was made of a light but strong balsa wood sandwich. Timber was used during the war because it was easier to obtain than metal and so furniture factories were able to build aircraft.

SD   CP   E   RF
C   WC   RFE

THEATRE
MALTINGS ART THEATRE
The Maltings, St. Albans AL1 3HL
Tel: (01727) 844222   Fax: (01727) 836616

CP   RE   ED   INT – Box Office
Counter   widths   L   AUD
B/R

STEVENAGE

There are both old and new towns, the latter, spacious, modern and well-planned and the old retaining its charm and historical interest with many old cottages and houses now turned into shops.

STEVENAGE SHOP MOBILITY
15 Queensway, Stevenage
Tel: (01438) 350300

HOTEL
NOVOTEL STEVENAGE
Knebworth Park
Stevenage SG1 2AX|
Tel: (01438) 742299   Fax: (01438) 723872
No. of Accessible Rooms: 2. Bath
Accessible Facilities: Lounge, restaurant.

WATFORD

Hertfordshire's largest town with a long, narrow high street leading to the river Colne that skirts the hills on which the town stands. C16th and C18th houses are still to be found, although the town is much modernised.

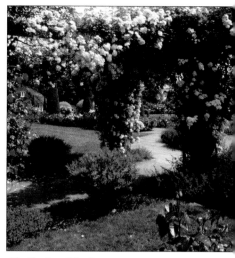

The Garden of the Roses.

ATTRACTION
WATFORD MUSEUM
194 High Street, Watford WD1 2HG
Tel/fax: (01923) 232297

A Watford Football Club display includes Elton John associations, historic printing presses, a reconstructed Victorian bar, and a collection of paintings and sculpture.

SD   CP   E   RF
L   C n/a   S   WC

WELWYN

Small old town with much charm: many of the houses are Georgian and the river Mimram runs through the village.

ATTRACTION
SHAW'S CORNER (NT)
Ayot St. Lawrence, Nr. Welwyn AL6 9BX
Tel/Fax: (01438) 820307

An Edwardian villa and home of playwright George Bernard Shaw. Presented much the way he left it to the NT. The ground floor (study, drawing room, dining room, kitchen) is level with wide doors. Outside, access to the garden is via the front door, down a ramp and through a side gate. Gravel paths and grassy slopes lead to the lawns.

CP   E   WC   G

ISLE OF MAN

ISLE OF MAN TOURISM
Sea Terminal Building, Douglas IM1 2RG
Tel: (01624) 686 766   Fax: (01624) 627 443
e-mail: tourism@gov.im
web: www.gov.im/tourism

MANX FOUNDATION FOR THE PHYSICALLY DISABLED
Marsham Court Day Centre, Victoria Avenue,
Douglas IM2 4AW
Tel: (01624) 628926   Fax: (01624) 670821

BALLAUGH

This is a large expanse of marshland in north of the island.

ATTRACTION
CURRAGHS WILDLIFE PARK
Ballaugh
Tel: (01624) 897323   Fax: (01624) 897327
A wide range of species of animals and birds in natural settings with large walk-through enclosures. Located midway between Kirkmichael and Ramsey.

SD [♿]   CP [🚶]   E [♿]   RF [♿]
C [♿]   S [♿]   WC [🚶]

DOUGLAS

Rather grand Victorian resort and the island's capital, with sweeping promenade, hotels, attractive quayside and yacht haven, entertainment and activities.

HOTEL
SEFTON HOTEL   [♿]
Harris Promenade, Douglas IM1 2RW
Tel: (01624) 645500   Fax: (01624) 676004
Web: www.seftonhotel.co.im
No. of Accessible Rooms: 3. Bath
Accessible Facilities: Lounge, restaurants (2), pool, sauna, whirlpool. Located on the promenade next to the Gaiety Theatre, with a wide range of facilities.

ATTRACTION
MANX MUSEUM AND NATIONAL TRUST
Douglas IM1 3LY
Tel: (01624) 648000   Fax: (01624) 648001
The Story of Man with a film portrayal of Manx history combined with gallery displays. NB: Entrance is stepped at 7.5cm from the pavement.

SD [♿]   CP [♿]   E [♿]   RF [♿]
L [♿]   C [🚶]   S [♿]   WC [♿]

Craggy Port Erin.

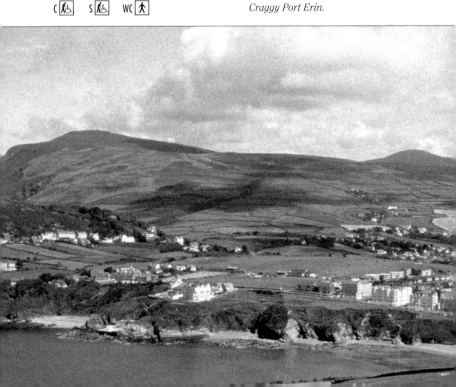

SELF-CATERING
KIONSLIEU FARM COTTAGES
Kionslieu Farm, Higher Foxdale IM4 3HB
Tel/Fax: (01624) 801349
No. of Accessible Units: 1 (Cottage No. 5).
Bath. No. of Beds per Unit: 4
Accessible Facilities: Open plan
kitchen/diner, sitting room. Combination
of newly built and renovated farm
buildings in a rural location about 10
minutes' drive from Douglas. Cottage 5
has been created from a former dairy and
is by a wooded area.

PORT ERIN
Located in south-west region with rocky
inlets, lovely beaches and a beach
lighthouse.

SELF-CATERING
THE CHERRY ORCHARD APARTMENTS
Port Erin IM9 6AN
Tel: (01624) 833811   Fax: (01624) 835060
e-mail: enquiries@cherry-orchard.com
web: www.cherry-orchard.com
No. of Accessible Units: 1. Roll-in Shower.
No. of Beds per Unit: 4
Accessible Facilities: Lounge, dining
room, pool, Jacuzzi, bar. Situated near the
lovely bay at Port Erin, 200m from the
beach.

SANTON

HOTEL
MOUNT MURRAY HOTEL
AND COUNTRY CLUB
Santon IM4 2HT
Tel: (01624) 661111   Fax: (01624) 661116
e-mail: mountmurray@advsys.net
web: www.mountmurray.com
No. of Accessible Rooms: 8. Bath
Accessible Facilities: Lounge, restaurants,
not all tables in bistro are accessible.
Sports hall, driving range.
Modern hotel in 200 acres overlooking the
island's newest golf course with an
extensive leisure complex.

ISLES OF SCILLY
An Area of Outstanding Beauty, an
archipelago of granite islands and outcrops,
five of which are inhabited, concentrated
mainly on St. Mary's. The islands are
famous for bird life and seals, particularly
on the more remote spots. There is a
flourishing flower industry, notably
narcissi, with about 30 million blooms
harvested from October to March and
shipped worldwide. The Gulf Stream
ensures the Scillies enjoy the mildest UK
climate, although Atlantic winds mean
considerable rainfall.

ST. MARY'S
The largest island with nine miles of
coastline. Hugh Town has most amenities,
including the famous Mermaid pub.

TOURIST INFORMATION CENTRE
Old Wesleyan Chapel, Well Lane, Hugh Town,
St. Mary's TR21 0JD
Tel: (01720) 422536   Fax: (01720) 422049
e-mail: steve@scilly.demon.co.uk

TAXIS
No taxis are licensed on the islands, The
matter is in the hands of solicitors!

FERRIES
Isles of Scilly Steamship Co.
Tel: (01736) 362009
Foot passengers only, wheelchairs carried
as cargo.

WHEELCHAIR HIRE
Round Table: Tel: (01720) 422786
Buckaboo Bike Hire: Tel: (01720) 422289

SELF-CATERING
ALTAMIRA FLATS
Porthlow Farm, St. Mary's TR21 0NF
Tel: (01720) 422636
No. of Accessible Units: 1
No. of Beds per Unit: 6
Accessible Facilities: Kitchen,
lounge/diner. Close to Porth Loo Beach
and under a mile to Hugh Town.

ISLE OF WIGHT

ISLE OF WIGHT TOURISM
Westridge Centre, Brading Road,
Ryde PO33 1QS
Tel: (01983) 823873
e-mail: post@isle-of-wight-tourism.gov.uk
web: www.isle-of-wight-tourism.gov.uk

DIAL Isle of Wight
Riverside Centre, The Quay, Newport PO30 2QR
Tel: (01983) 522823

BUSES
Southern Vectis: Tel: (01983) 827005
Some low-floor buses.

TAXIS
Able Taxis: Tel: (01983) 522968
One adapted minibus.
Norman Bakers Taxis: Tel: (01983) 403545
Two adapted vehicles.

TRAINS
Island Line: Tel: (01983) 812591
Accessible for wheelchairs, ring in advance.

FERRIES
Red Funnel, a car ferry from Southampton,
and Wightlink, a passenger ferry from
Portsmouth and Lymington. See under
Ferries in the Introduction.

CAR PARKING
Tel: (01983) 522823
Free unlimited orange badge parking.

ALUM BAY
Home to amazing multi-coloured cliffs and
the Needles.

ATTRACTION
NEEDLES PLEASURE PARK
Alum Bay PO39 0JD
Tel: (01983) 752401   Fax: (01983) 755260
Family attraction with rides and
entertainment plus a chairlift to the beach
to see the unique coloured sands.

SD   CP   E   RF
C   S   WC

BINSTEAD
Village two miles west of Ryde.

ATTRACTION
BRICKFIELDS HORSECOUNTRY
Newnham Road, Binstead PO33 3TH
Tel: (01983) 566801   Fax: (01983) 562649
e-mail: brickfields@binsteadiow
web: www.brickfields.co.uk
Shire horses, miniature ponies, heritage
and carriage collections. Most is outside
over several acres, flat and unobstructed,
except where ramped for bar/restaurant.
The restaurant ramp gradient is 1:5.

SD   CP   E   C n/a
S   WC   RFE

BRADING
One of the oldest towns on the island, and
an ancient port with the remains of an
extensive Roman villa built AD300 and a
C12th parish church.

ATTRACTION
OASIS
Carpenters Road, Brading PO36 0QA
Tel: (01983) 613760   Fax: (01983) 615335
World of indoor living with a delightful
range of arts and crafts shops.

SD n/a   CP   E   RF
C   S   WC

COWES
Located on the northern tip of the island.
Linked with sailing and boatbuilding and a
mecca for yachtsmen, particularly during
the international festival of Cowes Week
during the first week of August.

TOURIST INFORMATION CENTRE
The Arcade, Fountain Quay, Cowes PO31 3AR
Tel: (01983) 291914   Fax: (01983) 280078

SELF-CATERING
NEW STABLE COTTAGE
Little Thorness Farm, Nr. Cowes PO31 8NG
Tel: (01983) 297863
No. of Accessible Units: 1. Bath
No. of Beds per Unit: 2
Accessible Facilities: Dining room.
The cottage is central to the working farm

here. In summer the beach is accessible by car for accompanied wheelchair users.

ATTRACTION
ISLE OF WIGHT MODEL RAILWAYS
The Parade, Cowes PO31 7QJ
Tel/Fax: (01983) 280111

Not just a model railway layout, but a view of the world in miniature. A large diorama gives a picture of the English countryside as many different toy and model trains from the turn of the century onwards run. A delightful experience. Changes of level are by ramps at 1:18 and the exhibition can be seen from all view points.

SD n/a   CP 🚻♿   E ♿   RFE 🚻♿

OSBORNE HOUSE
York Avenue, East Cowes PO32 6JY
Tel: (01983) 200022   Fax: (01983) 281380

Designed by Prince Albert, and built between 1845/48 to resemble an Italian villa. This was Queen Victoria's favourite home. It is untouched, the state and family apartments are open to the public and the grounds are full of English trees, a miniature fort and a Swiss cottage. NB: The car park is 300m. from house and so is inaccessible.

SD ♿   CP n/a   E 🚻♿   RF ♿
C ♿   S ♿   WC 🚹

NEWPORT
The island's capital was originally an inland port, located in the centre of the island with some attractive old quays.

TOURIST INFORMATION CENTRE
The Car Park, South Street,
Newport PO30 1JU
Tel: (01983) 525450   Fax: (01983) 822929

ATTRACTIONS
CARISBROOKE CASTLE (E.H.)
Carisbrooke, Newport PO30 1XY
Tel: (01983) 529130   Fax: (01983) 528632

This is the only medieval castle on the island. It has Elizabethan and Jacobean additions, and Charles I was a prisoner here in 1647. NB. Entrance ramped at a gradient of 1:11

SD ♿   CP n/a   E 🚹   RF ♿   C ♿
S 🚹   WC 🚹

GUILDHALL MUSEUM
High Street, Newport PO30 1TY
Tel: (01983) 823366   Fax: (01983) 823841

Explore the island's history in this new museum using touch-screen computer technology, hands-on exhibits, microscopes, quizzes and games.

SD ♿   CP n/a   E ♿   RF ♿
S ♿   WC 🚹

Carisbrooke Castle. The enforced home of Charles I – for a while.

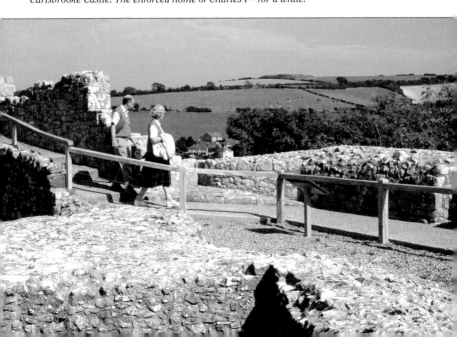

RYDE

The Island's largest town with six miles of sandy beaches stretching from west of the pier through to Springvale, and excellent leisure facilities.

TOURIST INFORMATION CENTRE
81-83 Union Street, Ryde PO33 2LW
Tel: (01983) 562905   Fax: (01983) 567610

BED AND BREAKFAST
SEAWARD GUEST HOUSE 　　　　　　[🏃]
14-16 George Street, Ryde PO33 2EW
Tel/Fax: (01983) 563168
No. of Accessible Rooms: 1. Bath
Accessible Facilities: Dining room on first floor (no lift) but meals can be served in rooms. Located very close to all the major transport and entertainment centres plus shopping, cafes and restaurants.

ATTRACTIONS
L.A.BOWL
The Pavilion, The Esplanade, Ryde PO33 2EL
Tel: (01983) 617070   Fax: (01983) 611581
web: www.wight-ads.co.uk/labowl
This family entertainment centre incorporates tenpin bowling, a children's indoor adventure play area and restaurants. The centre is open plan, on one level with a shallow ramp to the bowling lanes. Special equipment allows wheelchair users to enjoy bowling, including specially designed launching chutes and small ramps to gain access to the approaches (a small step of 5cm).
SD [♿] 　CP [♿] 　E [♿] 　RF [♿]
C [♿] 　WC [♿]

WALTZING WATERS
Westridge, Brading Road, Ryde PO33 1QS
Tel/Fax: (01983) 811333
An elaborate and exciting water, light and music production with thousands of dazzling patterns of moving water synchronised with music.
SD [♿] 　C P [♿] 　E [♿] 　RF [♿]
S [♿] 　WC [🏃] 　RFE [♿]

SANDOWN

A holiday resort bay with a fine sandy beach and a pier packed with amusements.

TOURIST INFORMATION CENTRE
The Esplanade, Sandown, PO36 8DA
Tel: (01983) 403886   Fax: (01983) 406482

SELF-CATERING
BARN and MIDDLE BARN 　　　　　[🏃]
Knighton Farm, Newchurch,
Sandown PO36 0NT
Tel/Fax: (01983) 865349
No. of Accessible Units: 2. Bath
No. of Beds per Unit: Barn-4, Middle Barn-5
Accessible Facilities: Living/dining room, kitchen. Small sheep farm in a lovely area between Ryde and Newchurch to the south of the Downs. Two cottages of three in a C17th listed barn, 50m from the farmhouse. Surrounded by a large lawn with delightful views of the countryside.

ATTRACTION
FRONT LINE AND AVIATION MUSEUM
Sandown Airport, Sandown PO36 0JP
Tel: (01983) 404448
90 years of aviation history from Louis Bleriot's flight across the Channel in 1909, and the Red Baron's triplane, to the jet age, displayed in two hangars.
SD [♿] 　CP [♿] 　E [♿] (entrance from rear car park direct into hangers, opened when required).
RF [♿] 　C- [♿] 　S [♿] 　WC [🏃] 　RFE [♿]

AMAZON WORLD
Watery Lane, Newchurch,
Nr. Sandown PO36 0LX
Tel: (01983) 867122   Fax: (01983) 868560
Over 200 different species of rare and exotic animals, birds, reptiles and insects set in a natural jungle environment that recreates the story of the rainforest.
SD [♿] 　CP [♿] 　E [♿] 　RF [♿] 　C [♿]
S [♿] 　WC [🏃] 　RFE [♿]

SHANKLIN

A popular family resort, Shanklin offers a sandy beach, safe bathing and entertainment, and a charming older village with a collection of lovely thatched cottages, antique shops and fragrant gardens.

TOURIST INFORMATION CENTRE
67 High Street, Shanklin PO38 6JJ
Tel: (01983) 862942   Fax: (01983) 863047

TOTLAND BAY
Quiet sandy beach with pier, promenade and restaurant in the west of the Island.

HOTEL
COUNTRY GARDEN
Church Hill, Totland Bay PO39 0ET
Tel/Fax: (01983) 754521
No. of Accessible Rooms: 4
Accessible Facilities: Lounge, restaurant. Charming small hotel in lovely grounds.

VENTNOR
Mediterranean in ambience and style, this Victorian spa town is built on terraces that climb steeply towards St. Boniface Down where there are superb views across the bay.

TOURIST INFORMATION CENTRE
34 High Street, Ventnor PO38 1RZ
Tel: (01983) 853625   Fax: (01983) 856232

ATTRACTION
BLACKGANG CHINE FANTASY PARK
Glackgang, Nr. Ventnor PO38 2HN
Tel: (01983) 730330   Fax: (01983) 731267
Set in 40 acres of cliff-top gardens. Rides and attractions include Maritime World, a Pirate Ship, a wild west town, dinosaurs, troublesome goblins and a sawmill.

SD CP E RF C S WC RFE

ISLE OF WIGHT OWL AND FALCONRY CENTRE
Appledurcombe House, Wroxall,
Nr. Ventnor PO38 3EQ
Tel: (01983) 852484
Baroque elegance is evident in this partly restored building aided by Capability Brown ornamental gardens and 11 acres of grounds containing the Falconry Centre. The house is surrounded by level flagstones and there is good access inside with no more than a couple of steps. The cellars are not accessible. Impacted gravel paths in the grounds are difficult for wheelchairs. Cars with disabled visitors should report to the shop from where they can proceed to the house. Assistance is available in Falconry Centre if requested.

SD CP E RF C S WC RFE

RARE BREEDS AND WATERFOWL PARK
Undercliff Drive (A3055),
St. Lawrence, Ventnor PO38 1UW
Tel: (01983) 852582
75% ACCESSIBLE BUT TELEPHONE IN ADVANCE.
One of largest survival collections with over 40 rare breeds of cattle, deer, sheep, pigs, ponies, miniature horses, llamas, owls and other species. Natural streams, ponds and lakes house waterfowl and poultry: lovely picnic areas and aviaries. Separate entrance from lower car park avoids some of the worst gradients. The key to this entrance is available on request from the main entrance.

SD CP E RF C S WC RFE

YARMOUTH
Not an over-populated area with rolling countryside and breathtaking views, Yarmouth is the main town in West Wight with a pretty harbour and a castle built by Henry VIII.

TOURIST INFORMATION CENTRE
The Quay, Yarmouth PO41 4PQ
Tel: (01983) 760015   Fax: (01983) 761047

ATTRACTION
FORT VICTORIA MODEL RAILWAY
Fort Victoria, Westhill Lane,
Yarmouth PO41 0RR
Tel: (01983) 761553
This is the largest and most advanced model railway layout in Britain. Both the Model Railway and Maritime Museum here are accessible. The Boathouse Cafe, Planetarium, Aquarium and Country Park are not accessible.

SD CP E- RF C n/a S WC RFE

149

KENT

DISABILITY INFORMATION SERVICES
20 Cheriton Gardens, Folkestone CT20 2AP
Tel: (01303) 226464 Fax: (01303) 226312
Local, regional and national information for those with a disability or their carers and families on a wide range of subjects including domestic and international holidays.

PUBLIC TRANSPORT HELPLINE
Tel: (08457) 696996

ASHFORD
A changing market town, once a major rail works and now an embarkation point for Eurostar services to France and Belgium. The town holds a regular cattle auction, one of the oldest of its kind in the country. The largest factory shop outlet in Europe is near the station.

TOURIST INFORMATION CENTRE
18 The Churchyard, Ashford TN23 1QG
Tel: (01233) 629165 Fax: (01233) 639166

ATTRACTIONS
BEECH COURT GARDENS
Challock, Nr. Ashford TN25 4DJ
Tel: (01233) 740735 Fax: (01233) 740842
Unbordered woodland garden where the discovery of Roman artefacts suggests the site is ancient. Developed to harmonise with the seasons and produce interest and colour throughout the year.

SD ♿ CP 🚶 E ♿ RF ♿
C 🚶 S 🚶 WC 🚶 G ♿

SOUTH OF ENGLAND RARE BREEDS CENTRE
Woodchurch, Ashford TN26 3RJ
Tel: (01233) 861493 Fax: (01233) 861457
The farm is owned and run by Canterbury Oast Trust, a charity providing homes, training and supported work experience for learning and physically disabled adults. All staff are experienced in understanding the needs of disabled people. The farm is home to 44 rare British farm breeds with plenty of hands-on experience.

SD ♿ CP ♿ E ♿ RF ♿ C ♿
S ♿ WC 🚶

RFE- Outdoor open farm with park surfaces varying in quality and construction. Most is accessible, although some is bumpy. Paths vary from brick and concrete to dirt and grass. Woodland inaccessible.

BEXLEY/BEXLEYHEATH
HOTEL
SWALLOW HOTEL ♿
1 Broadway, Bexleyheath DS6 7JZ
Tel: (020) 8298 1000   Fax: (020) 8298 1234
No. of Accessible Rooms: 2. Bath
Accessible Facilities: Lounge, restaurant, disabled lift for access to Leisure Club and hoist into pool, bar.

FORTE POSTHOUSE BEXLEY 🚶
Black Prince Interchange, Southwold Road, Bexley DA5 1ND
Tel: (01322) 526900   Fax: (01322) 526113
No. of Accessible Rooms: 1
Accessible Facilities: Lounge, restaurant, lift. A mile from Bexleyheath town centre, this is convenient for visitors to Greenwich, Leeds Castle and the Thames Barrier and is 35 minutes by train to central London.

BIRCHINGTON

ATTRACTION
QUEX HOUSE and GARDENS and POWELL-COTTON MUSEUM
Quex Park, Birchington CT7 0BH
Tel: (01843) 842168   Fax: (01843) 846661
Built as a Regency gentleman's country residence with oriental and period furniture on display, themjuseum has eight galleries with an amazing variety of items and the walled gardens have been returned to their Victorian splendour.

SD ♿ CP ♿ E ♿ RF ♿ C ♿
S ♿ WC 🚶

Features. Museum floors are level except between galleries 2 and 3 where there is a mobile ramp. Ramped also between the museum and the house. Gardens are gravelled but surface changes are planned.

CANTERBURY
A beautiful and picturesque city, most famous for its cathedral to which Chaucer's pilgrims and many others came to visit the

shrine of Thomas à Becket, murdered here in the C12th. The city is the centre of Christianity in England. Half the city's medieval walls, dating back to the C13th and C14th, stand. St. Martin's is probably the oldest church in England still in use.

CANTERBURY, HERNE BAY and WHITSTABLE TOURISM
c/o Canterbury City Council, Military Road, Canterbury CT1 4YW
Tel: (01227) 763763   Fax; (01227) 763727
web: www.canterbury.gov.uk

TOURIST INFORMATION CENTRES
34 St. Margaret's Street, Canterbury CT1 2TG
Tel: (01227) 766567   Fax: (01227) 459840

Coach Car Park, Kingsmead, Canterbury
Tel: (01227) 451096

BUSES
Stagecoach East Kent: Tel: (01227) 472082
No low-floor buses in Canterbury
Kent County Council Transport Services:
Tel: (01622) 605022/605098

TAXIS
Cabco: Tel: (01227) 455455
11 adapted vehicles.
Lynx Taxis: Tel: (01227) 464232
Eight adapted vehicles.
Procab: Tel: (01227) 478338
Five adapted vehicles.

TRAINS
Connex South Eastern: Customer Services:
Tel: (0870) 6030405   Fax: (0870) 6030505

CAR PARKS
The city centre is pedestrianised. Orange badge holder parking in Watling Street; behind Woolworth's in Canterbury Lane; behind the Library in Orange Street (specifically for O.B.H.)

HOTEL
HOLIDAY INN EXPRESS
Upper Harbledown,
Canterbury CT2 9HX
Tel: (01227) 865000   Fax:

The Black Prince's effigy.

(01227) 865100
No. of Accessible Rooms: 5
Accessible Facilities: Lounge, restaurant. Modern business-style property located on A2, four miles east of the city centre.

BED AND BREAKFAST
DELIGHTFUL B & B
1 Dryden Close, off Pilgrim Way,
Canterbury CT1 1XW
Tel: (01227) 764799
No. of Accessible Rooms: 1 - single. Shower
Accessible Facilities: Dining room, garden. Charming property with glorious garden in quiet cul-de-sac a short distance from the city centre. Owners are very welcoming and experienced in respite care.

ATTRACTIONS
ASH COOMBE VINEYARD
Coombe Lane, Ash, Canterbury
Tel: (01304) 813396
Small family-owned vineyard with grass path. WC facility within the family home. Experience with PHAB groups.

SD ♿	CP ♿	E ♿	RF ♿
S ♿	WC ♿	RFE ♿	

CANTERBURY CATHEDRAL
The Precincts, Canterbury CT1 2EH
Tel: (01227) 762862   Fax: (01227) 865222
e-mail: visits@canterbury-cathedral.org
Mother church of the Anglican community, dominating the city. A centre of pilgrimage for many centuries, the Shrine of Thomas à Beckett is a main attraction. The treasures of the shrine were carried off during the Dissolution and of the original cathedral nothing remains, but there is a great deal to see and much of its medieval design, including fine stained glass and central Bell Harry Tower remain. The C15th nave is high, narrow and awe-inspiring. Only one English king, Henry IV, is buried here, lying beside his queen, Joan of Navarre in Trinity Chapel. Access is by the NW door, lift into the quire. The crypt is ramped at 1:7, and together with Corona and Martyrdom are not accessible.

SD ♿	CP ♿	E ♿
RF ♿	L ♿	Cn/a
	S ♿	WC ♿

CANTERBURY TALES VISITOR ATTRACTION
St. Margarets Street, Canterbury CT1 2TG
Tel: (01227) 454888 Fax: (01227) 765584
Fine reconstruction of the C14th world of
Chaucer's famous pilgrims as they journey
from the Tabard Inn, London towards the
shrine of St. Thomas à Becket at Canterbury
Cathedral. Medieval streets, houses and
markets, together with Becket's shrine.
SD/CP n/a Nearest parking in Watling Street.
E 🦽 RF 🦽 L 🦽 C 🦽
S 🦽 WC 🚶 RFE 🦽

HOWLETTS WILD ANIMAL PARK
Bekesbourne, Canterbury CT4 5EL
Tel: (01303) 264647 Fax: (01303) 264944
Home to a famous breeding colony of
captive lowland gorillas, African elephants,
tigers, lemurs, deer, antelope, snow leopards
and more in natural style surroundings.
SD 🦽 CP 🦽 E 🦽 RF 🦽 C 🦽
S 🦽 WC 🚶

PARSONAGE FARM RURAL HERITAGE CENTRE
North Elham, Canterbury CT4 6UY
Tel: (01303) 840766 Fax: (01303) 840183
Family-run for over 100 years, this working
farm in situated in heart of the Elham valley
on the north Downs. Part of the farmhouse
dates from medieval times. Explore 600
years of history following trails around the
farm with old and rare animal breeds. Plants,
butterflies typical of the area. There is a
little museum in the farmhouse and visitors
can browse around the barns.
SD 🦽 CP 🦽 E 🦽 RF 🚶
C 🦽 S 🦽 WC 🚶

ST. AUGUSTINES ABBEY (EH)
Longport, Canterbury CT1 1TF
Tel/Fax: (01227) 767345
Explore the abbey founded in 598 by St.
Augustine after he was sent by Pope Gregory
from Rome to convert pagan King Ethelbert
of Kent. The abbey served for 1,000 years
until the Dissolution. This is one of the
most important religious sites in England.
Remarkable artefacts have been uncovered
during archaeological digs on the site.
A Batteridar is available free of charge.
**SD/CP n/a Nearest parking is at the corner of
Longport and Lower Chantry Lane.**
E 🦽 RF 🦽 S 🦽 WC 🦽 RFE 🦽

WINGHAM BIRD PARK
Rusham Road, Wingham, Canterbury CT3 1JL
Tel: (01227) 720836 Fax: (01227) 722452
Delightful park with a variety of purpose-
built environments, including walk-through
orchard aviary, pet village, landscaped
lakes and exhibition room.
SD 🦽 CP 🦽 E 🦽 RF 🦽 C 🦽
S 🦽 WC 🚶 RFE 🦽

THEATRE
MARLOWE THEATRE
The Friars, Canterbury
Tel: (01227) 787787
A side entrance is ramped. Bell for quick
access through the door. There is a
platform to the booking office.

CHATHAM
A busy commercial town where Charles
Dickens spent some of his boyhood. The
gates to the docklands are worth seeing,
and there are good parks and gardens.

ATTRACTION
ROYAL ENGINEERS MUSEUM OF MILITARY ENGINEERING
Brompton Barracks, Chatham ME4 4UG
Tel: (01634) 406397 Fax: (01634) 822371
e-mail: remuseum.rhgre@gtnet.gov.uk
Government designation as museum with
outstanding collection. Displays of
equipment, working models, costumes and
curios from around the world.
SD 🦽 CP 🦽 E 🦽 C 🚶
S 🚶 WC 🦽

DOVER
Famous for its castle begun in 1168 and
used as a military base until the 1980s, its
white cliffs and as a major Channel port.

TOURIST INFORMATION CENTRE
Townwall Street, Dover CT17 1JR
Tel: (01304) 205108 Fax: (01304) 225498

HOTEL
THE PLOUGH TRAVEL INN 🚶
Folkestone Road, Dover CT15 7AB
Tel: (01304) 213339
No. of Accessible Rooms: 4

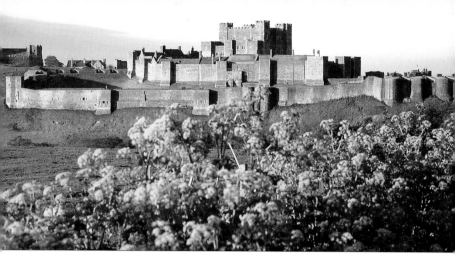

Dover Castle. The first view of England for many would-be invaders.

Accessible Facilities: Lounge, restaurant. Located on the B2011 between Dover and Folkestone.

ATTRACTIONS
DOVER CASTLE
Castle Hill Road, Dover CT16 1HU
Tel: (01304) 211067   Fax: (01304) 214739
Standing on a high hill, dominating the town and harbour, the castle was a military headquarters until the 1960s. Today much of its 2,000 year history can be experienced by visitors. Its underground tunnel system that was a command centre where many important decisions of WWII were made, is now open to the public.

SD   CP   E   C
S [♿]   WC [♿]   F [♿]

DOVER OLD TOWN GAOL
Biggin Street, Dover CT16 1DL
Tel: (01304) 202723   Fax: (01304) 201200
AV and talking TV heads take visitors back to Victorian England to experience the horrors of life behind bars. Reconstructed courtroom, exercise yard and cells.

SD [♿]   CP [♿]   E [♿]   S [♿]

THE WHITE CLIFFS EXPERIENCE
The Market Square, Dover CT16 1PB
Tel: (01304) 210101   Fax: (01304) 212057

e-mail: tourism@doveruk.com
Three floors tell the story of Dover since prehistoric times, using original artefacts, fine art and graphics. Roman Encounters and Our Finest Hours relive those periods.

SD [♿]   CP [♿]   E [♿]   RF [♿]
L [♿]   C [♿]   S [♿]   WC [♿]   RFE [♿]

Early immigration officer at the White Cliffs experience

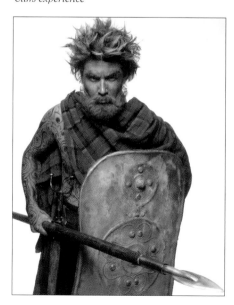

FAVERSHAM

ATTRACTION
FARMING WORLD
Nash Court, Boughton, Faversham ME13 9SW
Tel: (01227) 751144 Fax: (01795) 520813
e-mail: farmingworld@freeserve.co.uk
Traditional farm animals, rare breeds, heavy horses, farming bygones in the shape of machinery and methods and seasonal fruit are part of this charming attraction.

SD 🚹 CP 🚹 E 🚹 RF 🚹 C 🚹
S 🚹 WC 🚹 RFE 🚹

FOLKESTONE
A popular seaside resort with Victorian hotels and guest houses on the front. Old buildings are towards the harbour with some fine paths in and around the town with extensive views of the white cliffs.

TOURIST INFORMATION CENTRE
Harbour Street, Folkestone CT20 1QN
Tel: (01303) 258594 Fax: (01303) 259754
Covers The Garden Coast of Folkestone, Hythe and Romney Marsh.

HOTEL
GARDEN LODGE 🚶
324 Canterbury Road, Densole,
Folkestone CT18 7BB
Tel/Fax: (01303) 893147
e-mail: gardenlodge@tritontek.com
No. of Accessible Rooms: 1
Accessible Facilities: Lounge, restaurant, indoor pool with four steps. Attractive family hotel in extensive gardens with pets' corner, barbecue and patios. Three miles from Folkestone and 12 from Canterbury.

GILLINGHAM
Prehistoric and Roman traces have been found in this modern town.

ATTRACTION
ROYAL ENGINEERS MUSEUM
Prince Arthur Road, Gillingham ME4 4UG
Tel: (01634) 406397 Fax: (01634) 822371
Displays of equipment, working models, and a costume and curio collection.

SD CP E RF
C 🚶 S 🚹 WC 🚶

LYDD
Noted for the pinnacled tower of its parish church of the 13 and 15th centuries.

ATTRACTION
DUNGENESS RSPB NATURE RESERVE
Boulderwall Farm, Dungeness Road
Lydd TN29 9PN
Tel: (01797) 320588 Fax: (01797) 321962
This is a coastal reserve of over 2,000 acres of shingle beach and flooded pits, famous for rare migrants and permanent species. The two-mile nature trail can be traversed by wheelchair, although the shingle surfaces may prove difficult. Four of five bird-watching hides have low windows for wheelchair visitors, and may be reached by car on request.

SD 🚹 CP 🚹 E 🚹 RF 🚹
C 🚶 S 🚶 WC 🚶 RFE 🚹

MAIDSTONE
County town with many C14th buildings, parks and gardens all worth visiting.

TOURIST INFORMATION CENTRE
The Gatehouse, The Old Palace Gardens,
Mill Street, Maidstone ME15 6YE
Tel: (01622) 602169 Fax: (01622) 673581

SELF-CATERING
COURTLODGE COTTAGES
West Peckham, Maidstone ME18 5JN
Tel/Fax: (01622) 812529
Two accessible cottages:
STAPLE COTTAGE 🚹
No. of Accessible Units: 1. Bath
No. of Beds per Unit: 6
Accessible Facilities: Lounge, dining room.
LIME TREE COTTAGE 🚶
No. of Accessible Units: 1. Bath
No. of Beds per Unit: 3
Accessible Features: lounge, dining room. In a quiet village with little traffic, both cottages are full of character and many original features. A pub with food that welcomes wheelchair users is 50m away on a hard surface.

ATTRACTIONS
BEARSTED VINEYARD
24 Caring Lane, Bearsted,

154

Maidstone ME14 4NJ
Tel/Fax: (01622) 736974
e-mail: enquiries@bearstedwines.co.uk
web: www.bearstedwines.co.uk

Produces award-winning English wines from fresh grapes grown in the open. White, red and rose wines are made in the on-site winery.

SD ♿   CP ♿   Entrance ♿   C n/a   Shop ♿
Wine is sold to callers from the house. Groups are given tastings at the winery and can buy wine there.

WC ♿   Almost Cat.1 (apart from g horizontal support rail position from centre of seat).

Features ♿ . Winery is level except for one small area.

LEEDS CASTLE
Maidstone ME17 1PL
Tel: (01622) 765400   Fax: (01622) 735616
e-mail: enquiries@leeds-castle.co.uk
web: www.leeds-castle.co.uk

Located on two small islands in the middle of an encircling lake, this most English of castles was the home of the manor of the Saxon royal family in the C9th. The castle has been a Norman stronghold, a royal residence for six of England's medieval queens and a palace for Henry VII. Now restored, it offers collections of paintings, furnishings and tapestries. In the 500-acre park are woodlands, lakes, waterfalls, and gardens. There is an accessible route that includes a Stannah Stair Lift between the Heraldry Room and a corridor to main visitor route. The castle provides a comprehensive leaflet for visitors with disabilities. The entrance is ramped at gradient of 1:8 with a threshold of 20cm. Well worth the effort. Free wheelchair loan available.

SD ♿   CP ♿   E- (ramped at 1:8)
RF ♿   L--Wheelchair lift.   C ♿
S 🚶   WC 🚶

MUSEUM OF KENT LIFE – COBTREE
Lock Lane, Sandling, Maidstone ME15 9UY
Tel: (01622) 763936   Fax: (01622) 662024

Open-air working farm and social history museum of 50 acres with many farm and domestic buildings of various vintages. Other attractions include herb, hop and vegetable gardens.

SD ♿   CP ♿   E ♿   RF ♿
C ♿   S ♿   WC 🚶   RFE ♿

Leeds Castle is stunning for all visitors.

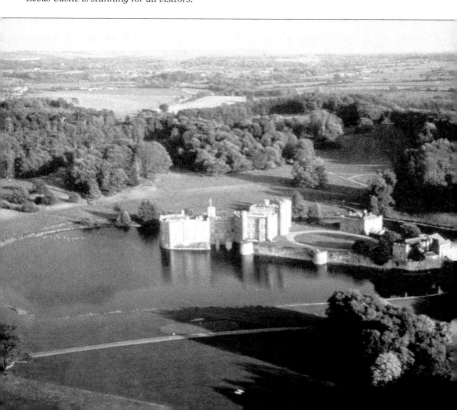

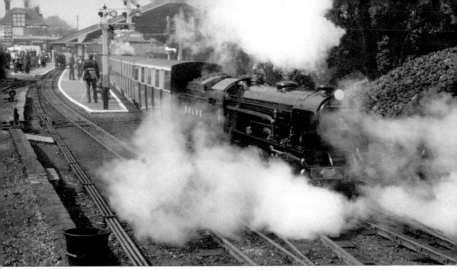

Letting of steam at the Romney Hythe and Dymchurch Railway.

NEW ROMNEY

One of the original Cinque Ports although now a mile from the sea. The church, once lapped by the sea, has fine stained-glass windows and is in the Norman style.

TOURIST INFORMATION CENTRE
(Summer months only)
Magpies, Church Approach,
New Romney TN28 8QT
Tel: (01797) 364044 Fax: (01797) 364194

BED AND BREAKFAST
DOLLY PLUM COTTAGE
Burmarsh Road, Burmarsh,
Romney Marsh TN29 0JT
Tel: (01303) 874558
No. of Accessible Rooms: 1
Accessible Facilities: Dining room
Idyllic cottage in lovely countryside location, a short distance from Channel access and a few minutes from nearest beach.

ATTRACTION
ROMNEY, HYTHE AND DYMCHURCH RAILWAY
New Romney TN28 8PL
Tel: (01797) 362353 Fax: (01797) 363591
e-mail: RHDR@dels.demon.co.uk
A mainline railway built for a millionaire racing driver in the 1920s with all locomotives and carriages one third full size. It runs from Hythe, via Dymchurch, St. Mary's Bay and New Romney to fishermen's cottages at Dungeness.

TRAIN – 1 disabled coach taking three wheelchairs and four helpers. Coach has on-board ramps, panoramic windows and large sliding doors.
NB. ADVANCE NOTICE REQUIRED.

SD ⬚ CP ⬚ E ⬚ C ⬚
S ⬚ WC ⬚

RAMSGATE

Refined seaside resort and working port with Channel access to France/Belgium. Victorian redbrick houses on the cliff top have sweeping roads down to the seafront.

TOURIST INFORMATION CENTRE
Queen Street, Ramsgate CT11 8HA
Tel: (01853) 591086

ATTRACTION
SPITFIRE and HURRICANE MEMORIAL BUILDING
The Airfield, Manston Road,
Ramsgate CT12 5DF
Tel: (01849) 821940
Situated on the site of one the very few surviving airfields that participated in the Battle of Britain. This was the closest airfield to the enemy coast and bore the brunt of Luftwaffe attacks in 1940. Fine examples of these two WWII fighter aircraft, now written in the folklore of Britain, are permanently housed here.

SD ⬚ CP ⬚ E ⬚ RF ⬚
C ⬚ S ⬚ WC ⬚ RFE ⬚

SANDWICH

Delightful old town with lovely walls. Pleasant paths along the river Stour and an old moat.

TOURIST INFORMATION SERVICE
Guildhall, Sandwich CT13 9AH
Tel/Fax: (01303) 613565

SELF-CATERING
THE OLD DAIRY
Updown Park Farm, Eastry, Nr. Sandwich
Bookings through Mrs. J. R. Montgomery,
Little Brooksend Farm,
Birchington Kent CT7 0JW)
No. of Accessible Units: 2
No. of Beds per Unit: 4-6: 7
Accessible Facilities: Kitchen/lounge.
21 holiday homes set in 30 acres of secluded parkland, approached via private roadway.

SEVENOAKS

Located 25 miles from London. Sadly lost all but one of its ageing oaks in the 1987 hurricane. Access point for Knole.

ATTRACTIONS
EMMETTS GARDEN (NT)
Ide Hill, Sevenoaks TN14 6BA
Tel: (01732) 750367   Fax: (01732) 868193
Standing on one of highest spots in Kent with fine views over the unspoilt Weald, this charming garden was laid out in the late C19th with exotic and rare trees and shrubs. There are formal, rock, south and north gardens, a bluebell bank and woodlands that surrounds the garden.

SD [⌘]   CP [⌘]   E [⌘]   RF [⌘]
C [⌘]   S [⌘]   WC [⌘]   G [⌘]

SEVENOAKS WILDFOWL RESERVE
Bradbourne Vale Road, Sevenoaks TN13 3DH
Tel: (01732) 456407
First example in Britain of a gravel-pit being developed for nature conservation. 135 acres of equal proportions of water and land. Ponds and reedbeds combine with woodland. There is access to visitor centre, except one first-floor display, and three bird-watching hides. 50% of the nature trail is accessible by car.

SD [⌘]   CP [⌘]   E [⌘]   RF [⌘]
C [⌘]   S [⌘]   WC [⌘]   RFE [⌘]

SITTINGBOURNE

Situated in the Medway and Maritime area, between Whitstable and Chatham.

BED AND BREAKFAST
PALACE FARMHOUSE   [⌘]
Chequers Hill, Doddington,
Sittingbourne ME9 0AU
Tel: (01795) 886820
No. of Accessible Rooms: 1.
Accessible Facilities: Lounge, dining room
Early Victorian farmhouse set in orchards on the edge of the village of Doddington.

ATTRACTION
THE DOLPHIN SAILING BARGE MUSEUM
Crown Quay Lane, Sittingbourne
Tel: (01795) 423215
History of the Thames sailing barge with large display of tools, models, plans and photographs. Inlet alongside the museum usually contains at least one vessel brought to the yard for restoration, including the *Cambria*, launched in 1906. She was the last vessel in the UK to carry commercial cargo under sail. Shipwright's shop, forge and barge are on the level: The sail loft is up a flight of stairs.

SD [⌘]   CP [⌘]   E [⌘]   RF [⌘]
S [⌘]   WC [⌘]   RFE [⌘]

157

STAPLEHURST
ATTRACTION
BRATTLE FARM MUSEUM
Brattle Farm,
Staplehurst TN12 0HE
Tel: (015980) 891222
Privately owned, unique country collection dealing with agricultural bygones, showing country life, skills and tools from rural trades and crafts of the past two centuries. Housed in old cowsheds and oast house of the farm. NB. By appointment only. The first floor is not accessible.

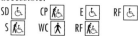

SD [⌘]   CP [⌘]   E [⌘]   RF [⌘]
S [⌘]   WC [⌘]   RF [⌘]

TENTERDEN

A charming town, its high street lined with shops and houses still retaining their original facades from Elizabethan to Georgian times. Many antique shops.

HOTEL
LITTLE SILVER COUNTRY HOTEL
Ashford Road, St. Michaels,
Tenterden TN30 6SP
Tel: (01233) 850321   Fax: (01233) 850647
No. of Accessible Rooms: 3. Bath
Accessible Facilities: Lounge, restaurant.
Charming country house hotel with a personal touch. Victorian style conservatory and delightful gardens.

TUNBRIDGE WELLS

Forest until discovered in 1606, this is a tranquil country town with much charm and taste in its architecture, parks and gardens.

TOURIST INFORMATION CENTRE
The Old Fish Market, The Pantiles,
Tunbridge Wells TN2 5TN
Tel: (01892) 515675   Fax: (01892) 534660
Produces *Access in Tunbridge Wells*.

BUSES
Arriva Kent and Sussex: Tel: (01634) 281100
Some low-floor routes.

TAXIS
Goodfellows Taxis (Paddock Wood):
Tel: (01892) 837799
Five adapted vehicles.
Kent and Sussex Cars: Tel: (01892) 513377
Three adapted vehicles.

TRAINS
Connex South Eastern: Customer Services:
Tel: (0870) 6030405   Fax: (0870) 6030505
Minicom: (01233) 617621

CAR PARKS
Free orange badge parking in all borough council car parks.

SHOPMOBILITY
Lower Mall, Royal Victoria Place.
Tel: (01892) 544355

HOTELS
THE SPA HOTEL
Mount Ephraim, Royal Tunbridge Wells TN4 8XJ
Tel: (01892) 520331   Fax: (01892) 510575
e-mail: info@spahotel.co.uk
web: www.spahotel.co.uk/
No. of Accessible Rooms: 1. Bath
Accessible Facilities: Lounge, restaurant, pool, sauna, gardens. Built in 1766 this is a family owned hotel set in 15 acres of fine gardens overlooking the town.

JARVIS INTERNATIONAL HOTEL
8 Tonbridge Road, Pembury,
Tunbridge Wells TN2 4QL
Tel: (01892) 823567   Fax: (01892) 823931
No. of Accessible Rooms: 2. Bath
Accessible Facilities: Lounge, restaurant, steam and beauty rooms.
Quality modern hotel on the east of town.

ATTRACTIONS
TUNBRIDGE WELLS MUSEUM AND GALLERY
Civic Centre, Mount Pleasant,
Royal Tunbridge Wells TN1 1JN
Tel: (01892) 526121   Fax: (01892) 534227
Museum displays local and natural history, archaeology and agricultural artefacts: the art gallery has changing exhibitions.
SD | CP | E | L | Thyssen Stairlift
S

SISSINGHURST CASTLE GARDEN
Sissinghurst, Cranbrook TN17 2AB
Tel: (01580) 715330   Fax: (01580) 713911
Transformed by Vita Sackville-West and Harold Nicholson in the 1920s into one of the finest gardens in the country. Each area is planted with colour or seasonal theme, notably White and Cottage Gardens.
Located 12 miles east of town.
SD | CP | E | RF | C
S | WC | G

BEWL WATER
Lamberhurst, Tunbridge Wells TN3 9JH
Tel: (01892) 890661   Fax: (01892) 890232
Largest area of inland water in the south east, with 21kms of shore line to explore.
SD CP E C
S   WC   RFE

LANCASHIRE

DIAL WEST LANCS
Skelmersdale Library, Skelmersdale
Tel: (01695) 51819

GENERAL INFORMATION ON ALL TRANSPORT
Tel: (0870) 6082608
Minicom: (01257) 241693

ST. HELENS DISABILITY NETWORK
64/66 Bickerstaff Street, St. Helens
Tel: (0500) 827463

WARRINGTON DISABLED LIVING CENTRE
Beaufort Street, Warrington
Tel: (01925) 240064

SPECIALIST OUTDOOR ACTIVITIES
NEW HORIZONS
Bookings: 2 Fishers Bridge, Hayfield, High
Peak SK22 2JZ
Tel: (01663) 742796)
Information: 63 Carver Road, Marple,
Stockport, Gtr. Manchester, SK6 7PS
Tel: (0161) 449 7787
Canal boat trips and cruises designed for
disabled people navigated by skipper and
volunteer crew. The narrow boat is fully
accessible with boarding ramp and lift, fully
accessible WC, raised open viewing deck at
front. The Cheshire Canal Ring serves
Manchester as a vast water pleasure ground,
and New Horizons is based in Marple, 11
miles SE of Manchester's city centre.

ACCRINGTON
Originally an East Lancashire Mill town,
now without the chimneys or the smoke.

LANCASHIRE'S HILL COUNTRY TOURISM
Freepost NWW8077, Accrington BB5 0ZZ
Tel: (01254) 380678   Fax: (01254) 380600
e-mail: lhc@hyndburnbc.gov.uk

TOURIST INFORMATION CENTRE
Town Hall, Blackburn Road,
Accrington BB5 1LA
Tel: (01254) 386807   Fax: (01254) 380291

ATTRACTION
OSWALDTWISTLE MILLS
Moscow Hill, Collier Street, Oswaldtwistle,
Accrington BB5 3HL
Tel: (01254) 871025   Fax: (01254) 770790
A family attraction, set within one of the
very few remaining Victorian mills still
producing cotton fabric and owned by the
same family since 1847. Start in the
handloom weaver's cottage of 1700 and
learn about the Industrial Revolution. Also
includes reconstructed Victorian factory
yard, craft workshops, traditional sweet
factory, gardens and wildfowl preserve. An
excellent day out.

SD 🚻   CP 🚻   E 🚶   C 🚶
S 🚶   WC 🚶   RF 🚶

BLACKBURN
Deeply involved in the Industrial Revolution,
this old mill town has, in recent years, seen
much development and re-planning.

TOURIST INFORMATION CENTRE
King George Hall, Northgate,
Blackburn BB2 1AA
Tel: (01254) 53277   Fax: (01254) 683536

BED AND BREAKFAST
MYTTON FOLD HOTEL AND GOLF COMPLEX 🚶
Whalley Road, Langho, Blackburn BB6 8AB
Tel: (01254) 240662   Fax: (01254) 248119
e-mail: Hotel@virgin.net
web: SmoothHound.co.uk/hotels/mytton.html
No. of Accessible Rooms: 3
Accessible Facilities: Lounge, restaurant,
gardens. Independent hotel run by third-
generation family at the gateway to Ribble
Valley. Lovely gardens from where to enjoy
views of Pendle Hill, guardian of C17th
secrets of the famous Pendle witches.

ATTRACTION
WAVES WATER FUN CENTRE
Nab Lane, Blackburn BB2 1LN
Tel: (01254) 511111   Fax: (01254) 268801
Tropical water park with shipwreck slide,
hot tub, alien encounter, white knuckle
ride, and disabled sessions.

SD 🚻   CP 🚻   E 🚻   RF 🚻   L 🚻
C 🚻   S 🚻   WC 🚶

SPORTING VENUE
BLACKBURN ROVERS FOOTBALL AND ATHLETIC PLC
Ewood Park, Blackburn BB2 4JF
Tel: (01254) 698888   Fax: (01254) 671042
Booking: Telesales (01254) 296100
Ticket Office: (01254) 296214
Minicom: (01254) 668008
Facility complies with Part M, Building Regulations. Trophy awarded by Minister for Sport in 1988 for Best Disabled Facilities in the Premier League.
CP | RE | ED | INT
L | WC | (20 units located in all stands)
SS | From designated entrance gate on level, unobstructed route to designated spaces at ground floor level.   B/R – Lift Access.

BLACKPOOL
An extremely popular holiday resort stretching along the Lancashire coast, with every conceivable form of entertainment. Its landmark tower offers an outstanding view. Trams run along the promenade and its famous Christmas illuminations are spectacular, as is its Pleasure Beach.

TOURIST INFORMATION CENTRES
1 Clifton Street, Blackpool FY1 1LY
Tel: (01253) 478222/477477
Fax: (01253) 478210
e-mail: blackpool.tourism@dial.pipex.com
Publishes *Special Needs Guide to Blackpool*.

Blackpool Pleasure Beach, Unit 11, Ocean Boulevard, Blackpool FY4 1PL
Tel: (01253) 403223   Fax: (01253) 408718

BLACKPOOL TRANSPORT
Tel: (01253) 473001
General information for Blackpool.

BUSES
Easy Access Handy Bus: Tel: (01253) 473000

TAXIS
Blacktax: Tel: (0585) 175321 (mobile), (07930) 578401 (mobile)
'C' Cabs: Tel: (01253) 62201
10 adapted vehicles.
Radio Cabs: Tel: (01253) 293222
Four adapted vehicles.

TRAINS
First North Western: Special Needs: Tel: (0845) 6040231
Northern Spirit: Special Needs: Tel: (0845) 6008008
Virgin Trains: Special Needs: Tel: (0845) 7443366
Minicom: (0845) 7443367

CAR PARKS
Municipal surface car parks – three hours free orange badge parking, thereafter normal rates apply.
Tel: (01253) 291091

SHOPMOBILITY
Winifred Street, Blackpool FY1 4ST
Tel: (01253) 753331

HOTEL
BOND HOTEL
120 Bond Street, South Shore, Blackpool FY4 1HG
Tel: (01253) 341218   Fax: (01253) 394952
No. of Accessible Rooms: 19. Roll-in Shower Accessible Facilities: Lounge, dining room, bar, sun roof. Award winning hotel for able-bodied and disabled guests. Located

Blackpool tram and the famous tower.

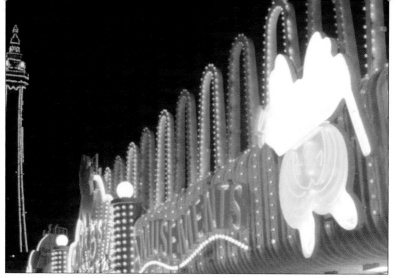

The lights of Blackpool. Not quite Vegas, but more accessible for most.

close to the promenade, Pleasure Beach and Sandcastle Leisure Complex. The Lido Swimming Pool that is equipped for disabled visitors is also close by.

SHELLARD HOTEL 🏠
18-20 Dean Street, South Shore,
Blackpool FY4 1AU
Tel/Fax: (01253) 342679

No. of Accessible Rooms: 10. Roll-in Shower Accessible Facilities: Lounge, restaurant, bar. Both disabled and able-bodied guests are welcome here in a hotel very close to the Pleasure Beach, Sandcastle Leisure Centre and Granada Studios.

ATTRACTIONS
BLACKPOOL PLEASURE BEACH ARENA
Ocean Boulevard, Blackpool FY4 1EZ
Tel: (01253) 341033   Fax: (01253) 405467

Over 145 rides and attractions, plus spectacular shows. The Accessibility Guide Book is comprehensive and worth obtaining from the number above. For full details of catering and shopping facilities, plus rides, check the guide.

SD 🦽   CP 🚹   E 🦽   WC 🚹

BLACKPOOL ZOO
East Park Drive, Blackpool FY3 8PP
Tel: (01253) 765027 Fax: (01253) 798884

Wheelchair access throughout on tarmac paths with no major slopes or gradients .

32-acre park, its population divided into weather-orientated regions from tropical forest and hot grasslands and desert through to winter regions, water world, farming and domestic exhibits.

SD 🦽   CP 🚹   E 🦽   RF 🦽   C 🦽
S 🦽   WC 🦽   RFE 🦽

BURNLEY
TOURIST INFORMATION CENTRE
Burnley Mechanics, Manchester Road,
Burnley BB11 1JA
Tel: (01282) 455485   Fax: (01282) 457428

ATTRACTION
TOWNELEY HALL ART GALLERY AND MUSEUMS
Burnley BB11 3RQ
Tel: (01282) 424213   Fax: (01282) 436138

Home of the Townley family from C14th until 1902, offering a glimpse of how the family lived. Original period rooms include the Elizabethan long gallery and Regency rooms, Victorian kitchen together with fine glass, ceramic and oak furniture collections. The Museum of Local Crafts and Industries tells the story of the inhabitants at home and at work. Together with the Natural History Centre, this is a wonderful day out.

NB. Accessible entrance at rear by request.

SD 🦽   CP 🚹   E 🦽   RF 🦽
C 🦽   S 🦽   WC 🚹   RFE 🦽

CLITHEROE

A very old Ribble Valley town with pleasant country atmosphere and lovely walks. The C12th. castle, set on limestone crag, is a dominant landmark and much of its grounds are part of a recreational area.

TOURIST INFORMATION CENTRE
12-14 Market Place, Clitheroe BB7 2DA
Tel: (01200) 425566   Fax: (01200) 426339

SELF-CATERING
HIGHER GILLS FARM
Rimington, Clitheroe BB7 4DA
Tel: (01200) 445370
No. of Accessible Units: 1. Bath
No. of Beds per Unit: 3 – 4
Accessible Facilities: Lounge, dining room, kitchen, patio and lawn. Working farm with sheep and cows with two apartments. Situated at the foot of Pendle Hills, offering fine views of western Yorkshire Dales and Trough of Bowland.

LANCASTER

Surrounded by superb moorland where Lancashire and Yorkshire meet, the history of the town dates back 7.5 centuries, some buildings still survive from this period.

TOURIST INFORMATION CENTRE
29 Castle Hill, Lancaster LA1 1YN
Tel: (01524) 32878   Fax: (01524) 847472
Web: www.lancaster.gov.uk

LANCASTER CITY COUNCIL
Tel: (01524) 582000
Minicom: (01524) 582175/582875
Produces *Lancaster, Morecambe and District Access Guide*.

DISC (Disablement Information Support Centre)
Trinity Community Centre,
Middle Street, Lancaster LA1 1JZ
Tel: (01524) 34411/32660
e-mail: disc@lancasterdisc.free-on-line.co.uk
People with disabilities providing information and support for others.

BUSES
Lune Valley Transport: Tel: (01524) 844944
Operate a semi-scheduled service, but need 48hrs' notice.
Stagecoach: Tel: (01772) 886633

TAXIS
Beatstream: Tel: (01524) 32090
Five adapted vehicles.
D & c Taxis: Tel: (01524) 69824
One adapted vehicle.
Westgate Taxis: Tel: (01524) 412781

TRAINS
First North Western: Special Needs:
Tel: (0845) 6040231
Virgin Trains: Special Needs:
Tel: (0845) 7443366
Minicom: (0845) 7443367

HOTELS
LANCASTER HOUSE HOTEL
Green Lane, Ellel, Lancaster LA1 4GJ
Tel: (01524) 844822   Fax: (01524) 844766
e-mail: lanchouse@elh.co.uk
No. of Accessible Rooms: 4
Accessible Facilities: Lounge, restaurant, limited access because on split levels with pillars. Pre-book for accessible area, bar. Prestigious property located close to the city, and three minutes from the M6.

THURNHAM MILL HOTEL
Thurnham, Lancaster LA2 0BD
Tel: (01524) 752852   Fax: (01524) 752477
No. of Accessible Rooms: 4. Bath
Accessible Facilities: Lounge, restaurant
Historic C16th converted mill beside a canal, close to the remote Forest of Bowland with high moorland and fine views over the Flyde Coast and Lune Valley. For nearly 100 years the mill was driven by canal water, whereas most mills are driven by rivers.

ATTRACTIONS
LANCASTER MARITIME MUSEUM
Custom House, St. George's Quay,
Lancaster LA1 1RB
Tel: (01524) 64637   Fax: (01524) 841692
Discover Lancaster's seafaring history spanning 2,000 years from Roman harbour to major C18th port for the West

Indies. This waterfront museum occupies the historic Custom House of 1764 with modern displays, reconstructions, sound effects and even authentic smells!

SD ♿ CP ♿ E ♿ RF ♿
L ♿ C 🚶 S ♿ WC 🚶

PETER SCOTT GALLERY
Lancaster University, Lancaster LA1 3HB
Tel: (01524) 593057   Fax: (01524) 592603
e-mail: m.p.gavagan@lancaster.ac.uk
Although not as accessible as we would wish, this gallery houses the University's fine art collection including contemporary British artists from the St. Ives School such as Barbara Hepworth, and examples of Inuit, African ands far eastern art and ceramics.

SD ♿ CP 🚶 E 🚶 L ♿ stair lift

WILLIAMSON PARK AND BUTTERFLY HOUSE
Williamson Park, Lancaster LA1 1NX
Tel: (01524) 33318 Fax: (01524) 848338
e-mail: office@williamsonpark.u-netcom
See the colourful world of the butterfly.

SD ♿ CP ♿ E ♿ RF ♿
L ♿ C 🚶 S ♿ WC ♿

LYTHAM ST. ANNES
Some half-timbered buildings mingle pleasantly with peaceful parks and gardens. Known for its championship golf course.

TOURIST INFORMATION CENTRE
290 Clifton Drive South, Lytham FY8 1LH
Tel: (01253) 725610   Fax: (01253) 713754

HOTEL
CHADWICK HOTEL ♿ 🚶
South Promenade, Lytham St. Annes FY8 1NP
Tel: (01253) 720061 Fax: (01253) 714455
No. of Accessible Rooms: 12 (1 is Cat.1)
Accessible Facilities: Lounge, restaurant. Family owned and managed since 1947. Sea front position overlooking the Ribble Estuary and the Irish Sea.

MORECAMBE
Originally an ancient fishing village and now a popular holiday resort.

TOURIST INFORMATION CENTRE
Old Station Buildings, Marine Road Central, Morecambe LA4 4DBA
Tel: (01524) 582808   Fax: (01524) 582663

SELF-CATERING
MORECAMBE BAY BUNGALOW ♿
6 Marine Drive, Hest Bank, Morecambe LA4
Tel: (01524) 412498
No. of Accessible Units: 1
No. of Beds per Unit: 2
Accessible Facilities: Lounge, kitchen.

ORMSKIRK
Located a few miles inland of the north-east coast, south of Southport, long associated with the Stanley family, Earls of Derby from Knowsley Hall.

HOTEL
BEAUFORT HOTEL 🚶
High Lane, Burscough, Ormskirk L40 7SN
Tel: (01704) 892665   Fax: (01704) 895135
e-mail: info@beaufort.co.uk.com
web: www.Beaufort.uk.com
No. of Accessible Rooms: 1
Accessible Facilities: Lounge, restaurant, bar. Smart, modern, commercial hotel.

ATTRACTION
THE WILDFOWL and WETLANDS TRUST – MARTIN MERE
Burscough, Nr. Ormskirk L40 0TA
Tel: (01704) 895181   Fax: (01704) 892343
e-mail: Eileen.beesley@WWT
376 acres of wetlands with swan, flamingo, African, Siberian and Australasian goose and oriental and North and South American species. Special leaflet, *Access the Wild Side*, is very helpful.

SD ♿ CP ♿ E ♿ RF ♿ C ♿
S ♿ WC ♿ RFE ♿ 6 wheelchairs available.

PRESTON
Site of the Battle of Preston in 1648 and centre of the Industrial Revolution in the C18th, today the city is the legal, commercial and administrative capital of the county. Surrounded by breathtaking countryside.

TOURIST INFORMATION CENTRE
Guildhall Arcade,
Lancaster Road,
Preston PR1 1HT
Tel: (01772) 253731

HOTEL
NOVOTEL PRESTON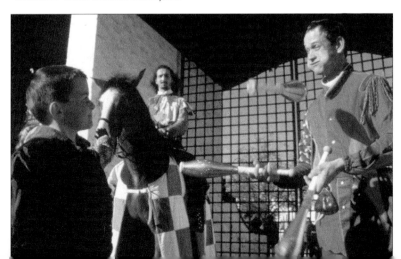
Reedfield Place,
Walton Summit,
Preston PR5 6ABA
Tel: (01772) 313331   Fax: (01772) 627868
No. of Accessible Rooms: 2. Bath
Accessible Facilities: Lounge, restaurant,
Outdoor Pool. Modern quality hotel
situated at motorway junctions 29 (M6),
(M61) and (M65): useful stop-over en route
to Wales, Scotland, midlands or southern
England.

THE GIBBON BRIDGE HOTEL
Chipping, Preston PR3 2TQ
Tel: (01995) 61456   Fax: (01995) 61277
No. of Accessible Rooms: 2, Roll-in shower
Accessible Facilities: Lounge, dining room.
Country hotel set in the Forest of Bowland.

ATTRACTIONS
ASTLEY HALL MUSEUM and ART GALLERY
Astley Park,
off Hallgate,
Chorley,
Nr. Preston PR7 1NP
Tel: (01257) 515555 Fax: (01257) 515556
400-year-old Grade 1 listed building with
much original furniture and decoration.

Ground floor accessible but Art Gallery on
first floor, with changing exhibitions is
NOT ACCESSIBLE. Video guide to upper
floors and exhibitions is available.

SD | CP | E
RF | S | WC

CAMELOT THEME PARK and RARE BREEDS FARM
Charnock Richard,
Chorley,
Preston PR7 5LP
Tel: (01257) 453044   Fax: (01527) 452320
Over 100 rides, shows and attractions on
Arthurian theme, including Merlin's Magic
Show and live jousting tournament plus
petting area in Rare Breeds Farm.

SD | CP | E | RF
C | S | WC | RFE

LONGTON BRICKCROFT NATURE RESERVE
off Liverpool Road, Longton,
Preston PR4 5YY
Tel: (01772 611497)
Covering over 11 hectares this is a wetland
reserve in two distinct areas – the southern
area set aside for recreation such as fishing
and picnics. The northern area is
established as a nature reserve with wildlife
conservation the main priority. Good range
of semi-natural habitats supporting an
extensive number of birds, mammals,
insects, wild flowers and pond life. The
visitor centre contains informative
environmental displays. NB: No shop/
catering facility on site.

CP | E | WC | RFE

'Westworld' at the Camelot theme park.

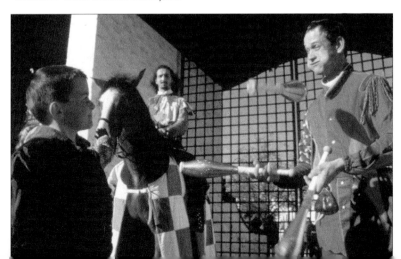

LEICESTERSHIRE AND RUTLAND

LEICESTERSHIRE AND RUTLAND GUILD OF THE DISABLED
The Guild Hall, Colton Street,
Leicester LE1 1QB
Tel: (0116) 2515565   Fax: (0116) 2519969
Minicom: (0116) 2511009

BRITISH RED CROSS
Leicestershire and Rutland Branch
244 London Road, Leicester LE2 1RN
Tel: (0116) 2705087

HINCKLEY
HOTEL
HANOVER INTERNATIONAL HOTEL   [♿]
A5 Watling Street, Hinckley LE10 3JA
Tel: (01455) 631122   Fax: (01455) 634536
Web: www.hanover-international.com
No. of Accessible Rooms: 8
Accessible Facilities: Lounge, restaurant,
bar. Extremely modern large hotel with
lovely lake running alongside, seconds
from the M69 (J1).

BED AND BREAKFAST
WOODSIDE FARM GUESTHOUSE   [♿]
Ashby Road, Stapleton, Nr. Hinckley LE9 8JF
Tel: (01455) 291929   Fax: (01455) 292626
No. of Accessible Rooms: 1. Bath
Accessible Facilities: Lounge, dining
room. Country guest house five miles
from Hinkley.

LEICESTER
Largely modern city dating back over
2,000 years with Celtish and Roman
history. The castle, built in 1088, has a
beautiful church, St. Mary de Castro, with
a superb 700-year-old font.

TOURIST INFORMATION CENTRE
7-9 Every Street, Town Hall Square,
Leicester LE1 6AG
Tel: (0116) 2998888

LEICESTERSHIRE CENTRE FOR INTEGRATED

LIVING
Tel: (0116) 2510330   Fax: (0116) 2515052
Provides general information on access to
and in the city.

BUSES
Access Bus: Tel: (0116) 2657311/2657248
Single decker following timetabled route,
but will stop on request.

TAXIS
Colemans of Leicester:
Tel: (0116) 2856126/2912317
Variety of adapted vehicles.
Kings Taxis: Tel: (0116) 2425260
Three adapted vehicles.
Gold Line Cabs: Tel: (0116) 2731110

TRAINS
Central Trains: Assistance:
Tel: (0845) 7056027
Web: www.centraltrains.co.uk
Midland Mainline: Special Needs:
Tel: (0114) 2537654
Minicom: (0845) 7078051

SHOPMOBILITY
Level 2, Shires Car Park, High Street,
Leicester and Charles Bus Station:
Tel: (0116) 2532596

HOTELS
THE RED COW   [♿]
Hinckley Road, Leicester Forest East LE3 3PG
Tel: (0116) 2387878   Fax: (0116) 2386539
No. of Accessible Rooms: 1
Accessible Facilities: restaurant
An historic inn with a thatched roof and ivy
covered frontage, recently refurbished. 31
rooms and an attractive garden. Located
close to the M1/M69 junction at Leicester.

FIELD HEAD HOTEL   [🚶]
Markfield Lane, Markfield, Leicester LE67 9PS
Tel: (01530) 245454   Fax: (01530) 243740
No. of Accessible Rooms: 1. Bath
Accessible Facilities: Lounge, restaurant
Built from local stone and in the style of its
original farmhouse building of 1672.
Situated on the edge of Charnwood Forest,
eight miles from Leicester.

LOUGHBOROUGH

Second largest town in the county with a Thursday market that began in 1206. Known for its university, and so is lively, with plenty of shops and entertainment.

HOTEL
QUALITY HOTEL ⬜🚹
New Ashby Road, Loughborough LE11 0EX
Tel: (01509) 211800   Fax: (01509) 211868
e-mail: admin@gb613.u-net.com
web: www.choicehotelseurope.com
No. of Accessible Rooms: 1. Bath
Accessible Facilities: Lounge, restaurant
Located five minutes from the M1 (J23), between Leicester and Nottingham, a good base for touring the Peak District. In the other direction are Burghley House and the lovely Georgian town of Stamford.

MARKET BOSWORTH

Village with lovely thatched cottages, a red brick and white stone hall of the English renaissance period and a Tudor grammar school where Samuel Johnson taught as second master.

BED AND BREAKFAST
BOSWORTH FIRS ⬜🚹
Bosworth Road,
Market Bosworth CV13 0DW
Tel: (01455) 290727
No. of Accessible Rooms: 1
Accessible Facilities: Lounge, dining room. Small, chalet-style dorma bungalow in pleasant, rural location surrounded front and back by fields, a mile from town.

ATTRACTION
BOSWORTH BATTLEFIELD VISITOR CENTRE
Sutton Cheney CV132 0AD
Tel: (01455) 290429   Fax: (01455) 292841
Historic site of the Battle of Bosworth Field where in 1485 King Richard 11 lost his crown and his life to the future Henry V11. Discover the sights, sound and smells of long ago in the Exhibition and Film Theatre plus 1.75 mile Battle Trail with illustrated boards detailing each stage of the battle. A useful map of the Battle Trail is available. It is a circular route, one

small section has a gradient of 1:8. This is avoidable if you take the same route to and from King Richard's Field via Ambion Wood and Henry's Lines. Battle re-enactments held annually, ring for dates.

SD ⬜ CP ⬜ E ⬜ RF 🚹 C 🚹
S 🚹 WC 🚹 RFE 🚹 Battle Trail, garden

MARKET HARBOROUGH

On Northamptonshire border, created by Henry II especially to be a market. Historically important as HQ of Royalist army on the eve of the defeat at the Battle of Naseby in 1645.

TOURIST INFORMATION CENTRE
Adam & Eve Street,
Market Harborough LE16 7AG
Tel: (01858) 821270   Fax: (01858) 821144

HOTEL
HOTHORPE HALL ♿
Theddingworth LE17 6QX
Tel: (01858) 880257   Fax: (01858) 880979
No. of Accessible Rooms: 9. Roll-in shower.
Accessible Facilities: Lounge, restaurant, lift. Primarily a Christian conference centre that also takes families and groups for holidays. Large country house in 12 acres of ground located between the M1 (J20) and Market Harborough.

OADBY

Peaceful village and suburb of Leicester, three miles from the city centre.

REGAL HERMITAGE HOTEL ⬜🚹
Wigston Road, Oadby LE2 5QE
Tel: (0116) 2569955   Fax: (0116) 2720559
Web: www.corushotels.com
No. of Accessible Rooms: 1. Bath
Accessible Facilities: Lounge, bar.
Originally a private house, now an attractive red-brick modern hotel.

ATTRACTION
FARMWORLD
Stoughton Farm Park, Gartree Road, Oadby
LE2 2FB
Tel: (0116) 2710355   Fax: (0116) 2713211

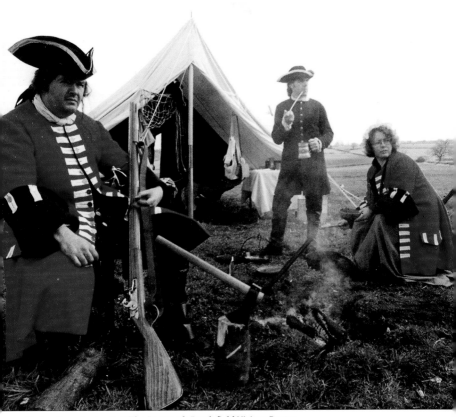

Re-inactment groups at The Bosworth Battlefield Visitor Centre.

Working farm with Children's Farmyard, Edwardian ale-house and craft shops.

SD ♿   CP ♿   E ♿   RF ♿   C ♿
S ♿   WC 🚶   RFE 🚶

UNIVERSITY OF LEICESTER BOTANIC GARDENS
Beaumont Hall, Stoughton Drive South, Oadby LE2 2NA
Tel: (0116) 2717725

The grounds of four houses, not open to the public, make up the grounds of this 16-acre garden. A wide variety of plants in many different settings. The garden is on a south-facing slope with gravel paths throughout. The herb, limestone and sunken gardens and east lawn of the hall are inaccessible.

SD ♿   CP 🚶

OAKHAM

Home of the infamous Titus Oates, this is a pleasant town with an old Butter Cross in the market place.

ATTRACTION
OAKHAM CASTLE
Market Place, Oakham
All enquiries to Rutland Co. Museum, Catmos Street, Oakham LE15 6HW
Tel: (01572) 723654   Fax: (01572) 757576

C12th fortified manor house with superb Norman Great hall. Earthworks and medieval sculptures on display.

SD ♿   CP ♿   E ♿

LINCOLNSHIRE

NORTH LINCOLNSHIRE TOURISM UNIT
The Angel, Market Place,
Brigg DN20 8LD
Tel: (01724) 297351   Fax: (01724) 297500
web: www.northlincs.gov.uk
www.barton-net.org

SOUTH WEST LINCOLNSHIRE
Guildhall Arts Centre, St. Peter's Hill,
Grantham NG31 6PZ
Tel: (01476) 590191   Fax: (01476) 591810

**LINCS. ASSOCIATION OF PEOPLE WITH
DISABILITIES**
Beech House, Witham Park,
Waterside South, Lincoln LN5 7JH
Tel: (01522) 574194   Fax: (01522) 534575

LINCOLNSHIRE COUNTY COUNCIL
City hall, Lincoln LN1 1DN
Tel: (01522) 552222   Fax: (01522) 553149
Minicom: (01522) 552055

BRIGG
Small brick town on the river Ancholme.
The mill at nearby Wrawbry is the last
working post mill in the north of England.

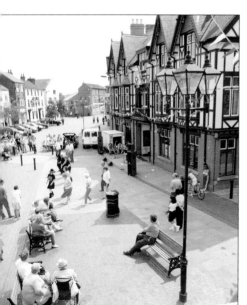

Brigg Market Place.

ATTRACTION
ELSHAM HALL COUNTRY AND WILDLIFE PARK
Elsham, Nr. Brigg DN200QZ
Tel: (01652) 688698 Fax: (01652) 688240
Miniature zoo and children's farmyard;
garden and design centre; craft and
exhibition centres; carp feeding jetty; wild
butterfly garden walkway; arboretum and
woodland garden, children's animal farm,
falconry and conservation centre.

SD [&]   CP [&]   E [&]   S [&]
WC [大]   RFE [&]

CLEETHORPES
Family resort, famous for miles of golden
sands, lovely parks and peaceful gardens.
Has one of England's few remaining piers,
now totally refurbished.

ATTRACTION
HUMBER ESTUARY DISCOVERY CENTRE
Lakeside, Kings Road,
Cleethorpes DN35 0AG
Postal address: c/o Civic Offices, Knoll Street,
Cleethorpes DN35 8LN
Tel: (01472) 323232 Fax: (01472) 323233
Combination of aquarium displays with a
state-of-the-art exhibition.

SD [&]   CP [&]   E [&]   RF [&]   L [&]
C [大]   S [&]   WC [&]   RFE [&]

GAINSBOROUGH
Britain's most inland port with attractive
an shopping centre and a fine Georgian
parish church.

SELF-CATERING
BLACK SWAN GUEST HOUSE   [大]
21 High Street, Marton,
Gainsborough DN21 5AH
Tel/Fax: (01427) 718878
No. of Accessible Units: 1. Roll-in Shower
No. of Beds per Unit: 2
Accessible Facilities: Open plan
sleeping/living/dining/kitchenette, plus
lounge in guest house. Originally part of
an C18th coaching inn, believed to have
provided accommodation to Oliver Cromwell
during the Battle of Gainsborough in 1643.

This complex of farm buildings offers one accessible unit from several around an attractive courtyard.

ATTRACTION
GAINSBOROUGH OLD HALL (EH)
Parnell Street, Gainsborough DN21 2NB
Tel: (01427) 612669 Fax: (01427) 612779
e-mail: cumminsh@lincolnshire.gov.uk
One of best preserved medieval manor houses in Britain, built by Sir Thomas Burgh c1460. Little has changed architecturally in this timber-framed building with its characteristic striped appearance. At its centre is the Great Hall where Richard III and Henry VIII once banqueted. The kitchens remain unchanged and the room settings provide historic impressions. NB. The ground floor only is accessible. Experience the upper floor through an interactive AV presentation in the shop.

SD ♿ CP n/a (nearest 200m with designated parking).
E ♿ RF ♿ C ♿ S ♿ WC n/a

GRANTHAM
Interesting red brick and stone town with a high steepled parish church. Once an important staging post on the Great North Road, now famous because Lady Thatcher was born here, and because Sir Isaac Newton was born at nearby Woolsthorpe Manor.

HOTEL
KINGS HOTEL
130 North Parade, Grantham NG31 8AU
Tel/Fax: (01476) 590800
No. of Accessible Rooms: 3. Bath
Accessible Facilities: Lounge, restaurant. Originally a Victorian gentleman's residence now well refurbished, this small, privately owned hotel is on the main northern route out of Grantham to the A1.

SWALLOW HOTEL
Swingbridge Road, Grantham NG31 7XT
Tel: (01476) 593000 Fax: (01476) 592592
No. of Accessible Rooms: 2. Bath
Accessible Facilities: Lounge, restaurant, pool (three steps). Opened in 1992, this quality courtyard-style hotel is just off the A1 near Grantham. Actively promotes its disabled facilities.

GRIMSBY
Surrounded by beautiful countryside with easy access to miles of sandy beaches, Grimsby is famous for its fishing industry.

ATTRACTION
NATIONAL FISHING HERITAGE CENTRE
Alexandra Dock, Grimsby DN31 1UZ
Tel: (01472) 323345 Fax: (01472) 323355
Fascinating history of the British fishing industry through Grimsby's vision. Experience life at sea on a trawler, hearing, smelling and touching recreated environments.

SD ♿ CP ♿ E ♿ RF ♿ L ♿
C ♿ S ♿ WC ♿ RFE ♿

LINCOLN
Few cathedrals are as awe inspiring as Lincoln's, dominating the skyline here at the top, or upper part of the city. And following the heritage trail around uphill Lincoln is a good way of discovering the city's history. The trail does need a good pusher, but the streets between the accessible attractions below are a delight. Downhill offers a medieval high bridge with half-timbered buildings and a river cruise.

TOURIST INFORMATION CENTRES
9 Castle Hill, Lincoln LN1 3AA
Tel: (01522) 873700/873703

The Cornhill, Lincoln LN5 7HB
Tel: (01522) 873703

ACCESSABILITY LINCOLN
TEL: (01673) 861556
General information for people with disabilities.

LINCOLN TIMETABLE HOTLINE
Tel: (01522) 553135
web: www.lincscc.u-net.com/bus.htm
Information on all aspects of bus and train travel in Lincoln and beyond.

BUSES
See Lincoln Timetable Hotline.
Some low-floor buses, some with tailifts.

TAXIS
Bob's Taxis: Tel: (01522) 688151
One adapted vehicle.

Ken Taylor: Tel: (0850) 479160
2 adapted vehicles.
Ted Charles: Tel: (0378) 430612
2 adapted vehicles.

TRAINS
Central Trains: Assistance:
Tel: (0845) 7056027
web: www.centraltrains.co.uk
Northern Spirit: Special Needs:
Tel: (0845) 6008008

CAR PARKS
Free orange badge spaces in all council-owned car parks and some on-street parking, map available from TIC.

SHOPMOBILITY
Tentercroft Street Car Park.

HOTEL
DAMON MOTEL   ⟨♿⟩
997 Doddington Road, Lincoln LN6 3SE
Tel: (01522) 887733   Fax: (01522) 887734
No. of Accessible Rooms: 3. Bath
Accessible Facilities: Lounge, restaurant.
Purpose-built, quality motel on Lincoln
by-pass in the south-west area of the city.

MOOR LODGE HOTEL   ⟨♿⟩
Sleaford Road, Branston, Lincoln LN4 1HU
Tel: (01522) 791366   Fax: (01522) 794389
No. of Accessible Rooms: 3. Bath
Accessible Facilities: Lounge, restaurant.
Michelin-recommended country hotel in a
village three miles south of Lincoln.

ATTRACTION
HARTSHOLME COUNTRY PARK
Skellingthorpe Road, Lincoln LN6 0EY
Tel/Fax: (01522) 686264
100 acres of heath, lawns and woodland
surrounding a large lake. Educational
visitor centre, aviary and nature trails.

| SD- ♿ | CP ♿ | E ♿ | RF ♿ |
| C ♿ | WC ♿ | | |

LINCOLN CATHEDRAL
Minster Yard, Lincoln LN2 1PX
Tel: (01522) 544544   Fax: (01522) 511307
e-mail: john.campbell13@virgin.net
This is the third largest cathedral in
England after York and St. Paul's. It was
rebuilt in 1192 in the Early English style,
enduring today, although much is Gothic,
from the C13th and C14th. The vast
interior is reached through the arch of
Exchequergate at the west front. Attractive
features include the magnificent open
nave, St. Hugh's choir, the angel choir and
the beautiful stained glass windows, the
wooden-roofed cloisters and the ten-sided
chapter house.
NB: Enter at the west front Entrance
where the external ramp is 1:7, the internal
is 1:15. Good pusher needed. The chapter
house entrance from inside the cloister is
1:26. The entrance to the choir north is
1:8, and from the nave to the choir aisle is
1:13. A motorised wheelchair is available.

| SD ♿ | CP n/a | E n/a | RF ♿ |
| C ♿ | S ♿ | WC ♿ | |

LINCOLN CASTLE
Castle Hill, Lincoln LN1 3AA
Tel: (01522) 511068   Fax: (01522) 512150
One of the first great castles built by
William the Conqueror, this was begun in
1068. For 900 years the castle has been
used as a court and a prison. Many original
features still stand, although the wall walks
are not accessible. A major highlight is the
ten-year Magna Carta exhibition that is
now in its seventh year. This document,
almost 800 years old, one of four surviving
originals sealed by King John at
Runnymede in 1215, is housed within the
exhibition. Originally every county had its
own copy. To see the real thing is an
overwhelming experience.
NB: Use Eastgate car park and entrance.

| CP ♿ | E ♿ | RFE ♿ | C ♿ |
| S ♿ | WC ♿ | G ♿ | |

MUSEUM OF LINCOLNSHIRE LIFE
Burton Road, Lincoln LN1 3LY
Tel: (01522) 528448   Fax: (01522) 521264
Award-winning social history museum
housed in extensive barracks built for
Royal North Lincoln Militia in 1857. Varied
displays depict many aspects of
Lincolnshire life including the schoolroom,
chapel, wagon and wheelwright's workshop
among many others. A delightful museum.

| SD ♿ | CP ♿ | E ♿ | RF ♿ |
| C ♿ | S ♿ | WC ♿ | |

USHER GALLERY
Lindum Road, Lincoln LN2 1NN
Tel: (01522) 527980   Fax: (01522) 560165

Lincolnshire's main visual arts venue with a permanent collections of C20th work by L S Lowry, John Piper and Walter Sickert, and topographical works depicting the county including Turner watercolours. These are combined with fine porcelain and jewellery in excellent collection.

SD ♿ CP 🚶 E ♿ (via street level entrance intercom to reception, then lifts to ground and first floors)
RF ♿ L ♿ C ♿ S 🚶 WC 🚶

RAF DIGBY SECTOR OPERATIONS ROOM MUSEUM
RAF Digby, Lincoln LN4 3LH
Tel: (01526) 327503   Fax: (01526) 327560

Just outside Sleaford, beneath a mound, is an operations room restored and refurbished to represent it as it was during WWII. RAF stations like Digby were in the front line during the war when teenage airmen took to the skies in Hurricanes, Spitfires and Lancasters. The museum was founded to commemorate their bravery.

SD ♿ CP ♿ E ♿ RF ♿ WC 🚶

MARKET RASEN

Traditional small market town with Georgian and Victorian buildings, and original shop fronts.

SELF-CATERING
ROSE COTTAGE
Ivy House, Osgodby, Market Rasen LN8 3PA
Tel/Fax: (01673) 828539
e-mail: hrosser@compuserve.com

No. of Accessible Units: 1
No. of Beds per Unit: 2
Accessible Facilities: Open plan lounge/diner/ kitchen. Own garden and patio. Delightful cottage at the rear of Ivy House garden, independent of, but close to, the main house. Own garden area with fruit trees, parking directly outside and family sheep in an adjacent field. Owned by a charming couple who will assist if necessary. Osgodby is at the foot of the Lincolnshire Wolds, four miles NW of Market Rasen. There is a pub, a shop and post office.

MININGSBY

A small village off the beaten track surrounded by quiet country lanes.

SELF-CATERING ACCOMMODATION
STAMFORD FARM HOUSE
Miningsby PE22 7NW
Tel: (01507) 588 682

No. of Accessible Units: 1. Roll-in shower
No. of Beds per Unit: 1S/1D
Accessible Facilities: Lounge, dining room, kitchen. Victorian farmhouse in village between Lincoln and Spilsbury.

SCUNTHORPE

Garden town that has evolved from five small villages in line with the development of the steel industry. Fine parklands.

ATTRACTION
NORMANBY HALL COUNTRY PARK
Normanby, Nr. Scunthorpe DN15 9HU
Tel: (01724) 720588   Fax: (01724) 721248

Sadly the hall is not accessible, it has four steps, but the remainder is good with a very pro-active principal keeper. There is a delightful Victorian walled garden, specialising in period varieties of fruit, vegetables and flowers with wide gravel, paving paths and small, fascinating museum exhibits on the life of gardeners. A farming museum with exhibits on rural trades and crafts is also accessible by a newly installed lift to the first floor. 300 acres of parkland surrounding the hall include lovely trails, impressive main lawns outside the hall and duck ponds and a deer park. A perfect place to unwind.

SD ♿ CP ♿ E ♿ RF ♿ C ♿
S ♿ WC ♿ (at car park)
L ♿ (farming museum) G ♿

SKEGNESS

Family seaside resort with six miles of sandy beaches and many attractions.

HOTEL
THE CHATSWORTH HOTEL 🚶
North Parade, Skegness PE25 2UB
Tel: (01754) 764117   Fax: (01754) 761173
e-mail: Altipper@aol.com

web: www.travelfirst.co.uk/main
/area/emid/lincolnshire/linchot/chats.htm
No. of Accessible Rooms: 1. Bath
Accessible Facilities: Lounge, restaurant,
chair lift situated in a good position on the
seafront.

THE SAXBY HOTEL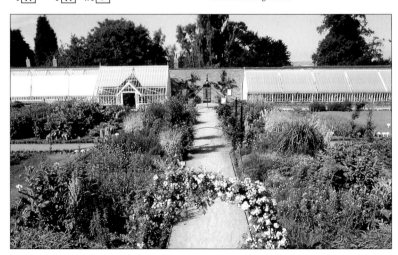
12 Saxby Avenue, Skegness PE25 3lg
Tel/Fax: (01754) 763905
No. of Accessible Rooms: 1. Bath
Accessible Facilities: Lounge, restaurant,
south-facing garden. Close to the beach
and to local amenities.

SELF-CATERING
KINGS CHALET PARK
Trunch Lane, Chapel-St-Leonards, Skegness.
Book through Grooms Holidays
No. of Accessible Units: 1
No. of Beds per Unit: 8
Accessible Facilities: Kitchen/diner, lounge.
Chalet overlooking lush green lawns in a
chalet park a few minutes away from a
picturesque village and close to Skegness
on the east Lincolnshire coast.

ATTRACTION
CHURCH FARM MUSEUM
Church Road South, Skegness PE25 2HF
Tel/Fax: (01754) 766658
e-mail: willsf@lincolnshire.gov.uk
Stroll into a bygone era in a period
furnished farmhouse, traditional farm
buildings, a thatched cottage with nurtured
flower beds and the sound of farm animals.

SD 🚹 CP 🚶 E 🚹 RF 🚹
C 🚶 S 🚶 WC 🚹

SKEGNESS NATURELAND SEAL SANCTUARY
North Parade, Skegness PE25 1DB
Tel/Fax: (01754) 764345
Known for its seal rescue centre, rearing
and returning to their natural
environment abandoned bay seal pups.
Also an aquarium, pets' corner, floral
palace and tropical house. The tropical
house is the only inaccessible area.

SD 🚻 E 🚹 RF 🚹 C 🚻
S 🚹 WC 🚹

SPALDING
A peaceful town at the centre of the flower
industry. Georgian terraces front the tree-
lined river Welland with many buildings
showing a Dutch influence.

TOURIST INFORMATION CENTRE
Ayscoughfee Hall, Churchgate,
Spalding PE11 2RA
Tel: (01775) 725458

ATTRACTION
THE BUTTERFLY and WILDLIFE PARK
Long Sutton, Spalding PE12 9LE
Tel: (01406) 363833   Fax: (01406) 363182
Utterly captivating attraction of 12 acres
that includes superb tropical house where
hundreds of butterflies enchant in natural
surroundings of pathways, bridges and

*The splendid walled garden at Normamby
Hall Country Park.*

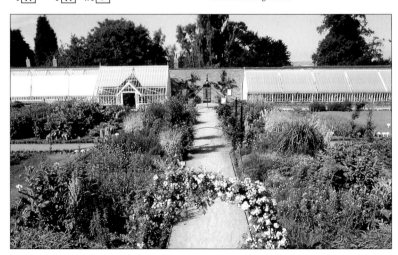

pools. In the famous Ant Room see leaf-cutting ants at work and visit the Insecteria. Bird of prey exhibits include an American bald eagle, a trained vulture and charming owls, including the Barn and Tawny species. There is a lovely café with a picnic area. Wheelchairs available. Owned and run by charming couple, this is a must.

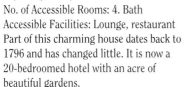

STAMFORD
The town still retains its medieval street pattern of narrow passageways and cobbled streets opening out into spacious squares. Superb historical architecture remains, most of the town is devoid of C20th or Victorian buildings. The water meadows are right in the centre of the town.

HOTEL
GARDEN HOUSE HOTEL
St. Martins, Stamford PE9 2LP
Tel/Fax: (01780) 763359
No. of Accessible Rooms: 4. Bath Accessible Facilities: Lounge, restaurant Part of this charming house dates back to 1796 and has changed little. It is now a 20-bedroomed hotel with an acre of beautiful gardens.

ATTRACTION
BURGHLEY HOUSE
Stamford PE9 3JY
Tel: (01780) 752451   Fax: (01780) 480125
e-mail: burghley@dial.pipex.com
Built between 1565/87 by William Cecil, Elizabeth I's trusted adviser, this remains his descendants' family home and contains a fine collection of C17th Italian paintings, a Breughel and a Gainsborough, wood-carvings by Grinling Gibbons and Japanese ceramics. A new sculpture garden and a Capability Brown park complement the house. The first-floor state rooms are accessed by a Stannah chairlift, so there is limited access to this and the restaurant.

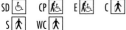

LIVERPOOL AND MERSEYSIDE

A fishing village that grew into one of the world's largest ports, trading in slaves, freight and emigration until the middle of this century, Liverpool's legacy is manifest is some fine buildings, two cathedrals and the city's mercantile history that is well displayed in museums. The rejuvenation of the Albert Docks and the Beatles connections ensure there is some life in the old dog yet.

TOURIST INFORMATION CENTRES
Merseyside Welcome Centre, Clayton Square Shopping Centre, Liverpool L1 1QR
Tel: (0151) 7093631   Fax: (0151) 7080204

Atlantic Pavilion, Albert Dock, Liverpool L3 4AE
Tel: (0151) 7088854   Fax: (0151) 7093350

BUSES
Merseytravel, 24 Hatton Garden, Liverpool L3 1AN
Tel: (0151) 2367676
Produces an Access Guide.

TAXIS
City Council: Tel: (0151) 2273911
1,400 taxis, most able to carry wheelchairs. There are ranks all over city including at Lime Street station.

TRAINS
Central Trains: Assistance:
Tel: (0845) 7056027
web: www.centraltrains.co.uk
First North Western: Special Needs:
Tel: (0845) 6040231
Merseyrail: Special Needs:
Tel: (0151) 7022071 (minicom available)
Northern Spirit: Special Needs:
Tel: (0845) 6008008
Virgin Trains: Special Needs:
Tel: (0845) 7443366
Minicom: (0845) 7443367
Wales and West: Special Needs:
Tel: (0845) 3003005
Minicom: (0845) 7585469
Portable ramps are available at Liverpool Moorfields and Southport Stations.

CAR PARKS

Orange badge holders may park on-street or in Pay & Display parks free of charge with no time limit.

SHOPMOBILITY

48a Clayton Square, Liverpool L11 0QR
Tel: (0151) 7089993   Fax: (0151) 7080775

HOTELS

LIVERPOOL MOAT HOUSE

Paradise Street, Liverpool L1 8JD
Tel/Fax: (0151) 7092706

No. of Accessible Rooms: 1. Bath
Accessible Facilities: Restaurant
Large, modern and centrally located hotel close to Albert Dock and Tate Gallery with fine views across the Mersey.

TRAVEL INN LIVERPOOL WEST DERBY

The Stag & Rainbow Beefeater, Queens Drive, West Derby, Liverpool L13 0DL
Tel: (0151) 2284724   Fax: (0151) 2207610
web: www.travelinn.co.uk

No. of Accessible Rooms: Unknown
Accessible Facilities: Unknown
A508, left past the Esso Garage, travelling towards Bootle on the NE side of the city.

ATTRACTIONS

CROXTETH HALL AND COUNTRY PARK

Croxteth Hall Lane, Liverpool L12 0HB
Tel: (0151) 2285311   Fax: (0151) 2282817

Former home of the Earls of Sefton, the rooms are furnished in Edwardian period pieces. The grounds contain a Victorian walled garden, a collection of rare-breed animals and a miniature railway.

SD   CP   E   RF   L
C   S   WC
RFE-Building, Garden

LIVERPOOL FOOTBALL CLUB MUSEUM AND TOUR CENTRE

Anfield Road, Liverpool L4 0TH
Tel: (0151) 2606677   Fax: (0151) 264 0149

The museum is accessible, the tour is not. For grounds see sporting venue below.

SD   CP   E   L   S
WC   RFE

MERSEYSIDE MARITIME MUSEUM

Albert Dock, Liverpool L3 4AQ

Tel: (0151) 4784507   Fax: (0151) 4784590

History of the great port of Liverpool, its ships and its people. *Titanic* and *Lusitania* exhibits and others on emigration to the new world. Visit the Transatlantic Slavery Gallery to learn of the origins of slavery and its legacy. Pass through a reconstruction of a slave ship. Lifeline galleries display WWII exhibits. The HM Customs & Excise National Museum is located within this museum, where you can enter a world of secret cargoes, concealment and smuggling

SD   CP   E   RF
L   C   S   WC

METROPOLITAN CATHEDRAL OF CHRIST THE KING

Mount Pleasant, Liverpool L3 5TQ
Tel: (0151) 7099222   Fax: (0151) 7087274
e-mail: met.cathedral@cwcom.net

Modern Roman Catholic cathedral, consecrated in 1967. Renowned for glass designs by John Piper.

SD   CP   E (disabled entrance accessed via underground car park)   RF
L   C-   S   WC   RFE

MUSEUM OF LIVERPOOL LIFE

Pierhead, Liverpool L3 1PZ
Tel: (0151) 4784507   Fax: (0151) 4784090

Mersey culture, Liverpool's sporting life and industrial development, trade union and women's suffrage displays and a local perspective on the 1981 Toxteth Riots.

SD   CP   E   RF   S   WC

SPEKE HALL (NT)

The Walk, Speke, Liverpool L24 1XD
Tel: (0151) 4277231   Fax: (0151) 4279860

Famous half-timbered house, built in 1490. The interior is of many periods, Victorian, Jacobean, Tudor. Delightful restored garden.

SD   CP   E   C
S   WC   RFE

TATE GALLERY LIVERPOOL

Albert Dock, Liverpool L3 4BB
Tel: (0151) 7093223   Fax: (0151) 7093122
e-mail: liverpool.info@tate.org.uk

Fine examples of the national collection of C20th art from private and public collections.

SD   CP n/a   E   L
C   S   WC

WALKER ART GALLERY

William Brown Street,
Liverpool L3 8EL
Tel: (0151) 4784199 Fax: (0151) 4784190

Superb collection of European paintings and sculpture, plus temporary exhibitions throughout the year. Adjacent to the main entrance is an adapted door that opens electronically.It is operated by pressing a large button 85cm off the floor. Car parking is in William Brown St, 50m from the gallery.

SD ♿ CP 🚶 E ♿ RF ♿
L ♿ C ♿ S ♿ WC ♿

SPORTING VENUE

LIVERPOOL FOOTBALL CLUB
Anfield Road, Liverpool L4 0TH
Admin: Tel: (0151) 2632361
Fax: (0151) 2608813
Booking: General: (0151) 2608680
CC: (0151) 2635727 Fax: (0151) 2611415

Complies with Part M, Building Regulations.

CP ♿ (for annual pass holders only.)
P 🚶 (public parking at nearby Anfield Comprehensive School, Utting Avenue) RE ♿
ED ♿ (except non-automatic)
INT ♿ L ♿
WC ♿ (16 adapted throughout stadium)

SS ♿ 82 designated positions through dedicated entrance door for wheelchair and helpers only.
B/R ♿

THEATRE/CONCERT HALL

PHILARMONIC HALL
Hope Street, Liverpool L1 9BP
Admin: (0151) 2102895
Fax: (0151) 2102902
Booking-Box Office: (0151) 7093789

Complies with Part M, Building Regulations.

SD ♿ CP ♿ Public CP-Caledonia Street
Nearest taxi rank is outside the main entrance
RE ♿ ED ♿ INT ♿ L ♿
WC ♿ (rear of auditorium next to lift)
AUD ♿ B/R ♿
Lift from foyer to rear stalls, slight incline to box seats, slight decline to stalls.

MERSEYSIDE

LIVERPOOL-MERSEY TOURISM
5th Floor, Cunard Building, Pier Head,
Liverpool L3 1ET
Tel: (0151) 2272727 Fax: (0151) 2272325
e-mail: tourism@cybase.co.uk
tourism@cybase.co.uk
web: www.merseyside.org.uk

The modern Metropolitan Cathedral of Christ the King.

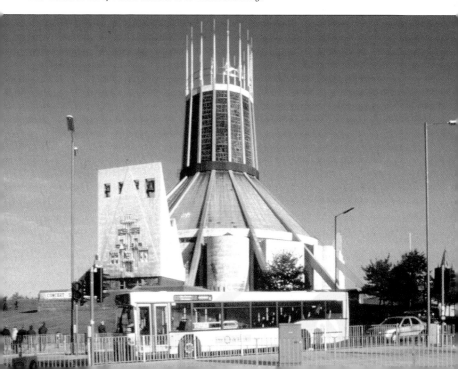

LIVERPOOL ASSOCIATION OF DISABLED PEOPLE
Lime Court Centre, Upper Baker Street,
Liverpool L6 1NB
Tel: (0151) 2638366

DISABLEMENT RESOURCE UNIT
Mount Vernon Green, Hall Lane,
Liverpool
Tel: (0151) 7090990

MERSEY VOLUNTEER BUREAU
35 Lime Street, Liverpool
Tel: (0151) 7071113

WIRRAL ASSOCIATION OF DISABLED PEOPLE
Shopmobility Centre, 5 St. John Street,
Birkenhead
Tel: (0151) 6476162

DISABILITY INFORMATION CENTRE
Poole Centre, New Grosvenor Road,
Ellesmere Port
Tel: (0151) 3568253

WHEELCHAIR REPAIRS
Mobility Shop
143 Thomas Lane, Broadgreen,
Liverpool L14 5NT
Tel: (0151) 734 4728

BIRKENHEAD

Situated near the head of the Wirral
peninsula. Considerable residential and
shopping development in recent years.

SPORTS/LEISURE
EUROPA POOLS
Conway Street, Birkenhead, Wirral L41 6RN
Tel: (0151) 6474182 Fax: (0151) 6474178

SD 🚫 CP 🚫 E 🚫 RF 🚫 L 🚫
C 🚫 S 🚫 WC 🚫 RFE 🚫

PORT SUNLIGHT

A garden village on Liverpool's outskirts
created in 1888 by industrialist William
Hesketh Lever for his soap factory employees.

ATTRACTION
LADY LEVER ART GALLERY
Port Sunlight Village, Bebington L62 5EQ
Tel: (0151) 4784136 Fax: (0151) 4784140

Collection of mainly C18th and C19th
paintings, ceramics, furniture and
sculpture, and is notable for pre-Raphaelite
pictures.

SD 🚫 CP 🚫 E 🚫 RF 🚫 L 🚫
C 🚶 S 🚫 WC 🚫

SOUTHPORT

Pleasant resort, notable for Lord Street, a
boulevard lined with elegant shops
running parallel to the coast for 1.5
miles.

TOURIST BOARD
SOUTHPORT TOURIST INFORMATION CENTRE
112 Lord Street, Southport PR8 1NY
Tel: (01704) 533333 Fax: (0151) 9342418

ACCESSIBLE TOILETS
The RADAR National Key Scheme.
Keys obtainable from the Tourist
Information Centre, 112 Lord Street, at the
corner with Eastbank Street. Available at
the Floral Hall, Promenade Central, Princes
Park, Hill Street, Market Street and Queen
Anne St.

ACCESSIBLE PARKING
On-street disabled parking available in
Chapel Street and both sides of Lord
Street.

ACCESSIBLE TAXIS

YELLOW TOP CABS
Tel: 531 000
Three specially adapted to accommodate
wheelchairs.

WHEELCHAIR HIRE
BRADLEYS CHEMIST
34 Shakespeare Street, Southport
Tel: (01704) 532326

HOTELS
SANDPIPERS (Winged Fellowship)   🚫
Fairway, Southport PR9 0LA
Tel: (01704) 538388 Fax: (01704) 549764
No. of Accessible Rooms: All (24). Roll-in
Shower
Accessible Facilities: Lounge, restaurant,
bar, grounds, including sun deck.

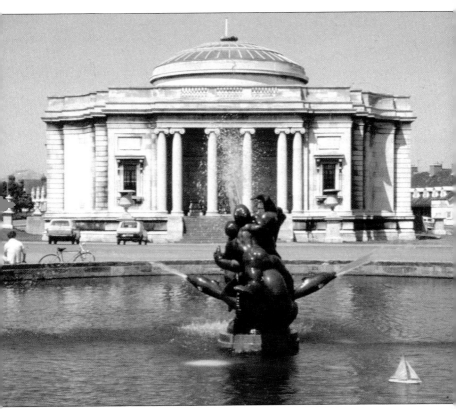

There must have been money in soap! The Lady Lever Art Gallery at the wonderfully eclectic Port Sunlight.

A holiday centre for those with physical disabilities. Located on sand dunes on the edge of the town's Marine Lake with easy beach access .

THE ROYAL CLIFTON HOTEL (BEST WESTERN)
The Promenade, Southport PR8 1RB
Tel: (01704) 533771 Fax: (01704) 500657
No. of Accessible Rooms: 3. Bath
Accessible Facilities: Lounge, restaurant
Quality hotel in front of Lord Street.

BED AND BREAKFAST
SANDY BROOK FARM
Wyke Cop Road, Scarisbrick,
Southport PR8 5LR
Tel: (01704) 880337
No. of Accessible Rooms: 1. Bath
Accessible Facilities: Lounge, dining room. Converted farm building on a small arable farm 3.5 miles from Southport.

SELF-CATERING
SANDY BROOK FARM
As above. The Dairy
No. of Accessible Units: 1. Roll-in shower.
No. of Beds per Unit: 2/4
Accessible Facilities: Open plan lounge/dining/kitchen. C18th barn converted into five holiday apartments, The Dairy being specially designed. Many of the barn's original features have been retained.

ATTRACTION
SOUTHPORT ZOO AND CONSERVATION TRUST
Princes Park, Southport PR8 1RX
Tel: (01704) 538102 Fax: (01704) 548529
Family-owned zoo with a varied collection of animals living in family groups. The emphasis is on breeding.

SD	CP	E	RF
C	S	WC	RFE

LONDON (GREATER)

CENTRAL INNER LONDON POSTAL CODES: E1, E2, E9, EC1, EC2, EC3, EC4, N1, NW1, NW8, SW1, SW3, SW5, SW7, SW10, SE1, SE11, SE17, WC1, WC2, W1, W2, W6, W8, W9, W10, W11, W14. GREATER LONDON – ALL OTHER CODES:

GREATER LONDON ASSOCIATION OF DISABLED PEOPLE (GLAD)
336 Brixton Road, London SW9 7AA
Tel: (020) 7346 5800

LONDON TOURIST BOARD AND CONVENTION BUREAU
Glen House, Stag Place, London SW1E 5LT
Tel: (020) 7932 2000   Fax: (020) 7932 0222
web: www.londontown.com

CITY OF LONDON SOCIAL SERVICES DEPARTMENT
Access Officer, Milton Court, Moor Lane, London, EC2Y 9BL
Tel: (020) 7332 1995   Fax: (020) 7332 3398

TAXIS
Computer Cab, Taxis House,
7 Woodfield Road, London W9 2BA
Tel: (020) 7286 6070
London Taxi company with a number of accessible vehicles.

TRAINS
Central Trains: Assistance:
Tel: (0845) 7056027
web: www.centraltrains.co.uk
Chiltern Railways: Mobility Impaired:
Tel: (01296) 332113/4
web: www.chilternrailways.co.uk
Connex: Customer Services:
Tel: (0870) 6030405
Fax: (0870) 6030505
Minicom: (01233) 617621
First Great Eastern: Special Needs:
Tel: (0845) 9505050
Minicom: (0845) 9606099
First Great Western: Special Needs:
Tel: (0845) 7413775
Great North Eastern Railway:
Special Needs: Tel: (0845) 7225444
Minicom: (0191) 2330173

London Transport: Special Needs:
Tel/Minicom: (01702) 357640
Midland Mainline: Special Needs:
Tel: (0114) 2537654
Minicom: (0845) 7078051
Silverlink: Special Needs:
Tel: (01923) 207818   Fax: (01923) 207023
Minicom: (01923) 256430
Thameslink: Special Needs:
Tel: (020) 7620 6333
Minicom: (020) 7620 5561
Stationlink bus:
Tel: (0207) 9183312
Virgin Trains: Special Needs:
(0845) 7443366
Minicom: (0845) 7443367
Wales and West: Special Needs:
Tel: (0845) 3003005
Minicom: (0845) 7585469
West Anglia Great Northern:
Special Needs (0345) 226688
Minicom: (0345) 125988

CITY PARKING
Parking Services, City Engineer's Dept.
2 White Lyon Court, Barbican,
London, EC2Y 8PS
Tel: (020) 7332 1548   Fax: (020) 7332 1557
Because of the pressure on parking, the national Orange Badge Scheme does not apply in central London, including the City of London. There is, however, 150 specific parking provisions for visitors within the square mile for those with disabilities. Streets with designated bays for orange badge holders are:
Aldermanbury, America Square, Bartholomew Close, Basinghall Street, Bridewell Place, Bury Street, Carmelite Street, Cloak Lane, Coleman Street, Creechurch Lane, Crosswall, Crutched Friars, Deans Court, Devonshire Square, Dowgate Hill, Eastcheap, Eldon Street, Farringdon Street, Fetter Lane, Finsbury Circus, Fore Street, Furnival Street, Godliman Street, Gravel Lane, Gt. Tower Street, Gt. Winchester Street, Gresham Street, Gutter Lane, Harrow Place, High Timber Street, Houndsditch, Jewry Street, John Carpenter Street, Laurence Poutney Hill, Little Britain, Little New Street, Little Trinity Lane, Liverpool Street, Lloyds Avenue, Lower Thames Street, Tower, Mark Lane, Middlesex Street, Mincing Lane, Minories, Monument Street, Moor Lane, Mumford Court, Muscovy Street, New Fetter Lane, Noble Street, Old Jewry, Pepys Street, Plumtree Court, Queen Victoria Street, Salisbury Court, Savage Gardens, Seething Lane,

Shoe Lane, Silk Street/Barbican, Snow Hill, St. Andrews Hill, St. Bride Street, St. Mary at Hill, Staining Lane, Temple Avenue, Thavies Inn, Trump Street, Tudor Street, Watergate, Watling Street, West Smithfield, Whitefriars Street, Wood Street.

Apply in writing to parking services above for permission to park while in the City.

WHEELCHAIR-ACCESSIBLE WCs

With RADAR key:

West Smithfield, opposite St. Bartholomew's Hospital. St. Paul's Churchyard, between the coach park and New Change. Fenchurch BR Station, take the lift to the first floor. City Thameslink BR Station, Ludgate Hill, through the ticket barrier on the ground floor. Liverpool Street BR Station, in the ticket office.

<u>Other wheelchair accessible public toilets</u>

Barbican Centre. Pit floor (level 2),
Mezzanine (only during performances),
Library floor (level 2), Conference floor (level 4),
Stalls floor (level 1).
Guildhall. Ground and 4th floors of north block,
2nd floor of west wing.
Museum of London. level 4.
Exchange Square, Broadgate. Ring the bell at the entrance to request entry.
Tower Hill. In Tower Place, unisex.
Tower of London. Behind the Jewel House.

MUSEUM AND GALLERIES DISABILITY ASSOCIATION - MAGDA

C/o Saffron Walden Museum, Museum Street, Saffron Walden, Essex CB10 1JL
Tel: (01799) 522836 Fax: (01799) 510333
Promotes access to museums for visitors with disabilities.

HOTELS
COPTHORNE TARA
Scarsdale Place,
off Kensington High Street W8 5SR
Tel: (020) 7937 7211 Fax: (020) 7937 7100
No. of Accessible Rooms: 10
Accessible Facilities: Lounge, restaurant
Large hotel in a residential area off Kensington High Street with a smart atmosphere. Highly recommended for visitors with mobility difficulties.

THISTLE MARBLE ARCH
Bryanston Street W1A 4UR
Tel: (020) 7629 8040 Fax: (020) 7499 7792
No. of Accessible Rooms: 10. Roll-in

Shower. Accessible Facilities: Lounge, restaurant. The award-winning rooms for disabled guests are among the very best. Situated in the heart of the West End, where Park lane meets Oxford Street.

THE BONNINGTON IN BLOOMSBURY
Southampton Row WC1B 4BH
Tel: (020) 7242 2828 Fax: (020) 7831 9170
No. of Accessible Rooms: 4. Bath
Accessible Facilities: Lounge, restaurant, lift. Late Edwardian hotel with good access to central London theatreland.

COLUMBIA HOTEL
95-99 Lancaster Gate W2 3NS
Tel: (020) 7402 0021 Fax: (020) 7706 4691
No. of Accessible Rooms: 1. Bath
Accessible Facilities: Lounge, restaurant
Originally five large Victorian town houses. Located a mile from Marble Arch on the north side of Hyde Park, overlooking the park and Kensington Gardens. Lively Queensway with ethnic restaurants, cafes and multi-storey shopping is very close. The hotel supplied considerable detail on its accessible room and has a pro-active and positive policy.

THE BARBICAN THISTLE HOTEL
120 Central Street, Clerkenwell,
London EC1V 8DS
Tel: (020) 7251 1565 Fax; (020) 7253 1005
No. of Accessible Rooms: 1
Accessible Facilities: Open plan on ground floor. On the edge of the City of London.

THE FORUM HOTEL
97 Cromwell Road SW7 4DN
Tel: (020) 7370 5757 Fax: (020) 7373 1448
No. of Accessible Rooms: 2
Accessible Facilities: Lounge, restaurant
London's tallest hotel with rooms offering panoramic views over the capital.

THE SELFRIDGE THISTLE HOTEL
Orchard Street, London W1G 0JS
Tel: (020) 7408 2080 Fax; (020) 7409 2295
No. of Accessible Rooms: 1
Accessible Facilities: Lounge, restaurant on the 1st floor, accessed by a lift. Elegant hotel located behind Selfridges department store in heart of the West End.

179

LONDON HILTON

22 Park Lane W1Y 4BE
Tel: (020) 7493 8000   Fax: (020) 7208 4142
No. of Accessible Rooms: 3. Roll-in Shower.
Accessible Facilities: Lounge, restaurants
(except Trader Vics), lift. Well-established
property, always buzzing with activity, with
sweeping views of Hyde Park.

NOVOTEL LONDON WATERLOO

113 Lambeth Road SE1 7LS
Tel: (020) 7793 1010   Fax: (020) 7793 0202
No. of Accessible Rooms: 10. Roll-in
Shower. Accessible Facilities: Lounge,
restaurant, fitness area. Close to Waterloo
International Station.

TOWER THISTLE HOTEL

St. Katherine's Way E1 9LD
Tel: (020) 7481 2575   Fax: (020) 7488 4106
e-mail: Tower.BusinessCentre@Thistle.co.uk
No. of Accessible Rooms: 3. Roll-in Shower
Accessible Facilities: Lounge, restaurants
(2), two on the ground floor, one via an
accessible lift.
Situated next to Tower Bridge and the
Tower of London, the hotel is in unique
location overlooking St. Katherine's Dock
with yachts, shops, walkways and bridges.

WESTLAND HOTEL

154 Bayswater Road W2 4HP

London's very own eye-full.

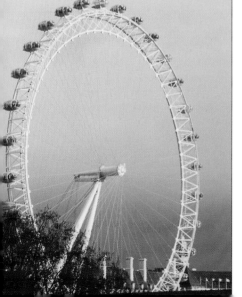

Tel: (020) 7229 9191   Fax: (020) 7727 1054
No. of Accessible Rooms: 3. Bath
Accessible Facilities: Lounge, restaurant.
Located directly opposite Kensington Palace,
five minutes from Whitleys Shopping Centre.

THE BERNERS HOTEL

Berners Street W1A 3BB
Tel: (020) 7666 2000   Fax: (020) 7666 2001
e-mail: berners@berners.co.uk
web: www.thebernershotel.co.uk
No. of Accessible Rooms: 6. Bath
Accessible Facilities: Lounge, dining room,
lift. Relatively small but gracious property
with personal ambience. In a very central
location behind Oxford Street, between
Oxford Circus and Tottenham Court Road.

THE DORCHESTER

Park Lane W1A 2HJ
Tel: (020) 7629 8888   Fax: (020) 7409 0114
No. of Accessible Rooms: 2. Bath
Accessible Facilities: Lounge, restaurants
(4), lift, sauna and spa, (three steps,
landing, two steps).
Renowned Mayfair hotel facing Hyde Park.

ATTRACTIONS

BRITISH AIRWAYS LONDON EYE

Jubilee Gardens, County Hall, SE1 1GZ
Tel: Bookings: (0870) 5000 600
Groups: (0870) 4003 005
web:www.ba-londoneye.com
Largest observation wheel in the world at
450ft high. Overhanging the Thames on
the South Bank between Westminster and
Hungerford Bridges. 32 capsules carrying
passengers on a 35 minute journey taking
in some of the best London views,
spanning 25 miles. NB. Set down in
Belvedere Road, with entrance via Jubilee
Gardens – distance 70m. The Wheel:
wheelchairs are limited to one per capsule
and a maximum of four per revolution.
The wheel is stopped with a special ramp
coming down to make entrance level to
each capsule.

SD ♿   P N/A   E ♿   RF ♿
C ♿   S ♿   WC ♿

BETHNAL GREEN MUSEUM OF CHILDHOOD

Cambridge Heath Road, London E2 9PA
Tel: (020) 8980 5200   Fax: (020) 8983 5225

Parking Access-Tel: (020) 8983 5205
web: www.vam.ac.uk

One of the largest toy collections in the world, a branch of the Victoria and Albert Museum. Children's interests and experiences also are explored through their playthings, clothes and furniture. Most of the toys are in the lower galleries and on the upper gallery follow the path from Birth and Infancy through Early Years to Breaking Away. A charming museum for adults and children alike. Telephone in advance. Park at the rear entrance in Victoria Park Square, where a small curb cut leads directly to the new lift, and to the ground, first and upper floors. Base to ground is always controlled by a staff member, first and upper floors lift access. From first to ground apart from the lift there is also a ramp with a gradient of 1:12.

SD n/a   CP 🚾   E 🚾   RF 🚾   L 🚾
C 🚾   S 🚾   WC 🚾   Radar key from reception.

BRITISH MUSEUM
Great Russell Street, London WC1B 3DG
Tel: (020) 7323 8599   Fax: (020) 7323 8616
e-mail: info@british-museum.ac.uk
web: www.british-museum.ac.uk
Recorded information for disabled visitors:
Tel: (020) 7637 7384
Minicom: (020) 7323 8920

Founded in 1753, this is the oldest museum in the world. Collections include prehistoric and Roman Britain, medieval, renaissance and modern objects, ancient Egyptian, western, Asian, Greek, Roman and oriental art. Highlights include the Elgin Marbles, Lindow Man, Egyptian mummies and the Lindisfarne Gospels.

The Great Court will open in November 2000 and access will be disrupted until then. The main foyer is noisy and crowded while the Great Court is being built. Ultimately there will be two lifts with independent access located on left hand side of the main entrance, close to disabled parking, and one assisted lift on the right hand side of entrance. Access to the upper floors from the main entrance is by a stair lift next to the restaurant. The north lift, from the Montague Place entrance, allows access to the Japanese galleries, the prints and drawing gallery, the Arts of Korea

exhibition, and the Hotung oriental gallery. Level access from this section to the rest of the museum is on Level 3. The Great Court will house a centre for education, galleries, exhibition space and a restaurant. Complimentary wheelchairs are available at both entrances.

CP 🚾 MUST ADVISE WELL IN ADVANCE – TEL. AS ABOVE
E 🚾   RF 🚾   L 🚾   S 🚾   WC 🚾

BANKSIDE GALLERY
48 Hopton Street SE1 9JH
Tel: (020) 7928 7521
Fax: (020) 7928 2820
e-mail: re&rws@bankside-gallery.demon.co.uk

Home of the Royal Watercolour Society and Royal Society of Painter-Printmakers with changing contemporary exhibitions.

SD 🚾   CP n/a   E 🚹   RF 🚾   S 🚾   WC n/a

BUCKINGHAM PALACE
1. THE STATE ROOMS
The Visitor Office, Buckingham Palace, SW1A 1AA
Tel: (020) 7839 1377   Fax: (020) 7930 9625
Ticket Office: (020) 7321 2233 credit card bookings.
e-mail: information@royalcollection.org.uk
web: www.royal.gov.uk

Buckingham Palace is again welcoming visitors to the summer opening, and a chance to see the memorable State Rooms with their treasures before they close to the public on October 3rd 2000. Here you are caught up in the echoes of history. Characters from Britain's past appear about to step out of the paintings in the long Portrait Gallery. Beauty and colour everywhere turns your head and eye for a lingering look at silk-lined walls, exquisite furniture, sculptures, fabled ornaments and the diamond-dazzle of chandeliers. Disabled access is excellent, so too is the disabled toilet. Alongside a privileged parking spot. a stair rider is manipulated in the hands of well-practised staff. From there a lift takes you to the sweep of the majestic west-facing rooms overlooking lawns and lake. Entry for designated parking is at North Centre Gate. Electric chairs are not allowed inside, but six wheelchairs are available for loan. The wheelchair access route uses a vertical lift. NB. PRE-BOOKING ESSENTIAL.

SD [♿]　　CP – Vehicles with a disabled driver or passenger may apply for permission to park right inside the Palace grounds. It is essential that you phone the Special Access Officer (020 7839 1377) or write to Royal Collection Enterprises, The Visitor Office, Buckingham Palace, London SW1A 1AA　　E- [♿] Stair rider L [♿] (Stair lift)　　S [♿]　　wc [♿]

2. THE ROYAL MEWS

The monarch's magnificent gilded state carriages and coaches, including the unique Gold State Coach, are housed here together with their horses and state liveries. Accessible with fully accessible WC. Open all year, on Monday, Tuesday, Wednesday, and Thursday.

3. QUEEN'S GALLERY

Major restoration to be completed in spring 2000. All facilities advised as accessible, but pre-check.

CABINET WAR ROOMS
Clive Steps, King Charles Street SW1A 2AQ
Tel: (020) 7930 6961　Fax: (020) 7839 5897
web: www.iwm.org.uk
Rooms used by Winston Churchill and his chiefs of staff during WWII.

SD [♿]　　CP n/a　　E [♿]　　L [♿]　　C n/a
S [🚶]　　WC [🚶]

CHELSEA PHYSIC GARDEN
66 Royal Hospital Road SW3 4HS
Tel: (020) 7352 5646　Fax: (020) 7376 3910
Founded in 1673 by the Society of Apothecaries, this is one of Europe's oldest botanic gardens. Its 3.5 acres contain a garden showing the history of medicinal plants and an ethnobotanical garden of world medicines: There is also a very old rock garden (1773), and many rare and tender plants including the largest outdoor olive tree in Britain.

SD [♿]　　CP [♿]　　E [🚶]　　C [🚶]
S [🚶]　　WC [🚶]　　G [🚶]

COMMONWEALTH INSTITUTE AND EXPERIENCE
Kensington High Street, London W8 6NQ
Tel: (020) 7603 4535　Fax: (020) 7602 7374
e-mail: cburkitt@commonwealth.org.uk
A museum dedicated to exploring the diverse history and culture of over 40 Commonwealth countries with an amazing range of displays and exhibits. Truly fascinating.

SD [♿]　　CP [♿]　　E [♿]　　RF [♿]　　L [♿]　　WC [🚶]

CRAFT COUNCIL GALLERY
44 Pentonville Road, London N1 9BY
Tel: (020) 7806 2542
Fax: (020) 7837 0858
e-mail: crafts@craftscouncil.org.uk
web: www.cragtscouncil.org.uk
Within a neo-classical facade this gallery contains fine collections of contemporary British crafts plus changing temporary displays. Between January and September 2000 there is a special season of three exhibitions, each showing new bodies of work by three people.

SD n/a　　CP [♿]　　E [♿]　　L [♿]　　C [♿]
S [🚶]　　RFE [♿] Gallery.

DESIGN MUSEUM
Shad Thames, London SE1 2YD
Tel: (020) 7403 6933　Fax: (020) 7378 6540
A museum devoted to design for mass production. A first floor gallery is dedicated to Modern Britain 1929/29, with both historical and artistic exhibits. The second floor collections illustrate modern design in its social and economic context. A shop and café are on the ground floor. Galleries are accessed only by an attended lift.

SD [♿]　　CP n/a　　E [♿]　　RF [♿]　　L [♿]
C [♿]　　S [♿]　　WC [🚶]　　RFE [♿]

THE GEFFRYE MUSEUM
Kingsland Road, London E2 8EA
Tel: (020) 7739 9893　Fax: (020) 7729 5647
e-mail: info@geffrye-museum.org.uk
web: www.geffrye-museum.org.uk
Set in the former almshouses of the Ironmonger's Company, a delightful C18th building with attractive gardens and mature trees. The museum presents the changing style of the domestic interior, a walk through time from the C17th, past the refined splendour of the Georgian period and high style of the Victorians, to C20th modernity seen through a 1930s flat, a mid-century room in the contemporary style, and a late C20th living space in a converted warehouse.

SD [♿]　　CP-0 (2 orange badge bays outside the main entrance),　E [♿] (through small gate to L of main entrance in Kingsland Road)　　RF [♿]　　L [♿]
C [♿]　　S [♿]　　WC [🚶] RFE n/a (Gardens)

THE GUILDHALL
PO Box 270, Aldermanbury, London EC2P 2EJ
Tel: (020) 7 332 1462
web: www.cityoflondon.gov.uk
Home to the Corporation of London, Guildhall has been the seat of municipal government since the C12th and its ancient walls have twice survived catastrophic fire, in 1666 in the Great Fire of London, and in 1940 during the Blitz. This is a Grade 1 listed building and a rare example of mediaeval architecture. The Great Hall is the setting for ceremonial and civic occasions. Recent events of significance have included 1995 VE Day celebrations and the bestowing of the Honorary freedom of the City on Nelson Mandela in July 1996. There is a high-level security check. Access to the Great Hall is by a back entrance between the hall and the catering department, ramped and then level. The new library and art gallery building connected to the old library avoids stairs.

SD ♿ (Roadside onto pavement and into Guildhall Yard, always free)   E ♿   RF ♿   S 🚶
WC ♿   RFE ♿

HAYWARD GALLERY
Belvedere Road, South Bank Centre, London SE1 8XX
Tel: (020) 7928 3144   Fax: (020) 7921 0830
Modern, concrete venue for large art exhibitions of classical and contemporary work with the accent on modern British art. NB: Ramps here can be steep but there is always a guard on duty who will help.

SD ♿   CP ♿   E ♿   RF ♿   L ♿
C 🚶   S ♿   WC 🚶

HOUSES OF PARLIAMENT
Palace of Westminster, London SW1A 0AA
Tel: Serjeant at Arms: (020) 7219 3050
Fax: (020) 7799 2178
Rebuilt in the 1830s after a disastrous fire, this Gothic-style building is 310m long, covers eight acres and includes 1,100 apartments along two miles of passages. Telephone Black Rod's Office or Serjeant at Arms' Office WELL IN ADVANCE. Dispensation entrance is from Black Rod's Garden using the sovereign's lift in the House of Lords up to the Principal Floor, then following the normal line of route until returning to the Member's Lobby in the House of Commons. There is space for four wheelchairs at the back of the Strangers Gallery where visitors listen to debates. Access to the gallery is by No 1 lift from the Principal Floor. There is a comprehen-sive leaflet for those with mobility problems.

SD ♿   CP n/a   E ♿   S ♿   WC n/a

IMPERIAL WAR MUSEUM
Lambeth Road SE1 6HZ
Tel: (020) 7416 5000   Fax: (020) 7416 5374
e-mail: mail@iwm.org.uk
web: www.iwm.org.uk
Display of modern warfare plus exhibits relating to the social effect of C20th wars and period art, films and photographs. First and Second World War exhibitions, and the Blitz Experience. Galleries on all four levels are accessible.

SD n/a   CP ♿   RF ♿   L ♿
C 🚶   S 🚶   WC 🚶

KENSINGTON PALACE STATE APARTMENTS and ROYAL CEREMONIAL DRESS COLLECTION
Kensington Gardens, London W8 4PX
Tel: (020) 7937 9561   Fax: (020) 7376 0198
web: www.hrp.org.uk
Displays of court uniforms and protocol from c1760, including dresses of the present royal family. NB: There is no vehicular access or disabled parking in the Orangery Gardens. ADVANCE BOOKING ON THE ABOVE NUMBER IS ESSENTIAL. The Royal Ceremonial Dress Collection is on the Garden Floor.
NB: There is no access to state apartments.

SD ♿   CP n/a   E ♿   C 🚶
S 🚶   WC 🚶   RFE ♿

LONDON AQUARIUM
County Hall, Riverside Building, Westminster Bridge SE1 7PB
Tel: (020) 7967 8000 Fax: (020) 7967 8029
A voyage of discovery through the waters of the world with hundreds of live specimens in superb underwater scenes, aided by touchtanks and educational, inter-active displays. Car parking is available in Jubilee Gardens or at the Shell Building. There is a pathway past the BA Eye along a wide walkway on the south bank of the Thames.

Two floors are accessed by lift with disabled WC on both. The wheelchair/pushchair route is well signed throughout from the lift exit on each floor. There is a shallow exit ramp. The Ray Touchpool is too high to touch but the Sea Shore Touchpool at 64cm high, is accessible.

SD N/A CP [♿] E [♿] RF [♿] L [♿]
S [♿] WC [♿] RFE [♿]

LONDON CANAL MUSEUM
12-13 New Wharf Road N1 9RT
Tel: (020) 7713 0836
e-mail: martins@dircon.co.uk
web: www.charitynet.org/~LCanalMus

Here is the story of London's canal development, particularly of Regent's Canal with exhibits on vessels, people and trade, notably the import of ice from Norway, all housed in a former ice warehouse and stables. On two floors, the majority of the ground floor gallery is accessible. The first floor is accessed via stairs, but as part of the historic fabric, there is a ramp designed for horses! This can be used to assist wheelchair users who must have two fit and strong people to assist. A very positive attitude everywhere.

SD [♿] CP [🚶] E [♿] C n/a
S [♿] WC [♿]

LONDON DUNGEON
28-34 Tooley Street SE1 2SZ
Tel: (020) 7403 7221 Fax: (020) 7378 1529

Historic death, torture and witchcraft brought vividly to life in sights and sounds. Some passageways are quite narrow and dark. A companion is recommended.

SD [♿] CP n/a E [♿] RF [♿] C [♿]
S [♿] WC [♿] RFE [♿]

LONDON PLANETARIUM
Marylebone Road NW1 5LR
Tel: (020) 7487 0200 Fax: (020) 7465 0862
e-mail: chris.rhodes@madame

Two inter-active space zones, plus 30-minute Planetary Quest star show under the green dome – educational and fascinating.

SD [♿] CP n/a E [♿] RF [♿] L [♿]
C n/a S [♿] WC [🚶] RFE [🚶]

LONDON TRANSPORT MUSEUM
Covent Garden Piazza, London WC2E 7BB
Tel: (020) 7379 6344 Fax: (020) 7565 7254

e-mail: contact@ltmuseum.co.uk
web: www.ltmuseum.co.uk

The story of travel since 1800 told through wonderful displays of old trams, buses, the Tube and posters. Hands-on fun with buses and train simulators and working models. A must!

SD [♿] CP n/a E [♿] RF [♿] L [♿]
C [♿] S [♿] WC [🚶]

LONDON ZOO
Regent's Park, NW1 4RY
Tel: (020) 7449 6551 Fax: (020) 7449 6579

Houses 8,000 species of animals, insects, reptiles and fish. Captive breeding programmes include the rare Asiatic lion and black rhinos. There is also a Children's Zoo and activities. The zoo grounds are level except at the entrances/exits to two tunnels leading from one area to another. These are steeper than 1:10 and are about 15-20m long. There is level or short-ramped access into the animal houses except at the Aquarium that has three steps, but volunteers assist via a side, level door. The Moonlight World is not accessible: and there's a steep ramp to the elephant house.

SD [♿] CP n/a E [♿] RF [♿] C [🚶]
S [🚶] WC [🚶] RFE [♿] [🚶]

MADAME TUSSAUD'S
Marylebone Road NW1 5LR
Tel: (020) 7935 6861 Fax: (020) 7465 0862

This world-famous waxwork collection, where visitors can mix with the famous and notorious, includes a re-vamped Chamber of Horrors. NB. All areas are accessible except Superstars and the continuous Dark Ride. Entrance is via a ticket-holders entrance in Marylebone Road. Wheelchair visitors are limited to three at any one time so phoning in advance is strongly recommended. Catering has a steep ramp and help is needed from staff. The shop is accessed by a stair lift, operated by staff, that takes a wheelchair.

SD [♿] CP n/a E [♿] RF [♿] C [🚶]
S [🚶] WC [♿] L [♿]

NATIONAL GALLERY
Trafalgar Square
London WC2N 5DN
Tel: (020) 7747 2885 Fax: (020) 7747 2423

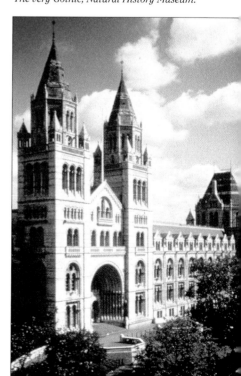

e-mail: :information@ng-london.org.uk

One of the country's great galleries, the neo-classical building houses paintings from all the great periods of western European art from 1260-1900. The Sainsbury Wing, opened in 1991, contains early renaissance works from 1260-1510. Level entrance is gained from both the Sainsbury Wing and the Orange Street entrances, though the former is specifically accessible. The SW lift accesses all five levels of the wing, including the main floor from which there is a direct, level and very wide corridor joining the remaining wings of the gallery. All gallery rooms are very spacious with ample room to view. There is one disabled parking space at the Orange Street entrance that should be booked in advance. Wheelchairs are available here also and throughout the gallery. The WCs are Radar operated, a key is obtainable from the warder on each floor. The gallery provides detailed information on access, which is very useful.

SD ♿ CP ♿ E ♿ RF ♿
L ♿ C- ♿ S ♿ WC ♿

NATIONAL PORTRAIT GALLERY
St. Martin's Place, London WC2H 0HE
Tel: (020) 7306 0055   Fax: (020) 7306 0056
web: npg.org.uk

British history seen through portraits of the famous and infamous from the medieval period to present day. Undergoing extensive rebuilding work as part of the NPG 2000 Masterplan Millennium project. The needs of disabled visitors are under discussion. Telephone for further information.

NATURAL HISTORY MUSEUM
Cromwell Road, SW7 5BD
Tel: (020) 7938 9123   Fax: (020) 7938 9066
Web: www.nhm.ac.uk

Covering four acres, this superb nature museum includes the new Earth Gallery. Wheelchair entrance is at the Earth Gallery Exhibition Road by the Museum car park, reserve a space in advance. There is unreservable on-street orange badge parking, or general parking. The entrance is through glass swing doors. A lift takes you to the mezzanine level WC. All areas are linked by lifts or ramps (some steep). The Earth Sculpture is accessed by escalator but the Earth Lab exhibit is not accessible. Galleries are linked on the ground floor through Waterhouse Way, through the main entrance with the famous dinosaurs and onwards. The gallery shop and bookshop, the gallery restaurant and the Waterhouse Coffee Bar are all on this access route.

SD ♿ CP ♿ E ♿ RF ♿ L ♿
C ♿ & ♿ S ♿ WC ♿ RFE ♿

ROYAL ACADEMY OF ARTS
Burlington House, Piccadilly, London W1V 0DS
Tel: (020) 7300 8000   Fax: (020) 7300 8001

Founded in 1768, Britain's oldest fine arts institution is known for its permanent and important temporary art exhibitions. Famous among permanent sculpture is the Michaelangelo relief of the Madonna and Child outside the Seckler Galleries. WARNING: ACCESS ONLY IN ELECTRIC WHEELCHAIR. GALLERIES ACCESSED BY LIFT AND STANNAH STAIR LIFT.

SD n/a   CP ♿   E ♿ (electric/ramped at 1:5 - 1:10)
RF ♿   L ♿   C ♿ (main restaurant ramped at 1:10, courtyard cafe level)   S ♿ (lift access)
WC ♿ (would be 1, but positioned adjacent to gents, and constant traffic makes access difficult)

The very Gothic, Natural History Museum.

ST. BRIDE'S CHURCH
Fleet Street, London EC47 8AU
Tel: (020) 7353 1301   Fax: (020) 7583 0239
e-mail: info@stbrides.com

This famous Wren church, just off Fleet Street, is a traditional venue for memorials to journalists. Wall plaques commemorate them and printers. Its wonderful octagonal spire, added to the church in 1703, has been a model for tiered wedding cakes since. Bombed in 1940, the interior has been fully restored.

SD 🚻 CP n/a E 🚻 (Fleet St. entrance, 4/5 steps, use Salisbury Court level entrance.

RF 🚹 S 🚻

ST. GILES and ST. LUKE CRIPPLEGATE
c/o St. Giles Rectory, 4 The Postern,
Wood Street, London EC2Y 8BJ
Tel/Fax: (020) 7638 1997
e-mail: stgiles@globalnet.co.uk
web: www.users.globalnet.co.uk

Only the tower survives from the original St Giles of 1550, now the parish church for the Barbican. Oliver Cromwell was married here and John Milton is buried here.

SD 🚻 CP 🚹 E 🚻 RF 🚻 WC 🚻

ST. JAMES, PICCADILLY
197 Piccadilly, London W1V OLL
Tel: (020) 7734 4511   Fax: (020) 7734 7449

A major Wren church, built in 1684 and bombed in 1940, it retains its essential features, tall arched windows, an ornate C17th Grinling Gibbons screen behind the altar, carvings above the organ and his marble font. William Blake and Pitt the Elder were baptised here. A busy urban church welcoming all.

SD n/a CP 🚹 E 🚻 C 🚹 Franchise adjacent.
RFE 🚻 Church itself.

ST. KATHERINE'S DOCK
Taylor Woodrow Property Co. Ltd
International House,
1 St. Katherine's Way, London E1 9TW
Tel: (020) 7488 0555   Fax: (020) 7481 4515
e-mail:mark.heran@taywood.co.uk

Since the C10th St. Katherine's Dock has played an important part in the life of London. During WWII the docks suffered appalling damage and although commerce continued here, container shipping became too massive for the old docks, which were closed in 1968, the other docks also closing by 1983. It has now been completely renovated and is one of the city's most successful and attractive commercial, residential and entertainment facilities. The yacht basin buzzes with activity of cafes, restaurants, shops and the continual throb of shipping. Set down in St. Katherine's Way, a small left hand side turning onto a service road. An NCP car park is 100m. further on, but trhere is no designated parking. All areas are connected by wide, planked or pavemented pathways, with only the bridge dividing the central and eastern basins being rather narrow and inaccessible.

SD 🚻 CP 🚻 E 🚻 C 🚻
S 🚻 WC 🚻 Radar Key

ST. MARTIN-IN-THE-FIELDS
Trafalgar Square, London WC2N 4JJ
Tel: (020) 7930 0089   Fax: (020) 7839 5163

The present church is the fourth to stand on this site. Completed in 1726 by James Gibbs, the fine facade was a new style, with its huge Corinthian columns, a great tower and graceful steeple, topped with a gilt crown. Notable in the interior are delicate Italian scrolls and cherubs on the ceiling, but it is the essential being of St.Martin's, a church in the middle of a lively city, which emanates. The church is indeed in-the - fields, working with all who fall outside the social net of urban life, with a busy Social Care Unit attending to the homeless or less fortunate. There are free lunchtime concerts several days each week. The crypt, with cafe and brass rubbing centre is, unfortunately, not accessible. Set down in Adelaide Street, level onto pavement and go through a small market with large, level flagstones, to a ramp at a side entrance.

SD 🚻 CP n/a E 🚻 RF 🚻 WC 🚹

ST. PAUL' S CATHEDRAL
Ludgate Hill, London EC4
Tel: (020) 7236 4128

The present St. Pauls, designed by Sir Christopher Wren, and built between 1675 and 1710, is the fifth cathedral to stand on the hill that dominates the ancient City of London. Built in the shape of a cross, with one of the largest cathedral domes in the

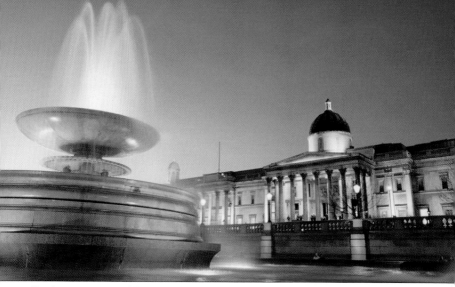

Keeping an eye on Trafalgar Square, The National Gallery with its imposing portico.

world, its sheer scale and grandeur are quite overwhelming. Europe's largest crypt contains the tombs of the Duke of Wellington, Nelson and Wren and also houses a cafe, refectory, shop and WC facilities. The Whispering Gallery, quire and American Memorial Chapel in the apse behind the high altar, are not accessible. Disabled access is on the south transept, a short walk through the churchyard from Ludgate Hill. An accessible lift connects the crypt and the main floor, alternately there is a stair lift. There is an NCP car park in Paternoster Row, to the west of the cathedral, but no designated parking spaces, and the surface is cobbled.

SD ♿ CP n/a E ♿ RF ♿
L ♿ WC ♿ C ♿ S ♿

SCIENCE MUSEUM
Exhibition Road, South Kensington, London
Tel: (020) 7938 9841 Fax: (020) 7938 9804
e-mail: control@nmsi.ac.uk
web: www.nmsi.ac.uk

Seven floors of items taken from every area of experimental science. Power, Space and Transport; Space Gallery; Launch Pad; Food for Thought; Challenge of Materials; Science and Art of Medicine; Navigation and Surveying; and Land Transport to name a few. An absolute must.

SD ♿ CP n/a E ♿ RF ♿ L ♿
C ♿ S ♿ WC ♿

THE SERPENTINE GALLERY
Kensington Gardens, London W2 3XA
Tel: (020) 7402 6075 Fax: (020) 7402 4103
web: www.serpentinegallery.org

Temporary exhibitions of contemporary painting and sculpture in a former tea pavilion built in 1912. Located in SE corner of Kensington Gardens.

SD ♿ CP n/a E ♿ RF ♿ S ♿ WC ♿

TATE GALLERY
Millbank, London SW1P 4RG
Tel: (020) 7887 8000 Fax: (020) 7887 8007
e-mail: information@tate.org.uk

National Collection of British art from C16th to present day in a family of Tates including Bankside, Liverpool and St. Ives. Millbank includes the Turner Bequest, Hogarth, Constable, Spencer and much controversial contemporary art. Not to be missed. NB: An accessible entrance is on Clore Street. A comprehensive access guide is available.

SD ♿ CP ♿ E ♿ L ♿
C ♿ S ♿ WC ♿

TOWER OF LONDON
Tower Hill, London EC3N 4AB
Tel: (020) 7709 0765
web: www.hrp.org.uk

Probably the most famous castle in the world, and an amazing example of Norman military architecture. Frequently used as a state prison, two of Henry VIII's wives were executed here and during both world wars German prisoners were housed here. Yeoman Warders or Beefeaters are keepers of The Tower. They are welcoming while also protecting the Crown Jewels.

NB: Set down/parking is at the WEST GATE. Wheelchair access is very limited, only the Jewel House is really accessible, but an excellent access guide is available.

General:

SD ♿   P 🚶♿   E 🚶♿   RF 🚶♿   C 🚶♿
S n/a   WC 🚶   L n/a   RFE 🚶♿
Jewel House: E ♿   S ♿
Education Centre: E 🚶♿   RF 🚶♿
Chapel: E 🚶

VICTORIA & ALBERT MUSEUM
Cromwell Road SW7 2RL
Tel: (020) 7942 2000   Fax: (020) 7942 2524
e-mail: postmaster@vam.ac.uk
web: www.vam.ac.uk

Probably the world's finest museum of decorative arts with several miles of galleries of ancient and modern displays, including the national collection of John Constable, plus special exhibitions. The wheelchair entrance is on Exhibition Road, opposite the Natural History museum with non-reservable orange badge parking spaces on the road. WC access is by ramp. Steep temporary ramps lead to some galleries and galleries 2-7, 40a, 43, 11-117 are not wheelchair accessible.

SD ♿   CP 🚶   E ♿   L ♿
C 🚶♿   S ♿   WC ♿   RFE 🚶♿

WESLEY'S CHAPEL, HOUSE AND MUSEUM
49 City Road, London EC1Y 1AU
Tel: (020) 7253 2262   Fax: (020) 7608 3825

John Wesley (1703-91), founder of Methodism, built this chapel as his London base. Built in 1779, it is one of London's undiscovered jewels. The museum houses a fine collection of Wesleyan ceramics and Methodist paintings. The whole building has a calm, welcoming ambience. The chapel and museum are accessible, the house is not.

SD ♿   E ♿   RF ♿   L ♿
C ♿   S ♿   WC ♿

SUTTON HOUSE (NT)
2 and 4 Homerton High Street, London E9 6JQ
Tel: (020) 8986 2264   Fax: (020) 8533 0556
e-mail: tshrbd@smtp.ntrust.org.uk

In the City's East End, a rare example of a Tudor red-brick house, built in 1535 for Henry VIII with C18th alterations and later

The Tower of London with all its history.

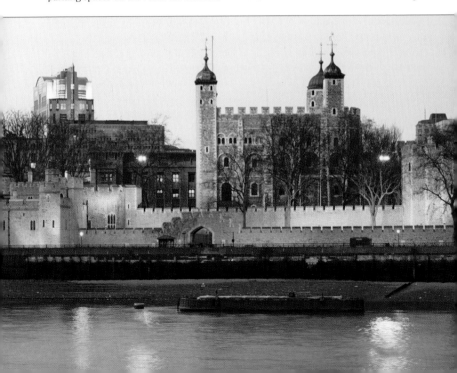

additions. Many early details are displayed, plus an exhibition on the history of the house and a multi-media presentation of local archive material. There are changing shows of contemporary arts and sculpture. Only the ground floor is accessible.

SD [♿] CP n/a E [♿] RF [♿]
C [♿] S [♿] WC [🚶]

WESTMINSTER ABBEY
Dean's Yard, London SW1P 3PA
Tel: (020) 7222 7100   Fax: (020) 7233 2072
e-mail: press@westminster-Abbey.org
web: www.westminster-abbey.org

Consecrated in 1065, although the present building was improved by Henry III in the C13th. The Abbey has been the setting for every coronation since 1066 and has the tallest Gothic nave in Britain. The royal families of England and many famous people are buried here, including Chaucer and others in Poets Corner. The Abbey produces a useful access leaflet. The entrance, through the North Door, has a small step, but is ramped. Cloisters are accessible via Dean's Yard. Little Cloister with a C17th fountain court is accessible. The College Garden, open on specific days, is accessible. The Lady Chapel, Queen Elizabeth and Queen Mary Chapels, Chapter House, Library and Pyx Chamger are not accessible. Disabled parking is in Dean's Yard by permit only and must be applied for in advance. The nearest adapted WC is in the nearby Queen Elizabeth II Conference Centre.

SD n/a CP [♿] E [♿] RF [🚶] C n/a
S [🚶] WC n/a

WHITECHAPEL ART GALLERY
80-82 Whitechapel High Street, London E1 7QX
Tel: (020) 7522 7888   Fax: (020) 7377 1685

An art nouveau facade leads into light, spacious galleries of contemporary art. Frequent exhibitions reflect local community cultural origins. David Hockney had his first exhibition here. The shop and gallery are on the ground floor: the café and upper galleries are accessed by lift.

SD [♿] CP [♿] E [♿] RF [♿]
L [♿] (goods lift, attended) C [♿] WC [🚶]
S [♿] RFE [♿]

EAST OF THE CENTRE

GREENWICH
GREENWICH TOURISM
151 Powis Street, Woolwich SE18 6JL
Tel: (020) 8855 6130   Fax: (020) 8317 2822

GREENWICH ASSOCIATION OF DISABLED PEOPLE (GAD)
Centre for Independent Living, Christchurch Forum, Trafalgar Road, London SE10 9QE
Tel: (020) 8305 2221

One of pioneering organisations of the independent-living movement. Runs training courses for disabled people wishing to live independently.

ATTRACTIONS
CUTTY SARK CLIPPER SHIP
King William Walk, Greenwich SE10 9HT
(020) 8858 3445   Fax: (020) 8853 3589
e-mail: info@cuttysark.org.uk

Built in 1869, this was the fastest of all the tea clippers. Now preserved in a dry dock, dominating the riverside at Greenwich, with exhibitions and a video telling its story.

SD/A & CP – work in progress, check
E [♿] C n/a S n/a WC n/a
RFE – Access to Tween deck only.

MILLENNIUM DOME
Greenwich Peninsula, Drawdock Road, Greenwich SE10 0BB
Tel: (020) 8293 8134
e-mail: info@newmill.co.uk
web: www.dome2000.co.uk

It's all been said already! 14 exhibition zones, aerial and acrobatic displays in the central arena and an exterior Skyscape cinema. Large choice of food and drink outlets and souvenir shops. Tickets must be booked in advance from National Lottery retailers, Dome Ticket Line Tel: (0870) 6062000, Dome website, travel agents, or rail and coach companies. For free wheelchair loan tel: (0870) 2410540. Parking available only for orange badge holders and coaches, 200m from the entrance, farther away than ideal. Entrance booths are sufficiently wide. The ground floor zones have good access. There is long, shallow ramping with many rest areas from the ground floor to the central walkway around the arena with three spacious designated wheelchair viewing areas.

SD n/a   CP ♿   E ⬚   RF ♿   L ⬚
C ⬚   S ⬚   WC ⬚   RFE ♿

NATIONAL MARITIME MUSEUM
Greenwich, London SE10 9NF
Tel: (020) 8312 6603   Fax: (020) 8312 6521
e-mail: rscates@nmm.ac.uk
web: www.nmm.ac.uk

The story of Britain and the sea, including exhibitions on the C20th, sea power and, of course, on Nelson.

SD ⬚   CP ♿   E ⬚   RF ⬚
L ♿   C ♿   S ♿   WC 🚶

ROYAL OBSERVATORY GREENWICH
Greenwich Park, Greenwich, London SE10 9NF
Tel: (020) 8858 4422   Fax: (020) 83126632
e-mail: bookings@nmm.ac.uk
web: www.nmm.ac.uk

The meridian (0 degrees longitude) dividing earth's eastern and western hemispheres, passes through here and in 1884 Greenwich Mean Time was established. The original building, Flamsteed House, was designed by Sir Chritopher Wren, and was the government observatory from 1675 until 1948 when London lights became too strong and astronomers moved to Sussex. Access to the facilities is level, but is over a cobbled courtyard and paving slab. Wheelchair access to Royal Observatory is limited to courtyard, part of Meridian Building and shop. Flamsteed House entrance has five steps.

SD ⬚   CP ♿   E ⬚   S 🚶   WC ⬚

NORTHWEST OF THE CENTRE

HENDON
ROYAL AIR FORCE MUSEUM
Grahame Park Way, Hendon, London NW9 5LL
Tel: (020) 8204 2266   Fax: (020) 8200 1751
e-mail: richard.tweed@rafmuseum.org.uk

Fine range of aeroplanes and extensive galleries tell the story of flight through the ages and its impact on transport and communication. The excellent Battle of Britain experience includes Tornado flight simulator and touch-and-try Jet Provost.

SD ⬚   CP ♿   E ⬚   RF ♿   L ♿
C ⬚   S ⬚   WC ♿   RFE ♿

SOUTH OF THE CENTRE
CROYDON
This is a bustling borough that has grown incredibly fast with numerous tall modern buildings. Good, traffic-free shopping precinct. Good access to centre of the town.

TOURIST INFORMATION CENTRE
Katherine Street, Croydon, Surrey CR9 1ET
Tel: (020) 8253 1009

HOTEL
HILTON NATIONAL CROYDON   🚶
101 Waddon Way, Purley Way,
Croydon CR9 4HH
Tel: (020) 8680 3000   Fax: (020) 8681 6171
No. of Accessible Rooms: 2. Bath
Accessible Facilities: Lounge, restaurant, pool, sauna, whirlpool. A modern hotel located on the A23.

THEATRE
FAIRFIELD HALLS
Park Lane, Croydon CR9 1DG
Tel: (020) 8681 0821   Fax: (020) 8760 0835
Box Office: (020) 8688 9291

Complies with Part M, Building Regulations - Y

SD ⬚   CP ⬚ (book in advance) Nearest taxi rank – taxi telephone on premises.   RE ⬚
ED ⬚   INT ⬚   L ⬚   WC 🚶
AUD ♿   B/R ⬚ (foyer coffee shop)
Lift to 2nd floor Concert Hall.
Lift to ground floor Aschcroft Theatre.

MORDEN
ATTRACTION
MORDEN HALL PARK (NT)
Morden Hall Road, Morden, Surrey SM4 5JD
Tel: (020) 8648 1845   Fax: (020) 8687 0094

A green oasis in this London suburb, this former deer park with waterways, hay meadows and old estate buildings, has craft workshops and a newly restored rose garden. An excellent information sheet and map for visitors in wheelchairs is provided. And wheelchairs available.

SD ⬚   CP 🚶   E ⬚   RF ⬚
C ⬚   ⬚    🚶

SOUTHWEST OF THE CENTRE

HAMPTON WICK

ATTRACTION
HAMPTON COURT PALACE
Hampton Wick, Nr. Kingston-upon-Thames,
Surrey KT8 9AU
Tel: (020) 8781 9500   Fax: (020) 8781 5362
Started in early C16th by Cardinal Wolsey, extended by Henry Vlll himself and in 1690s, by William and Mary who employed Sir Christopher Wren. His influence particularly noticeable in the Baroque landscaped gardens. As a historic Royal Palace, Hampton Court bears witness to all kings and queens of England from Henry Vlll to Elizabeth ll. The Great Hall, Tudor Court, Clock and Fountain Courts and Queen's Gallery are among notable areas of the Palace. NB: For parking in main Entrance (West Front), please notify in advance. There are cobbled stones in both Tudor courtyards. All rooms with incline have ramps. Lift access to all State Apartments. Electrical and mechanical chairs available at West Front entrance, where electric buggies also available for gardens. 3 of 4 shops accessible - kitchen shop is not.

WEST OF THE CENTRE

BRENTFORD

ATTRACTION
KEW BRIDGE STEAM MUSEUM
Green Dragon Lane, Brentford,
Middlesex TW8 0EN
Tel: (020) 8568 4757   Fax: (020) 8569 9978
Housed in C19th Pumping Station, a fine collection of water pumping machinery. Many engines in steam every weekend, including the largest working beam engine in the world – the Cornish grand Junction 90. In the Water for Life Gallery learn about water supply in London from Roman times to the Thames Water Ring Main (you can walk through a slice of it) and about life and disease in the sewers. Also a waterworks railway.

CHISWICK
HOGARTH'S HOUSE
Hogarth Lane, Great West Road, Chiswick,
London W4 2QN
Tel: (020) 8994 6757
Very small Georgian house, home of William Hogarth, with fine permanent display of artist's famous black and white engravings. Ground floor rooms accessible, upper rooms are not. Curator happy to bring a particular picture downstairs.

SD n/a   CP   E   S   WC

LONDON HEATHROW AIRPORT

TRAINS
Heathrow Express: Disabled Assistance:
Tel: (020) 7313 1041

HOTEL
NOVOTEL HEATHROW
Cherry Lane, West Drayton, Middlesex UB7 9HB
Tel: (01895) 431431   Fax: (01895) 431221
No. of Accessible Rooms: 5. Bath
Accessible Facilities: Lounge, restaurant, Pool. Located four miles from Airport at M4 (J4) with shuttle bus service to/from the airport.

RICHMOND
Situated on a delightful stretch of the River Thames, a mile upstream from Kew, rich in parks and gardens. Richmond Park, once the hunting ground of Charles I, is Europe's largest city park, famous for its deer.

ATTRACTION
ROYAL BOTANIC GARDENS, KEW
Richmond TW9 3AB
Tel: (020) 8940 1171   Fax: (020) 8332 5197
On a first visit you must see the famous Palm House and the Princess of Wales Conservatory, then explore either the East or North sections. There is much to see here.

RFE   Entire site has level tarmac paths.
Kew operates a 'Discovery' mobility bus for groups with special needs with space for two permanent wheelchair users. Must pre-book.

CONCERT HALLS
ROYAL ALBERT HALL
Kensington Gore, London SW7 2AP
Tel: (020) 7589 3203   Fax: (020) 7823 7725
e-mail: admin@royalalberthall.com

Huge concert hall, a London landmark, modelled on the Roman amphitheatre and completed in 1871. Famous as home of the Proms concerts, but also used for major boxing matches and other events. NB: Use the West Car Park, almost completely designated for disabled users. Entrance ramped at 1:16.

SD ♿ CP ♿ E ♿ RF ♿ L ♿
C ♿ S n/a WC 🚹

ROYAL FESTIVAL HALL
Belvedere Road, South Bank Centre,
London SE1 8XX
Tel: (020) 7921 0926   Fax: (020) 7921 0607
e-mail: customer@rfh.org.uk

First major public building in London after WWII, a major concert venue, with sweeping staircases leading up from foyer.

SD ♿ CP ♿ E ♿ RF ♿ L ♿
C ♿ S ♿ WC 🚹 RFE 🚹

WIGMORE HALL
36 Wigmore Street, London W1H 0BP
Tel: (020) 7486 1907   Fax: (020) 7224 3800
Box Office: Tel: (020) 7935 2141
Fax: (020) 7935 3344

Complies Part M, Building Regulations. NB. Nearest Public car park, NCP Cavendish Square and Marylebone Lane. Access straight in from foyer to rear of auditorium to wheelchair spaces.

SD ♿ CP 🚹 E ♿ RF ♿
L ♿ WC ♿ C ♿

THEATRES. FOR FULL DETAILS CONTACT ARTSLINE – LONDON'S LEADING CHARITY FOR INFORMATION ON DISABLED ACCESS TO ALL ARTS VENUES.
ARTSLINE
54 Chalton Street, London NW1 1HS
Tel/Minicom: (020) 7388 2227
Fax: (020) 7388 2653
e-mail: artsline@dircon.co.uk
web: dircon.co.uk/artsline

All listed offer designated seats and accessible WC facilities. All require an able-bodied companion.

ADELPHI
The Strand WC2E 7NA
Tel: Ticketmaster: (020) 7344 0055
BARBICAN THEATRE
Barbican Centre, Silk Street EC2Y 8DS
Tel: (020) 7638 8891
Minicom: (020) 7382 7297
Fax: (020) 7382 7270
CAMBRIDGE THEATRE
Earlham Street WC2 9HU
Box Office through Stoll Moss:
Tel: (020) 7494 5470   Fax: (020) 7494 5147
COLISEUM
St. Martin's Lane EC2N 9HU
Tel: (020) 7632 8300
Minicom: (020) 7836 7666
CRITERION
Piccadilly Circus W1V 9LB
Tel: (020) 7839 8811
DRURY LANE
Theatre Royal, Catherine Street WC2B 5JF
Tel: Stoll Moss (020) 7494 5470
Fax: (020) 7494 5154
HER MAJESTY'S
Haymarket SW1 4QR
Tel: Stoll Moss: (020) 7494 5470
Fax: (020) 7494 5154

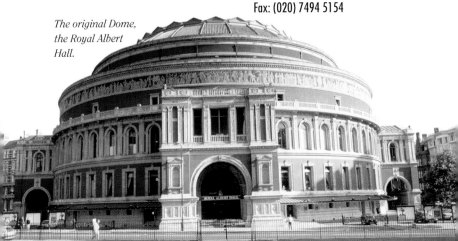

The original Dome, the Royal Albert Hall.

LONDON PALLADIUM
Argyll Street W1V 1AD
Tel: Stoll Moss: (020) 7494 5470
Fax: (020) 7494 5154
LYCEUM
Wellington Street WC2E 7DA
Tel: (020) 7420 8112 Fax: (020) 7240 4346
LYRIC
Shaftesbury Avenue W1V 7HA
Tel: Stoll Moss: (020) 7494 5470
Fax: (020) 7494 5154
NATIONAL THEATRE
South Bank SE1 9PX
Three auditoria housed in one building.
Tel: (020) 7928 2252
Minicom: (020) 7928 1963
Information Desk: (020) 7633 0880
OLD VIC
Waterloo Road SE1 8NB
Tel: (020) 7928 7616 Fax: (020) 7928 3608
OPEN AIR
Inner Circle, Regent's Park NW1 4NP
Tel: (020) 7486 2431 Fax: (020) 7487 4562
PALACE
Shaftesbury Avenue W1V 8AY
Tel: (020) 7434 0909 Fax: (020) 7734 6157
PHOENIX
Charing Cross Road WC2H 0JP
Tel: (020) 7465 0211 Fax: (020) 7465 0212
THE PLAYERS' THEATRE
The Arches, Villiers Street, Strand WC2N 6NG
Booking: (020) 7839 1136 Fax: (020) 7839 8067
e-mail: THEPLAYERS@aol.com
Not covered by Artsline.
Access: Cars drop passengers at entrance to
Arches in Villiers Street (40m. on flat). Taxis
can also be called to this spot. Route to
Entrance is level: Main entrance accessible,
although with manual door: Interior doors
75cm wide and corridors 120cm: Adapted
unisex WC on entrance level (Access to three
dispersed designated wheelchair spaces with
companion spaces adjacent, through front
entrance. Level access Restaurant and Bar
THE PLAYHOUSE
Northumberland Avenue WC2N 5De
Tel: (020) 7839 4401 Fax: (020) 7839 1195
PRINCE EDWARD
Old Compton Street W1V 6HS
Tel: (020) 7447 5400
ROYAL COURT THEATRE DOWNSTAIRS
(Duke of York's)
St. Martin's Lane WC2N 9HN

Tel: (020) 7565 5000 Fax: (020) 7565 5001
SAVOY
The Strand WC2R 0ET
Tel: (020) 7836 8888
VICTORIA PALACE
Victoria Street SW1E 5EA
Tel: (020) 7834 1317

SPORTING VENUES

ARSENAL FOOTBALL CLUB
Arsenal Stadium, Highbury, London N5 1BU
Tel: (020) 7704 4000 Fax: (020) 7704 4001
web: www.arsenal.co.uk
Booking: as above.
CP [♿] (Elwood Street) RE [♿] ED [♿] INT [♿]
L [♿] WC [♿] (10 units in various locations)
SS [♿] (Direct access to enclosure) B/R [♿]

ALL ENGLAND LAWN TENNIS AND CROQUET
CLUB (WIMBLEDON)
Church Road, Wimbledon, London SW19 5AE
Tel: (020) 8944 1066 Fax: (020) 8947 8752
Booking: Only by public Ballot
Facility complies with Part M, Building
Regulations. 'Wheelchair Users Guide to
the Championships' brochure available.
Wheelchair spaces: Centre & No. 1 Courts – ticket holders
only. Courts 6, 13, 14, 15, 18, 19 – unreserved space.
CP [♿] RE [♿] ED (On-the-day sales) [♿]
L [♿] WC [♿] (5 units) SS [♿] B/R [♿]

WEST HAM UNITED FOOTBALL CLUB
Boleyn Ground, Green Street, Upton Park,
Plaistow, London E13 9az
Admin. & Box Office: Tel: (020) 8548 2748
Fax: (020) 8548 2758
Web: www.westhamunited.co.uk
Complies with Part M, Building Regulations
CP [♿] RE [♿] ED [♿] (except door non-
automatic) INT [♿] L [♿] WC [♿]
SS [♿] (5 separate wheelchair locations) B/R [♿]

WIMBLEDON FOOTBALL CLUB
Selhurst Park Stadium, South Norwood,
London SE25 6PY
Tel: (020) 8771 2233 Fax: (020) 8768 0641
Booking: Tel: (020) 8777 8841
Fax: (020) 8653 4708
Tailor made area, Holmesdale Stand with
steward on duty.
CP [♿] ED [♿] WC [♿] (2 sites within disabled area)
SS [♿] B/R [♿]

MANCHESTER
(GREATER)

GREATER MANCHESTER HIGHWAYS AND ACCESS DISABILITY GROUP
Tel: (0161) 246 8323

GREATER MANCHESTER COALITION OF DISABLED PEOPLE (GMCDP)
CarisBrooke, Wenlock Way, Gorton, Manchester M12 5LF
Tel: (0161) 273 5154

GREATER MANCHESTER COUNCIL FOR VOLUNTARY SERVICE
St.Thomas Centre, Ardwick Green North, Manchester M12 6FZ
Tel: (0161) 273 7451

BOLTON

Fine industrial heritage and Victorian architecture situated in the lee of the West Pennine Moors, with excellent shopping, large selection of mill shops and diverse range of attractions.

TOURIST INFORMATION CENTRE
Town Hall, Victoria Square, Bolton BL1 1RU
Tel: (01204) 364333 Fax: (01204) 398101

HOTEL
BOLTON MOAT HOUSE ♿
1 Higher Bridge Street, Bolton BL1 2EW
Tel: (01204) 879988 Fax: (01204) 280777
No. of Accessible Rooms: 2
Accessible Facilities: Lounge, Restaurant, Lift, Pool, Sauna, Spa. Premier hotel set within former church in heart of town centre. Promotes welcome to wheelchair users travelling independently.

MANCHESTER

Fast becoming one of the UK's most dynamic cities with a rich combination of arts, entertainment, heritage, leisure activities and shopping.

TOURIST INFORMATION CENTRE
Town Hall Extension, Lloyd Street, Manchester M60 2LA
Tel: (0161) 234 3157/3158
Tel: (0891) 715533 (24 hour)
Fax: (0161) 236 9900

THE ACCESS UNIT
GMPTE, 9 Portland Street, Piccadilly Gardens, Manchester M60 1HX
Tel: (0161) 242 6243
Produces comprehensive *Rough Guide* for people with disabilities, covering Central Greater Manchester and surrounding area.

BUSES
GMPTE enquiry line: Tel: (0161) 2287811 - textphone available)
Some low-floor buses.
Metrolink: tel: (0161) 2052000
Fully accessible tram.

TAXIS
Taxi Licensing officer: Tel: (0161) 2344956
Mantax: Tel: (0161) 2365133
702 adapted vehicles.

TRAINS
First North Western: Special Needs:
Tel: (0845) 6040231
Virgin Trains: Special Needs:
Tel: (0845) 7443366
Minicom: (0845) 7443367
Wales & West: Special Needs:
Tel: (0845) 3003005
Minicom: (0845) 7585469
Piccadilly Station: Tel: (0345) 697275
Victoria Station: (0845) 6040231

CAR PARKS
Free unlimited parking in pay and display car parks:
Tel: (0161) 234 4039

SHOPMOBILITY
Unit 129, Market Way, Upper Mall, Arndale Centre, Manchester M4 2EA
Tel: (0161) 839 4060
Fax: (0161) 839 5110
Minicom: (0161) 839 6050

HOTELS
COPTHORNE MANCHESTER ♿
Clippers Quay, Salford Quays, Manchester M5 2XP
Tel: (0161) 873 7321 Fax: (0161) 873 7318

No. of Accessible Rooms: 1. Bath Accessible Facilities: Lounge, Restaurant. Modern hotel with fine waterfront location in unique setting of Salford Quays.

RENAISSANCE (RAMADA) HOTEL
Blackfriars Street, Manchester M3 2EQ
Tel: (0161) 835 2555   Fax: (0161) 833 0731
No. of Accessible Rooms: 2. Bath Accessible Facilities: Lounge, Restaurant, Bar. Quality city centre hotel, modern and bright with large bedrooms.

LE MERIDIEN VICTORIA & ALBERT HOTEL
Water Street, Manchester M3 4JQ
Tel: (0161) 832 1888   Fax: (0161) 834 2484
No. of Accessible Rooms: 2. Bath Accessible Facilities: Lounge, Restaurant. Listed building of mellowed brickwork and exposed beams, standing on banks of River Irwell.

NOVOTEL MANCHESTER WEST
Worsley Brow, Worsley, Manchester M22 5WP
Tel: (0161) 799 3535 Fax: (0161) 703 8207
No. of Accessible Rooms: 2. Bath Accessible Facilities: Lounge, Restaurant, Pool. Modern hotel located west of city near M62.

RADISSON SAS HOTEL MANCHESTER AIRPORT
Chicago Avenue, Manchester M90 3RA
Tel: (0161) 490 5000 Fax: (0161) 490 5095
Web: www.radisson.com.manchesteruk
No. of Accessible Rooms: 18. Roll-in Shower. Accessible Facilities: Lounge, Restaurant. Situated between Terminals 1 and 2 and the railway station and directly connected to these by a Skylink walkway.

CROWNE PLAZA THE MIDLAND
Peter Street, Manchester M60 2DS
Tel: (0161) 236 3333 Fax: (0161) 9324100
web: www.crowneplaza.com
No. of Accessible Rooms: 1. Bath Accessible Facilities: Lounge (ramped), Restaurants (2 of 3 -Nico's not accessible), Health Centre (Pool-2 steps).
Large, quality hotel of grand Edwardian architecture, built in 1903, in city centre. Venue of first meeting between Messrs Rolls and Royce in 1904.

JURYS MANCHESTER INN
56 Great Bridgewater Street, Manchester M1 5LE
Tel: (0161) 9538888 Fax: (0161) 9539090
e-mail: enquiry@jurys.com
web: www.jurys.com
City centre location

MANCHESTER AIRPORT MOAT HOUSE
Altrincham Road, Wilmslow SK9 4LR
Tel: (01625) 889988 Fax: (01625) 531876
No. of Accessible Rooms: 2
Accessible Facilities: Lounge, Restaurant. Conveniently situated for the Airport and M6.

THISTLE MANCHESTER
Portland Street, Manchester M1 6DP
Tel: (0161) 2283400 Fax: (0161) 2286347
e-mail: sales.manchester@thistle.co.uk
No. of Accessible Rooms: 1
Accessible Facilities: Lounge, Restaurant
Quality hotel in central location

ATTRACTIONS
GRANADA STUDIOS
Water Street, Manchester M60 9EA
Tel: (0161) 832 4999   Fax: (0161) 834 3684
For more than 4 decades Granada Television has been one of the world's busiest studios, and now offers themed attractions, from the thrills of Robocop, through the glamour of a backstage tour, sets from Coronation Street and the inter-action of Cracker.

SD | CP | E- | L
C | S | WC | RFE

Pint please, Natalie!

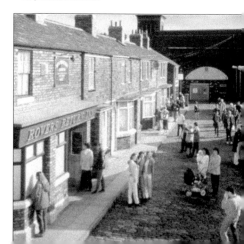

MUSEUM OF TRANSPORT
Boyle Street, Cheetham, Manchester M8 8UL
Tel/Fax: (0161) 2052122
Travel through the ages here with over 70 buses and other vehicles from the city's past.

SD ♿   CP ♿   E ♿   RF ♿   C ♿
S ♿   WC ♿   RFE ♿

THE PUMP HOUSE: PEOPLE'S HISTORY MUSEUM
Left Bank, Bridge Street, Manchester M3 3ER
Tel: (0161) 839 6061   Fax: (0161) 839 6027
The Museum houses the galleries of the National Museum of Labour History, and tells the story of the ordinary people of Britain and how they organised together to change society. Displays and reconstructions recreate day to day lives.

SD ♿   CP ♿   E ♿   C ♿
S ♿   WC ♿   L ♿

TRAFFORD ECOLOGY PARK
Lake Road, Trafford Park, Manchester M17 1TU
Tel: (0161) 873 7182   Fax: (0161) 876 0523

SD ♿   CP ♿   E ♿   C & S n/a   WC ♿
Features: Some tree roots grow across park which may obstruct. 50% of the park is grass covered making chair movement difficult in places.

Sensory Garden ♿   Picnic Area ♿
Bird Hide ♿   Bee observation Hide ♿
Ponds ♿

MANCHESTER CITY ART GALLERY
Mosley Street, Manchester M2 3JL
Tell: (0161) 236 5244   Fax: (0161) 236 7369
Closed until 2001. New gallery will be fully accesible with ramps throughout and lifts to all floors.

THEATRE
MANCHESTER OPERA HOUSE
Quay Street, Manchester M3 3HP
Tel: (0161) 8341787   Fax: (0161) 834 5243

SD ♿
CP ♿ Nearest Public CP: Haldman Street
Nearest Taxi Rank: Byron Street.
RE ♿   ED ♿
INT ♿ Box Office Counter widths ♿
WC ♿   AUD ♿

The Manchester Opera House. Built when cotton was king.

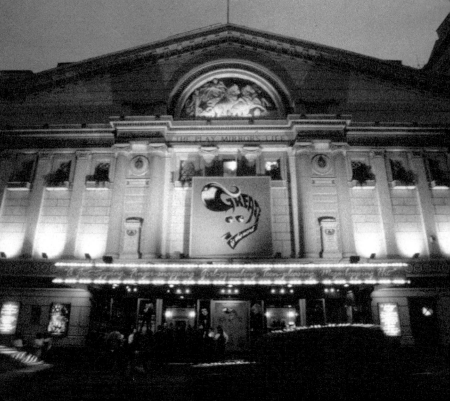

STOCKPORT

Originally a market centre with its own bridge across the River Mersey in the 13thC, it developed during the Industrial Revolution.There are mills, great chimneys and a fine 19thC railway viaduct.

TOURIST INFORMATION CENTRE

Graylaw House, Chestergate, Stockport SK1 1NH
Tel: (0161) 4743320/3321
Fax: (0161) 4296348

BUSES

GMPTE: Tel: (0161) 2287811
All information on local bus & train services.

TAXIS

Rank at railway Station
Hackney Taxis: Tel: (0161) 4801236
5 adapted vehicles
1919 Taxis: Tel: (0161) 4941919
1 adapted minibus
Metro Taxis: Tel: (0161) 4773633
6 adapted vehicles
Teletaxis: tel: (0161) 4804864
24 adapted vehicles

TRAINS

First North Western: Special Needs:
Tel: (0845) 6040231
Wales & West: Special Needs:
Tel: (0845) 3003005
Minicom: (0845) 7585469

CAR PARKS

Orange badge parking provided both on- and-off -street.
Tel: (0161) 480 4949

SHOPMOBLITY
Level 2, Merseyway Car Park,
Stockport SK1 1PD
Tel: (0161) 6661100
Fax: (0161) 6661101

HOTELS

THE SAXON HOLME   ⟨🕴⟩
230 Wellington Road North, Stockport SK4 2QN
Tel: (0161) 432 2335 Fax: (0161) 431 8076
No. of Accessible Rooms: 29. Shower
Family owned hotel on outskirts of town
within easy reach of the Peak District,

North Wales, Lakes and Yorkshire Dales
(close to Chatsworth, Styal and Lyme Hall)

COUNTY HOTEL   ⟨🕴⟩
Bramhall Lane, South Bramhall,
Stockport SK7 2EB
Tel: (0161) 4559988 Fax: (0161) 4408071
No. of Accessible Rooms: 1
Accessible Facilities: Lounge, Restaurant.
Modern and comfortable property located in village of Bramhall, a few miles from Stockport, in pleasant countryside.

WIGAN

Interesting blend of picturesque countryside and hidden villages, award winning shopping centres and some heritage and culture. Originally important for its coal production.

TOURIST INFORMATION CENTRE

Trencherfield Mill, Wallgate, Wigan WN3 4EL
Tel/Fax: (01942) 825677

HOTEL

WIGAN/STANDISH MOAT HOUSE   ⟨🕴⟩
Almond Brook Road, Standish,
Nr. Wigan WN6 0SR
Tel: (01257) 499988 Fax: (01257) 427327
No. of Accessible Rooms: 2. Bath
Accessible Facilities: Reception, Lounge,
Restaurant, Bar (2 steps)
Modern, light and airy property within easy reach of Manchester and Blackpool.

ATTRACTION

WIGAN PIER 'The Way we Were' MUSEUM
Wallgate, Wigan WN3 4EU
Tel: (01942) 323666 Fax: (01942) 322031
Recreation of Lancashire life at the turn of the century through series of set and exhibits. On 3 floors with passenger lift. 8 wheelchairs available. The Engine Room in Trencherfield Mill houses world's largest original mill steam engine ñ accessed by lift. Waterbuses around the Pier complex offer wheelchair lifts on ëEmma' and ëNetta' but with Pier wheelchairs only. Canal-side towpaths are not accessible. Useful Access leaflet.

SD ⟨♿⟩ CP ⟨♿⟩ E ⟨♿⟩ RF ⟨♿⟩ L ⟨♿⟩ WC ⟨🕴⟩

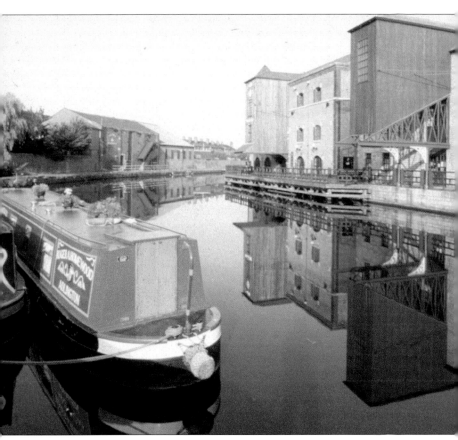

Wigan Pier. No sign of 'Our Gracie'.

WIGAN PIER 'Museum of Memories'
Address as above.

Opened in May 1999, this is a visual journey through Wigan's social history from Victorian times to present day. Re-creation of shops and evocative displays, all aspects of daily life are explored.

SD n/a   CP   E   RF   C
S [&]   WC [大]

WIGAN COUNTRYSIDE SERVICES
1-3 Worlsey Terrace, Standish Gate, Wigan
Tel: (01942) 828906

Accessible countryside.
Pennington Flash. Tel: (01942) 605253
Turn of the century mining subsidence and flooding now developed in park with 180 acre lake focal point surrounded by wetland, attracting many bird species. Ramped bird hides placed around well-maintained circular footpath. Paths are double width for wheelchair access, but in some parts a pusher needed.
Very accessible.

Leeds-Liverpool Canal
Tel: (01942) 242239

Part of Wigan's industrial heritage, the canal and locks provide varied scenery. Blocked paved stretches provide good surfaces although some gradients around the locks need pusher. Top Lock at New Springs well worth a visit.
Assistance required in places.

The Three Sisters
Tel: (01942) 720453

Reclaimed from 3 huge colliery tips, this recreation area offers family fun. Accessible footpath encircling lake. Very accessible.

NORFOLK

NORFOLK DISABILITY INFORMATION SERVICE
The Vauxhall Centre, Johnson Place, Vauxhall
Street, Norwich NR2 2SA
Tel: (01603) 763295   Fax: (01603) 610632
e-mail: ndis@gtnet.gov.uk
NDIS newsletter published regularly.

CASTLE ACRE
Conservation village 4 miles north of
Swaffham. Straddled by ancient Roman
road, the Peddlars Way, with 15thC
church, the village has two EH sites: ruins
of 11thC castle built by son in law of
William the Conqueror, and remains of
12thC Cluniac priory. Full of Restaurants,
pubs, antique and craft shops.

SELF-CATERING
CHERRY TREE COTTAGE
Wellington House, Back Lane, Castle Acre,
Kings Lynn PE32 2AR
Tel/Fax: (01760) 755000
E-mail: boswell@paston.co.uk
boswell@paston.co.uk
No of Accessible Units: 1. Roll-in Shower
No. of Beds per Unit: 6
Accessible Facilities: Lounge, Dinging
Room, Kitchen. One of a pair of traditional
Norfolk brick and flint cottages of 19thC
on the periphery of the village.

CROMER
Victorian seaside town, once a renowned
port with the tower of St. Peter & St. Paul
standing 55m tall.

TOURIST INFORMATION CENTRE
Cromer Bus Station, Prince of Wales Road,
Cromer NR27 9HS
Tel: (01263) 512497

HOTEL
ROMAN CAMP INN
Holt Road, Aylmerton, Nr. Cromer NR11 5QD
Tel: (01263) 838921   Fax: (01263) 837071
No. of Accessible Rooms: 2. Shower
Accessible Facilities: Lounge, Conservatory

Restaurant, Landscaped Gardens.
Fine old fashioned rural inn atmosphere,
with lovely gardens, located between
Sheringham and Cromer, close to
Norfolk's highest point, Beacon Hill.

DEREHAM
Busy market town originally established as
a religious community by the daughter of a
Saxon king. It has a Grade II listed
windmill and a quaint local history
museum housed in the16thC Bishop
Bonner's cottages.

TOURIST INFORMATION CENTRE
The Bell Tower, Church Street, Dereham
Tel: (01362) 698992

SELF-CATERING
DAIRY FARMHOUSE COTTAGES
Bittering, Dereham NR19 1QU
Tel/Fax: (01362) 687687
No. of Accessible Units: 2. Roll-in Shower
No. of Beds per Unit: 6. Accessible
Facilities: Lounge, Dining Room, Kitchen,
Garden, Garden furniture, Games Room.
2, of 3 properties, situated in peaceful
rural surroundings with private garden.
Bittering is a small hamlet centrally placed
for touring Kings Lynn, Cromer, Broads
and Norwich. Nearest beaches at Holkham
and Wells-30 minutes drive.

MOOR FARM STABLE COTTAGES
Moor Farm, Foxley, Dereham NR20 4QN
Tel/Fax: (01352) 688523
e-mail: moorfarm@aol.com
No. of Accessible Units: 2. Shower
No. of Beds per Unit: 2
Accessible Facilities: Lounge, Dining
Room, kitchen, 2 , of 7 converted stable
cottages a courtyard. Situated on a
working farm in village between Fakenham
and Dereham.

ATTRACTION
NORFOLK RURAL LIFE MUSEUM
Beech House, Gressenhall, Dereham NR20 4DR
Tel: (01362) 860563
200 years of Norfolk's rural history with
displays which include a typical farm
labourer's home at the turn of the century,

a working farm with machinery used before the age of the tractor and farm trail and woodland.

SD ♿   CP ♿   E ♿   RF ♿
C ♿   S ♿   WC ♿   RFE ♿

DISS
ATTRACTION
BRESSINGHAM STEAM MUSEUM TRUST & GARDENS
Bressingham, Diss IP22 2AB
Tel: (01379) 687386
Fax: (01379) 688085

Gardens: The steam trains run through 2.5 miles of Europe's largest hardy plant nursery. The Dell Garden has wonderful species of perennials and alpines: Foggy Bottom has panoramas, pathways, trees and shrubs. Trains: Entrance and area for 40m beyond are level: thereafter the site sits on gentle gradient of 1:55. The features of the site include 3 ramps: 1) over level crossing, avoidable by path around outside of adjacent building): 2) Ramp to another level crossing of 1:20: 3) Ramp up from same level crossing of 1:10. Ramps 2 and 3 lead to the gardens. Level crossings themselves are smooth. The Nursery Railway, the main railway feature, has specially converted carriage to carry wheelchairs and boarding is via a wide and level gangplank. Access to Waveney Railway is more difficult, unless able to transfer from wheelchair to train seat. The miniature Garden railway is not accessible. All the railways can be watched easily from almost anywhere on the site.

SD ♿   CP   E ♿   RF ♿
C ♿   S   WC ♿   RFE

FAKENHAM
Thriving market town in lovely countryside. Famous for one of finest National Hunt courses in the country.

TOURIST INFORMATION CENTRE
Red Lion House, Market Place, Fakenham
Tel: (01328) 851981

SPORTING VENUE
FAKENHAM RACEOURSE
Fakenham NR21 7NY
Admin & Booking-Box Office:
(01328) 862388   Fax: (01328) 855908

CP ♿   RE ♿   ED ♿   INT ♿
WC ♿   B/R ♿

GREAT YARMOUTH
Situated where three Rivers, the Bure, Waveney and Yare, converge to find their way into the North Sea, this watery surrounding gives the town a character similar to that of Dutch and Flemish cities. Busy harbour, market town and popular seaside resort.

HOTEL
HORSE & GROOM MOTEL
Main Road, Rollesby, Gt. Yarmouth NR29 5ER
Tel: (01493) 740624   Fax: (01493) 740022
No. of Accessible Rooms: 1. Bath
Accessible Facilities: Restaurant.
Located 6 miles from Gt. Yarmouth.

BURLINGTON & PALM COURT HOTELS ♿
North Drive, Great Yarmouth NR30 1EG
Tel: (01493) 844568   Fax: (01493) 331848
No. of Accessible Rooms: 5. Bath
Accessible Facilities: Lounge, Restaurant, Pool (3 steps). Family owned and managed adjacent hotels facing the seafront

ATTRACTION
THRIGBY HALL WILDLIFE GARDENS
Thrigby, Great Yarmouth NR29 3DR
Tel: (01493) 368256   Fax: (01493) 369477
e-mail: thrigby@globalnet.co.uk
web: www/optpoint.co.uk/thrigby

Home to the animals of Asia. Tropical bird house, blue willow-patterned garden, tree walk and summerhouse. Jungle swamp hall has underwater viewing of crocodiles.

SD ♿   CP ♿   E ♿   RF ♿   C ♿
S ♿   WC ♿   RFE ♿

HOLT
Site of the famous Greshams School, founded in 1555, the town has pleasant buildings.

TOURIST INFORMATION CENTRE
3 Pound House, Market Place, Holt
Tel: (01263) 713100

HOTEL
THE PHEASANT HOTEL ♿
The Coast Road, Kelling, Nr. Holt NR25 7EG
Tel: (01263) 588382   Fax: (01263) 588101
e-mail: stay@hotel-pheasant.co.uk
web: www.hotel-pheasant.co.uk
No. of Accessible Rooms: 5. Bath
Accessible Facilities: Lounge, Restaurant.
Attractive country hotel situated on the
coast road in a delightful setting, midway
between Blakeney and Sheringham.

ATTRACTION
THE MUCKLEBURGH COLLECTION
Weybourne Military Camp, Weybourne,
Holt NR25 7EG
Tel: (01263) 588210   Fax: (01263) 588425
e-mail: Jenny@Muckleburgh.demon.co.uk
Large military collection with 3000
exhibits including restored tanks and
artillery of WW11, Falklands and Gulf War
equipment and model displays and
dioramas, and much more.

HORNING
Well-known Broadland centre on River
Bure, with picturesque cottages and
attractive glimpses of the River from the
main street.

SELF-CATERING
LADY LODGE
HORNING LODGES 1, 2 & 3
KINGS LINE CRUISES
Ferry View Estate, Horning, Norwich NR12 8PT
Tel: (01692) 630297   Fax: (01692) 630498
e-mail: kingline@norfolk-braods.co.uk
web: www.norfolk-broads.co.uk
No. of Accessible Units: 4.
Lady & Lodge 3 - Roll-in Shower.
Lodge 1 & 2. -Shower.
No. of Beds per Unit: Lady -1D/1T
Horning 1-1D/1T: Horning 2 & 3-2T/1D
Accessible Facilities: Lounge, Kitchen.
Family owned and operated cottages on
Norfolk Broads. Superb location with

frontage on the River Bure, about 10 miles
from Norwich.

HORSEY
Only a barrier of sand dunes separates this
Broad from the North Sea, and the seepage
of seawater makes this the most brackish of
all the Norfolk Broads. As a result, bird and
insect life is particularly interesting.

BED & BREAKFAST
THE OLD CHAPEL
Horsey Corner, Horsey NR29 4EH
Tel: (01493) 393498   Fax: (01493) 393444
No. of Accessible Rooms: 3. Shower
Accessible Facilities: Dining Room
Located 12 miles NE of Norwich close to
the coast. Boat trips available at Hickling
for wheelchair users. Park & Ride facilities
into Norwich for wheelchair users at
Postwick

HUNSTANTON
Facing into the Wash, on the west coast of
Norfolk, there is a vast shingle and sand
beach backed by cliffs. Much of the town is
Victorian, built simultaneously with the
railway line.

TOURIST INFORMATION CENTRE
The Green, Hunstanton PE36 6BQ
Tel: (01485) 532610

HOTEL
GOLDEN LION HOTEL
The Green, Hunstanton PE36 6BQ
Tel: (01485) 532688 Fax: (01485) 535310
No. of Accessible Rooms: 3. Bath
Accessible Facilities: Lounge, Restaurant
Hunstanton's oldest building, constructed
in 1846 of red brick and recently
refurbished, is the hub of much of
Hunstanton's social activity.

ATTRACTION
NORFOLK LAVENDER
Caley Mill, Heacham, Nr. Hunstanton PE31 7JE
Tel: (01485) 570384 Fax: (01485) 571176
e-mail: admin@norfolk-lavender.co.uk
Caley Mill, originally a water mill for
grinding corn, and now set in the Lavender

Gardens, which hold the National Collection of Lavenders. Each of the 50 variety or species has its own bed. Also Herb Garden, Fragrant Meadow Garden and Plant Centre.

SD ♿ CP ♿ E ♿ RF ♿
C ♿ S 🚶 WC 🚶 RFE ♿

KING'S LYNN

Originally a walled city of considerable importance, much of the wall remains in this busy town, seaport and agricultural centre.

TOURIST INFORMATION CENTRE
The Old Gaol House, Saturday Market Place, King's Lynn
Tel: (01553) 763044

HOTEL
FFOLKES ARMS HOTEL 🚶
Lynn Road, Hillington, King's Lynn PE31 6BJ
Tel: (01485) 600210 Fax: (01485) 601196
No. of Accessible Rooms: 10. Roll-in Shower
Accessible Facilities: Lounge, Restaurant. Constructed over 300 years ago, the hotel became well known as a coaching inn, and has been completely modernised without losing any of its original charm. Located 6 miles from nearest town or railway station.

SELF-CATERING
PARK COTTAGE ♿
Narford Road, Narborough, King's Lynn PE32 1HZ
Tel: (01760) 337220
No. of Accessible Units: 1
Accessible Facilities:
Peaceful Bungalow in 3 acres of garden and woodland in village near town.

NORTH WALSHAM
Located between Cromer and Great Yarmouth.

TOURIST INFORMATION CENTRE
Brentnall House, 32 Vicarage Street,
North Walsham
Tel: (01692) 407509

SELF-CATERING
DAIRY FARM COTTAGES ♿
Manor Farm, Dilham, North Walsham NR28 9PZ

Tel: (01692) 535178 Fax: (01692) 536723
e-mail: JAPdilman@farmline.com
No. of Accessible Units: 2
No. of Beds per Unit: 3. Roll-in Shower
Accessible Facilities: Kitchen/Living area combined. 2 of 6 cottages converted from farm buildings, facing south across large grassed area. Each has a patio. Small traditional farm in peaceful rural setting, surrounded by woodland. Dilham is in the heart of the Norfolk Broads, 5 miles from North Walsham.

NORWICH
The capital of Norfolk, a beautiful city developed by a large double bend in the River Wensum and within its medieval walls. Its lack of industrialisation and geographical position have help to preserve many of the city's older buildings, with Colman's mustard the only large industrial company here. It is hilly and the Saxon street layout is disorientating but the landmarks of Cathedral and Norman castle stand out.

TOURIST INFORMATION CENTRE
The Guildhall, Gaol Hill, Norwich NR2 1NF
Tel: (01603) 666071 Fax: (01603) 765389
e-mail: tourism.norwich@gtnet.gov.uk

NORWICH ACCESS GROUP
22 Brecon Road, Brooke, Norwich NR15 1HS
Tel/Fax: (01508) 550116
e-mail: sash@paston.co.uk

BUSES
Bus Information Centre: Tel: (0500) 626116
Publishes information on services and park & ride.

TAXIS
Rank at station
Express Taxis: Tel: (01603) 767626
20 adapted vehicles.

TRAINS
Anglia Railways: Assistance:
Tel: (01473) 693333
Minicom: (01603) 630748 or (0845) 6050600

CAR PARKS
Car Park services: Tel: (01603) 212420
Green badge scheme for residents and
visitors -apply in advance at above tel.no.

SHOPMOBILITY
2 Castle Mall, Norwich NR1 3DD
Tel: (01603) 766430

WHEELCHAIR HIRE
New Life: Tel: (01603) 623200
Hires wheelchairs to all.

HOTEL
ASHWELLTHORPE HALL HOTEL ♿
Ashwellthorpe, Norwich NR16 1EX
Tel: (01508) 489324   Fax: (01508) 488409
No. of Accessible Rooms: 19. Roll-in
Shower
Accessible Facilities: Lounge, Restaurant,
Games & TV Rooms. 8 miles south of
Norwich, an Elizabethan manor house set
in 15 acres of easily accessible grounds.
Fully accessible and equipped for disabled
people, whilst maintaining hotel ambience
and suitable for non-disabled guests also.

THE BEECHES HOTEL ♿
4-6 Earlham Road, Norwich NR2 3DB
Tel: (01603) 621167   Fax: (01603) 620151
E-mail: reception@beeches.co.uk
No. of Accessible Rooms: 1. Bath
Accessible Facilities: Lounge, Dining
Room. Set in a 3-acre garden 0.5 mile from
city centre.

THE OLD RECTORY 🚶
North Walsham Road, Crostwick,
Norwich NR12 7BG
Tel: (01603) 738513 Fax: (01603) 738712
No. of Accessible Rooms: 1.Bath
Accessible Facilities: Lounge, Restaurant,
Bar, Garden, Outdoor Pool.
Original building dates back to mid 18thC
to which 13 lovely rooms have been added.
Located 4 miles north of Norwich

SELF-CATERING
THE HIDEAWAY 🚶
C/o Heath Bungalow, Woodbastwick Road,
Blofield Heath, Nr. Norwich NR15 4AB
Tel: (01603) 715052
No. of Accessible Units: 1. Shower

No. of Beds per Unit: 1
Accessible Facilities: Lounge, Dining
Room, Kitchen. Holiday flat adjoining
owner's home, in village about 7 miles
east of city centre on A27.

ATTRACTIONS
SAINSBURY CENTRE FOR VISUAL ARTS
University of East Anglia, Norwich NR4 7TJ
Tel: (01603) 593199   Fax: (01603) 259401
e-mail: scva.@uea.ac.uk
European art of 19th and 20thCs on
display together with African tribal
sculpture and North American and pre-
Colombian art. Antiquities from Egypt,
Asia and Europe also on show.

SD ♿   CP ♿   E ♿   RF ♿
L ♿   C 🚶   S ♿
WC ♿   (horizontal support rail 57cm from seat centre.)
RFE ♿

**THE FAIRHAVEN TRUST WOODLAND & WATER
GARDEN**
School Road, South Walsham,
Nr. Norwich NR13 6DZ
Tel/Fax: (01603) 270449
Delightful gardens with splendid array of
shrubs and plants leading to private Broad
with boat trips. I visited in late spring
when rhododendrons and candelabra
primulas at their finest. Long walk from
CP to gardens themselves, but wide paths
are grassy and solid earth. River launch
cruises around south Walsham Broads or
explore River Bure and view ancient St.
Benet's Abbey ruins. Although boat staff
happy to assist in swinging from chair
onboard, there is a ramp over the 2 steps
and handrail, ramp height adjusted to tide
and sufficient space inside.

CP ♿   E - Direct access from CP
RF ♿   C ♿   S 🚶   WC 🚶
RFE ♿   BOAT ♿

FELBRIGG HALL (NT)
Felbrigg, Norwich NR11 8PR
Tel: (01263) 837444   Fax: 01263 837032
Fine 17thC house with outstanding library
and Grand Tour paintings. Restored Walled
garden with small orchard. Park of fine
trees.

SD ♿   CP 🚶   E 🚶   RF 🚶
C 🚶   S 🚶   WC 🚶

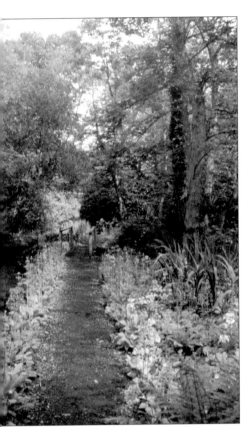

Fairhaven Woodland and Water Gardens can be reached via its own private Broad.

SANDRINGHAM

Famous for Sandringham House, residence of the Royal Family. The estates are extensive and include several parishes and farms, woodlands and other agricultural activities.

HOTEL
PARK HOUSE ⌖
Sandringham, PE35 6EH
Tel: (01485) 543000 Fax: (01485) 540663
No. of Accessible Rooms: All 16
Accessible Facilities: Lounge, Dining Room, Grounds (terraced patio, raised flower beds, wheelchair paths leading through trees), Outdoor Pool with hoist (May-Sept). Adapted Vehicles for area visits to places of interest. Birthplace and childhood home of the late Diana, Princess of Wales, this impressive Victorian country house is set in its own grounds amidst the trees and parkland of the Sandringham Royal Estate. Leased from Her Majesty the Queen by Leonard Cheshire, a leading disability care charity, and converted in a unique purpose-built hotel for people with disabilities and their companions or carers.

ATTRACTION
SANDRINGHAM HOUSE, GROUNDS & MUSEUM
Estate office, Sandringham PE35 6EN
Tel: (01553) 772675 Fax: (01485) 541571
Norfolk country retreat of HM the Queen. The imposing house was built in 1870 and all main rooms used by the Royal Family are open to the public. The 60 acres of grounds are full of shrubs, trees and flowers and the museum contains exhibits of memorabilia of the Royal Family.

CP ⌖   E ⌖   RF ⌖   C ⌖
S ⌖   WC ⌖   RFE ⌖

SWAFFHAM

Elegant town, once a fashionable centre for the Norfolk gentry in the 18thC. Today the triangular market place with its 'market cross' retains a number of fine Georgian houses.

TOURIST INFORMATION CENTRE
Market Place, Swaffham
Tel: (01760) 722255

BED & BREAKFAST
CORFIELD HOUSE ⌖
Sporle, Nr. Swaffham PE32 2EA
Tel: (01760) 723636
e-mail: corfield-house@virgin
No. of Accessible Rooms: 1
Accessible Facilities: Lounge, Dining Room. Family run guest house in peaceful village of Sporle. Accessible room overlooks half-acre of gardens and open fields.

GLEBE BUNGALOW ⌖
8a Princes Street, Swaffham PE37 7BP
Tel: (01760) 722764
No. of Accessible Rooms: 3. Bath
Accessible Facilities: Dining Room, Garden, Patio. Situated on northern edge of the market town of Swaffham, a comfortable home.

SELF-CATERING
HALL BARN COTTAGES
Old Hall Lane, Beachamwell,
Nr. Swaffham PE37 8BG
Tel: (01366) 328794
No. of Accessible Units: 1
Accessible Facilities:
1 of 5 architect designed cottages created
from 17thC barn. Set in five acres of
grounds, each cottage has its own terrace
and shares a lovely walled garden. Cowslip
Cottage has levelled and ramped access and
stairlift to first floor.

THETFORD
Small market town on River Thet,
centrally placed at the junction of eight
main roads. Its most famous citizen was
Thomas Paine, author of *The Rights of
Man* written in 1791. A town full of
interesting streets and buildings.

TOURIST INFORMATION CENTRE
Ancient House Museum,
21 White Hart Street, Thetford
Tel: (01842) 752599

Royal retreat of Sandringham House.

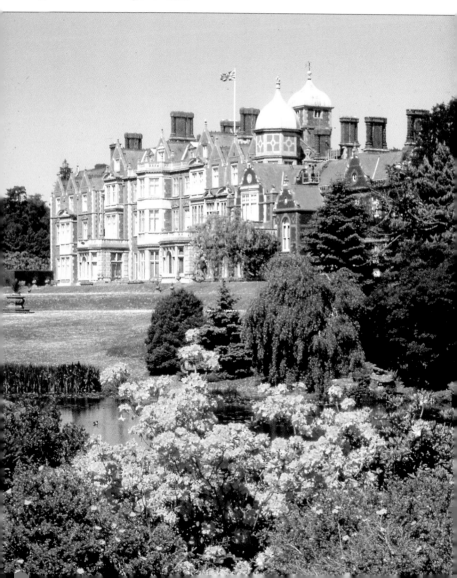

HOTEL
POUND GREEN HOTEL 🚶
Pound Green Lane, Shipdham,
Thetford IP25 7LS
Tel: (01362) 820940 Fax: (01562) 821253
e-mail: poundgreen@aol.com
web: www.poundgreen.co.uk
No. of Accessible Rooms: 5. Bath
Accessible Facilities: Lounge, Restaurant.
Recently refurbished, attractive property
set in 1 acre of own grounds in peaceful
village.

BED & BREAKFAST
JUNIPERS 🚶
18 South Street, Hockwold,
Nr. Thetford OP26 4JG
Tel: (01842) 827370
No. of Accessible Rooms: 1
Accessible Facilities: Dining Room
Spacious bungalow in walled half-acre
garden in quiet village location.

UPPER SHERINGHAM
A village built on the hillside above the
coastal strips. All Saints Church is mainly
perpendicular with a fine 15htC screen
and overhang.

TOURIST INFORMATION CENTRE
Railway Approach, off Station Road,
Sheringham NR26 8RA
Tel: (01263) 824329

BED & BREAKFAST
THE BAY LEAF GUEST HOUSE 🚶
10 Saint Peters Road, Sheringham NR26 8QY
Tel: (01263) 823779 Fax: (01263) 820041
No. of Accessible Rooms: 2
Accessible Facilities: Dining room
Delightful Victorian B & B in central
location for amenities and seafront.

ATTRACTION
SHERINGHAM PARK (NT)
Upper Sheringham NR26 8TB
Tel: (01263) 823778 Fax: None
Woodland park of over 700 acres SW of
the town designed by Humphry Repton,
particularly notable for rhododendrons
and azaleas in late spring. Stunning
views of coast and countryside from

viewing towers.

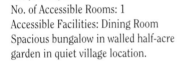

SD ♿   CP ♿   E ♿   RF ♿
C- Outside kiosk   WC ♿
RFE ♿ boarded walkway from car park to viewpoints.
Self-drive vehicle and wheelchair available on request.

WALTON HIGHWAY
4 miles SW of Wisbech and 9 miles SW of
King's Lynn, with much to do in the area.

BED & BREAKFAST/SELF-CATERING
STRATTON FARM B & B: ♿   S/C: ♿
West Drove North, Walton Highway PE14 7DP
Tel: (01945) 880162
B & B: No. of Accessible Rooms: 1. Bath
Accessible Facilities: Lounge, Dining
Room
S/C: No. of Accessible Units: 1. Bath
No. of Beds per Unit: 4
Accessible Facilities: Open Plan
Kitchen/Diner, Lounge. Spacious farm
bungalow and self-catering unit
(Carysfort) set amidst 22 acres of
grassland, grazed by Beef Shorthorn
cattle. There is a lake.

WICKMERE
Quiet agricultural hamlet in heart of
North Norfolk, a few miles SW of Cromer.
Located in rural Conservation Area lying
between Aylsham and coast.

MEADOW COTTAGE 🚶
Church Farm, Wickmere, Norfolk NR11 7NB
Tel: (01263) 577332
e-mail: churchfarm@csma-netlink.co.uk
web: www.csma-netlink.co.uk/users/
churchfarm/welcome.html
No. of Accessible Units: 1
No. of Beds per Unit: 6
Accessible Facilities: Open plan
Living/Dining/ Kitchen, Large private
garden. Meadow Cottage is 1 of 2 lovely
barn conversions forming the wings of
traditional Norfolk bullock yard,
surrounded by fields on 3 sides.

WROXHAM
Busy yachting centre which has grown up
on either side of River Bure. Wroxham

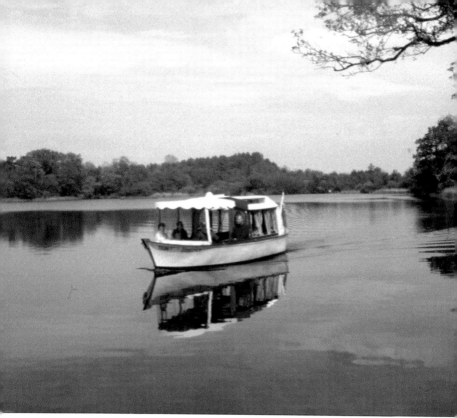

Messing around in boats. The Broads can be peaceful, if you're lucky.

Broad, although quite small, is very popular.

SELF-CATERING
BROOMHILL ♿
Station Road, Hoverton, Wroxham
Book through Grooms Holidays
No. of Accessible Units: 2. Roll-in Shower
No. of Beds per Units: 8
Accessible Facilities: communal Garden.
Quality apartments set in quiet village of
Hoveton on Wroxham Broad, close to
shops.

ATTRACTION
THE SARAH ROSE II
Book through Grooms Holidays
21m. long wide Beam Barge providing day
trips or cruising holidays on the Norfolk
Broads. She sleeps 8, has a hoist on board
and shower with chair. Qualified Dept. of
Transport Boat Master on board at all
times. There are 2 lifts.

WYMONDHAM
A busy market town lying on the main
London/Norwich road, subject to quite
heavy traffic. Fine Abbey Church of St.
Mary & St. Thomas of Canterbury. There
are also several timbered houses and
fascinating local inns.

ATTRACTION
WYMONDHAM HERITATE MUSEUM
10 The Bridewell, Norwich Road,
Wymondham NR18 0NS
Tel: (01953) 600205
The Bridwell was built in 1785 as a model
prison after John Howard's instigation of the
Prison Reform Acts 1782/85. This Museum
tells the story of this historic building from
original Elizabethan foundation to its
"reformed" prison in 1785 and beyond. Also
travel through Wymondham's growth.
Excavation in rear garden is not accessible,
but viewable from its edge.

| SD ♿ | CP n/a | E ♿ | RF ♿ |
| C ♯ | S | WC ♯ | |

NORTHAMPTONSHIRE

NORTHAMPTONSHIRE COUNCIL FOR THE DISABLED
13 Hazlewood Road, Northampton NN1 1LG
Tel: (01604) 624088   Fax: (01604) 605124

KETTERING
An industrial town set in lovely countryside: of architectural interest are the Victorian and Edwardian buildings centred around the church, reached by narrow, twisting high street and large market place.

ATTRACTION
ALFRED EAST ART GALLERY
Sheep Street, Kettering NN16 0AN
Tel: (01536) 534381   Fax: (01536) 534370
Fine arts, crafts and photography in changing temporary exhibitions. Entrance to the Gallery is via the Library. Both are ground floor buildings connected by a corridor. Visitors can park by the Library front door and go directly in, although the road (tarmac) does slope slightly.
SD 🦽   CP 🦽   E 🦽

NORTHAMPTON
Large town merging into countryside with several interesting Victorian and Georgian buildings and probably the largest market square in England.

BUSES
Gas Bus: Tel: (01604) 751431
Some low floor buses.

TAXIS
Take 6 Taxis: Tel: (01604) 764678
2 adapted vehicles
Hackney carriages: Tel: (01604) 638888
77 adapted vehicles
Door to Door: Tel: (01604) 466669
3 adapted minibuses, operate in Northampton only

TRAINS
Connex South Central & South Eastern:
Customer Services:
Tel: (0870) 6030405 Fax: (0870) 6030505
Minicom: (01233) 617621
Silverlink: Special Needs:
Tel: (01923) 207818   Fax: (01923) 207023
Minicom: (01923) 256430

CAR PARKS
Orange badge holders park free up to 4 hours in short stay parks, all day in long term parks.
Tel: (01604) 238515

HOTEL ACCOMODATION
NORTHAMPTON MOAT HOUSE   🧍
Silver Street, Northampton NN1 2TA
Tel: (01604) 739988 Fax: (01604) 230614
No. of Accessible Rooms: 2
Accessible Facilities: Lounge, Restaurant
City centre hotel with smart public areas.

SWALLOW HOTEL   🧍
Eagle Drive, Northampton NN4 7HW
Tel: (01604) 768700 Fax: 901604) 769011
No. of Accessible Rooms: 2. Bath
Accessible Facilities: Lounge, 2 Restaurants. Modern hotel on the edge of town.

THEATRE
THE ROYAL THEATRE
Guildhall Road, Northampton NN1 1EA
Admin: (01604) 638343
Fax (01604) 602408
Booking--Box Office: (01604) 632533
Minicom/Fax: (01604) 233095.
Leaflet available on access.
SD 🦽   CP 🧍 Nearest Public CP at St. Johns.
Nearest Taxi Rank: 200m.
RE 🦽   ED 🧍   INT 🧍   WC 🧍
AUD 🦽   B/R unknown
Stalls accessed by ramp into Royalties CafÈ-Bar and into Stalls.

NORTHUMBERLAND

HADRIAN'S WALL TOURISM PARTNERSHIP
Eastburn, South Park, Hexham NE46 1BS
Tel: (01434) 602505   Fax: (01434) 601267
e-mail: info@hadrians-wall.org
web: www.hadrians-wall.org

ALNWICK

Narrow streets, cobblestones and passageways, sturdy grey buildings and monuments. Situated on the River Aln, there is also a fine castle, outwardly barely changed since the 14thC.

TOURIST INFORMATION CENTRE
2 The Shambles, Alnwick NE66 1TN
Tel: (01665) 510665

SELF-CATERING
CRASTER PINE LODGES
9 West End, Craster, Alnwick NE66 3TS
Tel/Fax: (01665) 576286
No. of Accessible Units: 1. Roll-in Shower.
No. of Beds per Unit: 6
Accessible Facilities: Open plan Lounge/Kitchen. Located on edge of small village of Craster, near picturesque harbour.

VILLAGE FARM
Town Foot Farm, Shilbottle, Alnwick NE66 2XR
Tel/Fax: (01665) 575591
e-mail: crissy@villagefarm.demon.co.uk
web: www.villagefarm.demon.co.uk
No. of Accessible Units: 4
No. of Beds per Unit: 6/7
Accessible Facilities: all open plan Lounge/Kitchen/Diner.
Coquet Lodge: Danish chalet.
Pantile Cottage: old stone farm building.
Cedar & Pine Chalets: 4 of 8 units around 17thC farmhouse with Scandinavian chalets and cosy cottages. 3 miles from Alnwick between A1 and Northumbrian coast.

BAMBURGH

No Castle could look more imposing than Banburgh, a magnificent red sandstone mass, a startling sight from all approaches. The road takes motorists directly under its walls on the land side, whilst on the other it towers over the sea from a 50m precipice. The village itself is tiny, very close to two fine sandy beaches.

SELF-CATERING
POINT COTTAGES
39 The Wynding, Bamburgh NE69 7DD
Tel: (0191) 266 2800   Fax: (0191) 215 1630
No. of Accessible Units: 1
No. of Beds per Unit: 2 - 5
Accessible Facilities: Living Room, Open-plan Kitchenette. Shared Garden. Cluster of cottages in superb location at the end of the Wynding, next to a lovely golf course. Adjacent to, and overlooking sandy beaches with views to Lindisfarne and Bamburgh Castle.

BERWICK-UPON-TWEED

Originally Berwick was one of the 4 ancient Scots royal burghs, the largest town in Scotland and its greatest seaport. From 1296 it changed hands 14 times during 3 centuries of Anglo-Scots warfare. The only town in GB whose walls (Elizabethan) remain intact. At 8pm the curfew stills rings a reminder of the times when the town gates were securely locked at night.

TOURIST INFORMATION CENTRE
The Maltings, Eastern Lane, Berwick upon Tweed TD15 1DT
Tel: (01289) 330733

BED & BREAKFAST
MEADOW HILL GUEST HOUSE CAT2
Duns Road, Berwick-upon-Tweed TD15 1UB
Tel/Fax: (01289) 306325
web: www.secretkingdom.com/meadow/hill.htm
No. of Accessible Rooms: 2.
Roll-in Shower
Accessible Facilities: Lounge, Dining Room. Approximately 170 yrs old, the house is situated on the edge of town at the foot of Halidon hill-site of the battle of 1333 when Edward lll took Berwick and re-drew the English/Scots border. Wonderful views of the River Tweed, to the east Berwick and across the coast to Lindisfarne and south to the Cheviots.

CORNHILL-ON-TWEED
HOTEL
THE COACH HOUSE   ♿
Crookham, Cornhill-on-Tweed TD12 4TD
Tel: (01890) 820293   Fax: (01890) 820284
No. of Accessible Rooms: 3. Roll-in Shower
Accessible Facilities: Lounge, Dining
Room. Warm stone building around an
ancient courtyard.

GREENHEAD
SELF-CATERING
HOLMEAD FARM   ♿
Hadrian's Wall, Greenhead,
Nr. Carlisle CA6 7HY
Tel: (016977) 47402
No. of Accessible Units: 1
No. of Beds per Unit: 4
Accessible Facilities: Open plan
Lounge/Kitchen
On Hadrian's Wall, near Haltwhistle.

210

Those Romans got everywhere.

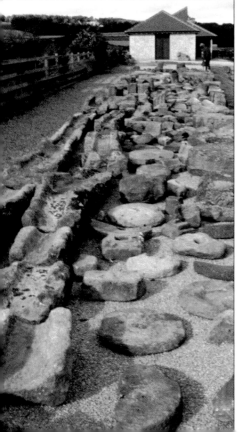

HEXHAM
Good base for exploring Hadrian's Wall,
this is an attractive market town with a
fine C11th. Abbey.

TOURIST INFORMATION CENTRE
The Manor Office, Hallgate, Hexham NE46 1XD
Tel: (01434) 605225

SELF-CATERING
CONHEATH COTTAGE   🚶
Blakelaw Farm, Bellingham,
Hexham NE48 2EF
Tel/Fax: (01434) 220250
No. of Accessible Units: 1. Bath
No. of Beds per Unit: 5
Accessible Facilities: Living room,
Kitchen/Diner, Walled garden with
barbecue and furniture. Lovely stone
semi-detached holiday cottage in the
North Tyne Valley, 1.5 miles from
Bellingham. Bed-rooms are upstairs,
accessed by stair lift.

GIBBS HILL FARM COTTAGES   🚶
Once Brewed, Bardon Mill, Hexham NE47 7AP
Tel/Fax: (01434) 344030
No. of Accessible Units: 1
No. of Beds per Unit: 2
Stone cottages on working organic family
farm near Hadrian's Wall. Fine views and
5 minutes from main Roman sites.

ROSE COTTAGE   🚶
Falstone, Nr., Hexham NE48 1AA
Tel: (0191) 285 4643
Bookable through: Mrs. Winternitz, 20
Sheldon Grove, Kenton Park, Newcastle-upon-
Tyne NE43 4JP. Tel: (0191) 285 4643
No. of Accessible Units: 1
No. of Beds per Unit: 2
Accessible Facilities: Living Room,
Kitchenette. Garden Traditional, cosy
forestry worker's single storey-cottage
built in local stone in early 19thC. Garden
views up the valley toward forest and dam.
Falstone is quiet and unspoilt.

ATTRACTIONS
CHESTERS ROMAN FORT (EH)
Chollerford, Humshaugh, Hexham NE46 4EP
Tel: (01434) 681379
Remains of a Fort built for 500

cavalrymen including 5 gateways, barracks and fine military bath house.

SD 🚾   CP ♿   E ♿   RF 🚹 3
WC 🚹   RFE 🚹

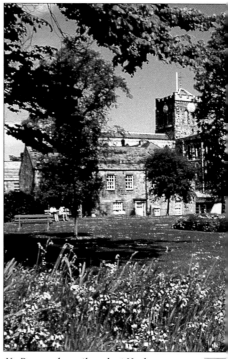

CORBRIDGE ROMAN SITE (EH)
Corbridge NE45 5NT
Tel: (01434) 632349
Archaeological site with uneven loose surfaces-access is limited. The Museum is accessible. Wheelchair available. Extensive remains include 2 large granaries, strongroom, fountain house and aqueduct.

SD 🚾   CP 🚹   E 🚹   RF 🚾   S 🚹   WC 🚹

KELSO
Situated in the Tweed Valley at junction of Rivers Tweed and Teviot, originally famous for its Abbey of 1128, now in poor state of ruin. Attractive Square with neo-classical town hall and 18th and 19thC pastel buildings.

KELSO RACES
Office: 18-20 Glendale Road, Wooler NE71 6DW
Admin & Booking-Box Office: (01668) 281611
Fax: (01668) 281113
Facility complies with Part M, Building Regulations

CP ♿   RE ♿   ED 🚾
WC ♿ (2 units, one in each enclosure)
SS 🚾   B/R 🚹

MORPETH
Attractive town in a U-shaped bend of the River Wansbeck with plentiful trees and parks. Gateway to the moors, hills and coast of Northumberland.

TOURIST INFORMATION CENTRE
The Chantry, Bridge Street, Morpeth NE61 1PD
Tel: (01670) 511323

HOTELS
LINDEN HALL HOTEL & HEALTH SPA   🚹
Longhorsley, Morpeth NE65 8XF
Tel: (01670) 516611
Fax: (01670) 788544
No. of Accessible Rooms: 1. Bath
Accessible Facilities: Lounge, Restaurant
Grade II listed Georgian country house

No Romans here, though at Hexham Abbey.

hotel set in 450 acres of private park and woodland. Much of the interior has been restored since it was built in 1812

WHITTON FARMHOUSE HOTEL   🚹
Whitton, Rothbury, Morpeth NE65 7RL
Tel/Fax: (01669) 620811
No. of Accessible Rooms:1. Bath
Accessible Facilities: Lounge, Restaurant, Bar. Built in 1829 in traditional Northumbrian style, farmhouse and buildings converted to charming small hotel located on the edge of the Northumberland National Park, overlooking Coquet Valley.

THE SWAN   🚹
Choppington, Nr. Morpeth NE62 5TG
Tel: (01670) 826060
No. of Accessible Rooms: 1. Bath
Accessible Facilities: Restaurant, Conservatory.

SELF-CATERING
DENE HOUSE FARM COTTAGES ♿
Dene House Farm, Longframlington ,
Morpeth NE65 8EE
Tel: (01665) 570549
No. of Accessible Units: 4. Roll-in Shower
No. of Beds per Unit: 4
Accessible Facilities: Open plan
Lounge/Kitchen. (Only 1 kitchen
accessible). 4 cottages a mile from the
village designed for disabled access.
Previous Holiday Care Award winner.

OAK & ELM COTTAGES ♿
Beacon Hill Farm, Longhorsley,
Morpeth NE65 8QW
Tel/Fax: (01670) 788372
E-mail: alun@beacon-hill.demon.co
web: www.beacon-hill.demon.co.uk
No. of Accessible Units: 2. Bath, Shower.
No. of Beds per Unit: 1D 7 1T
Accessible Facilities: Open Plan Kitchen &
Lounge. Beacon Hill is a 350 acre farm
deep in unspoilt countryside between
Cheviot Hills and Northumbrian coastline.
There are 10 stone cottages with gardens.

ATTRACTION
THE WHITEHOUSE FARM CENTRE
North Whitehouse Farm, Morpeth
Tel: (01670) 789571
Fax: (01670) 789113
A good day out for adults and children -
learn how a farm works, see guinea pigs,
rabbits, chicks, ducks and exotic animals.

| SD ♿ | CP ♿ | E ♿ | RF ♿ |
| C ♿ | S ♿ | WC 🚶 | RFE ♿ |

PONTELAND
Located just NW of Newcastle Airport, a
small village.

ATTRACTION
BELSAY HALL, CASTLE & GARDENS (EH)
Belsay, Nr. Ponteland NE20 0DX
Tel: (01661) 881636
Fax: (01661) 881043
Neo-classical Regency hall which is empty
and unreal. 30 acres of landscaped gardens
and 14thC Castle. Long walk to Castle
through delightful woodland, with some
wheelchair adjusted paths, but worth it!

Visited on damp June morning, paths of
fairly firm gravel.

| SD ♿ | CP ♿ | E ♿ | RF ♿ |
| C ♿ | S ♿ | WC ♿ | RFE ♿ |

PRUDHOE
Occupying a bank of the River Tyne,
consisting mainly of long terraces of
houses on steep river bank. Prudhoe
Castle is situated on a wooded spur
overlooking river. There is a legend that
Prudhoe is connected to Bywell Castle –
situated several miles away – by a special
underground passage.

SPORTS/LEISURE/TOURIST
INFORMATION CENTRE
PRUDHOE WATERWORLD
Front Street, Prudhoe NE42 5DQ
Tel: (01661) 833144
Fax: (01661) 833885
Lovely leisure pool. On Wednesday
evenings there is "Be Able Disabled"
session in the pool.

| SD ♿ | CP ♿ | E ♿ | RF 🚶 |
| C 🚶 | S 🚶 | RFE – Pool – Direct access |
via Shower Chair into water via beach area.
WC – Dryside 🚶   Wetside ♿

WARKWORTH
Village set in the loop of the River
Coquet, a famous castle at its head. Used
by Harry Hotspur, hero of the Battle of
Otterbun in 1402, by Great Earl of
Warwick in 1462 as a base to attack the
Borders castles. The area has wonderful
beaches and landscapes - northwards to
Holy Island and the Farne Islands and to
the west the Rolling Hills.

HOTEL
WARKWORTH HOUSE ♿
16 Bridge Street, Warkworth NE65 0XB
Tel: (01665) 711276   Fax: (01665) 713323
No. of Accessible Rooms: 2. Roll-in
Shower.
Accessible Facilities: Lounge, Restaurant.
This hotel carries a specific brochure and
map of its disabled ground floor rooms.
Built in 1830 and family owned, it is
located in the village centre.

NOTTINGHAMSHIRE

EDWINDSTOW

Lying at the edge of spacious common, leading to Birklands and Bilhagh, two of the most beautiful parts of Sherwood Forest. Also close to Warsop on the River Maun, in whose church Robin Hood and Maid Marian are said to have been married.

ATTRACTION
SHERWOOD FOREST COUNTRY PARK & VISITOR CENTRE
Edwinstow NG21 9HN
Tel/Fax: (01623) 823202
View over 450 acres of Robin Hood's original forest with waymarked paths, including the famous Major Oak. VC shows exhibition on Robin Hood

SD ♿ CP ♿ E ♿ RF ♿ (Visitor Centre)
C ♿ S ♿ WC ♿
RFE ♿ (Major Oak-Robin Hood hiding place)

MANSFIELD

TOURIST INFORMATION CENTRE
Old Town Hall, Market Place,
Mansfield NG18 1HX
Tel: (01623) 427770

ATTRACTION
MANSFIELD MUSEUM & ART GALLERY
Leeming Street, Mansfield NG18 1NG
Tel: (01623) 463088   Fax: (01523) 412922
3 permanent galleries tell Mansfield's story through displays of natural, industrial and social history with examples of fine and decorative arts of local significance. Also temporary exhibitions.

SD ♿ CP n/a E ♿ RF ♿
L ♿ C n/a S ♿ WC ♿

NOTTINGHAM

Famous for its association with Robin Hood, 13thC. outlaw, and for lace and (Boots has its HQ here) pharmacy, plus Luddites (pre-Union strikers). The Old Market Square remains the centre of the city, with the Lace Market close by. In 1840s the city introduced machined lace clothing and industry boomed until the end of WWI. There are Georgian and neo-classical buildings and Victorian warehouses.

TOURIST INFORMATION CENTRES
1-4 Smithy Row, Nottingham NG1 2BY
Tel: (0115) 9155330

County Hall, West Bridgford,
Nottingham NG2 7QP
Tel: (0115) 9773558   Fax: (0115) 9773886

BUSES
Nottingham City Transport:
Tel: (0115) 9503665
Some low floors, some raised kerbs
Park & Ride: Tel: (0115) 9240000 - accessible to folding chairs.

TAXIS
City Cabs: Tel: (0115) 9701701
120 adapted vehicles
Royal Cabs: Tel: (0115) 9608608
85 adapted vehicles

TRAINS
Midland Mainline: Special Needs:
Tel: (0114) 2537654
Minicom: (0845) 7078051
Robin Hood Line: Tel: (0115) 9240000
All trains carry ramps, but cannot take all powered wheelchairs because of limited space.
Assisted Travel Line: Tel: (0345) 056027

CAR PARKS
Orange badge spaces free for first 4 hours, thereafter chargeable - also some on-street parking.
Tel: (0115) 9158282

SHOPMOBILITY
Victoria Centre, off Woodborough Road, Broad Marsh Centre, Nottingham.
Tel: (0115) 9153888   Fax: (0115) 9155377
e-mail:
building.control@nottinghamcity.gov.uk

HOTEL

SKYLARKS (Winged Fellowship) ♿
Adbolton Lane, West Bridgeford,
Nottingham NG2 5AU
Tel: (0115) 9820962   Fax: (0115) 9824920
No. of Accessible Rooms: 31. Roll-in Shower.
Accessible Facilities: Lounge, Dining Room,
Indoor Pool, Rose Garden, Ornamental
Pond. Purpose- built holiday accommodation
located at city's edge, an ideal starting point
for trips to Sherwood Forest.

HOLIDAY INN GARDEN COURT 🚶
Castle Marina Park, Nottingham NG7 1GX
Tel: (0115) 9935000   Fax: (0115) 9934000
No. of Accessible Rooms: 3 Deluxe, 22
others.
Accessible Facilities: Lounge, Restaurant.
Award winning hotel within sight of the
castle on the new Marina.

THE NOTTINGHAM GATEWAY HOTEL 🚶
Nuthall Road, Nottingham NG8 6AZ
Tel: (0115) 9794949   Fax: (0115) 9794744
No. of Accessible Rooms: 5. Bath
Accessible Facilities: Lounge, Restaurant
Modern hotel located 3 miles from city
centre in suburbs.

NOTTINGHAM MOAT HOUSE 🚶
Mansfield Road, Nottingham NG5 2BT
Tel: (0115) 9359988   Fax: (0115) 9691506

No. of Accessible Rooms: 1. Bath
Accessible Facilities: Lift (to
accommodation on 1st floor), Lounge,
Restaurant, Bars. Modern hotel north of
city centre

NOTTINGHAM ROYAL MOAT HOUSE 🚶
Wollaton Street, Nottingham NG1 5RH
Tel: (0115) 9369988   Fax: (0115) 9475888
No. of Accessible Rooms: 2.
Accessible Facilities: Restaurants 2, Bars 2
Newly refurbished city centre hotel

ATTRACTION

MUSEUM OF NOTTINGHAM LIFE
Brewhouse Yard, Castle Boulevard,
Nottingham NG7 1FB
Tel: (0115) 9153600   Fax: (0115) 9153601
Nestled in the rock beneath Nottingham
Castle, the museum is housed in a group of
5 restored cottages built in 1675 for the
Castle servants. It presents a realistic
glimpse of everyday domestic and working
life in the city during the last 300 years. A
number of inter-active exhibits and wide
variety of displays are both enchanting and
educational. Behind the museum is a series
of caves set into the castle rock depicting
WWII and other displays. These are
accessible with fairly even brick floors.

SD ♿   CP ♿   E ♿   RF ♿
S ♿   WC 🚶   RFE ♿

The views from Nottingham Castle are spectacular, but you might not see Robin.

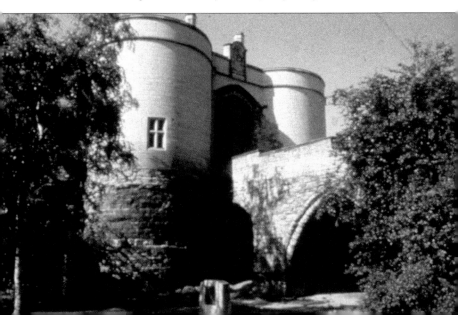

NOTTINGHAM CASTLE MUSEUM & ART GALLERY
Nottingham NG1 6EL
Tel: (0115) 9153700 Fax: (0115) 9153653
Interactive "Story of Nottingham" exhibition on city's history in 17thC building.

SD n/a   CP ♿   E ♿   RF ♿
L ♿   C ♿   S ♿   WC ♿

THEATRES
NOTTINGHAM PLAYHOUSE
Wellington Circus, Nottingham NG1 5AF
Admin: (0115) 9474361
Booking: Box Office: (0115) 9419419
Minicom: (0015) 9476100
Fax: (0115) 9241484

CP ♿ (North Circus St., East Circus St., Wellington Circus)
RE ♿   ED ♿   INT ♿   L ♿
WC ♿   AUD ♿ From entrance foyer lift to level 1 - enter stairs by side entrance on Row M where wheelchair seating located.   B/R ♿

THEATRE ROYAL
Theatre Square, Nottingham NG1 5ND
Part of Royal Centre, which includes Royal Concert Hall, also accessible.
Admin: (0115) 9895500
Booking: Box Office: (0115) 9895555
Minicom: (0115) 9470025
Fax: (0115) 9503476

CP ♿ (Disabled bays on Burton Street).
RE ♿   ED ♿ (except Manual Door)   INT ♿
WC ♿ (good, except WC seat 51cm above floor).
AUD ♿ (Stalls only - whole back row removed at 8.00pm).   Ends of all stalls rows A - V accessible for wheelchair transfer.
B/R ♿

OLLERTON
17 miles north of Nottingham, a small mining town at the junction of the Rivers Rainworth-Water and Maun.

TOURIST INFORMATION CENTRE
Sherwood Heath, Ollerton Roundabout, Ollerton NG22 9DR
Tel: (01623) 824545

ATTRACTION
RUFFORD COUNTRY PARK – ABBEY END
Ollerton NG22 9DF
Tel: (01623) 822944
NOTE: There are 2 entrances – take Abbey End, not Mill End. Rufford Abbey was founded as a Cistercian Monastery in 12thC. After Dissolution of Monasteries in 1536, Rufford passed to private hands and picturesque remains are still standing. There are large areas of woodland and parkland, a craft centre in the former stable block, a Gallery with changing exhibitions and Britain's first Ceramics Centre.

SD ♿   CP ♿   E ♿   RF ♿   L ♿
C ♿   S ♿   WC ♿   RFE ♿

SUTTON-IN-ASHFIELD
ATTRACTION
TEVERSAL VISITOR CENTRE
Carnarvon Street, Teversal, Sutton-in-Ashfield NG17 3HJ
Tel: (01623) 442021
Displays on wildlife and industrial heritage of Pleasley Trails network, now designated as local Nature Reserves. The Trails themselves, tranquil, through lovely countryside, include the old village of Teversal, one of most unspoilt in the country and with connections with Lord Carnarvon of Tutankhamun fame and D.S. Lawrence's "Lady Chatterley's Love."
Of 6 trails, Areas 1,2,3 and part of 5 are accessible.

NB: Entrance ramped at 1:10.

SD ♿   CP ♿   E n/a   RF ♿   C ♿
S ♿   WC ♿   RFE ♿

WORKSOP
TOURIST INFORMATION CENTRE
Public Library, memorial Avenue, Worksop S80 2BP
Tel: (01909) 501148

ATTRACTION
CRESSWELL CRAGS VISITOR CENTRE
Crags Road, Welbeck, Worksop S80 3LH
Tel: (01909) 720378 Fax: (01909) 724726
e-mail: heritage@cresswell.co.uk
Caves and rock shelters of the crags were used by Stone Age hunters and artefacts now in visitor centre whose exhibition and audio-visual displays explain life in prehistoric times.

SD ♿   CP ♿   E ♿   RF ♿
S ♿   WC ♿   RFE ♿

OXFORDSHIRE

ABINGDON

Lying near the water meadows of the River Thames where it is joined by the Little Ock, the town originally grew up around its Abbey and has some fine early timbered-framed houses and Georgian properties.

BED & BREAKFAST ACCOMMODATION
KINGFISHER BARN
Rye Farm, Culham, Abingdon OX14 3NN
Tel/Fax: (01235) 537538
e-mail: liz@kingfisherbarn.demon.co.uk
No. of Accessible Rooms: 10. Bath
Accessible Facilities: C17th renovated barn with adjacent stable buildings offering wide selection of activities in rural setting.

BANBURY

Flourishing community with one of the oldest breweries in the country and many fine old houses remain plus twisted medieval streets.

TOURIST INFORMATION CENTRE
Banbury Museum, 8 Horsefair,
Banbury OX16 0AA
Tel: (01295) 259855   Fax: (01295) 270556

ATTRACTION
UPTON HOUSE (NT)
Nr. Banbury OX15 6HT
Tel: (01295) 670266
e-mail: vuplan@smtp.ntrust.org.uk
Impressive late C17th house remodelled 1927 for the 2nd Viscount Bearsted. Fine painting collection includes El Greco, Bruegel, Bosch, Hogarth and Stubbs. Wide lawns and terraced herbaceous borders with the National Collection of Asters, descend to two lakes.

SD [&]   CP [&]   E [人] (Side Door)
C [人]   S [人]   WC [人]

SWALCLIFFE BARN MUSEUM
Swalcliffe, Nr. Banbury OX15 5DR
Tel: (01295) 788278
Swalcliffe Barn was built for the Rectorial Manor of Swalcliffe by New College, Oxford, who owned the manor. Constructed between 1400 and 1409 it retains much of its medieval timber half-cruck roof intact and is one of the finest medieval barns in the country. Collection of agricultural and trade vehicles.

SD [&]   CP [人]   E [&]   RF [&]   WC [&]

BURFORD

Lovely Cotswolds' town, with a wide High Street sloping down to the River Windrush, crossed by a narrow 3-arched bridge. Golden Cotswold stone houses everywhere.

TOURIST INFORMATION CENTRE
The Brewery, Sheep Street, Burford OX18 4LP
Tel: (01993) 823558   Fax: (01993) 823590

ATTRACTION
COTSWOLD WILDLIFE PARK
Burford OX18 4JW
Tel: (01993) 823006   Fax: (01993) 823807
Set in 160 acres of gardens and parklands around listed Victorian manor house.

Now remember, don't get out of the car.

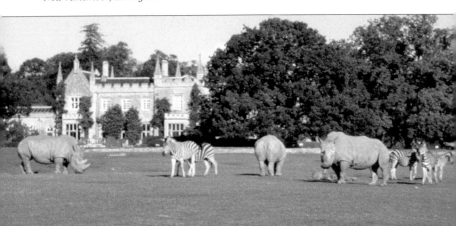

Several endangered species including Giant Tortoise and Red Panda with tropical birds, penguins and mammals in the walled garden, plus tropical and reptile houses, aquarium, insect house and fruit bats.

SD ♿	CP ♿	E ♿	RF ♿
C ♿	S ♿	WC 🚶	RFE ♿

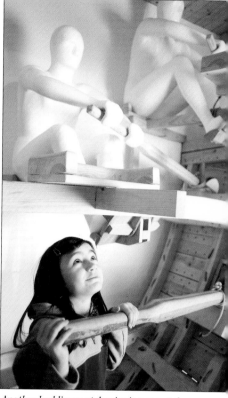

FARINGDON

On the edge of the Cotswolds between Oxford and Swindon. Historically famous for its Civil War stand against the Roundheads, the town is still a vibrant market centre.

HOTEL
SUDBURY HOUSE HOTEL ♿
56 London Street, Faringdon SW7 8AA
Tel: (01367) 241272 Fax: (01367) 242346
e-mail: sudburyhouse@cix.co.uk
No. of Accessible Rooms: 10. Bath Accessible Facilities: Lounge, Restaurant, Lift. Originally a fine Regency house, now extended to a fully equipped hotel. Set in 9 acres of secluded private grounds.

HENLEY-ON-THAMES.

Picturesque Thameside town, with Victorian houses, separated from the neighbouring county of Buckinghamshire by elegant C18th bridge spanning a wide stretch of the River.

Another budding match-winning cox at the River and Rowing Museum.

TOURIST INFORMATION CENTRE
Town Hall, Market Place, Henley RG9 2AQ
Tel: (01491) 578034 Fax: (01491) 411766

HOTEL
HOLMWOOD 🚶
Shiplake Row, Binfield Heath, Henley-on-Thames RG9 4DP
Tel: (0118) 9478747 Fax: (0118) 9478637
No. of Accessible Rooms: 2, via vertical (not stair) lift. Accessible Facilities: Lounge, Dining Room. Large secluded Georgian country house with impressive reception rooms and galleried hall. Set in 4 acres of lovely gardens with additional grounds of 26 acres of paddocks and woods. Extensive views of Thames Valley. Emily Tennyson spent the night here before her wedding to Alfred, Lord Tennyson and Algernon Charles Swinburne composed much poetry here.

ATTRACTION
RIVER AND ROWING MUSEUM
Mill Meadows, Henley-on-Thames RE9 1BF
Tel: (01491) 415600 Fax: (01491) 415601
e-mail: museum@rrm.co.uk
web: www.rrm.co.uk www.rrm.co.uk
Walk the length of River Thames from source to sea, exploring River's role through history from major trading route to boating paradise. Experience highs and low of international rowing with fascinating artefacts and memorabilia brought to life with archive film.

SD ♿	CP ♿	E ♿	RF ♿	L 🚶
C ♿	S 🚶	WC ♿		

OXFORD

Oxford University is the second oldest in Europe, whose fine buildings combine with many other outstanding architectural features. Little back streets and scenes of Christ Church meadows, where the River Isis becomes the Thames, produce a magical atmosphere.

TOURIST INFORMATION CENTRE
The Old School, Gloucester Green,
Oxford OX1 2DA
Tel: (01865) 726871   Fax: (01865) 240261

BUSES
Oxford Bus Company: Tel: (01865) 785410
Operate some low floor buses, including
Park & Ride, which are all low floor.
Stagecoach Oxford: Tel: (01865) 772250
Operate some low floor kneeling buses,
also the "Oxford Tube" to London
Thames Travel: Tel: (01491) 874216

TAXIS
ABC Taxis: Tel: (01865) 770077
20 adapted vehicles
City Taxis: Tel: (01865) 794000
20 adapted vehicles
Euro Taxis: Tel: (01865) 430430
20 adapted vehicles
Radio Taxis: Tel: (01865) 242424
20 adapted vehicles

TRAINS
Thames Trains: Special Needs:
Tel: (0118) 9083607
web: www.thamestrains.co.uk
Virgin Trains: Special Needs:
Tel: (0845) 7443366
Minicom: (0845) 7443367

Oxford Station has level access to both platforms from car parks, lifts to both platforms, disabled WC on concourse, helpline telephone on both platforms.

CAR PARKS
Orange badge spaces in all 4 Park & Ride car parks, also plenty of free on-street spaces.
Tel: (01865) 726871

SHOPMOBILITY
Level 1a, Westgate Car Park, Oxford
Tel: (01865) 248737   Fax: (01865) 249536
e-mail: robin@shopmo.oxford.demon.co.uk

HOTELS
WESTWOOD COUNTRY HOTEL
Hinksey Hill Top, Nr. Boars Hill,
Oxford OX1 5BH
Tel: (01865) 735408   Fax: (01865) 736536
e-mail: reservations@westwoodhotel.co.uk
web: westwoodhotel.co.uk
No. of accessible Rooms: 2. Roll-in Shower
Accessible Facilities: Lounge, Restaurant.
Charming property, privately owned, set in
3.5 acres of landscaped gardens, backing
onto 160 acres of woodland, 2.5 m. from
city centre.

BOWOOD HOUSE HOTEL
238 Oxford Road, Kidlington,
Oxford OX5 1EB
Tel: (01865) 842288   Fax: (01865) 841858
No. of Accessible Rooms: 1
Accessible Facilities: Lounge, Restaurant.
Comfortable, small hotel situated on the
A4260 in village of Kidlington, 3.5 m. from
city centre.

BED & BREAKFAST
BURLINGTON HOUSE
374 Banbury Road, Summerton,
Oxford OX2 7PP
Tel: (01865) 513513   Fax: (01865) 311785
e-mail: stay@burlington-house.co.uk
web: www.burlington-house.co.uk
No. of Accessible Rooms: 1. Roll-in Shower
Accessible Facilities: Lounge, Dining
Room
Large, detached Victorian merchant's
house, dating from 1889, situated in
premier residential area, 5 minutes from
centre of Oxford.

ATTRACTION
ASHMOLEAN MUSEUM
Beaumont Street, Oxford OX1 2PH
Tel: (01865) 278000   Fax: (01865) 278018
e-mail: name/dept@ashmus.ox.ac.uk
Oldest museum open to the public in
Britain and a fine example of neo-classical
architecture, containing the University's
collections of European and Near Eastern
Antiquities, Western and Eastern paintings
and sculptures, with ever changing
temporary exhibitions

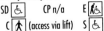

THEATRE
OXFORD PLAYHOUSE
Beaumont Street, Oxford OX1 2LW
Admin: (01865) 247134
Fax: (01865) 793748
Booking-Box Office: (01865) 798600
Minicom: (01865) 792196
Complies with Part M, Building
Regulations

| CP 🚶 | RE 🦽 | ED 🦽 (except Manual Door) |
| INT 🦽 | WC 🦽 | AUD 🦽 | B/R 🦽 |

WALLINGFORD

HOTEL
THE GEORGE 🚶
High Street, Wallingford OX10 0BS
Tel: (01491) 836665   Fax: (01491) 823359
No. of Accessible Rooms: 3. Bath
Accessible Facilities: Lounge, Restaurant.
Lovely hotel in centre of town, originally a
16thC coaching inn.

WITNEY
Situated on the River Windrush, on the
edge of the sheep-rearing area, the town's
fame for blanket-making is worldwide.
Mellowed stone-built town with wide
street, gradually narrowing and continuing
for almost 1 mile.

TOURIST INFORMATION CENTRE
51a Market Square, Witney OX8 6AG
Tel: (01993) 775802   Fax: (01993) 709261

HOTEL
FOUR PILLARS HOTEL 🦽
Ducklington Lane, Witney OX8 7TJ
Tel: (01993) 779777   Fax: (01993) 703467
e-mail: enquiries@four-pillars.co.uk
web: www.four-pillars.co.uk
No. of Accessible Rooms: 1. Bath
Accessible Facilities: Lounge, Restaurant,
Bar. Located 2 miles from centre of town,
this is a modern, very comfortable and
spacious hotel, built in traditional style
immediately off the A40 on A415

BED & BREAKFAST
CROFTERS GUEST HOUSE 🚶
29 Oxford Hill, Witney OX8 6JU

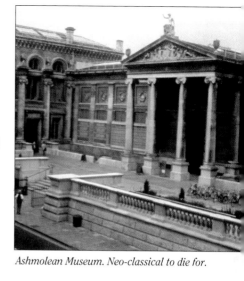

Ashmolean Museum. Neo-classical to die for.

Tel/Fax: (01993) 778165
No. of Accessible Rooms: 1. Bath
Accessible Facilities: Lounge, Conservatory
Breakfast Room. Family home bursting
with knick knacks, run by charming hosts
who hope their clients will arrive as "guests
and depart as friends". 1.5 miles from town
centre
A 2nd adaptive bedroom currently being
built.

WOODSTOCK
Lovely old country town bisected by a
handsome bridge over the River Glyme,
with many old stone houses and pleasant
streets which lead to the great Palace of
Blenheim.

TOURIST INFORMATION CENTRE
Oxfordshire Museum, Park Street,
Woodstock OX20 1SN
Tel: (01993) 813276   Fax: (01993) 813632
e-mail: oxonmuseum.occcs@dial.peipex.com

ATTRACTION
THE OXFORDSHIRE MUSEUM
(Tourist Information Centre) see above,
History of the people of Oxfordshire located
in charming townhouse.

| SD 🦽 | CP 🚶 | E 🦽 | RF 🦽 |
| C 🦽 | S 🚶 | WC 🦽 |

SHROPSHIRE

SHROPSHIRE TOURISM
Unit 12, Harlescott Barns, Harlscott,
Shrewsbury SY1 3SZ
Tel: (01743) 462462   Fax (01743) 462035
e-mail: shropshire.tourism@virgin.net
web:www.virtual-shropshire.co.uk

SPECIALIST OUTDOOR ACTIVITES
THE LYNEAL TRUST
The Shirehall, Shrewsbury SY2 6ND
Tel: (01743) 251000
The Llangollen Canal weaves across the
Cheshire/Shropshire borders through
wonderful canal-side country.
The Trust arranges canal based holidays on
two canal boats on a do-it-yourself basis, so
each party should include some able-
bodied adults. For day trips the Trust
provides a helmsman. Both boats carry
hydraulic lift, steering and ramps and the
larger has adapted WCs.

BRIDGNORTH
Both high and low town connected by
flights of steps and a railway with steepest
gradient in Britain. This setting, part
spread across the red sandstone ridge, part
at its foot, is unique in England with some
fine buildings in the town.

TOURIST INFORMATION CENTRE
The Library, Lidstley Street,
Bridgnorth WV16 4AW
Tel: (01746) 763257   Fax: (01746) 766625

HOTEL
THE OLD VICARAGE HOTEL
Worfield, Nr. Bridgnorth WV15 5JZ
Tel: (01746) 716497 Fax: (01746) 716552
e-mail: admin@the-old-vicarage.demon.co.uk
web: oldvicarageworfield.co.uk
No. of Accessible Rooms: 2. Roll-in Shower.
Accessible Facilities: Lounge, Restaurant,
Gardens via Croquet lawn
Privately owned 14 bedroomed property
full of antique furniture in lovely grounds.

ATTRACTION
DUDMASTON HALL (NT)

Quatt, Bridgnorth WV15 6QN
Tel: (01746) 780866   Fax: (01746) 780744
e-mail: mduefe@smtp.ntrust.org.uk
17thC. house with fine furniture,
contemporary paintings and sculpture and
lovely gardens.
NB: Entrance ramped at 1:10

| SD ♿ | CP n/a | E ♿ | RF ♿ |
| C ♿ | S ♿ | WC ⚖ | |

CHURCH STRETTON
Mary Webb country: she spent her
honeymoon here and the "Shepwardine" of
her novels is Church Stretton. The
surrounding hills and bleak, heathery Long
Mynd offer magnificent views.

TOURIST INFORMATION CENTRE
County Branch Library, Church Streeton SY6 6DQ
Tel: (01694) 723133

BED & BREAKFAST
JINLYE ⚖
Castle Hill, All Stretton, Church Stretton SY6 6JP
Tel/Fax: (01694) 723243
e-mail: kate@jinlye.freeserve.co.uk
No. of Accessible Rooms: 1. Roll-in Shower.
Accessible Facilities: Lounge, Dining
Room, Garden. Excellently situated guest
house standing in 15 acres of grounds
adjoining the Long Mynd - an area of great
beauty. Period furnishings and cottage
gardens.

LUDLOW
Historic market town, capital of the
Marches, with Broad Street described by
Nicholas Pevsner as 'the most beautiful
street in England'. To the south of its
Castle lies a medieval grid of streets mostly
rebuilt in 18thC. There are 500 listed
buildings in Ludlow, many half-timbered
Tudor and red-brick Georgian houses.

TOURIST INFORMATION CENTRE
Castle Street, Ludlow SY8 2AS
Tel: (01584) 875053 Fax: (01584) 877931

HOTEL
THE FEATHERS AT LUDLOW
The Bull Ring, Ludlow SY8 1AA

Tel: (01584) 875261   Fax: (01584) 876030
No. of Accessible Rooms: 9. Bath
Accessible Facilities: Lounge, Restaurant.
Historic hotel in town centre, this Grade I
listed building is the oldest timbered
faÁade in England. The New York Times
has described this inn as 'the most
handsome in the world.'.

BED & BREAKFAST
CORNDENE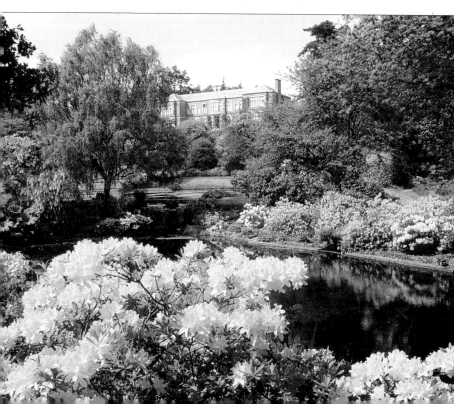
Coreley, Ludlow SY8 3AW
Tel/Fax: (01584) 890324
No. of Accessible Rooms: 3 - Oak room
Cat.1. Elm & Ash rooms Cat.2.
All have roll-in showers
Accessible Facilities: Lounge, Dining
Room, Garden, Terrace.
Originally the rectory for the small Parish
of Coreley, the core of the house is late
18thC with Victorian additions. Situated in
large grounds with pond, hay meadow,
small wood and many mature trees in the
south Shropshire hills. No evening meals,
but visitors kitchen is fully equipped.

THE GABLES
Broome, Craven Arms SY7 0NX
Tel: (01588) 660667   Fax: (01588) 660799

No. of Accessible Rooms: 3
Accessible Facilities: Dining Room
Lovely house and gardens in glorious
countryside

SELF-CATERING
HOLLY COTTAGE
Sutton Court Farm, Little Sutton, Ludlow SY8 2AJ
Tel: (01584) 861305 Fax: (01584) 861441
No. of Accessible Units: 1
No. of Beds per Unit: 2. Bath
Accessible Facilities: Lounge, Dining
Room, Kitchen, Garden. 1 of 6 holiday
cottages set in Corve Dale Valley. Located
5.5 miles from Ludlow.

SPORTING VENUE
LUDLOW RACECOURSE
Bromfield, Ludlow
Tel: (01981) 250052 Fax: (01981) 250192
Booking: No advance booking required.
Tel. above for information
CP   RE   ED   WC
SS n/a (CCTV in all bars)   B/R

221

*The superb landscape gardens of Hodnet
Hall, Market Drayton.*

MARKET DRAYTON

Home to gingerbread and Clive of India, with black and white half-timbered inns and bustling street markets, held here for over 750 years.

TOURIST INFORMATION CENTRE
49 Cheshire Street, Market Drayton TF9 1PH
Tel/Fax: (01630) 652139

BED & BREAKFAST
MICKLEY HOUSE [符]
Faulsgreen, Tern Hill, Market Drayton TF9 3QW
Tel: (01630) 638505
No. of Accessible Rooms: 2.
Accessible Facilities: Lounge, Dining Room
Victorian farmhouse, within 125 acre cattle farm, with oak beams and leaded windows situated between Market Drayton and Shrewsbury.

ATTRACTION
HODNET HALL GARDENS
Hodnet, Market Drayton TF9 3NN
Tel: (01630) 685202   Fax: (01630) 685853
60 acres of quite superb landscaped gardens with pools, lush plants and trees. Set down outside Victorian Tearoom.

SD [&]   CP [符]   RF [符]
C [符]   S [&]   WC [符]

SHIFNAL

In 1591 this small town was largely destroyed by fire, and its architecture is therefore very varied with some fine examples of both Norman and Georgian design.

ATTRACTION
WESTON PARK
Weston-under-Lizard, Nr. Shifnal TF11 8LF
Tel: (01952) 850207   Fax: (01952) 850430
Mansion built in 1671, surrounded by wonderful gardens and park designed by ëCapability' Brown with lakes, miniature railway and adventure playground.

SD [&]   CP [符]   E [&]   RF [&]   C [&]
S [&]   WC [符]   RFE [&]

ROYAL AIR FORCE MUSEUM COSFORD
Shifnal TF11 8UP
Tel: (01902) 376200 Fax: (01902) 376211

e-mail: rafmuseumcosford@compuserve.com
Large aviation collection including Spitfires and Hurricanes from WW11, Victor and Vulcan Bombers and British Airways exhibition hall

SD [&]   CP [符]   E [&]   RF [&]   C [&]
S [&]   WC [&]   RFE [符]

SHREWSBURY

One of the best preserved medieval towns in England, the spires of its 2 churches piercing the skyline and its town centre houses of beautiful timber-framing.

TOURIST INFORMATION CENTRE
The Music Hall, The Square, Shrewsbury SY1 1LH
Tel: (01743) 350761   Fax: (01743) 355323

SHREWSBURY & ATCHAM BOROUGH COUNCIL
Director of Health, Tourism & Leisure
Oakley Manor, Belle Vue Road,
Shrewsbury SY3 7NW
Tel: (01743) 231456   Fax: (01743) 271593

BUSES
First PMT: Tel: (01782) 207999
Buses throughout Shropshire & the Potteries.

TAXIS
Clare's Cab: Tel: (01743) 236900
1 adapted vehicle

TRAINS
Virgin Trains: Special Needs:
Tel: (0845) 7443366
Minicom: (0845) 7443367
Wales & West: Special Needs:
Tel: (0845) 3003005
Minicom: (0345) 585469
Shrewsbury Station is suitable for wheelchairs using ramp access.

CAR PARKS
Designated parking bays for disabled drivers all over the city -map available from Shopmobility as below.

SHOPMOBILITY
Level 1, Ground Floor, Ravens Meadows Car Park, Shrewsbury SY1 1PL
Tel: (01743) 236900

HOTEL
ALBRIGHT HUSSEY HOTEL
Ellesmere Road, Shrewsbury SY4 3AF
Tel: (01939) 290571   Fax: (01939) 291143
e-mail: abhotel@aol.com   abhotel@aol.com
web: www.albrighthussey.co.uk
No. of Accessible Rooms: 1
Accessible Facilities: Restaurant, Bar.
Lovely hotel, half timbered, recorded in
Domesday Book. Current building dates
from 1524, with original wall beams, an
architectural treasure. A garrison for
Royalist troops in the Civil War. Situated
in 4 acres of landscaped gardens in lovely
open countryside.

SELF-CATERING
NEWTON MEADOWS HOLIDAY COTTAGES
Wem Road, Harmer Hill,
Nr. Shrewsbury SY4 3DZ
Tel/Fax: (01939) 290346
No. of Accessible Units: 3. Roll-in Showers.
No. of Beds per Unit: 4/7
Accessible Facilities: Open plan
Lounge/Diner/Kitchen, Patio. 3 newly
renovated spacious adjoining cottages,
converted from old cow shed in rural
hamlet. 6 miles north of Shrewsbury with
country views.

ATTRACTIONS
ATTINGHAM PARK (NT)
Atcham, Shrewsbury
Tel: (01743) 709203
Elegant neo-classical mansions with 250
acres of superb parkland. Deer park,
woodlands and River.

SD ♿ CP ♿ E ♿ RF ♿ L ♿
C 🚶 S 🚶 WC 🚶

THE SHREWSBURY QUEST
193 Abbey Foregate, Shrewsbury SY2 6AH
Tel: (01743) 366355   Fax: (01743) 244342
Staff Training: Yes. The Benedictine Abbey
of St. Peter and St. Paul stood on this site
for 500 years. This is a re-creation of
mediaeval monastic life – the bustle of
tradespeople, delicate sounds of dulcimer,
harp and lute, barrels rolling into the great
store, bells proclaiming Vespers.

SD ♿ CP ♿ E ♿ RF ♿ L ♿
C ♿ S ♿ WC 🚶

TELFORD
Britain's first major new city, begun in
1963, comprised of Madely, Ironbridge,
Coalbrookdale, Wellington and Oakengates.
The name was chosen to commemorate
Thomas Telford whose bridges, viaducts,
canals and churches are endemic to
Shropshire.

TOURIST INFORMATION CENTRE
The Telford Centre, Telford TF3 4BX
Tel: (01952) 230032   Fax: (01952) 291723

HOTEL
HOLIDAY INN TELFORD/IRONBRIDGE
Telford International Centre, St. Quentin Gate,
Telford TF3 4EH
Tel: (01952) 292500   Fax: (01952) 291949
e-mail: holidayinn.telford@virgin.net
web: www.holiday
inn.com/hotels/telux/welcome.html
No. of Accessible Rooms: 2. Bath
Accessible Facilities: Lounge, Dining
Room. Modern low-rise property located
adjacent to Telford International Centre
with good access to M54 and town centre

TELFORD MOAT HOUSE
Foregate, Telford Centre, Telford TF3 4NA
Tel: (01952) 429988 Fax: (01952) 292012
No. of Accessible Rooms: 1
Accessible Facilities: Lounge, Restaurant,
Leisure Club. Large modern hotel just off
M54.

The monk's herb garden, Shrewsbury Quest.

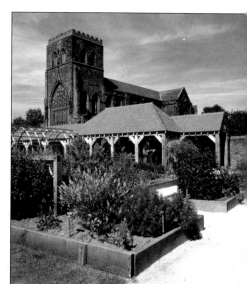

223

SOMERSET

SOMERSET TOURISM
web: www.somerset.gov.uk/tourism/default.htm

BATH & NORTHEAST SOMERSET COUNCIL
Trimbridge House, Trim Street, Bath BA1 2DP
Tel: (01225) 477000   Fax: (01225) 477637

BASONBRIDGE

Small inland village Close to Burnham -on-Sea, equidistant between Weston -super-Mare and Bridgewater with many places of interest within a short drive.

BED & BREAKFAST
MERRY FARM.
Basonbridge TA9 3PS
Tel: (01278) 783655
No. of Accessible Rooms: 1. Bath
Accessible Facilities: Lounge, Dining Room 300 year old farmhouse full of character and old beams, with private fishing on 600m of the River Brue.

BATH

Somerset's largest town and the most celebrated of England's spa towns. The main pool today is below the modern street level and open to the sky with original lead flooring and surrounding paving. Major association with the Romans who enjoyed the baths over 4 centuries. Majority of Bath now dates from Georgian times, when fashionable people came to "take the waters". The city still retains fine Georgian terraces and other buildings of mellow Bath stone and virtually all the streets are very attractive with stylish shops. The city has a rich cultural life with an arts festival every May.

TOURIST INFORMATION CENTRE
Abbey Chambers, Abbey Church Yard,
Bath BA1 1LY
Tel: (01225) 477101
e-mail: tourism@bathnes.gov.uk
web: www.visitbath.co.uk

BUSES
Bath Bus Company
1 Pierrepont Street, Bath BA1 1LB
Tel: (01225) 330444 Fax: (01225) 330727
Some low floor routes
First Badgerline: Tel: (01225) 466889
Some low floor/kneeling routes
Abus: Tel: (0117) 9776126
Based in Bristol, some low floor routes.

The Romans loved their baths. The water, unfortunately, is highly poisonous.

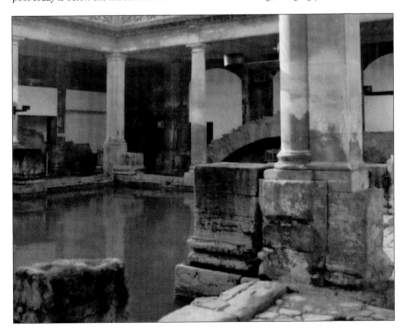

TAXIS
Taxi rank at station
Abbey Road Taxis: Tel: (01225) 444446
1 adapted vehicle
JD Cabs: Tel: (01225) 404162
2 adapted vehicles
Rainbow Taxis: Tel: (01225) 460606
2 adapted vehicles

TRAINS
First Great Western:
Special Needs: Tel: (0845) 7413775
Wales & West
Special Needs: (0845) 3003005
Minicom: (0845) 7585469

Bath Spa Station has level access to concourse with ticket counter, level tunnel to westbound platform via long ramp (1:12) and 1:11 to eastbound platform. Disabled WCs.

CAR PARKING
Free Orange badge parking in Council controlled car parks. Also considerable amount of on-street parking, free to Orange badge holders.
Tel: (01225) 477130

SHOPMOBILITY
4 Railway Street, Bath BA1 1PG
Tel/Fax: (01225) 481744
Minicom: (01225) 481773

HOTEL
HILTON NATIONAL
Walcot Street, Bath BA1 5BJ
Tel: (01225) 463411   Fax: (01225) 464393
No. of Accessible Rooms: 1
Accessible Facilities: Restaurant, Bar.
Modern hotel situated in city centre.

CENTURION HOTEL
Charlton Lane, Midsomer Norton,
Nr. Bath BA3 4BD
Tel: (01761) 417711 Fax: (01761) 418357
No. of Accessible Rooms: 2. Bath.
Accessible Facilities: Lounge, Restaurant (rear entrance).
Family run complex, including the Fosseway Country Club to which it is linked by the Restaurant with longish walk to club facilities.

Located 19 miles from Bath in fine setting midway between Bath and Wells.

ATTRACTION
BATH ABBEY
Bath BA1 1LT
Tel: (01225) 422462   Fax: (01225) 429990
C15th Perpendicular style Abbey church built on site of Saxon Abbey where coronation took place of England's first king, Edgar, in 973 AD.

SD | CP | E | RF
S | WC | RFE

MUSEUM OF COSTUME (NT)
Assembly Rooms, Bennett Street, Bath
Tel: (01225) 477789   Fax: (01225) 444793
e-mail: costume_enquiries@bathmus.gov.uk
Large and fine collection of fashionable dress from late C16th to present day, house in C18th Assembly Rooms.

SD | CP n/a | E | RF
L | S | WC

PRIOR PARK LANDSCAPE GARDEN (NT)
Ralph Allen Drive, Bath BA2 5AH
Tel: (01225) 833422
Fine example of C18th English landscape, a haven of peace and a work of art with panoramic views of the city. There is a Wilderness area of woodland, Serpentine Lake and natural springs, a Palladian Bridge created in 1755, lakes and dams and a Rock Gate.

SD | CP | E | RF
WC | RFE

THE ROMAN BATHS MUSEUM
Stall Street, Bath BA1 1LZ
Tel: (01225) 477785   Fax: (01225) 477743
e-mail: christine_mclean@bathnes.gov.uk
The baths, built by the Romans nearly 2000 years ago, served those who were ill and pilgrims who were visiting the adjacent Temple of Sulis Minerva.
Access for wheelchairs to inner and outer Terraces overlooking the Great Bath only. There are special access evenings when it is possible to take visitors down to the Museum - tel. above number.

SD | CP n/a | E | RF | C
S | WC | RFE

225

BRIDGWATER

Enterprising industrial town with both old and modern buildings. Castle Street, running down to the West Quay is a superb example of the C17th, whilst St. Mary's Church is C13th to C15th has some magnificent features.

BED & BREAKFAST ACCOMMODATION
BLACKMORE FARM
Cannington, Bridgwater TA5 2NE
Tel: (01278) 653442   Fax: (01278) 653427
e-mail: Dyerfarm@aol.com

No. of Accessible Rooms: 1. Roll-in Shower
Accessible Facilities: Lounge, Dining Room. Built in C14th and retains many of its period features including stone archways, garderobes and oak beams. The Stable is an annexe to the main house in a barn conversion with disabled facilities. The farm consists of 2 holdings extending to 750 acres, with both livestock and arable crops. Family owned and managed by the Dyers who have a fascinating history of the farm.

SELF-CATERING
THE GRANARY
5 Old Main Road, Pawlett, Bridgwater TA6 4RY
Tel: (01278) 684992

No. of accessible Units: 1. Bath
No. of Beds per Unit: 3
Accessible Facilities: Lounge/Diner. C17th stone barn situated in the centre of small village beside the post office and close to the local church and village green. The village of Pawlett is 2 miles from the M5 (J23) with access to many places of interest.

BRUTON

Picturesque small town on River Bruce, founded in Saxon times and retaining many intriguing glimpses of its past including Jacobean almshouses, Abbey remains, 15thC packhorse bridge, twin-towers church and famous dovecote.

SELF-CATERING
DISCOVE FARM
Bruton BA10 0NQ
Tel: (01749) 812284

The Dovecote:
Owl Barn:
No. of Accessible Units: 2. Roll-in Showers.
No. of Beds per Unit: Dovecote-2, Owl-4/5
Accessible Facilities: Lounge Dining Room, Kitchen, Garden with barbecue and picnic table, elevated level Sundeck. Purpose-built units for wheelchair users in peaceful countryside setting.

CASTLE CARY

Vibrant market town with winding main street of thatch and golden stone below Lodge Hill. On Bailey Hill stands the C18th 'pepper pot' lock up, one of only 4 in the country.

ATTRACTION
HADSPEN GARDEN & NURSERY
Castle Cary BA7 7NG
Tel/Fax: (01749) 813707

e-mail: hadspen@compuserve.com
five-acre garden noted for herbaceous borders and roses.

SD	♿	CP	♿	E	♿	RF	♿
C	♿	S	♿	WC	♿	RFE	♿

CHEDDAR

Pale-grey limestone cliffs rise vertically to 150m. on either side of the town, with spectacular views from the cliff top. Cheddar cheese has been made here in local farmhouses since the C12th, although its main industries are now market gardening (particularly strawberries), limestone quarrying and cheese straw making.

SELF-CATERING
THE HEATHERS
Westfield Lane, Draycott, Cheddar
Tel: (01934) 744187

No. of Accessible Units: 1. Roll-in Shower.
No. of Beds per Unit: 2
Accessible Facilities: Lounge, Dining Room, Kitchen, Garden.
A very private unit with wonderful views across the Cheddar Valley.

DULVERTON

Lies in the beautiful valley of the River Barle, in an area of densely wooded steep hillsides. There are narrow streets, live theatre, craft markets and special events, attracting artists and anglers particularly.

SELF-CATERING
NORTHMOOR HOUSE
Dulverton TA22 9QS
Tel: (01398) 323720
No. of Accessible Units: 1. Roll-in Shower.
No. of Beds Per Unit: 2
Accessible Facilities: Lounge, Dining Room. The House is arranged to accommodate up to 22 adults plus 3 cots and best suited for large parties where 1 or 2 people require wheelchair access. NB: The kitchen is not suitable for Cat. 2.

ATTRACTION
EXMOOR NATIONAL PARK
Exmoor House, Dulverton TA22 9HL
Tel: (01398) 323665   Fax: (01398) 323150
The rugged nature of Exmoor's 267 square miles of protected landscape, can seem challenging but the area's unique atmosphere is most enjoyable. Cool wooded valleys, flowing streams and wildlife, together with spectacular coastline of rugged cliffs, wild seas, high moorland and heather.

Visitor Centres at:
Combe Martin, Devon – Cross Street, Tel (01272) 883319
Lynmouth, Devon – The Esplanade, Tel: (01598) 752509
Dunster, Somerset – Dunster Steep, Tel: (01643) 821835
Dulverton, Somerset – Fore Street, Tel: (01398) 323841
Well worth visiting:
North West Exmoor: Barbrook, Blackmoor Gate, Brendon & Common,, Combe Martin, Heddon Valley, Holdstone & Trentishoe Downs, Lee Abbey Estate, Malmsmead, Oare & Doone Country, Martinhoe & Woody Bay, Parracombe, Valley of Rocks, Lynton, Lynmouth, Watersmeet, Countisbury Barna Barrow. Central & Southern Exmoor: Exford, Heasley Mill Nr. North Molton, Landacre

Bridge, Molland, Shoulsbarrow Common, Simonsbath, Tarr Steps, Wimbleball Lake, Winsford, Withypool.
North East Exmoor: Horner Water, Porlock Hill, Selworthy Beacon, Webber's Post, Yenworthy Common.

FROME

Long history from 685AD as market and agricultural town with many historic buildings, particularly around Cheap Street and the Catherine Hill areas. Notable C17th bridge, largely untouched over the past 200 years.

TOURIST INFORMATION CENTRE
The Round Tower, Black Swan, 2 Bridge Street, Frome BA11 1BB
Tel: (01373) 467271

BED & BREAKFAST
FOURWINDS GUEST HOUSE 🚶
Bath Road, Frome BA11 2HJ
Tel: (01373) 462618   Fax: (01373) 453029
Large, chalet style bungalow with amenities of a hotel, but friendly and informal. Lovely garden. Evening meals always available. Located 0.5 mile from Frome

GLASTONBURY

Famous for its connections with history of Christianity, the majestic ruins of its Abbey and its association with the legends of King Arthur, who with his wife, Guinevere, is reputed to be buried in the Abbey grounds. Many of the town centre shops are dedicated to the history, myth and legend which surround Glastonbury, producing a singular ambience.

TOURIST INFORMATION CENTRE
The Tribunal, 9 High Street, Glastonbury BA6 9DP
Tel: (01458) 832954

SELF-CATERING
HIGHLAND STUDIO ♿
Highlands Guest House, 21 Rowley Road, Glastonbury BA6 8HU
Tel/Fax: (01458) 834587
e-mail: highlands@eclipse.co.uk

Web: www.tavel-uk.net/highlands
No. of Accessible Units: 1. Roll-in Shower.
No. of Beds per Unit: 2 + child
Accessible Facilities: Open plan studio with bedroom/Lounge/kitchen, plus additional large hall with bed if needed. Double patio doors lead to lovely private wooden deck with patio furniture and barbecue. Contact bell for assistance. Located at the top of the town, up a steep drive equivalent to halfway up the Tor, facing west with wonderful views over the town, particularly the ruined Abbey, across the Somerset Levels to the Severn Estuary, Wales and Exmoor.

ATTRACTION
GLASTONBURY ABBEY
Abbey Gatehouse, Magdalene Street,
Glastonbury BA6 9EL
Tel/Fax: (01458) 832267
e-mail: glastonbury.abbey@dial.pipex.com
One of oldest religious foundations in Britain, steeped in history and legend. Extensive ruins in 36 acres in which Joseph of Arimathea is said to have stood his staff, which promptly sprouted. Descendants of that first tree still blooming twice a year in the Abbey grounds. Also home to legend of King Arthur and Queen Guinevere whose bodies were 'discovered' in Abbey cemetery in C12th. and re-interred in chancel in 1278. Destroyed in the Dissolution, the site is now marked by a plaque. Incredibly atmospheric ruins.
SD CP E RF S WC

HIGH LITTLETON
SELF-CATERING
GREYFIELD FARM COTTAGES
High Littleton BS18 5YQ
Tel: (01761) 471132
No. of Accessible Units: 3. 1 Cottage has roll-in Shower, 2 have Bath
No. of Beds per Unit: 4 + cot
Accessible Facilities: Lounge, Dining Room, Kitchen, Sauna, Jacuzzi, Spa bath. 4 accessible cottages, out of 5. Located 8 miles south of Bath.

MINEHEAD
Traditional seaside resort with a 1mile long seafront and fine curving stretch of sand.

Main shopping area close to colourful tree-lined avenue, numerous good walks and fine climate.

TOURIST INFORMATION CENTRE
17 Friday Street, Minehead TA24 5UB
Tel: (01643) 702624   Fax: (01643) 707166

ACCESSIBLE HOTELS
THE PROMENADE HOTEL
Grooms Holidays
The Esplanade, Minehead TA24 5QS
Tel/Fax: (01643) 702572
No. of Accessible Rooms: 8
Accessible Facilities: Lounge, Restaurant, Garden, Minibus with tail lift. Located beneath the North Hill on the seafront, overlooking the sea and local harbour. Excursions in minibus to local attractions.

PERITON PARK HOTEL
Middlecombe, Nr. Minehead TA24 8SW
Tel/Fax: (01643) 706885
No. of Accessible Rooms: 1
Accessible Facilities: Lounge, Restaurant. Located on northern edge of Exmoor National Park, in glorious countryside, the house was built in 1875 and retains the ambience of a gracious country house. Family owned and managed.

THE LANGBURY
Blue Anchor Bay, Nr. Minehead TA24 6LB
Tel/Fax: (01643) 821375
e-mail: langbury@globalnet.co.uk
Web: www.users.globalnet.co.uk/~langbury
No. of Accessible Rooms: 1. Shower
Accessible Facilities: Lounge/Bar, Restaurant. Small friendly hotel with fine sea views and the hills of Exmoor. Located 5 miles from Minehead and 3 from Dunster.

SELF-CATERING
PRIMROSE HILL

Wood Lane, Blue Anchor,
Nr. Minehead TA24 6LA
Tel: (01643) 821200
No. of Accessible Units: 4. Shower
No. of Beds per Unit: 2 - 3
Accessible Facilities: Lounge/Diner, Kitchen. A terrace of 4 brick bungalows, all accessible, with shared landscaped frontage, private back gardens with panoramic views.

Located 5 miles E of Minehead.

WESTERMILL FARM 🚶
Exford, Nr. Minehead TA24 7NJ
Tel: (01643) 831238 Fax: (01643) 831660
No. of Accessible Units: 2. Roll-in Shower/
Shower. No. of Beds per Unit: 4-8
Accessible Facilities: Lounge, Kitchen,
Garden furniture. Two Scandinavian log
cottages, Bracken and Molina, rebuilt for
disabled access on a 500 acre working farm
in centre of Exmoor National Park. Over 2
miles of shallow River Exe winds its way
through the farm, which won a 1997 David
Bellamy Gold conservation award.

ATTRACTIONS
DUNSTER CASTLE (NT)
Dunster, Nr. Minehead TA24 6SL
Tel: (01643) 821314 Fax: (01643) 823000
Situated on top of a wooded hill, with a
C13th gatehouse surviving amongst the
C17th new design of the house. Lovely
parkland.

SD ♿   CP 🚶   E 🚶   RF 🚶
S 🚶   WC ♿   RFE ♿

RODE
Pretty, rather unknown village. located
between Trowbridge and Frome

ATTRACTION
RODE BIRD GARDENS
Rode, Nr. Bath BA3 6QW
Tel: (01373) 830326 Fax: (01373) 831288
Outside attraction of 17 acres with a disabled
route marked out. Noted particularly for
conservation of exotic birds with over 200
species, there are also a miniature steam
railway, children's play area, pets corner,
woodlands & flowers, formal Victorian
gardens, ornamental lakes and streams.

SD ♿   CP 🚶   E ♿   RF ♿
C 🚶   S 🚶   WC 🚶

SOMERTON
C7th Royal Capital of Wessex, whose C17th
square, market cross, town hall and
elegant houses and inns create a most
attractive townscape of architectural and
historic interest.

LYTES CARY MANOR (NT)
Charlton Mackrell, Nr. Somerton TA11 7HU
Tel: (01985) 843600 Fax: (01985) 843624
Charming manor house, not accessible,
with attractive hedged garden full of typical
C16th plants and trees.
The garden only is suitable for wheelchairs

SD ♿   CP 🚶   S ♿
E 🚶 (Garden)   WC 🚶

STREET
Named after ancient causeway running
north across River Brue to Glastonbury. In
C19th tanning sheepskin was main trade,
prosperity much increasing when, in 1825,
C & J Clark founded their shoe factory here.

TOURIST INFORMATION CENTRE
Clark's Village, Farm Road, Street BA16 0BB
Tel: (01458) 447384

SHOPMOBILITY
Clark's Village as above.
Tel: (01458) 440155
Free loan of scooters, powerchairs and
manual wheelchairs.

ATTRACTION
CLARK'S VILLAGE
As above
Tel: (01458) 840064 Fax: (01458) 841132
Factory outlet shopping, with many retail
units offering discounts on well-known
products in charming surroundings.

SD ♿   CP ♿   E ♿   RF ♿
C ♿   S ♿ (all outlets)
WC 🚶   RFE ♿

TAUNTON
Prosperous town situated in the centre of
one of the country's most fertile plans. A
fine Georgian street of deep-red brick and
white porticoed houses combine with the
late C15th church of St. Mary Magdalene.

TOURIST INFORMATION CENTRE
The Library, Paul Street, Taunton TA1 2XZ
Tel: (01823) 336344 Fax: (01823) 340308
web: www.tauntondeane.gov.uk
Extremely helpful!

229

BUSES
First Southern National: Tel: (01823) 272033
Some low floor buses

TAXIS
A1 Taxis: Tel: (01823) 323323
7 adapted vehicles

TRAINS
First Great Western: Special Needs:
Tel: (0845) 7413775
Virgin Trains: Special Needs:
Tel: (0845) 7443366
Minicom: (0845) 7443367
Wales & West: Special Needs:
Tel: (0845) 3003005
Minicom: (0845) 7585469
Taunton Station accessible by lift.

CAR PARKS
Orange badge scheme. Tel: (01823) 356356

SHOPMOBILITY
1st Floor, Old Market Centre, Taunton
Tel: (01823) 327900

HOTEL
FORTE POSTHOUSE
Deane Gate Avenue, Taunton TA1 2UA
Tel: (01823) 332222   Fax: (01823) 332266
No. of Accessible Rooms: 2. Bath
Accessible Facilities: Lounge, Restaurant.
Modern property, close to numerous
attractions and with good access to Exmoor
National Park and Cheddar Gorge

BED & BREAKFAST
REDLANDS
Treble's Holford, Combe Florey, Taunton,
Somerset TA4 3HA
Tel: 01823 433159
e-mail: redlandshouse@hotmail.com
No. of Accessible Rooms: 1. Roll-in Shower
Accessible Facilities: Lounge, Dining Room
and areas of the Garden. The owner is
herself a wheelchair user. Set in quiet
country location by stream, adjacent to the
Quantock Hills. 8 miles from Taunton and
close to the preserved West Somerset
Railway. Both self-catering and b & b, the
latter in the Courtyard Room which is
accessible.

PROCTORS FARM
West Monkton, Taunton TA2 8QN
Tel: (01823) 412269
No. of Accessible Rooms: 2. Roll-in Shower
Accessible Facilities: Lounge, Dining
Room. C17th farmhouse with exposed oak
beams and log fires standing in own
grounds and surrounded by family-run
farm. Located 2 miles from Taunton

SELF-CATERING
HOLLY COTTAGE
Stoke St. Gregory, Taunton TA3 6HS
Tel: (01823) 490828   Fax: (01823) 490590
e-mail: robhembrow@btinternet.com
No. of Accessible Units: 1. Roll-in Shower.
No. of Beds per Unit: 4
Accessible Facilities: Lounge,
Kitchen/Diner. The Linny is 1 of 5 cottages
converted from stone barns built by
present owner's great grandfather. Holly
Farm is a traditional working farm in
peaceful rural countryside of Sedgemoor.

TEMPLECOMBE
HOTEL
FOUNTAIN INN MOTEL
High Street, Henstridge, Templecombe BA8 0RA
Tel: (01963) 362722
No. of Accessible Rooms: 1. Shower.
Accessible Facilities: Lounge, Restaurant.
Henstridge is on the Somerset/Dorset
border and overlooks the Blackmore Vale.

WATCHET
Busy small commercial port with attractive
harbour.

TOURIST INFORMATION CENTRE
The Esplanade, Watchet
Tel: as Minehead.

SELF-CATERING
ROSEVILLE
48A Brendon Road, Watchet TA23 0HT
Tel: (01984) 634199   Fax: (01984) 631572
No. of Accessible Units: 1. Bath
No. of Beds per Unit: 4 + 3 child.
Accessible Facilities: Lounge/Dining Room,
Kitchen. Large bungalow.

WELLS

England's smallest and Somerset's only city, with fine Cathedral The wells from which city derives its name rise in the grounds of the Bishop's Palace, producing an average 100 litres of water per second.

TOURIST INFORMATION CENTRE
Town Hall, Market Place, Wells BA5 2RB
Tel: (01749) 672552

ATTRACTION
THE BISHOP'S PALACE
The Henderson Rooms, The Bishop's Palace, Wells BA5 2PD
Tel/Fax: (01749) 678691
Medieval residence built by Bishop Jocelin in early C13th with undercroft still virtually intact. Fortified in the C14th there are several state rooms and a superb long gallery housing portraits of former Bishops. Access through C14th gatehouse only. Located next to Cathedral off Market Square.

SD 🚫 E 🧍 RF 🧍 C 🧍 WC 🧍

WOOKEY HOLE CAVES & PAPERMILL
Wookey Hole, Wells BA5 1BB
Tel: (01749) 677243   Fax: (01749) 677749
e-mail: witch@wookeyhole.demon.co.uk
Although no access to actual caves, worth visiting the Victorian Papermill-watch exquisite paper being made. In Mill also is Magical Mirror Maze and a typical Old Penny Arcade.

SD 🚫 CP 🧍 E 🚫 RF 🧍
C 🧍 S 🧍 WC 🧍 RFE 🚫

WESTON-SUPER-MARE

Somerset's largest seaside resort with fine wide sea-front roads, pavements and gardens.

HOTELS
MOORLANDS
Hutton, Weston-Super-Mare BS24 9QH
Tel/Fax: (01934) 812283
No. of Accessible Rooms: 1. Shower
Accessible Facilities: Lounge, Restaurant
Lovely Georgian house near centre delightful village of Hutton, standing in 2 acres of mature landscaped gardens and

paddock. The village lies under steep, wooded slopes of western Mendips. 10 minutes drive from Weston

LAURISTON HOTEL
6-12 Knightstone Road, Weston super Mare BS23 2AN
Tel: (01934) 620758   Fax: (01934) 621154
No. of Accessible Rooms: 2
Accessible Facilities: Lounge, Restaurant, Garden. Located opposite the beach, close to the sea front promenade and shopping precinct, this hotel caters specifically for visually impaired guests and most facilities accessible by wheelchair lift.

SELF-CATERING
HOPE FARM COTTAGE
Brean Road, Lympsham, Weston-Super-Mare BS24 0HA
Tel/Fax: (01934) 750506
No. of Accessible Units: 1. Bath.
No. of Beds per Unit: 4 + cot
Accessible Facilities: Open plan Lounge/Kitchen/Diner, Central Heating. Carthouse Cottage is 1 of 4 cottages set within a courtyard and backing onto open farmland. Located on outskirts of small village, 5 miles from Weston-super-Mare and close to Bath and Wells. Being within the Somerset Levels, much of the surrounding area is flat.

ATTRACTIONS
HELICOPTER MUSEUM
The Heliport, Lockine Hook Road, Weston-super-Mare BS22 8PL
Tel: (01934) 635227 Fax: (01934) 822400
Unique collection of over 60 helicopters with new large undercover displays including restoration hangar and how helicopters work.
Wheelchair available for loan.

SD ♿ CP ♿ E ♿ RF ♿
C ♿ S ♿ WC 🧍

TIME MACHINE MUSEUM
Burlington Street, Weston-Super-Mare BS23 1PR
Tel: (01934) 621028 Fax: (01934) 612526
e-mail: museum.service@n-somerset.gov.uk
Displays on the seaside holiday, apothecary shop, dairy and fountain with Victorian mosaics. Mendip mining and local

231

archaeology also on display.

SD 👤♿   CP n/a   E ♿   RF ♿

C ♿   S ♿   WC 🚹   RFE- ♿

aircrews train.

SD n/a   CP ♿   E ♿   RF ♿

L ♿   C 🚹   S 🚹   WC ♿   RFE ♿

YEOVIL

Major town in south Somerset situated in rolling fertile land beside the River Yeo.

TOURIST INFORMATION CENTRE
Petter's House, Petter's Way, Yeovil BA20 1SH
Tel: (01935) 471279

ATTRACTIONS
FLEET AIR ARM MUSEUM
RNAS Yeovilton, Ilchester, Nr. Yeovil BA22 8HT
Tel: (01935) 840565   Fax: (01935) 84020 8
e-mail: curator.@faam.org.uk

Leading aviation museum with impressive displays on both World Wars and recent conflicts such as Falklands and the Gulf and a Harrier Exhibition. The "Ultimate Carrier Experience", a flight deck built on land, offers special effects with sounds, smell and excitement of a big carrier on a mercy mission. Other attractions include model aircraft and ships, weapons, uniforms and airfield viewing galleries where visitors can watch modern Navy

MONTACUTE HOUSE (NT)
Montacute, Yeovil
Tel/Fax: (01935) 823289

Late C16th, this Elizabethan house was the location for the film ìSense & Sensibilityî. Features include Renaissance plasterwork, a long Gallery hung with Tudor and Jacobean court portraits, C17th and C18th furniture and a fine formal garden

SD ♿   CP 🚹   E ♿   C 🚹   S ♿   WC 🚹

HAYNES MOTOR MUSEUM
Sparkford, Nr. Yeovil BA22 7LH
Tel: (01963) 440804   Fax: (01963) 441004
e-mail: mike@gmpwin.demon.co.uk

Spectacular collection of over 250 cars from American monsters to marvellous Minis. A Hall of red sports cars including Ferarris and Cobras combines with Model T Ford of 1903 and the famous Duesenberg of 1931. Not a personal enthusiast, I was nevertheless captivated!

SD ♿   CP ♿   E ♿   RF ♿

C ♿   S ♿   WC ♿

See the British car industry before BMW at Haynes Motor Museum.

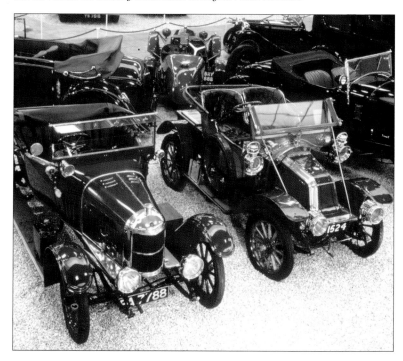

STAFFORDSHIRE

THE POTTERIES TOURISM
Civic Centre, Glebe Street,
Stoke-on-Trent ST4 1RP
Tel: (01782) 232701   Fax: (01782) 232910

ALTON
Stone-built village lying east of Cheadle on the rocky, wooded slopes of the Churnet Valley, all towers, turrets and spires. Alton is one half of the Rhineland of Staffordshire: every road and lane is a hill, every bend or gap in the trees or houses offers a central European view.

BED AND BREAKFAST
HANSLEY CROSS COTTAGE
Cheadle Road, Alton, Staffs ST10 4DH
Tel/Fax: (01538) 702189
No. of Accessible Rooms: 1. Roll-in Shower
Accessible Facilities: Lounge, Dining Room.
Country house near Alton Towers.

ATTRACTION
ALTON TOWERS
Alton ST10 4DB
Tel: (01538) 703344   Fax: (01538) 704097
web: www.alton-towers.co.uk
Theme park with a variety of rides, shows and attractions. Built into the landscape, the estate provides a delightful green, wooded backdrop. The park provides a guide to the rides for those with disabilities giving entrance details and any restrictions, but in the majority of cases, a companion must also come aboard. Nemesis and the Skyride are not accessible.

SD 👤	CP 👤	E 👤	RF 👤
C 👤 (Towers Family Restaurant particularly)			
S 👤	WC 👤 Wheelchairs available just inside entrance on right hand side.		

LEEK
Situated at the southern end of some of the most impressive scenery in the county.

BED AND BREAKFAST
CROFT MEADOWS FARM

Horton, Leek ST13 8QE
Tel: (01782) 513039
No. of Accessible Rooms: 1. Roll-in Shower
Accessible Facilities: Lounge, Dining Room.
Country Farmhouse.

LICHFIELD
From whichever direction one enters the city, the three magnificent spires of the cathedral can be seen. There is a cobbled market square, narrow streets and many links with Dr. Johnson, a statue of him is set in the square. Lichfield has long military associations, the Staffordshire Regiment being a famous aspect.

ATTRACTION
STAFFORDSHIRE REGIMENT MUSEUM
Whittington Barracks, Lichfield WS14 9PY
Tel: (0121) 311 3229   Fax: (0121) 311 3205
Regimental militaria including battle honours, trophies and uniforms.

SD n/a	CP 👤	E 👤	RF 👤
C 👤	WC 👤	RFE 👤	

STAFFORD
Birthplace of the world's most renowned angler, Izaak Walton and connections with the famous English playwright, Richard Brinsley Sheridan. The church of St. Mary, the High House, a four-storied timbered house where Charles I and Prince Rupert stayed in 1642, Royal Brine Baths, Church of St. Chad and Noel Almshouses in Mill Street, are all worth a view.

ATTRACTION
SHUGBOROUGH ESTATE (NT)
Shugborough, Milford, Nr. Stafford ST17 0XB
Tel: (01889) 881388   Fax: (01889) 881323
Truly superb estate built in the late C17th, enlarged c1750 and again at the turn of the C19th. Seat of the Earls of Lichfield and currently home to Patrick Lichfield, the well-known photographer. Now being restored as a C19th working estate. The house has a variety of collections plus original kitchens and laundry and working farm museum with educational programmes and demonstrations. The farmhouse has its original working mill,

used for grinding flour and providing the many estate animals' food. A great day out. Access to ground floor only of the house, but much to see and well worth while. Additional disabled parking at farmhouse. Accessible picnic tables.

SD ♿   CP 🚹   E ♿ (Stairclimber)
C 🚹   S ♿   WC ♿
RFE ♿ 3 self-drive Batri-cars available for park and garden, with instruction. (kept near museum)
5 wheelchairs available.

STOKE-ON-TRENT

Came into being in 1910 when Stoke-on-Trent was combined with five adjoining towns – Tunstall, Burslem, Hanley, Fenton and Longton. Today it is a large town renowned for its many potteries and ancient buildings.

TOURIST INFORMATION CENTRE
Quadrant Road, Hanley,
Stoke-on-Trent ST1 1RZ
Tel: (01782) 236000   Fax: (01782) 236005
Minicom: (01782) 236004
e-mail: stoke.tic@virgin.net

STOKE ON TRENT DEPARTMENT OF PLANNING
Building Advisory Service, PO Box 633,
Civic Centre, Glebe Street,
Stoke-on-Trent ST4 1RH
Tel: (01782) 234567
After hours: (01782) 232459
Fax: (01782) 236345
Minicom: (01782) 232331
Produces Guide to City Council Services for people with Disabilities.

BUSES
First PMT: Tel: (01782) 207999
Some low-floor buses.
Passenger Transport Team:
Tel: (01782) 234500
Staffordshire Busline: Tel: (01782) 206608

TAXIS
Roseville (Newcastle): Tel: (01872) 613456
Six adapted vehicles.
Scraggs Taxis: Tel: (01782) 265109
One adapted vehicle.

TRAINS
First North Western: Special Needs:
Tel: (0845) 6040231
Virgin Trains – Special Needs:
Tel: (0845) 7443366
Minicom: (0845) 7443367

CAR PARKS
Orange badge spaces in all council owned car parks. Some on-street parking in city centre.
Tel: (01782) 234567

SHOPMOBILITY
Level 1C, Potteries Shopping Centre Car Park,
Off Bryan Street, Stoke-on-Trent.
Tel: (01782) 233333 Fax: (01782) 233496
Minicom: (01782) 233334

HOTEL
STOKE-ON-TRENT MOAT HOUSE   🚹
Etruria Mall, Festival Way, Etruria,
Stoke on Trent ST1 5BQ
Tel: (01782) 609988   Fax: (01782) 284500
No. of Accessible Rooms: 3. Bath
Accessible Facilities: Lounge, Restaurant, Pool, Sauna, Whirlpool. The former home of Josiah Wedgwood, Etruria Hall is now a quality hotel.

ATTRACTION
ETRURIA INDUSTRIAL MUSEUM
Lower Bedford Street, Etruria,
Stoke-on-Trent ST4 7AF
Tel: (01782) 233144   Fax: (01782) 233145
Working forge and demonstrations of steam machinery, plus Britain's sole surviving steam powered potter's mill. Visitor Centre (i.e. entrance) is fully accessible: level access to Blacksmith's forge: no wheelchair access to Etruscan Bone Mill.

SD ♿   CP ♿   E ♿   RF ♿
L ♿   C 🚹   S ♿   WC ♿

GLADSTONE POTTERY MUSEUM
Uttoxeter Road, Longton,
Stoke-on-Trent ST3 1PQ
Tel: (01782) 311378   Fax: (01782) 598640
Cobbled yard within museum possibly problematical – bringing a companion will make it easier. The only remaining complete Victorian pottery. This unique

working museum allows visitors to see how potters worked. Traditional skills, original workshops, cobbled yard and huge bottle kilns create a real time-warp. Make your own pot or bone china flower.

SD ☐ CP ☐ E ☐ RF ☐ L ☐
C ☐ S ☐ WC ☐ RFE ☐

ROYAL DOULTON VISITOR CENTRE
Nile Street, Burslem, Stoke-on-Trent ST6 2AJ
Tel: (01782) 292434   Fax: (01782) 292424
e-mail: visitor@royal-doulton.com
New Centre combination of magic of Royal Doulton figures with treasures from the company's collection, including the biggest range of figurines in the world, displays of ceramic skills in the Royal Minton fine art studio where personal orders are all hand painted, sited on the ground floor of the original factory purchased in 1877. Visitor Centre accessible (Minton studio closed at weekends): video theatre with wheelchair spaces. Very civilised restaurant/museum. FACTORY TOURS NOT ACCESSIBLE.

SD ☐ CP ☐ E ☐ RF ☐
C ☐ S ☐ WC ☐ RF ☐

WEDGWOOD VISITOR CENTRE
Barlaston, Stoke-on-Trent ST12 9ES
Tel: (01782) 204141   Fax: (01782) 374083
Complex with art gallery of English paintings and re-construction of original C18th workshops. Demonstrations of traditional skills and museum with fine collection of Josiah Wedgwood's work from 1750. A video highlights history and craft of Wedgwood process.

SD ☐ CP ☐ E ☐ RF ☐
C ☐ S ☐ WC ☐ RFE ☐

UTTOXETER
Known mainly for its racecourse, reckoned to be the finest National Hunt Steeplechase course in the Midlands. The strangest thing about this small market town is its name, believed to derive from a form of Witta, a man's name and an old word for health.

SPORTING VENUE
UTTOXETER RACECOURSE
Wood Lane, Uttoxeter ST14 8BD
Admin & Booking-Box Office:

(01889) 562561   Fax: (01889) 562786
e-mail: info@uttoxeterracecourse.co.uk
web: www.uttoxeterracecourse.co.uk
CP ☐ RE ☐ ED ☐ INT ☐
L ☐ WC ☐ (except inward door opening).
3 units in main grandstand 7 in betting hall.
SS ☐ B/R ☐ Woodrows — all level, bistro style
☐ Platinum Suite — lift access, silver service.

WOLVERHAMPTON
(Staffs area)
See West Midlands for remainder.

ATTRACTION
MOSELEY OLD HALL (NT)
Moseley Old Hall Lane, Fordhouses,
Wolverhampton WV10 7HY
Tel: (01902) 782808
This is where Charles II hid after the Battle of Worcester. An exhibition retells the story of this dramatic escape from Cromwell's troops. The garden, recreated in C17th. style with formal knot garden, has varieties of herbs and plants of the period. Three rooms in the house, the exhibition and garden are accessible.

SD ☐ CP ☐ E ☐ RF ☐
C ☐ S ☐ WC ☐

235

The happy potter of Gladstone Pottery museum.

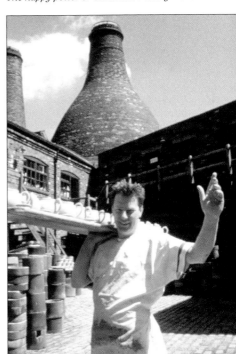

SUFFOLK

SUFFOLK TOURISM
web: www.suffolkcc.gov.uk
www.suffolkcc.gov.uk

TRAVELINE
Public Transport Group, Environment &
Transport Dept. Suffolk County Council, St.
Edmund House, County Hall, Ipswich IP4 1LZ
Tel: (0645) 583358
web: www.traveline.suffolkcc.gov.uk
For all information on bus, coach and rail
services within the county.

SPECIALIST OUTDOOR ACTIVITIES
WALDRINGFIELD BOATYARD LTD.
The Quay, Woodbridge IP12 4QZ
Tel/Fax: (01473) 736260.
Cruising on the River Deben through lovely
wooded country, from Felixstowe Ferry to
Woodbridge and Wilford Bridge. Organised
parties and individuals between May/October.
The *M.V. Jahan* is especially designed to
provide access for up to 12 disabled persons
with wide hatches and 2 hydraulic lifts.
Accessible WC on quay, but not on board.

ALDEBURGH
Quiet seaside resort of unspoilt charm with
an internationally famous Music Festival
(see BAFA in Intro.)

TOURIST INFORMATION CENTRE
Tel/Fax: (01728) 453637 (Seasonal)

HOTEL
UPLANDS HOTEL
Victoria Road, Aldeburgh IP15 5DX
Tel: (01728) 452420   Fax: (01728) 454872
No. of Accessible Rooms: 1
Accessible Facilities: Lounge, Restaurant,
Bar and TV Lounge (3 steps). Privately owned
Regency country house hotel in landscaped
gardens a short distance from the sea.

BUNGAY
Market town and yachting centre on the
River Waveney. Surrounded by sandy
beaches and unspoilt countryside.

ATTRACTION
NORFOLK AND SUFFOLK AVIATION MUSEUM
Flixton, Nr. Bungay NR35 1NZ
Tel: (01986) 896644
Living museum bursting with WW1 and
WW2 British, American and German civil
and military exhibits and personal
memorabilia amongst machinery and over
25 historic aircraft outside. This area of
Britain swarmed with aviation sites during
WW11 though many exhibits come from
farther afield. A must for both aviation fans
and laymen alike.

CP ♿   E ♿ (to hangars)
RF 🚹   C 🚹   S 🚹   WC 🚹

BURY ST. EDMUNDS
Began as Benedictine Abbey, founded in
945AD, becoming one of the richest in the
country prior to its dissolution in 1539. It
is known for its elegant Georgian streets
and flower gardens.

TOURIST INFORMATION CENTRE
6 Angel Hill, Bury St. Edmunds IP33 1UZ
Tel: (01284) 764667 Fax: (01284) 757084
Minicom: (01284) 757023
e-mail: appleby@burybo.stedsbc.gov.uk
web: www.stedmundsbury.gov.uk

BUSES
Suffolk Traveline: Tel: (0645) 583358
web: www.traveline.suffolkcc.gov.uk   Simonds
of Botesdale: Tel: (01379) 898202
R W Chenery: Tel: (01379) 741221
Operates London Service.
Whippet Coaches: Tel: (01480) 463792

TAXIS
No black cabs in Bury.
A1 Cars: Tel: (01284) 766777
2 adapted vehicles.

TRAINS
See Suffolk Traveline above.
Anglia Railways: Tel: (01473) 693333

CAR PARKS
Free orange badge spaces in all borough
council-owned car parks.
Tel: (01284) 763233

SHOPMOBILITY
The Old Bus Shelter, Angel Hill, Bury St.
Edmunds IP33 1XB
Tel/Fax: (01284) 757175
Minicom: (01284) 757023

ATTRACTION
ABBEY VISITOR CENTRE
Abbey Precinct, Abbey Gardens,
Bury St. Edmunds IP33 1RS
Tel: (01284) 763110   Fax: (01284) 757079
e-mail: blake@burybo.stedsbc.gov.uk
Local history museum housed in C11th.
Norman building with permanent
collections and temporary exhibitions and
Visitor Centre with hands-on activities and
interpretation of medieval life in the town.
Nearest car park at Manor House Museum
300m away.
SD ☐ CP n/a E ☐ RF ☐ S ☐ WC ☐

MOYSES HALL MUSEUM
Cornhill, Bury St. Edmunds IP33 1DX
Tel: (01284) 757489   Fax: (01284) 707079
e-mail: blake@burybo.stedsbc.gov.uk
Rare C12th. Norman house retaining many
original features. Houses an important
archaeology collection and many displays
on local history. Ground floor accessible.
SD ☐ CP ☐ E ☐ RF ☐ S ☐

FELIXSTOWE
Seaside resort with an important port. Its
pier, once 0.5 miles long, was shortened
after WWII, but there is an amusement
park and two miles of concrete promenade
plus a shingle beach with safe bathing.

TOURIST INFORMATION CENTRE
Tel: (01394) 276770   Fax: (01394) 277456

BED AND BREAKFAST
DORINCOURT GUEST HOUSE   ☐
41 Undercliffe Road West, Felixstowe IP11 8AH
Tel/Fax: (01394) 270447
No. of Accessible Rooms: 2. Bath
Accessible Facilities: Lounge, Dining
Room. Located on the seafront.

FRAMLINGHAM
Pleasant market town with attractive
architecture. 2 sets of Almshouses are

worth noting as are a number of shop
fronts on Market Hill and Castle Street.

ATTRACTION
FRAMLINGHAM CASTLE
Castle Street, Framlingham IP13 1BP
Tel: (01728) 724189 Fax: (01728) 621420
Built between 1177 and 1215, the castle
has fine curtain walls, 13 towers and many
Tudor chimneys. Wheelchairs available.
SD ☐   CP ☐   E ☐   RF ☐   S ☐

IPSWICH
Probably the first English town founded
by the Angles on the River Orwell.
Spectacular with a cluster of narrow
streets, open parks and dockland area.

TOURIST INFORMATION CENTRE
St. Stephen's Church, St. Stephen's Lane,
Ipswich UP1 1DP
Tel: (01473) 258070   Fax: (01473) 258072

IPSWICH BOROUGH COUNCIL
Tel: (01473) 262958
Access officer.
Produces Ipswich Access Guide.

BUSES
Ipswich Buses: Tel: (01473) 232600
Most low-floor buses with raised kerbs.

TAXIS
Anglia Taxis: Tel: (01473) 252222
Five adapted vehicles.
Avenue Taxis: Tel: (01473) 407777
Two adapted vehicles.

TRAINS
Anglia Railways: Assistance:
Tel: (01473) 693333
Minicom: (01603) 630748 or (0845)
6050600
Central Trains: Assistance:
Tel: (0845) 7056027
web: www.centraltrains.co.uk
First Great Eastern: Special Needs:
Tel: (0845) 9505050
Minicom: (0845) 9606099
Ipswich Station is NOT accessible to any
platform without assistance.

237

CAR PARKS

Ipswich main shopping streets now pedestrianised, but free 3-hour parking available on-street close by. Normal fee payable in most car parks for orange badge holders.
Tel: (01473) 738109.

SHOPMOBILITY

Buttermarket Centre, Buttermarket, St. Stephen's Lane, Ipswich.
Tel: (01473) 222225.

HOTELS
COURTYARD BY MARRIOTT

The Havens, Ransomes Europark, Ipswich IP3 9SJ
Tel: (01473) 272244   Fax: (01473) 272484
No. of Accessible Rooms: 2. Bath
Accessible Facilities: Lounge, Restaurant
Modern hotel on the east side of town centre. East on A14, first slip road after Orwell Bridge, signposted Nacton and Ransomes Europark. Good base for exploring Constable country and Suffolk Heritage Coast.

IPSWICH COUNTY HOTEL

London Road, Copdock, Ipswich IP8 3JD
Tel: (01473) 209988   Fax: (01473) 730801

No. of Accessible Rooms:1 . Bath.
Accessible Facilities: Lounge, Restaurant.
Comfortable hotel on old A12.

NOVOTEL IPSWICH

Greyfriars Road, Ipswich IP1 14P
Tel: (01473) 232400   Fax: (01473) 232414
No. of Accessible Rooms: 3. Bath
Accessible Facilities: Lounge, Restaurant, Bar. Located 0.5 mile from city centre.

SELF-CATERING ACCOMMODATION
STABLE COTTAGES

Chattisham Place, Nr. Ipswich IP8 3QD
Tel/Fax: (01473) 652210
e-mail: Margaret.Langton@talk21.com
No. of Accessible Units: 2
No. of Beds per Unit: 2 - 8
Accessible Facilities: Lounge/diner, Kitchen. Both have showers.
Converted individual farm buildings situated around south-east facing courtyard. Tennis and heated pool. Stable and Coachmans Cottages are accessible. Arable farm in small, quiet village near Constable country and Suffolk River valleys. Nearby towns of Kersey and Lavenham worth exploring.

BLACKSMITHS COTTAGE

Hall Farm, Hall Lane, Otley, Nr. Ipswich IP6 9PA
Tel/Fax: (01473) 890766

238

Out-of-steam visitor relaxes at Long Shop Steam museum.

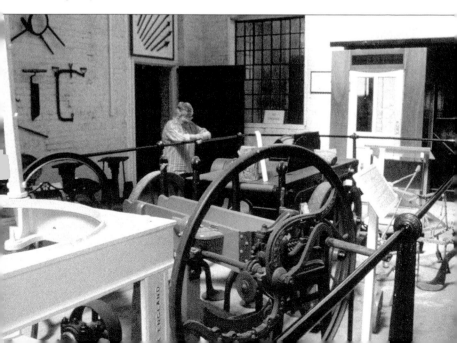

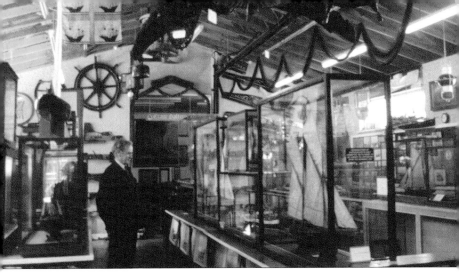

Landlubbers' delight at the excellent Lowestoft Maritime museum.

No. of Accessible Units: 2. Roll-in Shower.
No. of Bed per Unit:2
Accessible Facilities: Open plan
Kitchen/Lounge. Located in the heart of
rural Suffolk on a 200-acre working farm
on the outskirts of Otley village. Pubs
serving food close by.

LEISTON

Home of Leiston Abbey, probably the most
romantic ruin in the country.

ATTRACTION
LONG SHOP STEAM MUSEUM
Main Street, Leiston, Nr. Saxmundham IP16 4ES
Tel: (01728) 832189
web: www.suffolkce.gov.uk/libraries
The Long Shop was built in 1852 and was
one of Britain's first production lines for
steam engines. This award-winning
museum has a unique and fascinating
collection of exhibits. Travel back in time
and explore the industrial heritage of the
Victorians.

SD   [♿]   P   [♿]   E   [♿]   RF   [♿]
S   [♿]   WC   [♿]   RFE   [♿]

LOWESTOFT

Seaside town of some character which
pivots around the swing bridge.

TOURIST INFORMATION CENTRE
Tel: (01502) 523000
Fax: (01502) 539023

ATTRACTIONS
LOWESTOFT MARITIME MUSEUM
Sparrows Nest Park, Whapload Road,
Lowestoft NR32 1XG
Tel: (01502) 511260
Lively exhibition on the history of the
local fishing fleet from early sail to steam
and through to modern diesel vessels.
Displays on trawling and herring driftnet
fishing, plus the town's wartime
association with the Royal Navy.

SD [♿]   CP [♿]   RF [♿]   S [♿]

PLEASUREWOOD HILLS
Leisure Way, Corton, Lowestoft NR32 5DZ
Tel: (01502) 586000 Fax: (01502) 567393
e-mail: info@pleasurewoodhills.co.uk
web: www.pleasurewoodhills.co.uk
Family theme park with over 50 rides,
shows and attractions. The rides are mostly
ramped, but park staff not allowed (for
Health and Safety regulations) to assist
disabled guests, a companion is needed.
Some rides are inaccessible, and the
majority require guests to be able to sit
straight and hold onto any restraint on the
ride. Situated between Lowestoft and Great
Yarmouth just off the A12.

SD [♿]   CP [♿]   E [♿]   RF [♿]
C [♿]   S [♿]   WC [♿]   RFE [♿]

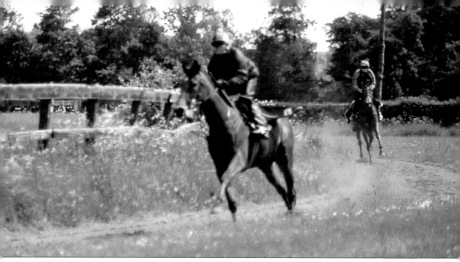

At the gallops, Newmarket is horse training.

SUFFOLK WILDLIFE PARK
Kessingland, Lowestoft NR33 7SL
Tel: (01502) 740291   Fax: (01502) 741105
Within 100 acres of parkland, wild cats, primates and other animals including the only aardvarks in the country living under natural conditions.

SD	CP	E	RF
C	S	WC	RFE

NAYLAND
A village set in beautiful country by the River Stour, at one time a busy cloth town. There is an obelisk milestone and a number of attractive cottages and inns.

SELF-CATERING
GLADWINS FARM
Harper's Hill, Nayland CO6 4NU
Tel: (01206) 62261   Fax: (01206) 263001
e-mail: GladwinsFarm@compuserve.co.uk
No. of Accessible Units: 2. Roll-in Shower
No. of Beds per Unit: Variable.
Accessible Facilities: Converted Tudor barn and stables. Gainsborough cottage has walk-in shower. Dedham and Hadleigh cottages also accessible. Located on the edge of Dedham Vale, famous for Constable and Gainsborough, in 22 acres of southern countryside overlooking the lovely Stour Valley.

NEWMARKET
On the border of Cambridgeshire and Suffolk. Newmarket has been the headquarters of British horseracing for nearly 400 years. With 3,000 acres of cultivated grassland, more than 2,700 racehorses are in training in 60 yards as well as 40 breeding studs.

TOURIST INFORMATION CENTRE
Tel: (01638) 667200 Fax: (01638) 660394

HOTEL
HEATH COURT HOTEL
Moulton Road, Newmarket CB8 8DY
Tel: (01638) 667171   Fax: (01638) 666533
e-mail: quality@heathcourt-hotel.co.uk
No. of Accessible Rooms: 48. Bath.
Accessible Facilities: Lounge, Restaurant.
Delightful property standing in its own grounds, 400m from the town centre, at the bottom of the famous Newmarket Heath where James I discovered that the heathlands were ideal for racing horses in 1605.

ATTRACTION
NATIONAL HORSERACING MUSEUM
99 High Street, Newmarket CB8 7JL
Tel: (01638) 560622 Fax: (01638) 665600
Watch horses on the gallops and in their swimming pool. Learn about racing and ask retired jockeys your questions.

SD	CP	E	RF	L
C	S	WC	RFE	

SAXMUNDHAM

The town straddles the main Ipswich/Lowestoft road, the main street beginning at the southern end with cottages and Georgian houses.

HOTEL
THE CROWN AT WESTLETON ♿
Westleton, Saxmundham IP17 3AD
Tel: (01728) 648777   Fax: (01728) 648239
No. of Accessible Rooms: 1. Bath
Accessible Facilities: Restaurant
A fine Inn, managed by owners with log fires and gardens. Located in delightful village midway between Southwold and Aldeburgh, with thatched C12th church, village green and duck pond.

SELF-CATERING
ROSE FARM ♿
Mill Street, Middleton,
Nr. Saxmundham IP17 3NG
Tel: (01728) 648456
No. of Accessible Units: 2. Roll-in Shower
No. of Beds per Unit: 1 - 3
Accessible Facilities: Lounge, Dining Room, Kitchen, Gardens, Barbecue.
Stable Cottage and Thatched Barn can sleep up to 6 and 2 respectively.
Located on the edge of rural Middleton, set on eight acres of land with open views across farm land. Approximately halfway between Aldeburgh and Southwold, ideal for exploring Suffolk's Heritage coast.

ATTRACTIONS
BRUISYARD VINEYARD & HERB CENTRE
Church Road, Bruisyard, Saxmundham IP17 2EF
Tel: (01728) 638281   Fax: (01728) 638442
e-mail: 106236.463@compuserve.com
Tour 10-acre vineyard and adjoining winery with audio/visual accompaniment followed by wine tasting and visit to tranquil herb and water gardens.

SD ♿	CP 🚶	E ♿	RF ♿
C ♿	S ♿	WC 🚶	
RFE- (Building) ♿	(garden) 🚶		

MINSMERE RSPB NATURE RESERVE
Westleton, Saxmundham IP17 3BY
Tel: (01728) 648281   Fax: (01728) 648770
e-mail: minsmere@interramp.co.uk
Reasonably firm paths lead to 4 hides overlooking famous Scrape with avocets and other waders- all accessible, some with special viewing places. Cars may be driven to hides by application to reception. Orange badge holders may drive within 400m of island Mere hide with ramped access. Batricar available free.

| SD ♿ | CP ♿ | E ♿ | RF ♿ |
| C ♿ | S ♿ | WC ♿ | RFE ♿ |

WOODBRIDGE

Originally a busy seaport now mainly a sailing centre with a winding channel emerging on the coast between Bawdsey and Felixstowe.

TOURIST INFORMATION CENTRE
Tel/Fax: (01394) 382240

HOTELS
GROVE HOUSE HOTEL ♿
39 Grove Road, Woodbridge IP12 4LG
Tel: (01394) 382202
No. of Accessible Rooms: 1.
Accessible Facilities: Dining Room
Newly renovated hotel with garden.

UFFORD PARK HOTEL 🚶
Yarmouth Road, Ufford, Woodbridge IP12 1QW
Tel: (01394) 383555   Fax: (01394) 383582
e-mail: uffordparkltd@btinternet.com
web: www.uffordpark.co.uk
No. of Accessible Rooms: 1
Accessible Facilities: Lounge, Restaurants (2), Leisure Centre.
Set in 120 acres of parkland, this is a modern hotel and leisure complex.

SELF-CATERING ACCOMMODATION
ST. PETER'S VIEW ♿
Book through Holidays for You & Me.
The Lodge, Monk Soham, Woodbridge IP12 7EN
Tel/Fax: (01728) 685358
No. of Accessible Units: 4. Shower
No. of Beds per Unit: 2 ñ 4
Accessible Facilities: Lounge, Dining Room, Kitchen.
4 cottages in grounds of the Hall.

SURREY

SURREY TOURISM
Room 391, County Hall
Kingston upon Thames KT1 2DT
Tel: (020) 8541 8092   Fax: (020) 8541 9172

DISS
Harrowlands, Harrowlands Park,
South Terrace, Dorking RH4 2RA
Tel: (01306) 875156
Operates a vast library of information on
all aspects of disability, including holiday
information.

WHEELCHAIR TRAVEL
1 Johnston Green, Guildford GU2 6XS
Tel: (020) 8233640   Fax: (020) 8237772
Provides independent transport for disabled
people on self-drive basis, plus taxi service.

SUTTON DISABILITY INFORMATION
C/o SCILL, 3 Robin Hood Lane, Sutton, SM1 2RJ
Tel: (020) 8770 4065   Fax: (020) 8770 4067.
e-mail: Sutton.Disability.Information@dial.pipex
Free, impartial and confidential
information on all aspects of life, including
employment, benefits, education, support
groups, equipment, access and holidays,
transport and recreation.

CAMBERLEY
Known for the Royal Staff College and
nearby Royal Military Academy, Sandhurst.

ATTRACTIONS
ROYAL LOGISTIC CORPS MUSEUM
Deepcut, Camberley GU16 6RW
Tel: (01252) 340871   Fax: (01252) 340875
e-mail: query@ricmuseum.freeserve.co.uk
The story of support to the Army in
transport, ordinance, pioneers, catering
and post in hands-on artefacts, hardware,
words and pictures. There is a large display
area, lecture room and seating areas.

| SD | ♿ | CP n/a | | E | ♿ | RF | ♿ |
| S | ♿ | | WC | ♿ | RFE | ♿ | |

BASINGSTOKE CANAL VISITOR CENTRE
Mytchett Place Road, Mytchett,

Nr. Frimley GU16 6DD
Tel: (01252) 370073   Fax: (01252) 371758
e-mail: cccspo@hants.gov.uk
Completed in 1794, 37 miles long with 29
locks, the canal survived through a series
of local developments, was privately owned
at one time and is now much restored.
From North Warnborough, through
Crookham Village, Fleet, Aldershot,
Pirbright, St. John's and West Byfleet, it
ends at Woodham. Displays on the sights
and sounds of Greywell Tunnel and the
lives of barge skippers over 100 years ago.
History, restoration and wildlife habitats of
the canal also on display.

| SD | ♿ | CP | ♿ | E | ♿ | RF | 🚶 | C | 🚶 |
| S | 🚶 | WC | 🚶 | RFE- (Exhibition) | ♿ | | | | |

FRIMLEY LODGE PARK
Sturt Road, Frimley Green,
Nr. Camberley GU16 6NG
Tel: (01252) 836970   Fax: (01252) 836970
Woodland and canalside walks, miniature
railway and play area.

| SD | ♿ | CP | ♿ | E | ♿ | RF | ♿ |
| C | ♿ | WC | 🚶 | RFE | ♿ | | |

CHERTSEY
FAMILY ATTRACTION
THORPE PARK
Staines Road, Chertsey KT16 8PN
Tel: (01932) 569393   Fax: (01932) 566367
e-mail:thorpepark@mail.bogo.co.uk
web: www.thorpepark.co.uk
Rides/attractions at large amusement park.

| SD | ♿ | CP | ♿ | E | ♿ | RF | ♿ |
| C | 🚶 | S | ♿ | WC | ♿ | RFE | ♿ |

DORKING
Ancient market town delightfully set
between Box Hill and the Downs rising to
the north.

SELF-CATERING ACCOMMODATION
BADGERHOLT   🚶
Bulmer Farm, Holmbury St. Mary,
Nr. Dorking RH5 6LG
Tel: (01306) 730210
No. of Accessible Units: 1. Bath
No. of Beds per Unit: 2
Accessible Facilities: Open plan

Lounge/Kitchenette, Garden. This is a working farm with the s/c units converted from original farm buildings. Holmbury is a lovely village with pubs, Victorian cottages and a famous church. Surrounded by the Surrey Hills.

ATTRACTION
POLESDEN LACEY (NT)
Great Bookham, Nr. Dorking RH5 6BD
Tel: (01372) 452048   Fax: (01372) 452023
Regency villa remodelled in 1906-9. Fine collection of paintings, furniture, porcelain and silver. Extensive grounds include walled rose garden and landscape walks through open countryside and woodland.

SD ♿ | CP ♿ | E ♿ | RF ♿ | C ♿ | S ♿
WC ♿ | RFE- ♿ (Landscaped walk of 1.5 miles)

BOX HILL (NT)
National Trust Information Centre, The Old Fort, Box Hill Road, Tadworth, Nr. Dorking KT20 7LB
Tel: (01306) 885502   Fax: (01306) 875030
Outstanding area of woodland and chalk downland with wonderful views toward South Downs. Access to summit area and slopes via wheelchair path to viewpoint.

SD ♿ | CP ♿ | E ♿ | RF ♿
C ♿ | S ♿ | WC ♿ | RFE ♿

EGHAM
Historic town skirted by the River Thames and the fields of Runnymede, scene of the signing of the Magna Carta in 1215.

HOTEL
RUNNYMEDE HOTEL AND SPA   ♿
Windsor Road, Egham tw20 0ag
Tel: (01784) 436171
Fax: (01784) 436340
e-mail: info@runnymedehotel.com
web: www.runnymedehotel.com
No. of Accessible Rooms: 47. Bath Accessible Facilities: Lift, Lounge, Restaurants (2), Spa (3 steps). Quality hotel on the banks of the River Thames, beside Bell Weir. Riverside gardens and lawns.

SAVILL COURT HOTEL   ♿
Wick Lane, Englefield Green, Egham TW20 0XN
Tel: (01784) 472000   Fax: (01784) 472200

No. of Accessible Rooms: 1. Bath Accessible Facilities: Lounge, Restaurant.
Jacobean style mansion set in 22 acres of secluded parkland. Located 5 minutes from M25 (J.13) and Heathrow airport.

ATTRACTION
THE SAVILL GARDEN
Windsor Great Park, Wick Lane, Englefield Green, Egham SL4 2HT
Tel: (01753) 847518
Fax: (01753) 847536
Within Windsor Great Park, 35 acres created to be the best and finest woodland garden for all seasons. Flower gardens blend with open vistas, secret glades and alpine meadows. Wheelchairs on site.

SD ♿ | CP ♿ | E ♿
RF ♿ | C ♿ | S ♿

EPSOM
15 miles south-west of London and home to the famous race course, Epsom Downs, and the English Derby.

ATTRACTION
HORTON PARK CHILDREN'S FARM
Horton Lane, Epsom KT19 8PT
Tel: (01372) 743984
Animals chosen for friendliness. Children can stroke and cuddle some of them, otherwise watch and talk to them. Farm walks, adventure play grounds and a new hands-on science exhibition.

SD ♿ | CP ♿ | E ♿ | RF ♿
C- ♿ | S ♿ | WC ♿

ESHER
Residential town on River Mole.

ATTRACTION
CLAREMONT LANDSCAPE GARDEN (NT)
Portsmouth Road, Esher KT10 9JG
Tel: (01372) 467806
Fax: (01932) 464394
e-mail: sclgen@smtp.ntrust.org.uk
Claremont was built for Clive of India. The Garden was laid out before 1720, and is the earliest known surviving

English landscaped garden with 50 acres including a lake, grotto and turf amphitheatre.

SD 👤	CP 👤	E 👤	RF 👤
C 👤	S 👤	WC 👤	RFE 👤

SPORTING VENUE
SANDOWN PARK RACECOURSE
Esher KT10 9AJ
Tel: (01372) 464348/463072
Fax: (01372) 465205

Booking: as above.

CP 👤	RE 👤	ED 👤 (except Manual Door)
INT 👤	L 👤	WC 👤 (2 units in main foyer

& near end of Surrey hall)

SS 👤 (follow signs to bottom of Grandstand)

B/R 👤 (lift access)

EWELL
ATTRACTION
BOURNE HALL MUSEUM
Spring Street, Ewell KT17 1UF
Tel: (020) 8394 1734

Low-lying circular modern building of 1960s, with open-plan galleries accessed by lift. Displays draws on a collection of over 5,000 items promoting area history, including collection of toys, old costume and medical items, a primitive fire engine and a hansom cab.

SD 👤	CP 👤	E 👤	RF 👤
L 👤	C 👤	S 👤	WC 👤

FARNHAM
Noted for its Georgian architecture, particularly in Castle and West Streets.

TOURIST INFORMATION CENTRE
Vernon House, 28 West Street,
Farnham GU9 7DR
Tel: (01252) 715109   Fax: (01252) 717377

BED AND BREAKFAST AND SELF-CATERING
AUDUBON HOUSE   👤
High Wray, 73 Lodge Hill Road,
Farnham GU10 3RB
Tel/Fax: (01252) 715589
e-mail: sdqq@dial.pipex.com
B & B: No. of Accessible Rooms: 1. Bath
Accessible Facilities: Lounge, Dining Room.

S/C: No. of Accessible Units: 2. Roll-in shower
No. of Beds per Unit: 2/5
Purpose-built flats for wheelchair users, a mile from town centre.

ATTRACTION
BIRDWORLD
Holt Pont, Farnham GU10 4LD
Tel: (01420) 22140   Fax: (01420) 23715

Wide variety of waterfowl and land birds in 18 acres of gardens and parkland. Meet the keepers in the Heron Theatre and enjoy a picnic in a covered area of the gardens.

SD 👤	CP 👤	E 👤	RF 👤
C 👤	S 👤	WC 👤	RFE 👤

GODALMING
An old town suffering from congested streets which contain several old buildings some dating back to the C16th. The first town in UK to have electric street lighting. Home of Charterhouse School, founded in 1611, now located on outskirts. Surrounded by open countryside and lovely villages.

On stage at Birdworld's Heron Theatre.

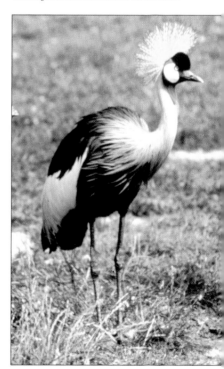

244

ATTRACTION
WINKWORTH ARBORETUM (NT)
Hascombe Road, Nr. Godalming GU8 4AD
Tel: (01483) 208477
Hillside woodland, created in C20th. with over 1,000 different shrubs and trees, many of them rare. Impressive displays in spring for azaleas and in autumn for amazing colours. 2 lakes and an abundance of wildlife. Located 2 miles SE of Godalming on E. side.

SD ⓖ   CP 🚹   E- ⓖ   RF ⓖ
C 🚹 /S 🚹 (combined)   WC 🚹   RFE 🚹

GUILDFORD
Historic old town rich in parks, gardens and open spaces. Natural amphitheatre close to town centre, used for open-air theatre. There is an attractive riverside along the River Wey, one of the first rivers to be converted to a navigable waterway.

TOURIST INFORMATION CENTRE
14 Tunsgate, Guildford GU1 3QT
Tel: (01483) 444333   Fax: (01483) 302046

GUILDFORD BOROUGH COUNCIL
Millmead House, Millmead,
Guildford GU2 5BB
Tel: (01483) 505050   Fax: (01483) 302221
web: www.guildfordborough.co.uk
Produce Access in Guildford.

BUSES
Arriva: Tel: (01483) 505693
Some low-floor buses.

TAXIS
Wheelchair Travel: Tel: (01483) 233640
36 adapted vehicles.

TRAINS
South West Trains: Special Needs:
Tel: (0845) 6050440
Minicom: (0845) 6050441
web: www.setrains.co.uk
Virgin Trains: Special Needs:
(0845) 7443366
Minicom: (0845) 7443367
Helpline: Tel: (01703) 213600
Guildford Station has level access from the street though not from Farnham Road:

platforms are accessible via the subway, standard-height (149cm) telephones, and a ramp for wheelchairs.

CAR PARKS
Free unlimited orange badge spaces in all borough council car parks, also some on-street parking.
Tel: (01483) 505050

SHOPMOBILITY
Level 3, Bedford Road Car Park,
Guildford GU1 4SA
Tel: (01483) 453993

HOTEL
FORTE POSTHOUSE GUILDFORD   🚹
Egerton Road, Guildford GU2 5XH
Tel: (01483) 574444   Fax: (01483) 302960
No. of Accessible Rooms: 1. Bath Accessible Facilities: Open plan public rooms. Modern property located 2 miles from town centre. Good location for Chessington and Thorpe Park.

ATTRACTIONS
CLANDON PARK (NT)
West Clandon, Nr. Guildford GU4 7RQ
Tel: (01483) 222482   Fax: (01483) 223479
Staff Training: No. The house contains spectacular ceilings, porcelain, furniture and tapestries, and the gardens include a parterre on the south side and a Maori house and sunken Dutch garden on the east side. The Queen's Royal Surrey Regiment Museum is in the basement.

SD ⓖ   CP 🚹 Entrance ♿ – an electric stair-climber is available to negotiate the few steps at the main entrance. Access generally easy apart from the first floor.
RF ⓖ   C ⓖ   S ⓖ   WC ♿
Wheelchairs and wheeled walkers/seats are available.

DAPDUNE WHARF (NT)
River Wey and Godalming Navigations,
Dapdune Wharf, Wharf Road,
Guildford GU1 4RR
Tel: (01483) 563189   Fax: (01483) 531667
A barge-building site on the river Wey. Navigations and parts of the wharf have been restored with stable, smithy, barge-building shed and original Wey barge. There are a series of exhibitions, models and displays which tell the story of the people

245

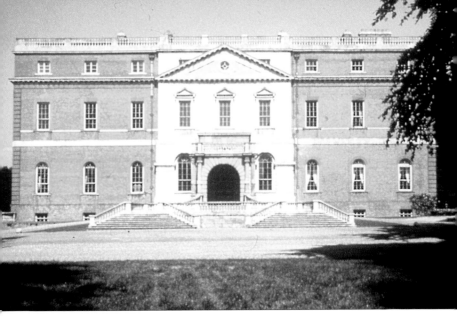

Clandon Park House has some wonderful exhibts.

who lived and worked on the river.

SD ♿		CP 🧍		E ♿		RF ♿
C 🧍		S 🧍		WC 🧍		RFE ♿

HORLEY
(GATWICK AIRPORT)
Small town close to West Sussex border with C14th church. Good access to M25 and A23.

HOTELS
CHEQUERS THISTLE HOTEL 🧍
Brighton Road, Horley RH6 8PH
Tel: (01293) 786992 Fax: (01293) 820625
No. of Accessible Rooms: 39. Bath
Accessible Facilities: Lounge.
Located close to Gatwick Airport

GATWICK MOAT HOUSE 🧍
Longbridge Roundabout, Horley RH6 0AB
Tel: (01293) 899988 Fax: (01293) 899904
No. of Accessible Rooms: 2 (2nd floor via accessible lift).
Accessible Facilities: Lounge, Restaurant (1st floor via lift)
Located close to Gatwick Airport

LEATHERHEAD
An old town home to the Royal School for the Blind established here in 1799.

ATTRACTION
BOCKETTS FARM PARK
Young Street, Fetcham,
Nr. Leatherhead KT22 9BS
Tel: (01372) 363764 Fax: (01372) 361764
Working family farm with old and modern animal breeds. Displays of agricultural bygones, outdoor paddocks and large covered areas. Farm Park area is flat earth.

SD ♿		CP ♿		E ♿		RF ♿
C ♿		S ♿		WC 🧍		RFE ♿

OXTED
BED AND BREAKFAST
ARAWA 🧍
58 Granville Road, Oxted RH8 0BZ
Tel/fax: (01883) 714107
e-mail: gibbsdj@compuserve.com
No. of Accessible Rooms: 1. Bath
Accessible Facilities: Lounge, Dining Room. Family home taking guests.

REDHILL
Part of the Borough of Reigate and almost a railway creation. Quickly grew in importance, outstripping its parent to become virtually the commercial centre of the borough, a role further increased by the creation of London Gatwick Airport three miles south.

HOTEL
CRABHILL HOUSE (Winged Fellowship)
Kings Cross Lane, South Nutfield,
Redhill RH1 5PA
Tel: (01737) 822221

In the heart of rural Surrey countryside,
within easy distance of Brighton and
London. All rooms have en-suite facilities
and hoist tracking and variable bed
heights. Indoor heated pool. Shop. Bar.
Library. Lounger. Conservatory. Lawns and
gardens. Adaptive transport.

ATTRACTION
THE OLD MILL
Outwood Common, Nr. Redhill RH1 5PW
Tel: (01342) 843644   Fax: (01342) 843458
e-mail: sheila@jimnutt.cix.co.uk

Oldest working windmill in England,
dating from 1665, and the best preserved.
Ground floor only is accessible.

SD 🚹   CP 🚹   E ♿
RF ♿   S 🚹   WC 🚹

WEYBRIDGE
An old town on the site where, according to
tradition, Julius Caesar crossed the Thames
in 55BC. Home to Brooklands Motor
Course.

ATTRACTION
BROOKLANDS MUSEUM
Brooklands Road, Weybridge KT13 7QN
Tel: (01932) 857381   Fax: (01932) 855465

Brooklands racing circuit was the home of
British motorsport and aviation. This
museum, on 30 acres of the original 1907
racing circuit, has many of the original
buildings, now restored, in which vehicles
and aircraft are displayed.

SD ♿   CP ♿   E ♿   RF ♿
C ♿   S ♿   WC ♿

WOKING
Comparatively new town, developed with
the railway line in the late 1830s.

ATTRACTION
RHS GARDEN WISLEY
Wisley, Woking GU23 6QB
Tel: (01483) 224234 Fax: (01483) 211750
e-mail: rhs@rhs.org.uk

Major experimental gardens of the Royal
Horticultural Society. 240 acres of both
gardens and vegetable gardens with
greenhouses and specialist areas with
many unusual plants and shrubs.

SD ♿   CP ♿   E ♿   RF ♿
C ♿   S ♿   WC 🚹

247

The house at Wisley in the experimental gardens of the Royal Horticultural Society.

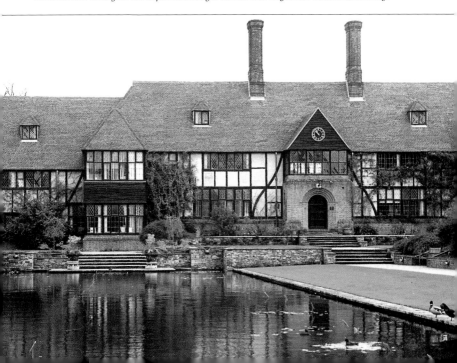

SUSSEX
EAST

ALFRISTON

Ancient town with first building to be acquired by the National Trust: the C14th Clergy House, and example of a pre-Reformation vicarage, purchased in 1896 for £10. The C15th Star Inn is one of the oldest in England.

ATTRACTION
DRUSILLAS PARK
Alfriston BN26 5QS
Tel: (01323) 870656   Fax: (01323) 870846
e-mail: drusilla@drusilla.demon.co.uk
Fine small zoo with wide variety of animals in naturalistic environments including a walk-through Bat Enclosure and Pet World. Children's activities include Playland, Train, Panning for Gold, Wacky Workshop, Maasai Exhibition and Animal Encounter sessions.

| SD ♿ | CP ♿ | E ♿ | RF ♿ |
| C ♿ | S ♿ | WC ♿ | RFE ♿ |

ENGLISH WINE CENTRE
Alfriston Roundabout, Alfriston BN26 5QS
Tel: (01323) 870164   Fax: (01323) 870005
e-mail: bottles@englishwine.co.uk
web: www.englishwine.co.uk
Wine tastings and tour of museum.

| SD ♿ | CP 🚶 | E ♿ | RF ♿ |
| C 🚶 | S 🚶 | WC 🚶 | RFE 🚶 |

BATTLE

Built on the site of the Battle of Hastings, the town contains many old buildings, some of C13th & C14th, but interest centres mainly around the abbey and the historic events of 1066.

TOURIST INFORMATION CENTRE
88 High Street, Battle, TN33 0AQ
Tel: (01424) 773721   Fax: (01424) 773436

ATTRACTION
BATTLEFIELD OF HASTINGS AND ABBEY RUINS (EH)
Battle Abbey, Battle TN33 0AD
Tel: (01424) 773792   Fax: (01424) 775059
Tour the battlefield and step back in time to October 1066. See interactive displays and exhibitions and audio-visual interpretation of the Battle. Of the abbey, the Great Gatehouse is the best preserved.

The original off-licence? No, not quite, it's the English Wine Centre at Alfriston.

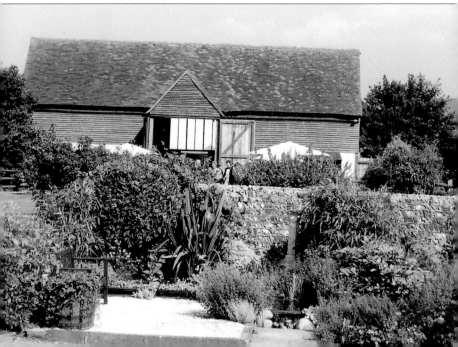

Separate entrance up a slight incline with York paving stones, through gate into abbey grounds.

SD CP E ♿ S ♿ F 🚶

BRIGHTON

Largest resort in the SE, combining gracious C18th architecture with modern amusements. Its wonderful Royal Pavilion, Palace Pier and an amble along the promenade sit rather oddly with an exploration of the famous Lanes, with restaurants and antique shops.

TOURIST INFORMATION CENTRES
10 Bartholomew Square, Brighton BN1 1JS
Tel: (01273) 292599
web: www.brighton.co.uk

Hove Town Hall, Church Road, Hove BN3 3BQ.
Telephone number as above

BRIGHTON AND HOVE FEDERATION OF DISABLED PEOPLE
Snowdon House, 3 Rutland Gardens, Hove BN3 5PD
Tel: (01273) 208934
Produces Access to Brighton & Hove.

BRIGHTON AND HOVE DISABILITY ADVICE CENTRE
Tel: (01273) 203016
Hire out wheelchairs.

BUSES
Brighton and Hove Bus Company:
Tel: (01273) 886200
Some low-floor buses.
Community Transport: Tel: (01273) 292599
Usually for residents, but do take visitors if space available.

TAXIS
Brighton Streamline Taxis:
Tel: (01273) 747474
10 adapted vehicles.
Brighton & Hove Radio Cabs:
Tel: (01273) 324245
1 adapted vehicle.
Hove Streamline Taxis: Tel: (01273) 202020
Southern Taxis: (01273) 205205
2 adapted vehicles.

TRAINS
Connex Southcentral: Disabled Traveline: Tel: (0870) 6030405
Fax: (0870) 6030505
Minicom: (01273) 617621
Thameslink: Special Needs: Tel: (0207) 6206333
Minicom: (0207) 6205561
Stationlink bus: Tel: (0207) 9183312
Virgin Trains: Special Needs: (0845) 7443366
Minicom: (0845) 7443367
Wales & West: Special Needs: Tel: (0845) 3003005
Minicom: (0845) 7585469
Brighton Railbus: Tel: (01273) 886200
Valid on all Brighton and Hove bus services within a given area.
Brighton Station is suitable for wheelchairs using ramp access.

CAR PARKS
Free unlimited orange badge spaces in Pay & Display and in council car parks.
Tel: (01273) 203016

WHEELCHAIR HIRE
Red Cross Medical Loans,
29-31 Prestonville Road, Brighton.

HOTELS
BRIGHTON OAK HOTEL 🚶
West Street, Brighton BN1 2RQ
Tel: (01273) 220033   Fax: (01273) 778000
No. of Accessible Rooms: 2. Roll-in Shower
Accessible Facilities: Lounge, Restaurant, Bar (3 steps). Modern hotel adjacent to the Conference Centre.

BRIGHTON THISTLE 🚶
Kings Road, Brighton BN1 2GS
Tel: (01273) 206700   Fax: (01273) 820692
No. of Accessible Rooms: 3.
Accessible Facilities: Public areas accessible by Lift. Quality hotel on the seafront.

DE VERE GRAND HOTEL 🚶
Kings Road, Brighton BN1 2PW
Tel: (01273) 321188   Fax: (01273) 202694
e-mail: general@grandbrighton.co.uk
No. of Accessible Rooms: unknown
Accessible Facilities: Ramped entrance, Lounge, Restaurant. Majestic property

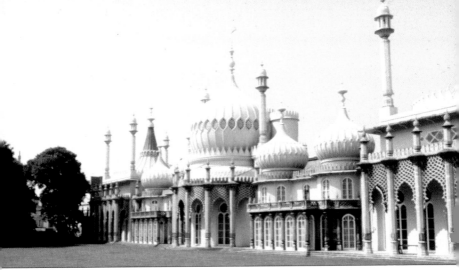

Now returned to its original palatial splendour, Brighton's Royal Pavilion.

designed in elaborate Italian Renaissance style, in commanding position on the seafront.

QUALITY HOTEL BRIGHTON

West Street, Brighton BN1 2RQ
Tel: (01273) 220033 Fax: (01273) 778000
e-mail: admin@gb057.u-net.com
web: www.choicehotelseurope.com
No. of Accessible Rooms: 2 (via accessible lift)
Accessible Facilities: all public areas (level or lift access).
Large modern hotel adjacent to the Conference Centre and close to seafront.

ACCESSIBLE ATTRACTION
BOOTH MUSEUM OF NATURAL HISTORY

194 Dyke Road, Brighton BN1 5AA
Tel: (01273) 292777 Fax: (01273) 292778
e-mail: boothmus@pavilion.co.uk
Creation of Victorian ornithologist Edward Booth, and built in 1874 to house his collection of stuffed British birds. The birds now share display with over half a million other specimens from the natural world - butterflies, beetles, skeletons, fossils, minerals and rocks, plants and microscope slides. Displays on taxidermy, flint knapping, fossil collecting and butterfly mounting etc. All galleries on one level.
SD   CP   E (via rear entrance)
S

THE ROYAL PAVILION

Brighton BN1 1EE
Tel:(01273) 290900 Fax:(01273) 2902821
Former seaside residence of George IV with domes and minarets and sumptuous interior. Recently undergone a massive structural restoration and a must to visit.
SD   CP (Book in advance in both cases)
E   C n/a   S   WC

BURWASH

Half way between Hastings and Tunbridge Wells, famous particularly as the home of Rudyard Kipling (Bateman's) but also worth a visit for its redbrick and weatherboard cottages.

ATTRACTION
BATEMAN'S (NT)

Burwash, Etchingham TN19 7DS
Tel: (01435) 882302 Fax: (01435) 882811
The home of Rudyard Kipling from 1902/1936, this is a delightful C17th ironmaster's house. Kipling's study is as it was, as is his 1928 Rolls-Royce. Lovely gardens with restored watermill. After reporting to the ticket office, those with mobility problems can drive down an alternative entrance, entering property by a path that, although of uneven stones, has no slope. House: Wheelchair access possible on ground floor of house and tea-room, but ambulant access only available to shop and

mill. Gardens: Garden paths have varying surfaces, and so a wheelchair access map is provided. Generally accessible.

SD 〔♿〕　CP 〔♿〕　E 〔♿〕　C 〔♿〕
S 〔♿〕　WC 〔♿〕　RFE 〔♿〕

EASTBOURNE

Much favoured by those in retirement, Eastbourne has a fine three-mile seafront, the coastline is dominated by miles of chalk cliffs and Beachy Head.

TOURIST INFORMATION CENTRE
3 Cornfield Road, Eastbourne BN21 4QL
Tel: (01323) 411400   Fax: (01323) 649574

TOURISM AND COMMUNITY SERVICES
College Road, Eastbourne, BN21 4JJ
Tel: (01323) 415437   Fax: (01323) 430093

ACCESS OFFICER
Department of Environmental Services, 68 grove Road, Eastbourne BN21 1DF
Tel: (01323) 415281   Fax: (01323) 415995
Minicom: (01323) 415111
Produces *Access*, information on all aspects of Eastbourne.

WHEELCHAIR/SCOOTER HIRE
Mobility Hire.
149 Tideswell Road, Eastbourne BN21 3RT
Tel: (01323) 721223/638046
Rental of Scooters and Electric and

Manual Wheelchairs.

BRITISH RED CROSS CENTRE
The Redoubt, Royal Parade, Eastbourne
Tel: (01323) 732471
Hires out wheelchairs as above.

BEACH LIFEGUARD STATION
Wish Tower, Eastbourne
Tel: (01323) 412290
Summer Season – a wheelchair available for daily hire and a Beach Wheelchair to help across shingle.

BUSES
Bus Stop Shops: Tel: (01323) 416416
Arndale Centre (Bankers Corner Entrance)
Railway Station for all bus information.

TAXIS
Town & Country Cabs: Tel: (01323) 727766
Nine adapted vehicles.
Ranks outside the station, the Pier, Bolton Road.

TRAINS
Connex Southcentral.
Disabled Traveline: Tel: (0870) 6030405
Fax: (0870) 6030505
Minicom: (01233) 617621
Eastbourne Station has a wheelchair ramp.

CAR PARKS
Some free orange badge spaces in council-

Poet's Corner, as Rudyard Kipling would have known it, Bateman's to us all.

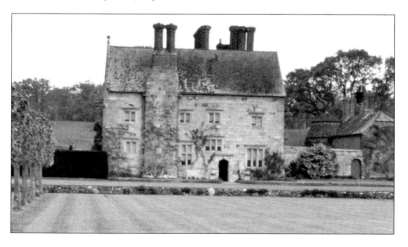

owned car parks, others are charged. On-street parking on yellow lines for 3 hours.
Tel: (01323) 415218

HOTELS
CONGRESS HOTEL
31-41 Carlisle Road, Eastbourne BN21 4LS
Tel: (01323) 732118   Fax: (01323) 720016
e-mail: Congresshotels@msn.co.uk
Congresshotels@msn.co.uk
No. of Accessible Rooms: 4. Bath
Accessible Facilities: Lounge/Bar
(ramped), Restaurant. Family owned and
managed hotel near town centre and
seafront.

HEATHERDENE HOTEL
26-28 Elms Avenue, Eastbourne BN21 3DN
Tel/Fax: (01323) 725811
No. of Accessible Rooms: 2
Accessible Facilities: Dining Room, Bar.
Privately owned attractive property in
pleasant avenue close to Grand Parade.

ATTRACTIONS

BEACHY HEAD COUNTRYSIDE CENTRE
Beachy Head, Eastbourne BN20 7YA
Tel: (01323) 737273
Innovative exhibition on local wildlife and
history with rock pool, mock cliff face,
micrarium, talking shepherd, Bronze Age
man and 3-D colour slide show.

SD   CP n/a   E   RF   C
S   WC   RFE

LIFEBOAT MUSEUM
King Edwards Parade, Eastbourne
Tel: (01323) 730717
Memorabilia and lifeboats models trace
the history of these sturdy vessels.
This is a very small museum and shop
with room for no more than 2
wheelchairs at a time. Lovely views onto
the beach and sea from the flat outside
area.

SD   CP   E

HAILSHAM
An important market town as far back as
Norman times and still has one of the
largest markets in East Sussex, covering
more than 3 acres.

ATTRACTION
CUCKOO TRAIL
Accessible route for wheelchairs through
attractive countryside following route
between Polegate and Heathfield. Stretch
between Polegate and Hailsham (3 miles)
particularly suitable for wheelchair users.

MICHELHAM PRIORY (EH)
Upper Dicker, Hailsham BN27 3QD
Tel: (01323) 844224   Fax: (01323)
844030
A moat and range of gardens surround
the medieval priory with Tudor additions.
Home to fascinating collection tracing
Michelham's religious origins, through
its life as a working farm to country
house. A watermill, Elizabethan barn and
imposing C14th gatehouse give further
evidence of the priory's importance. A
wonderful setting. Wheelchairs available
for hire.

SD   CP   E   RF
C   S   WC   RF

HASTINGS
Famous as the base from which William
the Conqueror set out to fight the Battle
of Hastings, there is an extensive shingle
beach and long pier supplying the usual
seaside amusements.

TOURIST INFORMATION CENTRE
Town Hall, Queens Road, Hastings TN34 1QR
Tel: (01424) 781111   Fax: (01424)
781186

HOTEL
GRAND HOTEL
Grand Parade, St. Leonards, Hastings TN8 0DD
Tel/Fax: (01424) 428510
No. of Accessible Rooms: 2. Bath
Accessible Facilities: Lounge, Restaurant.
Located within town, 200m from beach.

HERTSMONCEAUX
The castle, a fine example of a fortified
manor house, is home to the C15th Royal
Greenwich Observatory. The village is
noted for its woodcrafts, traditional in
this area.

BED & BREAKFAST
CONQUERORS
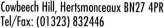
Cowbeech Hill, Hertsmonceaux BN27 4PR
Tel/Fax: (01323) 832446
No. of Accessible Rooms: 1. Roll-in Shower
Accessible Facilities: Lounge, Restaurant,
Gardens with horses, peacocks and sheep.
This is a working farm.

LEWES
Narrow and steep streets here, the High
Street has many Georgian buildings and
interesting little corners to delight the eye.

TOURIST INFORMATION CENTRE
187 High Street, Lewes BN7 2DE
Tel: (01273) 483448   Fax (01273) 484003
Car Parking – disability parking at precinct,
Cliffe High Street and Main High Street.

COMMUNITY TRANSPORT
Tel: (01273) 517 332
Car with ramped rear access available to
hire, accommodating 3 passengers,
including 1 in wheelchair. Minibus with
ramped rear access available for hire
carrying 16 passengers or 14 and 2 seated
in wheelchairs.

BUSES
CountyRider/Lewes Area Dial-a-Ride
wheelchair accessible transport, routes
vary on different days.
Contact: (01273) 478 007

TAXIS
Farmer/Saltdean Taxis
Tel: (01273) 307 827
7/8 seater minibus accommodating 2
wheelchairs.

Versacab, Hurstpierpoint
Tel: (01273) 832 832
6-seater taxi capable of being adjusted to
carry up to 2 wheelchairs.

ATTRACTION
TREKKERS DISABLED CYCLE CENTRE
Granary Barn
Seven Sisters County Park, Lewes
Tel: (01323) 870 310
Range of wheelchair and side by side tandem

bikes specially designed. These can be used
on paths and forest trails within the park.
There is disabled parking close to Hiring
Centre and an accessible WC and shower.

NEWHAVEN
Car Parking – disability parking in
Meeching Road and multi-storey car park.

PARADISE FAMILY LEISURE PARK
Avis Road, Newhaven BN9 0DH
Tel: (01273) 512123
Fax: (01273) 616005
e-mail: enquiries@paradisepark.co.uk
web: www.paradisepark.co.uk
Leisure and Botanic gardens, Planet Earth
Exhibition, including Dinosaur Museum,
Natural Science and History displays,
Maritime Museum and a play zone with
rides, railway, boats and pirate ship. A
great day out for all.

| SD 🦽 | CP 🦽 | E 🦽 | C 🦽 |
| S 🦽 | WC 🦽 | RFE 🦽 | |

NUTLEY
Small village in Ashdown Forest a short
drive from the south coast.

SELF-CATERING
WHITE HOUSE FARM HOLIDAY HOMES
Hornley Common, Nutley TN22 3EE
Tel/Fax: (01825) 712377
No. of Accessible Units: 1. Shower.
No. of Beds per Unit: 4
Accessible Facilities: Lounge/Diner,
Kitchen, Patio. 5 self contained single
storey cottages with views across Ashdown
Forest and undulating countryside.

PLUMPTON
SPORTING VENUE
PLUMPTON RACECOURSE
Plumpton BN7 3AL
Tel: (01273) 890383
Fax: (01273) 891557
Booking: as above.

CP 🦽	RE 🦽	ED 🦽 (except manual door)
INT 🚶	WC 🦽	(2 units on ground level)
SS 🚶	B/R 🚶	

RYE

Truly one of the most attractive towns in England which has managed to retain its ancient character despite the influx of visitors. Standing near the mouth of the River Rother, its hilly streets (many are cobbled, which can be tricky), there is a wealth of medieval, Tudor, Stuart and Georgian houses.

TOURIST INFORMATION CENTRE
The Heritage Centre, Strand Quay, Rye TN31 7AY
Tel: (01797) 226696   Fax: (01797) 223460

ACCESSIBLE ATTRACTIONS
GREAT KNELLE FARM
Beckley, Rye TN31 6UB
Tel: (01797) 260250   Fax: (01797) 260347
Working farm, encouraging visitors to hands-on-experience. Disabled fishing platforms for seasonal coarse fishing on River Rother. Woodland trail is the only area which is not hard surfaced and open to the vagaries of climate.
CP [♿] E [♿] C [♿] S [♿] WC [🚶] RFE [♿]

254

SEAFORD

Located on Sussex Downs on the coast between Newhaven and Eastbourne.

TOURIST INFORMATION CENTRE
Station Approach, Seaford BN25 2AR
Central location but small entrance step means access is difficult. Level promenade approximately 1.5 miles long, stretching from the Buckle to Splash Point. Disabled parking at Splash point in Esplanade car park. Viewing point allowing wheelchairs to get close to the sea at Splash Point.

ATTRACTION
SEVEN SISTERS COUNTRY PARK
Exceat, Seaford BN25 4AD
Tel: (01323) 870280   Fax: (01323) 871070
The park is 700 acres of open Downland, meadows, salt marsh, shingle beach and wetland, one of the few undeveloped valleys in the south east of the country. Within a site of Special Scientific Interest and an area of Outstanding Natural Beauty. At the valley bottom there is a

2km concrete track suitable for wheelchair users with resting places along main route.
SD [♿] CP [♿] E [♿] RF [♿] C [♿] S [♿] WC [🚶]
RFE [♿] Wheelchairs and two self-drive cars available.

UCKFIELD
ATTRACTIONS
BLUEBELL RAILWAY
Sheffield Park Station, Nr. Uckfield TN22 3QL
Tel: (01825) 723777   Fax: (01825) 724139
A leisurely journey through both the Sussex Weald and time, from the Victorian age at Sheffield Park, to the 1950s at Kingscote. Both stations accessible, although no parking at Kingscote and so it's more practical to begin and end at Sheffield Park. Intermediate station at Horsted Keynes not accessible. Sheffield Park is the HQ with a locomotive collection and a small museum.
SD [♿] CP [🚶] E [♿] RF [♿] C [♿] S [🚶]
WC [🚶] (located at Sheffield Park and Kingscote.)

HEAVEN FARM
Furners Green, Uckfield TN22 3RG
Tel: (01825) 790226   Fax: (01825) 790881
Buildings erected in early 1820s comprise the Farm Museum with cowshed, dairy, wood corners, oasthouse and cooling floor, These illustrate farming in that period. Sadly the wood parkland and waterside walks are undulating and hard work and therefore inaccessible.
SD [♿] CP [🚶] E [🚶] RF [🚶]
C [🚶] S [🚶] WC [🚶]

SHEFFIELD PARK GARDEN (NT)
Sheffield Park, Uckfield TN22 3QX
Tel: (01825) 790231   Fax: (01825) 791264
Four large lakes linked by cascades and waterfalls with rare shrubs and colourful flowers in this garden laid out by famous landscape gardener Capability Brown. WARNING: Unmade car park unsuitable, but disabled passengers can be set down directly at concrete ramps leading into the admissions area, before parking. If travelling alone, this option isn't feasible.
SD [♿] CP [♿] E [♿] RF [♿]
C [♿] (not NT but ramp & level access)
S [♿] WC [🚶] RFE [♿]

WEST

WEST SUSSEX TOURISM INITIATIVE
12 Steyne, Worthing BN11 3DU
e-mail: wsti@enta.net
web: www.westsussex.gov.uk

WEST SUSSEX ASSOCIATION FOR THE DISABLED
10 South Pallant, Chichester PO19 1SU
Tel: (01243) 774088

WEST SUSSEX TRAVELINE:
Tel: (0345) 959099

WEST SUSSX COUNTY COUNCIL.
Tel: (01243) 777100

ARUNDEL

Peaceful town nestles below the battlements of one of the most impressive castles in the country. Quaint narrow streets are brim-full of tearooms and antique shops. The warm stone of the castle stands over the red tiled roofs of the town rambling down to the river Arun.

TOURIST INFORMATION CENTRE
61 High Street, Arundel BN18 9AJ
Tel: (01903) 882258   Fax: (01903) 882419

BED AND BREAKFAST
MILL LANE HOUSE
Slindon, Arundel BN18 0RP
Tel: (01243) 814440   Fax: (01243) 814436
No. of Accessible Rooms: 2. Roll-in Shower
Accessible Facilities: Dining Room.
C17th house in National Trust downland village with superb views. Accommodation is in Coach House across drive from main house with own entrance. Breakfast can be taken in room or in main house (one step).

WOODYBANKS
Crossgate, Amberley, Nr. Arundel BN18 9NR
Tel: (01798) 831295
No. of Accessible Rooms: 2. Shower.
Accessible Facilities: Lounge, Dining Room, Low lying windows affording elevated views across the Wildbrooks of Amberely ranging for 10 miles. Amberley is a tranquil village nestling in the South Downs. The owners have a disabled daughter and sound extremely understanding and pleasant.

ATTRACTIONS
AMBERLEY MUSEUM
Amberley, Nr. Arundel BN18 9LT
Tel: (01798) 831370   Fax: (01798) 831831
Web: HYPERLINK
http://www.fastnet.co.uk/amberley.museum/
www.fastnet.co.uk/amberley.museum/
Established to preserve and record the working heritage of the South East, its collections include timber-working, brick-making, road-building, blacksmithing, pottery and recent histories of printing, mechanised transport and radio.

SD ♿	CP ♿	E ♿	RF ♿	C ♿
S 🚶	WC 🚶		RFE (AV Room) ♿	

DENMANS GARDENS
Denmans Lane, Fontwell,
Nr. Arundel BN18 0SU
Tel: (01243) 542808   Fax: (01243) 544064
3.5 acre site, gradually developed over the past 50 years to include a wonderful walled garden, bursting with perennials and old-fashioned roses: a gravel stream with a pond and grasses and a south garden with maple and cherry trees, plus rare species. There is a school of garden design in the clockhouse.

SD n/a	CP ♿	E ♿	RF ♿
C ♿	S 🚶	WC 🚶	RFE ♿

THE WILDFOWL AND WETLANDS TRUST
Mill Road, Arundel BN18 9PB

Arundel. A fine place for tea.

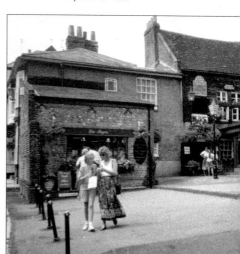

Tel: (01903) 883355 Fax: (01903) 884834
60 acres of ponds, lakes and reedbeds with thousands of tame and wild and migratory birds. Four activity stations spark interest and many birds can be hand fed.

SD ♿ CP ♿ E ♿ RF ♿ C ♿
S ♿ WC ♿ RFE ♿ G ♿

SPORTING VENUE
FONTWELL PARK RACECOURSE
Fontwell, Nr. Arundel BN18 0SX
Admin & Booking - Box Office:
(01243) 543335 Fax: (01243) 543904

CP ♿ (Orange badge parking on request)
RE ♿ ED ♿ (except Manual Door)
INT 🚶 L ♿
WC 🚶 (2 units, one in each enclosure)
SS n/a (No designated seating as such)

BOGNOR REGIS
Popular seaside resort with soft sands and calm seas. It lies in the lee of Selsey Bill and sheltered by the Isle of Wight and the South Downs.

TOURIST INFORMATION CENTRE
Belmont Street, Bognor Regis PO21 1BJ
Tel: (01243) 823140 Fax: (01243) 820435

HOTEL
THE ALDWICK HOTEL 🚶
Aldwick Road, Aldwick, Bognor Regis PO21 2QU
Tel: (01243) 821945 Fax: (01243) 821316
No. of Accessible Rooms: 1. Bath with Hydraulic Transfer Chair.
Accessible Facilities: Lounge, Restaurant.
Located 5 miles from Chichester close to the seafront and town centre.

SELF-CATERING
27 NELSON ROAD
Bognor Regis
Book through Grooms Holidays
No. of Accessible Units: 1
No. of Beds per Unit: 8
Accessible Facilities: Lounge, Kitchen, Diner. Specially designed, spacious house located in quiet residential area of town, 8 minutes' walk from seafront and shops.

BEACH LODGE
Flepham, Nr. Bognor Regis

Book through Grooms Holidays
No. of Accessible Units: 1
No. of Beds per Unit: 9
Accessible Facilities: Garden
Spacious, split level modern house on private seaside estate in small village. Located at entry to level promenade stretching for miles along sandy seafront.

CHICHESTER
Founded by the Romans c.AD70 who laid out the main street plan and built the original city walls, rebuilt in flint in medieval times. Notable now for its Georgian architecture, especially in the street Little London.

TOURIST INFORMATION CENTRE
29A South Street, Chichester PO19 1AH
Tel: (01243) 775888 Fax: (01243) 539449

BUSES
Stagecoach Coastline: Tel: (01243) 539953
No low-floor buses as yet.

TAXIS
Central Taxis: Tel: (0800) 789432
1 adapted vehicle.
Blueline Taxis: Tel: (01243) 774077
1 adapted vehicle.
Direct Line Taxis: Tel: (01243) 533335
3 adapted vehicles.
Many more available from ICIS:
Tel: (0800) 859929

TRAINS
Connex Southcentral. Disabled Traveline:
Tel: (0870) 6030405
Fax: (0870) 6030505
Minicom: (012333) 617621
Wales & West: Special Needs:
Tel: (0845) 30030005
Minicom: (0845) 585469
Chichester Station is suitable for wheelchairs using ramp access.

CAR PARKS
Orange badge spaces. Tel: (01243) 777100

HOTEL
CROUCHERS BOTTOM COUNTRY HOTEL

Birdham Road, Chichester PO20 7EH
Tel: (01243) 784995   Fax: (01243) 539797
e-mail: Crouchers_bottom@hantslife.co.uk
Crouchers_bottom@hantslife.co.uk
No. of Accessible Rooms: 2. Bath
Accessible Facilities: Lounge, Restaurant.
Early 1900s farmhouse converted to small
hotel with bedrooms in outside barn and
coach house and bar and restaurant in
main house. Situated between Chichester
Marina and Del Quay.

ST. ANDREWS LODGE ♿
Chichester Road, Selsey
Nr. Chichester PO20 0LX
Tel: (01243) 606899   Fax: (01243) 607826
No. of Accessible Rooms: 1. Roll-in Shower
Accessible Facilities: Lounge, Restaurant.
Family run hotel situated on the Manhood
Peninsula, 7 miles south of Chichester and
close to unspoilt beaches and countryside.

SELF-CATERING
SEAGULLS
Bill Point, Grafton Road, Selsey, Nr. Chichester
Book through Grooms Holidays
No. of Accessible Units: 1
No. of Beds per Unit: 6. Shower
Accessible Facilities: Garden. Ramp down
to the beach. Located on southernmost tip
of Selsey Bill, this lovely bungalow enjoys
panoramic view across English Channel.

TAMARISK
Farm Road, Bracklesham Bay,
Nr. Chichester
Book through Grooms Holidays.
No. of Accessible Units: 1. Shower
No. of Beds per Unit: 6
Accessible Facilities: Garden
New purpose-built bungalow a few minutes
from the sea. Bracklesham Bay has many
isolated havens.

SELSEY COTTAGE 🚶
Selsey, Nr. Chichester.
Bookings: Mrs. Sue Graves, 28 Wise Lane,
London NW7 2RE
e-mail: sue@suegraves.demon.co.uk
No. of Accessible Units: 1. Roll-in Shower
No. of Beds per Unit: 2
Accessible Facilities: Lounge, Dining
Room, Kitchen. Spacious seafront house

with fine views. Pets welcome. 20 minutes
from Chichester.

10 CULIMORE CLOSE 🚶
West Wittering, Chichester PO20 8HD
Tel: (01243) 672723
No. of Accessible Units: 1
No. of Beds per Unit: 2 + sofa-bed
Accessible Facilities: Lounge,
Kitchen/Diner, Private Garden.
Fully self-contained annexe of family home
in quiet cul-de-sac. 2 minutes from the sea
and village, 6 miles from Chichester.

ATTRACTIONS
EARNLEY GARDENS
133 Almodington Lane, Earnley,
Nr. Chichester PO20 7SR
Tel: (01243) 512637   Fax: (01243) 673658
Tropical butterflies, exotic birds. Theme
gardens, small animals, pottery, shipwreck
museum and Rejectamenta the Nostalgia
Museum, all under cover. Follow the
Butterflies & Gardens signs off the A286
Chichester/Witterings Road.

| SD ♿ | CP ♿ | E ♿ | RF ♿ |
| C ♿ | S ♿ | WC 🚶 | RFE ♿ |

GOODWOOD HOUSE
Goodwood, Chichester PO18 0PX
Tel: (01243) 755048   Fax: (01243) 755005
e-mail: debora@goodoowd.co.uk
Ancestral home of the Dukes of Richmond
for 300 years and now lived in by the Earl
of March and his family. Soon after
Napoleon's 1798 Campaign on the Nile, the
3rd Duke created his Egyptian State
Dining Room which has now been recreated
and open to the public together with the
other newly restored state apartments.

| SD ♿ | CP ♿ | E ♿ (Ballroom E.) | |
| RF ♿ | C ♿ | S ♿ | WC ♿ | RFE ♿ |

FISHBOURNE ROMAN PALACE
Salthill Road, Fishbourne,
Chichester PO19 3QR
Tel: (01243) 785859   Fax: (01243) 539266
Largest known Roman residence in Britain
with many original mosaic floors restored.
The museum relates the history of the
palace with full-size reconstruction of one
room and a museum of Roman gardening
and a reconstructed Roman garden.

257

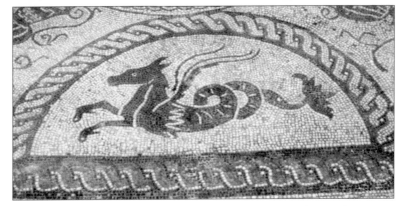

A floorcovering guaranteed to last a lifetime! A Fishbourne Roman Palace mosiac.

SD ♿ | CP ♿ | E ♿ | RF ♿ | C ♿
S ♿ | WC ♿ | RFE (Gardens) ♿

B/R ♿ (Access to all areas except Bentinck Bar in Richmond Enclosure)

MECHANICAL MUSIC AND DOLL COLLECTION
Church Road, Portfield, Chichester PO19 4HN
Tel: (01243) 372646   Fax: (01243) 370299
Rare barrel organs and musical boxes combine with fine examples of Victorian china and wax dolls housed in well-preserved Victorian church.

SD ♿ | CP ♿ | E ♿ | RF ♿ | S ♿ | RFE ♿

WEST DEAN GARDENS
West Dean, Chichester PO10 04Z.
Tel: (01243) 818201/811301
Fax: (01243) 811342
25 acres noted for a 100m long pergola. Newly restored walled garden contains Victorian glasshouses, large working kitchen garden and tool/mower collection. Glasshouses and pergola not suitable for wheelchairs.

SD ♿ | CP ♿ | E ♿ | C ♿
S ♿ | WC ♿ | RFE ♿

SPORTING VENUE
GOODWOOD RACECOURSE
Goodwood, Chichester PO18 9OS
Admin & Booking-Box Office: (01243) 755022
Fax: (01243) 755025
Credit Card bookings: (0800) 0818191
Wheelchair loan available.

CP ♿ (Park in CP 8 - need disabled sticker)
RE ♿ | ED ♿ | INT ♿ | L ♿
WC ♿ (5 units, in March Stand Floor, East & West. Sussex Stand Floor and Public Enclosure)
SS ♿ (Viewing ramps for access on Richmond Enclosure Lawn, Sussex Stand Lawn and Parade Ring (in Gordon Enclosure)

EAST GRINSTEAD
Notable for Sackville college in the High Street, Jacobean Almshouses founded in 1609 by Robert Sackville 2nd Earl of Dorset and still a home for the elderly.

ATTRACTION
STANDEN (NT)
West Hoathley Road,
East Grinstead RH19 4NE
Tel: (01342) 323029   Fax: (01342) 316424
e-mail: sstpro@smtp.ntrust.org.uk
Built in 1890s, a showpiece of the arts and crafts of the William Morris period. Hillside garden and wooded walks.

SD ♿ | CP ♿ | E ♿ | RF ♿
C ♿ | S ♿ | WC ♿

GATWICK AIRPORT
TRAINS
Connex: Customer Services:
Tel: (0870) 6030405
Fax: (0870) 6030505
Minicom: (01233) 617621
Gatwick Express: Assistance:
Tel/Minicom: (099) 301530
Thameslink: Special Needs:
Tel: (0207) 6206333
Minicom: (0207) 6205561
Stationlink bus: Tel: (0207) 9183312
Virgin Trains: Special Needs:
Tel: (0845) 7443366
Minicom: (0845) 7443367

HOTELS

COPTHORNE EFFINGHAM PARK
West Park Road,
Copthorne RH10 3EU
Tel: (01342) 714994 Fax: 901342) 716039
No. of Accessible Rooms: 1. Bath
Accessible Facilities: Lounge, Restaurant, Outdoor seating area. Fine modern hotel built around an historic country house in 40 acres of parkland and delightfully landscaped gardens.

COPTHORNE LONDON GATWICK
Copthorne Way, Copthorne RH10 3PG
Tel: (01342) 348800 Fax: (01342) 348833
No. of Accessible Rooms: 13. Bath
Accessible Facilities: Lounge, Restaurants (2). Built around a C16th farmhouse, set in 100 acres of wooded, landscape gardens in village of Copthorne. Very close to M23 (J10), close to Gatwick Airport.

HILTON LONDON GATWICK
South Terminal, Gatwick Airport RH6 0LL
Tel: (01293) 518080 Fax: (01293) 528980
No. of Accessible Rooms: 2. Roll-in Shower
Accessible Facilities: Lift (Cat.1), Lounge, Garden Restaurant, Pool, Sauna, Spa.

LE MERIDIEN LONDON GATWICK
North Terminal, Gatwick Airport RH6 0PH
Tel: (01293) 567070 Fax: (01293) 567739
No. of Accessible Rooms: 2. Bath
Accessible facilities: Lounge, Restaurant, Pool, Sauna, Spa.

HAYWARDS HEATH
Large market town with both urban and rural aspects as an important agricultural centre.

ATTRACTIONS
BORDE HILL GARDENS
Balcombe Road, Haywards Heath RH16 1XP
Tel: (01444) 450326 Fax: (01444) 440427
Web: www.bordehill.co.uk
Botanical and tranquil gardens with rich variety of seasonal colour set in 200 acres of parkland and woodland. Extensive planting with rose and herbaceous gardens.

SD   CP   E   RF
C   S   WC   RFE

NYMANS GARDEN (NT)
Handcross, Nr. Haywards Heath RH17 6EB
Tel: (01444) 400321 Fax: (01444) 400253
Flowering shrubs, roses, rare trees, a secret sunken garden and old walled orchard.

SD   CP   E   C   S   WC

WAKEHURST PLACE GARDEN
Royal Botanic Gardens, Ardingly, Haywards Heath EH17 6TN
Tel: (01444) 894049 Fax: (01444) 894069
web: www.rbgkew.org.uk
170 acres of gardens and woodlands contain many species not found at Kew Gardens. 4 national c ollections of birch, hypericum, southern beech and skimmia. Woodlands with temperate trees from 4 continents, Loder Valley Nature Reserve for conservation of plants and animals of the Sussex Weald. Winter Garden, Walled Gardens, Pinetum and Asian Heath Garden.

SD   CP   E   RF
C   S   WC   RFE

PETWORTH
The town has a number of very old houses, some timber-framed and many in narrow streets around the little market square, dating from Tudor to Georgian times.

TOURIST INFORMATION CENTRE
(Weekends only during winter)
Market Square, Petworth GU28 0AF
Tel: (01798) 343523 Fax: (01798) 343942

BED AND BREAKFAST
THE OLD RAILWAY STATION
Petworth GU28 0JF
Tel/Fax: (01798) 342346
e-mail: query@old-station.co.uk
web: www.old-station.co.uk
No. of Accessible Rooms: 1. Bath
Accessible Facilities: Lounge, Dining Room Colonial style splendour at Victorian station, a Grade 11 listed building. Pullman railway carriages are your home here. In summer take breakfast on the old platform.

ATTRACTIONS
THE DOLL HOUSE MUSEUM
Station Road, Petworth GU28 0BF

Tel: (01798) 344044 Fax: (01798) 343858

Amazing collection, mainly modern 1/12th scale showing present day life in all types of buildings, e.g. ballet boarding school, prison, log cabin, Shaker, Mozart Bicentenary. Also room and collection boxes and fully furnished house in 1/24th scale.

SD ♿ | CP 🚶 | E 🚶 | RF ♿
L ♿ | S ♿ | WC 🚶 | RFE ♿

PETWORTH HOUSE (NT)
Petworth GU28 0AE
Tel: (01798) 342207 Fax: (01798) 342963

Rebuilt in 1688 around the ancient manor house of the Percy family, Petworth houses the finest collection of paintings and sculpture in the care of the National Trust. Highlights include Turner oil paintings in Red Room and North Gallery, Van Dycks in Square and little Dining Rooms and Grinling Gibbon's limewood carvings in the Carved Room. Also a 30-acre woodland garden and 700-acre Petworth Park designed by Capability Brown and home to England's largest herd of fallow deer. All main showrooms, except chapel and some bedrooms are accessible.

SD ♿ | CP ♿ | E ♿ | RF ♿
C ♿ (wheelchair lift to C) | S ♿
WC 🚶 | RFE ♿

PULLBOROUGH
ATTRACTION
PARHAM HOUSE AND GARDENS
Parham Park, Nr. Pullborough
Tel: (01903) 742021 Fax: (01903) 746557
e-mail: Parham @dial.pipex.com

Major Elizabethan house, family-owned for many hundreds of years and containing a fine collection of paintings, furniture and carpets. Surrounded by 7 acres of gardens and C18th pleasure grounds with lake, and brick and turf maze. In turn surrounded by 875 acres of working agricultural and forestry land. Please give prior notice if entrance ramp is required.

SD ♿ | CP 🚶 | E ♿ | RF ♿
C ♿ | S ♿ | WC 🚶

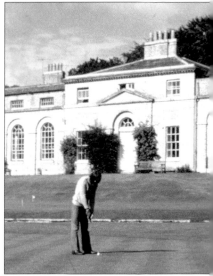

England's largest herd of deer are just out of this shot of this view of Petworth House.

PULLBOROUGH BROOKS RSPB NATURE RESERVE
Wiggonholt, Pullborough RH20 2EL
Tel: (01798) 875851 Fax: (01798) 873816

Excellent for viewing wintering and wading birds, with water meadows, ditches and pools, higher meadows, hedgerow and woodland. Nature trail on all-weather hardcore of 2 miles leading to 3 hides. Demanding journey for manual chair and requires pusher. Batricar available on loan, but cannot be taken into the hides.

SD ♿ | CP ♿ | E ♿ | RF ♿
C n/a | S ♿ | WC 🚶 | RFE ♿ & 🚶

SHOREHAM

Popular seaside resort and an ancient town. Old Shoreham lies north of the main centre, established by south Saxons in C5th. It is now separated from the sea by the Ader, the harbour and shingle of Shoreham Beach.

ATTRACTION
MUSEUM OF D-DAY AVIATION
Shoreham Airport, Shoreham BN43 5FJ
Tel: (01374) 971971

Aircraft engines for Hurricanes, Spitfires and Hawker Typhoons, plus Typhoon cockpit being restored. Unique collection of artefacts, uniforms, medals and photos.

SD ♿ | CP ♿ | E ♿ | RF ♿ | WC 🚶 | RFE ♿

STEYNING
ATTRACTION
STEYNING MUSEUM
Church Street, Steyning BN44 3YB
Tel: (01903) 813333
Celebration of Steyning's history, the
Normans and their successors established
the town. Exhibits on crafts and industries.

SD  CP E S WC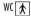

WORTHING
Popular seaside resort with extensive sands
and shingle beaches. The C19th pier is one
of the oldest. Several parks and gardens.

TOURIST INFORMATION CENTRES
Town Hall, Chapel Road, Worthing BN11 1HL
Tel: (01903) 210022   Fax: (01903) 236277
e-mail: wbctourism@pavilion.co.uk
web: www.worthing.gov.uk/wbc

Marine Parade, Worthing BN11 3PX
Tel: (01903) 210022
(Summer months only)
Produces a guide for disabled visitors.

WORTHING BOROUGH COUNCIL
Address as TIC. Tel: (01903) 239999

BUSES
Compass Travel: Tel: (01903) 233767
Stagecoach Coastline: Tel: (01903) 237661
Some low-floor buses.

TAXIS
Worthing Taxi Association:
Tel: (01903) 232523
One adapted vehicle, but has contact with
other firms.
Baz Cabs:Tel: (mobile) (07710) 992131
One adapted vehicle.

TRAINS
Connex South Central: Customer Services:
Tel: (0870) 6030405
Fax: (0870) 6030505
Minicom: (01233) 617621
Wales & West: Tel: Special Needs:
Tel: (0845) 3003005
Minicom: (0845) 7585469
Worthing Station is suitable for
wheelchairs using ramp access.

CAR PARKS
Free, unlimited parking in Pay & Display
car parks, Council-run car parks, also
many disabled parking bays around town.
Tel: (01903) 204436

SHOPMOBILITY
United Reform Church, Shelley Road,
Worthing BN11 1TT
Tel: (01903) 820980
Also has range of single and 2-seater
electric vehicles for hire: Towns to Downs.

HOTELS
BEACH HOTEL
Marine Parade, Worthing BN11 3QJ
Tel: (01903) 234001   Fax: (01903) 234567
e-mail: Thebeachhotel@Btinternet.com
No. of Accessible Rooms: 2. Shower
Accessible Facilities: Lounge, Restaurant,
all ground floor public rooms. Family
owned and managed for 40 years with
restaurant and rooms overlooking the sea.

BEST WESTERN BERKELEY HOTEL
86 - 95 Marine Parade, Worthing BN11 3GD
Tel: (01903) 820000   Fax: (01903) 821333
No. of Accessible Rooms: 1. Bath
Accessible Facilities: Lounge, Restaurant.
Seafront hotel overlooking promenade.

LANTERN HOTEL
54 Shelley Road, Worthing BN11 4BX
Tel: (01903) 238476   Fax: (01903) 602429
No. of Accessible Rooms: 13. Roll-in Shower
Accessible Facilities: All.
Hotel is owned by British Polio Fellowship.

KINGSWAY HOTEL
117 Marine Parade, Worthing BN11 3QQ
Tel: (01903) 237542   Fax: (01903) 204173
No. of Accessible Rooms: 2.
Accessible Facilities: Lounges (2), Bar,
Restaurant, Buttery. Family-owned,
seafront hotel .

WINDSOR HOUSE HOTEL
16 Windsor Road, Worthing
Tel: (01903) 239655   Fax: (01903) 210763
E-mail: thewindsorhotel@compuserve.com
No. of Accessible Rooms: 1. Shower
Accessible Facilities: Lounge, Restaurant
Refurbished in 1998.

TYNE AND WEAR

DISABILITY DIRECTORY
Tel: (01772) 631690
Covers the whole of the North East.

GATESHEAD
A fire in 1854 destroyed most of the historical buildings, and much is now modern. There are fine views of the famous five Tyne bridges linking Gateshead to Newcastle-upon-Tyne. Known for the superb MetroCentre shopping centre.

TOURIST INFORMATION CENTRE
Central Library, Prince Consort Road,
Gateshead NE8 4LN
Tel: (0191) 4773478

Gateshead Metrocentre, Portcullis,
7 The Arcade, MetroCentre NE11 9YL
Tel: (0191) 460 6345

HOTELS
NEWCASTLE/GATESHEAD MARRIOTT 🚶
Metro Centre, Gateshead NE11 9XF
Tel: (0191) 4932233
No. of Accessible Rooms: 2. Bath
Accessible Facilities: Lounge, Dining
Room, most of Bar.
Quality hotel by Metro Centre.

SWALLOW HOTEL 🚶
High West Street, Gateshead NE8 1PE
Tel: (0191) 4771105 Fax: (0191) 4787214
No. of Accessible Rooms: 1. Bath
Accessible Facilities: (Via accessible lift)
Lounge, Restaurant. Busy modern hotel
located a mile from Newcastle city centre.

JARROW
Part of the industrial Tyneside, lying at the Durham end of the Tyne tunnel. Intense poverty marked the closing of shipyards in 1933 followed by the famous hunger march that warned of dependence on one industry. Now new houses and flats replace slums and small factories and workshops have been introduced to prevent another civic crisis.

ATTRACTION
BEDE'S WORLD
Church Bank, Jarrow NE32 3DY
Tel: (0191) 4282106   Fax: (0191) 4282361
e-mail: visitor.info@bedesworld.co.uk
The Venerable Bede (AD673-735), early medieval Europe's greatest scholar, was the first to record the history of England, He lived and worked as a monk at Jarrow. Explore the golden age of saints and kings in Northumbria via an Anglo-Saxon Farm, Jarrow Hall Exhibition and St. Paul's Church and Monastic site where Bede spent much of his life. Great museum.

SD	♿	CP	♿	E	♿	RF	♿
L	♿	C	♿	S	♿	WC	🚶

NEWCASTLE-UPON-TYNE
A complex scene of blackened masses of old buildings, tall new blocks, the ornamental crown of St. Nicholas Cathedral, the pretty spire of All Saints, the square-shouldered castle keep, the quays, warehouses and industry. Main area for visitors is the square mile between the Riverside and the Town Moor. The Moor gives this highly industrialised city a unique breathing space of 927 windswept acres on which freemen can – and do – pasture cows.

TOURIST INFORMATION CENTRES
City First Stop and Information Centre,
City Library, Princess Square,
Newcastle upon Tyne NE99 1DX
Tel: (0191) 2610610

Main Concourse, Central Station, Newcastle
upon Tyne NE1 5DL
Tel: (0191) 2300300

Unit 1, Royal Quays Outlet Shopping Centre,
Coble Dene, North Shields NE29 6DW
Tel: (0191) 2005895

Museum and Art Gallery, Ocean Road,
South Shields NE33 1HZ
Tel: (0191) 4546612

BUSES
Arriva Northumbria: Tel: (0191) 2121313
Fax: (0191) 2818999

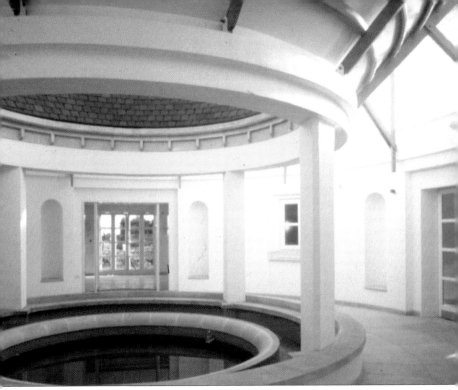

Bede's World, a worthy reminder of Britain's first historian.

web: www.arriva.co.uk
Some low-floor buses.
Stagecoach: Tel: (0191) 2761411
Some low-floor buses.

TAXIS
Metro Taxis: Tel: (0191) 2611891
50 adapted vehicles
Noda: Tel: (0191) 2221888
40 adapted vehicles outside Central
Station.
Transcab (South Shields):
Tel: (0378) 783614
3 adapted vehicles.

TRAINS
Great North Eastern Railway: Special Needs:
Tel: (0345) 225444
Minicom: (0191) 2330173
Virgin Trains: Special Needs:
Tel: (0845) 7443366
Minicom: (0845) 7443367

METRO
Tel: (0191) 2325325
ASSISTANCE REQUIRED

CAR PARKS
Free unlimited orange badge parking in
council-owned car parks.

SHOPMOBILITY
Eldon Square Shopping Centre, Eldon Court,
Percy Street, Newcastle upon Tyne NE1 7JB
Tel: (0191) 2611891
Fax: (0191) 2616340

HOTES
QUALITY FRIENDLY HOTEL
Witney Way, Boldon, Newcastle NE35 9PE
Tel: (0191) 5191999
No. of Accessible Rooms: 3
Accessible Facilities: Lounge, Restaurant.
Modern hotel located on junction of A19
and A184 east of Newcastle.

COPTHORNE NEWCASTLE
The Close, Quayside, Newcastle NE1 3RT
Tel: (0191) 2220333
Fax: (0191) 2301111
No. of Accessible Rooms: 1. Bath
Accessible Facilities: Lounge, Restaurant,
Bar. Quality hotel in city centre.

HOLIDAY INN [symbol]
Great North Road, Seaton Burn,
Newcastle NE13 6BF
Tel: (0191) 2019988 Fax: (0191) 2368091
No. of Accessible Rooms:
Accessible Facilities:
Purpose-built hotel located 3m west of
Tyne Tunnel toward Morpeth

NEWCASTLE AIRPORT MOAT HOUSE [symbol]
Woolsington, Newcastle NE13 8DJ
Tel: (0191) 4019988 Fax: (01661) 860157
No. of Accessible Rooms:
Accessible Facilities: Restaurant, Bar (lift)
Modern hotel within airport complex.

NOVOTEL NEWCASTLE [symbol]
Ponteland Road, Kenton, Newcastle 0633
Tel: (0191) 2140303
Fax: (0191) 2140633
No. of Accessible Rooms: 4. Bath
Accessible Facilities: Lounge, Restaurant,
Lift. Bright, modern hotel located off the
A1 western by-pass 4 miles from Newcastle
town centre.

ATTRACTIONS
MUSEUM OF ANTIQUITIES
University and Society of Antiquities,
Newcastle upon Tyne NE1 7RU
Tel: (0191) 2227849 Fax: (0191) 2228561
e-mail: m.o.antiquities@ncl.ac.uk
Main museum for Hadrian's Wall with
historical displays from prehistoric times.
SD [symbol]   CP [symbol]   E [symbol]   S [symbol]

SPORTING VENUE
NEWCASTLE UNITED FOOTBALL CLUB
St. James' Park, Newcastle NE1 4ST
Admin: (0191) 2018634
Booking: Box Office: (0191) 2018457 or
2611571
Fax: (0191) 2018609
web: www.nufc.co.uk
Complies with Building Regulations Part M.
CP [symbol]   RE [symbol]   ED [symbol]   INT [symbol]
L [symbol]   WC [symbol]   SS [symbol]   B/R [symbol]

THEATRE
THEATRE ROYAL
100 Grey Street, Newcastle NE1 6BR
Admin: (0191) 2320997
Booking: Box Office: (0191) 2322061

Fax: (0191) 2611906
CP [symbol]   RE [symbol]
ED [symbol] (Except for non-automatic door)
INT [symbol]   L [symbol]   WC [symbol]
AUD -. Alternative rear entrance leads past adapted WC to
back of stalls with wheelchair user positions.
B/R [symbol]

STOCKTON-ON-TEES
Famous for the open air market started in
1310 and still held twice weekly in the
broadest high street in England. History
was made here when the world's first
passenger railway steamed in on 27th
September 1825.

TOURIST INFORMATION CENTRE
Theatre Yard, off High Street,
Stockton on Tees TS18 1AT
Tel: (01642) 393936

SPORTING VENUE
SEDGEFIELD RACECOURSE
The Bungalow, Sedgefield,
Stockton-on-Tees TS21 2HW
Booking/Admin :Tel: (01740) 621925
Fax: (01740) 620663
CP [symbol] (pre-book)   RE [symbol]
ED [symbol] (except manual door)
INT [symbol]   L [symbol]
WC [symbol] (4 units situated on each level of pavilion and
first level of Fosters stand)
SS [symbol] (viewing area). Tarmac from turnstiles to
viewing area.
B/R [symbol]   Main bar ramped, lift to restaurant level

TYNEMOUTH
A walk along the 0.75mile North Tyne Pier
has been called a trip to sea without
leaving land. It is an excellent vantage
point for ship-watching and viewing the
priory ruins and coastline. Tynemouth
occupies the cliffs on the north side of the
river mouth and has been a seaside resort
for at least 200 years. There are fine sands,
overlooked by amusement centre and park.

ATTRACTION
TYNEMOUTH PRIORY AND CASTLE (EH)
East Street, Tynemouth,
North Shields NE30 4BZ

Tel: (0191) 2571090
Castle walls and gatehouse enclose
substantial remains of Benedictine priory
founded c1090 on a Saxon monastic site.

SD ♿   CP ♿   E ♿   RF ♿   S ♿

TYNEMOUTH SEA LIFE CENTRE
Grand Parade, Tynemouth,
North Shields NE30 4JF
Tel: (0191) 2581031   Fax: (0191) 2572116
Web: www.sealife.co.uk
Close encounters with marine life from
starfish to sharks, octopus to eels: feeding
demonstrations and touchpools in unique
aquariums.

SD ♿   CP ♿   E ♿   RF ♿
C ♿   S ♿   WC ♿   RFE ♿

WASHINGTON
A new town has risen on this former
colliery village, and streets of miners'
houses have been demolished. Pit-head
buildings are converted to a museum and
the pit heap moved away.

ATTRACTION
THE WILDFOWL AND WETLANDS TRUST
District 15,
Washington NE38 8LE
Tel: (0191) 4165454   Fax: (0191) 416801
e-mail: wetlands@globalnet.co.uk
Situated on north bank of the River Wear,
a 100 acre site, home to many exotic
wildfowl. Discovery centre, waterfowl
nursery and viewing gallery.
Wheelchairs available.

SD ♿   CP ♿   S ♿

WHITLEY BAY
Most popular of Northumbria's resorts, the
beach has grassy banks and runs the length
of the town. Fine lighthouse on St. Mary's
island lying off the north end of the bay.

TOURIST INFORMATION CENTRE
Park Road,
Whitley Bay NE26 1EJ
Tel: (0191) 2008535

HOTEL
YORK HOUSE HOTEL   ♿
28-32 Park Parade, The Promenade, Whitley

Bay NE26 1AP
Tel: (0191) 2528313   Fax: (0191) 2513953
No. of Accessible Rooms: 3. Shower.
Accessible Facilities: Lounge, Restaurant
Located in town centre.

BED AND BREAKFAST
MARLBOROUGH HOTEL   ♿
20- 21 East Parade,
Whitley Bay NE26 1AP
Tel: (0191) 2513628   Fax: (0191) 2525033
No. of Accessible Rooms: 2. Shower
Accessible Facilities: Lounge, Restaurant.
Entrance has ramped access.
Privately owned hotel overlooking beach.
Evening meals available but not at
weekends. Restaurant next door with two-
step access to the main door.

*Above us the waves, the amazing view at
Tynemouth sea life centre.*

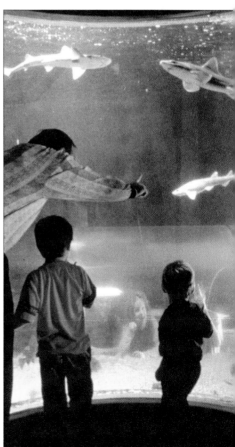

WARWICKSHIRE

SHAKESPEARE COUNTRY TOURISM
Conoco Centre, Warwick Technology Park,
Gallows Hill CV34 6DB
Tell: (01926) 404891   Fax: (01926) 404893
e-mail: info@shakespearecountry.co.uk

AVAILABLE FROM TICS.
Getting around in the West Midlands,
produced by Centro.
Tel: (0121) 2002700
Minicom: (0121) 2147777

ALCESTER
Small town 8 miles from Stratford at the
confluence of rivers Arrow and Alne.
Particularly attractive is the narrow Butter
Street, off the High Street, with its jumble
of ancient roofs.

ATTRACTION
RAGLEY HALL
Alcester B49 5NJ
Tel: (01789) 762090   Fax: (01789) 764791
Family home of the Marquis of Hertford
since it was built in 1680 and surrounded
by 27 acres of gardens, within vast parkland.
The house contains a fine collection of
treasures, particularly notable for James
Gibb's elegant baroque plasterwork. All
rooms are one floor, accessed by a lift close
to parking in right hand courtyard side of
main entrance. The Stables and Woodland
Walk reached along fairly steep gravel and
grass paths: slope uphill on the return. The
Rose Garden has steps and is not accessible.

ATHERSTONE
SELF-CATERING
HIPSLEY FARM COTTAGES
Hipsley Lane, Hurley, Atherstone CV9 2LR
Tel/Fax: (01827) 872437
No. of Accessible Units: 1
No. of Beds per Unit: 2
Accessible Facilities: Kitchen/Living
Room. Farm barns and a cowshed

converted to individual cottages with garden
and BBQ and garden furniture. Wainwright
Cottage is single-storey stone cottage.
Situated in rolling countryside, well placed
for Birmingham, National Exhibition Centre
and Stratford and Warwick.

ATTRACTION
TWYCROSS ZOO
Atherstone CV9 3PX
Tel: (01827) 880250   Fax: (01827) 880700
Run by a devoted crew specialising in
primates, there is an enormous variety of
species together with other animals
including lions and tigers, sealion and
penguin pools.

HATTON
Located between Warwick and Solihull on
A41/A4177 or M40 (Jct.15).

ATTRACTION
HATTON COUNTRY WORLD
Dark Lane, Hatton CV35 8XA
Tel: (01926) 843411 Fax: (01926) 842023
Rural crafts, farm park and shopping
village under one roof. A great deal to do,
see and to buy in 35 shops. Housed in
redundant farm buildings, access has been
made wherever possible. Farm park has
hard core pathways.

HUNTS GREEN
Tiny village between Birmingham and
Tamworth.

ATTRACTION
MIDDLETON HALL TRUST, WARWICKSHIRE.
(postal address is Staffordshire)
Middleton, Tamworth, Staffs B78 2AE
Tel: (01827) 283095 Fax: (01827) 285717
Originally built c1300, with an 11-bay
Georgian west wing and C16th Great hall,
restored in 1994. A display of 24 framed
embroideries depicting history of Sutton
Coldfield decorates the first-floor corridor.
Craft Centre in the former stable block.

Walled gardens plus nature reserve, orchard and woodland.

SD CP E RF
C [image] S [image] WC [image]

LAPWORTH
PACKWOOD HOUSE (NT)
Lapworth B94 6AT
Tel: (01564) 782024 Fax: (01564) 782912
Associated historically with both sides of the English Civil War in the mid 1600s. Much of the interior was designed this century as an idealised Elizabethan/Jacobean manor house. Despite lavish furnishings, it still retains intimate family ambience. Surrounded by delightful grounds.

SD [image] CP [image] E [image] RF [image] L n/a
C n/a S [image] WC [image] RFE [image]

LEAMINGTON SPA
Owes its being to the passion for taking the waters, following in the wake of Bath. Lovely Georgian, Regency and early Victorian terraced houses to be seen on the north side of the River Leam.

SHAKESPEARE COUNTRY TOURIST INFORMATION CENTRE
South Lodge, Jephson Gardens, Leamington Spa CV32 4AB
Tel: (01926) 311470 Fax: (01926) 881639

SELF-CATERING
HOME COTTAGE [image]
Knightcote Farm, Knightcote, Nr. Leamington Spa CV33 0SF
Tel: (01295) 770637 Fax: (01295) 770135
e-mail: fionawalker@mcmail.com
web: www.knightcotefarm@mcmail.com
No. of Accessible Units: 1. 2 Roll-in Showers.
How many Beds per Unit: 5
Accessible Facilities: Open plan Lounge/Diner, Kitchen, Patio garden with barbecue, Taxi service with wheelchair access, Local pubs with wheelchair access.
Award winning self-catering cottage with views of far stretching farmland. Located between Leamington Spa and Banbury,

STRATFORD-UPON-AVON
The least spoilt cult town. England's prime tourist centre outside London, its famous resident William Shakespeare is celebrated all over the town. Apart from the Shakespeare connections there is much to see. The canal wharf is lovely and the southern section of the Stratford-upon-Avon Canal has been completely restored by the National Trust.

STRATFORD-UPON-AVON TOURIST INFORMATION CENTRE
Bridgefoot, Stratford-upon-Avon CV37 6GW
Tel: (01789) 293127 Fax: (01789) 295262
CENTRO (Coventry): Tel: (024) 76 559559
web: www.centro.org.uk
All information on public transport in West Midlands.

BUSES
See Centro, some low-floor buses.

TAXIS
A & M Cars: Tel: (01926) 612487
Six adapted vehicles.
Mervs Taxis: Tel: (01789) 764981

TRAINS
Railtrack Property Major Stations: Tel: (0121) 6544288
Minicom: (0121) 6544292
Information on all stations on UK mainland.

Central Trains: Assistance:
Tel: (0845) 7056027
web: www.centraltrains.co.uk
Thames Trains: Special Needs:
Tel: (0118) 9083607
web: www.thamestrains.co.uk

CAR PARKS
Free unlimited orange badge parking in council car parks, 3 hours' parking in Sheep Street.
Tel: (01789) 260691

SHOPMOBILITY
Sheep Street, Stratford upon Avon CV37 6HX
Tel: (01789) 414534

HOTELS
FALCON HOTEL

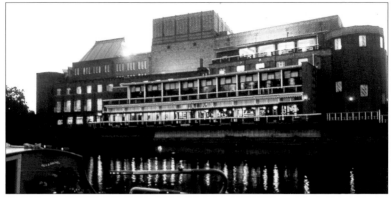

Royal Shakespeare Theatre. Luvvies' delight.

2 Chapel Street,
Stratford-upon-Avon CV37 6HA
Tel: (01789) 279953
No. of Accessible Rooms: 1
Accessible Facilities: Lounge, Restaurant
Delightful C16th inn right in centre of
town. There has been an alehouse on the
site since then.

GROVENOR HOUSE HOTEL 🚶
Warwick Road, Stratford-upon-Avon CV37 6YT
Tel: (01789) 269213
Fax: (01789) 266087
web: www.virtualhotels.com/grosvenor
No. of Accessible Rooms: 4. Bath
Accessible Facilities: Lounge, Restaurant
(ramped). Built between 1832/43 as private
homes in both Regency and Elizabethan
style, this Grade 11 listed hotel is within
two minutes of Stratford's high street.

STRATFORD MANOR 🚶
Warwick Road, Stratford-upon-Avon CV37 0PY
Tel: (01789) 731173
Fax: (01789) 731131
No. of Accessible Rooms: 5
Accessible Facilities: Lounge, Restaurant,
Pool, Sauna. Charming, modern hotel, set
in 21 acres of lovely countryside, 3 miles
from Stratford.

STRATFORD MOAT HOUSE 🚶
Bridgefoot, Stratford-upon-Avon CV37 6YR
Tel: (01789) 279988   Fax: (01789) 298589
No. of Accessible Rooms: 2
Accessible Facilities: Lounge, Restaurant,
Bar. Large modern hotel with attractive
setting on banks of River Avon.

WELCOME HOTEL 🚶
Warwick Road,
Stratford-upon-Avon CV37 0NR
Tel: (01789) 295252
No. of Accessible Rooms: 7
Accessible Facilities: Lounge, Restaurant.
Country house hotel; a spectacular C19th.
Jacobean-style mansion with many
original antiques. Set within 157 acres of
parkland and an 18-hole golf course.

BED AND BREAKFAST
CHURCH FARM 🚪
Dorsington, Stratford-upon-Avon CV37 8AX
Tel: (01789) 720471   Fax: (01789) 720830
No. of Accessible Rooms: 1
Accessible Facilities: Lounge, Dining
Room
Georgian farmhouse set in pretty and
quiet village, close to Stratford.

PENSHURST GUEST HOUSE 🚶
34 Evesham Place,
Stratford-upon-Avon CV37 6HT
Tel: (01789) 205259   Fax: (01789) 295322
e-mail: penshurst@cwcom.net
web: www.stratford-upon-
avon.co.uk/penshurst
No. of Accessible Rooms: 1. Roll-in
Shower.
Accessible Facilities: Dining room.
Holiday Care Service winner 1996.
Pretty Victorian townhouse 5 minutes
from town centre.

ATTRACTIONS
SHAKESPEARE BIRTHPLACE TRUST
The Shakespeare Centre, Henley Street,

Stratford-upon-Avon CV37 6QW
Tel: (01789) 204016   Fax: (01789) 296083
e-mail: info@shakespeare.org.uk
web: www.shakespeare.org.uk

The Trust manages the 5 Shakespeare houses in and around Stratford-upon-Avon. 3 in the town, The Birthplace, Nash's House and New Place and Halls' Croft: Anne Hathaway's cottage and Mary Arden's House a few miles outside. The houses do present some difficulties for disabled visitors, although in some cases ground floor rooms and gardens are accessible. Anne Hathaway's Cottage is not accessible. In all the 4 sites visited, we found the staff to be extremely helpful and attentive.The Birthplace Trust is in the process of improving the physical access to all the historic houses, with the help of consultation by South Warwickshire Access Group. These include detailed access guides, new exterior pathway surfaces, external entrances and exits, adaptive WC's where not yet in place, firm hand rails on ramps, wheelchair availability and more.

SHAKESPEARE'S BIRTHPLACE:

Born here in 1564, the tour begins in the very accessible Visitor's Centre exhibition, telling the story of Shakespeare's life and background with many original items and specially constructed scenes. The Birthplace is approached from the garden's wide paving stones, has one large step and one narrow doorway accessible by the site's own manual chair, but not by an electric wheelchair. Uneven flooring throughout, but ground floor rooms accessible. Plans to have CD on upper rooms for disabled only.

SD 🦽   CP 🦽   E 🦽   H 🚶   WC 🚶
S -Exhibition 🦽   House 🚶

NASH'S HOUSE & NEW PLACE
Chapel Street, Stratford-upon-Avon
Tel: (01789) 292325

Adjoins the site of New Place, Shakespeare's home for the last 18 years of his life. It belonged to Thomas Nash, who married Shakespeare's granddaughter in 1626, 10 years after the dramatist's death. The house, accessed by external and internal ramps, gradients 1:10, has notable oak furniture and paintings. Ground floor accessible. A passageway beyond the entrance hall leads to a small step onto the site and gardens of New Place, sadly no longer there. Paths in the first garden are too narrow for access, but the beautiful Great Garden beyond is accessible along Chapel Lane to the right of the entrance.

E 🚶   RF 🦽   WC 🚶

HALL'S CROFT
Old Town, Stratford-upon-Avon
Tel: (01789) 292107

Fine half-timbered, gabled house, owned by John Hall who married Shakespeare's daughter, Susanna, in 1607. Fine paintings inside and lovely walled garden. Entrance via stone step, ground floor mainly flat and level. Shop and restaurant via shallow ramp. Garden and seating area reached via flat access from house, lawn area ramped.

E 🚶   RF 🦽   C 🦽   S 🦽   WC 🦽   G 🦽

MARY ARDEN'S HOUSE
Wilmcote
Tel: (01789) 293455

Located 3 miles from Stratford-upon-Avon, this was probably the home of Shakespeare's mother before she married. It is a fine Tudor farmhouse with many old outbuildings, a delightful homestead and a

No mock-Tudor at Mary Arden's house.

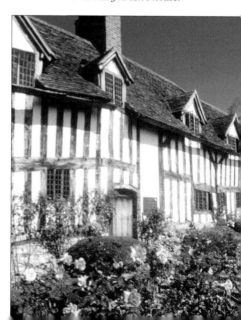

must to visit. Accessed in and out by shallow ramp, with flat and level access throughout most of the site although the house has some thresholds of 8cm. Flooring is stone flagging and there is room to manoeuvre between exhibits. 1 step into Glebe Farm and 1 step into the farming exhibit. Garden has flat picnic area. Wheelchair available for loan.

CP [♿] E [♿] RF [♿] C [♿] S [♿] WC [♿]

STRATFORD BUTTERFLY FARM
Swan's Nest Lane,
Stratford-upon-Avon CV37 7LS
Tel: (01789) 299288 Fax: (01789) 415878
Largest butterfly and insect exhibition in Europe with many of the world's most spectacular varieties of butterflies in tropical setting. Also Insect City and deadly spiders in Arachnoland.

SD [♿] CP [♿] E [🚶] RF [🚶] S [🚶]
WC n/a (Accessible WC 30m away-owned by council)
RFE [🚶]

THEATRE
ROYAL SHAKESPEARE COMPANY
Waterside, Stratford-upon-Avon
Admin-Minicom: (01789) 412658
Fax: (01789) 412639
Booking-Box Office: (01789) 295623,
Minicom/Fax: (01789) 261974
Complies with Part M, Building Regulations.
CP [♿] Public   CP-Market Place
Taxi Rank–200m or by phone in front of theatre.
RE [♿] ED [♿] INT [♿]
WC [♿] (ground floor) AUD [♿]   B [♿]

WARWICK
One of most unspoilt of all county towns, standing on a north rise from the river Avon, which is crossed by two bridges. Delightful pre-1694 houses in Castle Street. The castle itself is truly magnificent, but inaccurate.

WARWICK TOURIST INFORMATION CENTRE
Jury Street, Warwick CV34 4EW
Tel: (01926) 492212 Fax: (01926) 494?

HOTEL
CHARLECOTE PHEASANT COUNTRY HOTEL [🚶]
Charlecote CV35 9EW

Tel: (01789) 279954 Fax: (01789) 470222
No. of Accessible Rooms: 6
Accessible Facilities: Lounge, Restaurant.
Charming rural retreat converted from farm buildings, sitting alongside Charlecote Manor. Located in old village a short distance from both Warwick and Stratford-upon-Avon.

HILTON NATIONAL   [🚶]
WARWICK/STRATFORD
Stratford Road, Warwick CV34 6RE
Tel: (01926) 499555 Fax: (01926) 410020
No. of Accessible Rooms: 1
Accessible Facilities: Lounge, Restaurant
Located on M40 (J15).

BED AND BREAKFAST
WOODSIDE COUNTRY GUEST HOUSE   [🚶]
Langley Road, Claverdon, Warwick CV35 8PJ
Tel: (01926) 842446 Fax: (01926) 843697
No. of Accessible Rooms: 1. Bath.
Accessible Facilities: Lounge, Dining Room (2 step) – will lay up in Lounge.
Set in acres of English garden and woodland with lovely views. 4.5 miles from Warwick in attractive village overlooking former woodland of Arden, mentioned in Domesday Book, Anglo-Saxon in origin.

ATTRACTION
CHARLECOTE PARK (NT)
Warwick CV35 9ER
Tel: (01789) 470277 Fax: (01789) 470544
e-mail: vclgrismpt.ntrust. org
Strong associations with Elizabeth 1 and Shakespeare in this essentially Tudor house. Early Victorian interior and deer park designed by Capability Brown.

SD [♿] CP [🚶] E [♿] RF [♿]
C [♿] S [♿] WC [🚶] RFE – H & G [🚶]

HERITAGE MOTOR CENTRE
Banbury Road, Gaydon, Warwick CV35 0BJ
Tel: (01926) 641188 Fax: (01926) 641555
Largest purpose-built road transport museum in the UK, with the largest collection of historic British cars in the world. Directed at the whole family, displays include the Corgi collections and activities, and the quad bike circuit.

SD [♿] CP [♿] E [♿] RF [♿] L [♿]
C [♿] S [♿] WC [♿] RFE [♿]

WEST MIDLANDS

Tel: (0845) 30030005
Minicom:L (0845) 7585469
Centro Hotline: Tel: (0121) 2002700

BIRMINGHAM

Second largest city in Britain with a population of one million with a great concentration of industries, and their legacy of excellent heritage museums. Now a post-manufacturing centre, the city is dominated by wide roads, banked by large buildings with a shopping centre terraced beneath the flyovers. This area is traffic free and linked by subways.

TOURIST INFORMATION CENTRES
130 Colmore Row, Victoria Square,
Birmingham B3 3AP
Tel: (0121) 6936300   Fax: (0121) 6939600

2 City Arcade, Birmingham B2 4TX
Tel: (0121) 6432514   Fax: (0121) 6161038

CENTRO Hotline: Tel: (0121) 2002700
Minicom: (0121) 2147777
All information on buses in West Midlands.

BUSES
Easyrider: Tel: (0121) 3333108 (Birmingham North) : Tel: (0121) 4862663 (South).
Low steps, lifts, trained staff.

TAXIS
BB Cabs. Tel: (0121) 3032624
10 adapted vehicles
TOA: Tel: (0121) 4278888
300 adapted vehicles.

TRAINS
Central Trains: Assistance:
Tel: (0845) 7056027
web: www.centraltrains.co.uk
Chiltern Railways: Mobility Impaired:
Tel: (01296) 332113/4
web: www.chilternrailways.co.uk
Silverlink: Special Needs:
Tel: (01923) 207818
Fax: (01923) 207023
Minicom: (01923) 256430
Virgin Trains: Special Needs:
Tel: (0845) 7443366
Minicom: (0845) 7443367
Wales & West: Special Needs:

Birmingham New Street Station:
Tel: (0121) 6544288
Minicom: (0121) 6544292
Information covers whole of UK mainland.

CAR PARKS
3-hour free parking in council-owned car parks, some on-street parking.
Tel: (0121) 3033634

METRO
Tel: (0121) 2002700
Minicom: (0121) 2147777
All trams are easy access with ramps/lifts to platforms.

SHOPMOBILITY
The Central Library, Chamberlain Square,
Birmingham B3 3HQ
Tel: (0121) 6936613   Fax: (0121) 7850104

Birmingham Markets, Markets Customer Centre, Edgbaston Road, Birmingham B5 4RB
Tel: (0121) 6434130

HOTELS
COPTHORNE BIRMINGHAM
Paradise Circus, Birmingham BE 3HJ
Tel: (0121) 2002727 Fax: (0121) 2001197
web: www.mill-cop.com
No. of Accessible Rooms: 1
Accessible Facilities: Lounge, Restaurants 2.
Quality large city-centre hotel overlooking Centenary Square.

NOVOTEL BIRMINGHAM AIRPORT
Birmingham International Airport,
Birmingham B26 3QL
Tel: (0121) 7827000 Fax: (0121) 7820445
No. of Accessible Rooms: 6. Bath
Accessible Facilities: Lounge, Restaurant, Lift. Modern hotel with walkway connection to airport.

ATTRACTIONS
BIRMINGHAM BOTANICAL GARDENS
Westbourne Road, Edgbaston,
Birmingham B15 3TR
Tel: (0121) 4541860 Fax: (0121) 4547835

e-mail: admin@bham-bot-gdns.demon.co.uk

15 acres of ornamental gardens including Rock, Historic, Herb & Cottage and Themed Gardens, plus exotic birds in indoor and outdoor aviaries on the Loudon Terrace, cactus and succulent house and Japanese gardens.

SD | CP | E | RF | C
S | WC | RFE

SOHO HOUSE MUSEUM
Soho Avenue, Handsworth, Birmingham
Tel: (0121) 5549122 Fax: (0121) 5545929

Elegant home of industrial pioneer, Matthew Bolton from 1766 to 1809. Possibly the first centrally heated house since Roman times, it has been restored to its C18th appearance and contains original furniture. Also an opportunity to see products of his nearby factory where ormolu clocks and vases and Sheffield plate silverware were made, and where he developed the steam engine in partnership with James Watt. The VC is a community exhibition centre with changing programmes. The main entrance to the house has 2 steps of 5cm and 7cm, avoidable by portable ramp, or via ramped access at the side of the house. WC, shop and catering are in adjacent Visitor Centre (Cat. 3. as ramp is 1:11.2).

SD | CP | E | RF
L | C | S | WC

Could Matthew Bolton afford to leave the heating on all day at Soho House?

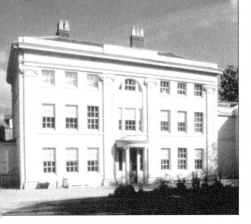

COVENTRY

A thriving city in which the legend of Godiva, who, it is said, rode naked through the city in order to obtain relief for the town from the taxes levied by her husband Leofric, is still part of its heritage. Much of the old city was devastated by the German air raid in November 1940, but the city centre is dominated by its new cathedral. Early wealth derived from textiles, but now is associated with car manufacture.

TOURIST INFORMATION CENTRE
Bayley Lane, Coventry CV1 5RN
Tel: (024) 76 832303

COVENTRY COUNCIL OF DISABLED PEOPLE
101 Broad Park Road, Henley Green,
Coventry CV2 1DB
Tel: (024) 76 61400

CENTRO Hotline: Tel: (024) 76 559559
All information on local trains, buses, metro.

BUSES
Easyrider: Tel: (024) 76 602293
Low steps, lifts, trained staff.

TAXIS
Alan's Taxis: Tel: (024) 76 555555
25 adapted vehicles.
Central Taxis: Tel: (024) 76 333333
80 adapted vehicles.
Lewis Taxis: Tel: (024) 76 666666
2 adapted vehicles.

TRAINS
Silverlink: Special Needs: (024) 76 207818
Fax: (024) 76 207023
Minicom: (024) 76 256430
Virgin Trains: Special Needs:
Tel: (0845) 7443366
Minicom: (0845) 7443367
Coventry Station accessible via level route.

CAR PARKS
Free unlimited orange badge parking in Pay & Display car parks.

SHOPMOBILITY
Barracks Car Park, Upper Precinct,
Coventry CV1 1DD
Tel: (024) 76 832020   Fax: (024) 76 832017

HOTELS

HILTON NATIONAL COVENTRY

Paradise Way, Walsgrave Triangle,
Coventry CV2 2ST
Tel: (024) 76 603000 Fax: (024) 76 603011
No. of Accessible Rooms: 2
Accessible Facilities: Open plan Public
Areas. Bright modern property situated just
outside Coventry.

NOVOTEL COVENTRY

Wilsons Lane, Longford, Coventry CV6 6HL
Tel: (024) 76 365000 Fax: (024) 76 362422
No. of Accessible Rooms: 2
Accessible Facilities: Lounge, Restaurant
(ramped access)
Modern bright hotel 11 miles from NEC
Birmingham. Located on M6 (J.3)

ATTRACTIONS

COVENTRY CATHEDRAL

Priory Street, Coventry
Tel: (024) 76 227597 Fax: (024) 76 631448
e-mail: information@coventrycathedral.org
The remains of the old cathedral, bombed
in 1940, have been preserved. The new
pink-sandstone cathedral, designed by Sir
Basil Spence and consecrated in 1962,
houses superb contemporary works
including John Piper's baptistery window,
tapestry by Graham Sutherland and
bronzes by Epstein.

| SD 🚾 | CP 🚹 | E 🚾 | RF 🚾 | L 🚾 |
| C 🚹 | S main n/a, bookstall 🚾 | | WC 🚹 | |

HERBERT ART GALLERY AND MUSEUM

Jordan Well, Coventry CV1 5QP
Tel: (024) 76 832381 Fax: (024) 76 832410
e-mail: coventry.museums@dial.pipex.com
History of Lady Godiva's city told through
interactive displays and paintings. Details
of Sutherland's design for the cathedral
also on display.

| SD 🚾 | CP 🚾 | E 🚾 | RF 🚾 | L 🚾 |
| C 🚾 | S 🚾 | WC 🚾 | RFE 🚾 | |

MUSEUM OF BRITISH ROAD TRANSPORT

Hales Street, Coventry CU1 1PN
Tel: (024) 76 832425 Fax: (024) 76 832465
web: www.mbrt.co.uk
Largest display of British-made road
transport in the world, under one
enormous roof. Explore Memory Lanes
display of Edwardian and vintage vehicles
set in period street scenes: trace the
progress of the cycle from Hobby Horse to
Mountain Bike: see old and new buses and
public vehicles: experience the Coventry
Blitz in an emotionally interpreted display.
A charming, easily accessible museum.

| SD 🚾 | CP 🚹 | E 🚾 | RF 🚾 |
| L 🚾 | C 🚾 | S 🚾 | WC 🚾 |

SPORTING VENUE

COVENTRY CITY FOOTBALL CLUB

Highfield Road Stadium, King Richard Street,
Coventry CV2 4FW
Admin: (024) 76 234000

Cathedrals old and new.

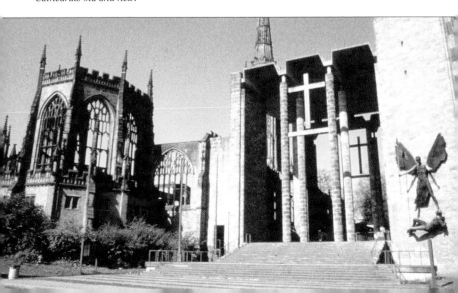

Fax: (024) 76 234099
web: www.ccfc.co.uk
Booking: Wheelchair spaces for car park
and viewing: (01203) 234020 for credit card
or by post.

CP ♿ RE ♿ ED ♿ (except manual door)
L ♿ WC ♿ (2 units)

SOLIHULL

A suburb of Birmingham with some Tudor
houses in the High Street.

HOTEL
SOLIHULL MOAT HOUSE 🚶
Homer Road, Solihull B91 3QD
Tel: (0121) 6239988 Fax: (0121) 7112696
No. of Accessible Rooms:
Accessible Facilities: Lounge, Bar, Restaurant
Modern hotel well located for NEC or
shopping centre very close by.

ATTRACTIONS
BADDESLEY CLINTON HALL (NT)
Knowle, Solihull
Tel: (01564) 783294 Fax: (01564) 782706
The written history of Baddesley began
long before the C13th when the Clintons
settled here, dug the moat and gave the
place their name. The house has grey stone
walls, tiled roofs and tall red-brick
chimneys emblazoned in trees in the
hollow of a park which has never been
formally planted or landscaped.

SD ♿ CP 🚶 E 🚶 RF ♿
C 🚶 S ♿🚶 WC 🚶 RFE 🚶

PACKWOOD HOUSE
Lapworth, Solihull B94 6AT
Tel: (01564) 782024 Fax: (01564) 782912
Cromwell's general, Henry Ireton, stayed
here before the Battle of Edgehill in 1642,
but many of the interiors were designed in
the 1920s and 30s as an idealised
Elizabethan or Jacobean manor and offer
great insight into the taste, rich decoration
and way of life of a wealthy amateur
connoisseur between the wars. The house
is surrounded by tranquil gardens.
NB: Access to ground floor only.

SD ♿ E 🚶 RF 🚶 C n/a S 🚶
WC 🚶 RFE 🚶 Wheelchairs and battery powered
vehicles available for hire.

STOURBRIDGE

Early importance as glass-making centre,
introduced by religious refugees from
Hungary in C16th. Situated on south
bank of river Stour on edge of the Black
Country.

ATTRACTION
BROADFIELD HOUSE GLASS MUSEUM
Compton Drive, Kingswinford,
Nr. Stourbridge DY6 9NS
Tel: (01384) 812745
Fax: (01384) 812746
Fine collection of C19th and C20th glass
cut in nearby Stourbridge. Ground floor
only is accessible.

SD ♿ CP 🚶 E ♿ RF ♿
C 🚶 S ♿ WC 🚶

WOLVERHAMPTON

Capital of the Black Country with many
striking buildings of Victorian civic
architecture, but little else.

HOTEL
NOVOTEL WOLVERHAMPTON ♿
Union Street, Wolverhampton WV1 3JN
Tel: (01902) 871199
Fax: (01902) 870054
No. of Accessible Rooms: 3. Bath
Accessible Facilities: Lounge,
Restaurant.
Located within easy reach of city centre.

ATTRACTION
WOLVERHAMPTON ART GALLERY
Lichfield Road, Wolverhampton WV1 1DU
Tel: (01902) 552055
Fax: (01902) 552053
e-mail: infor.wag@dial.pipex.com
web: artgall.scit.wlv.ac.uk
Changing art, sculpture and
photographic exhibitions throughout the
year, plus hands-on Ways of Seeing
Room, an exploration of art through
eyes, ears and hands. Very accessible
gallery.

SD ♿ CP ♿🚶 E ♿ RF ♿
L ♿ C ♿ S ♿ WC 🚶

WILTSHIRE

CHIPPENHAM

King Alfred spent much time here, hunting in the nearby forests. There is a C15th Town Hall and some attractive half-timbered houses, and others in stone dating from the C18th.

TOURIST INFORMATION CENTRE
The Citadel, Bath Road, Chippenham SN15 2AA
Tel: (01249) 657733   Fax: (01249) 460776

ATTRACTION
LACOCK ABBEY (NT)
Lacock, Chippenham SN15 2LG
Tel: (01249) 730227

Founded in 1232, Lacock became secular after the Dissolution of the Monasteries by Henry V111. The church was destroyed but fine medieval cloisters remain. In the mid C19th William Henry Fox Talbot remodelled south elevation and added 3 oriel windows. The abbey and most of the village was donated to the NT in 1944/46, and the village retains its unique mixture of architecture spanning 700 years. The museum commemorates the life and work of W H F Talbot who invented the positive/negative process in 1840, and was known as the Father of Modern Photography. Abbey is not accessible, but cloisters and museum are. Museum has stair lift to upper floor. The present cloisteral walkway is of C14th and C15th.

SD   ♿   CP ♿   E ♿   RF ♿
C ♿   S 🚶
WC ♿   (Radar key obtained from Stable Cafe)
RFE ♿

DEVIZES

An old market town with some C16th buildings, the town is particularly rich in C18th structures.

TOURIST INFORMATION CENTRE
39 St. John's Street, Devizes SN10 1BL
Tel: (01380) 729408

SELF-CATERING
ABBOTTS BALL FARM   🚶   275
Pound Hill, Worton Road, Potterne,
Devizes SN10 5PW

Laycock Abbey spans 700 years from monks to photography.

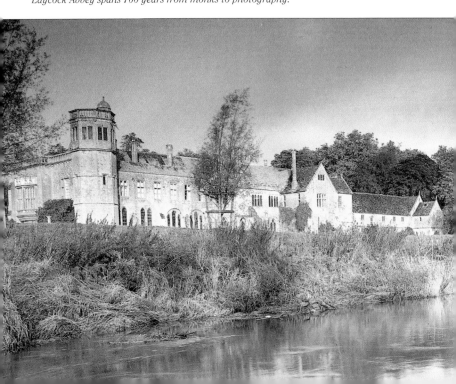

Tel: (01380) 721661
No. of Accessible Units: 1. Roll-in Shower
No. of Beds per Unit: 2D +1S.
Accessible Facilities: Lounge/diner, Kitchen,
Garden. The cottage is an annexe onto the
farmhouse on edge of village of Potterne
with far reaching views. 30 minutes from
Salisbury, Bath and Stonehenge.

MARLBOROUGH
Situated in the Kennet Valley and on a main
road, Marlborough was popular in coaching
times. Most of the older half-timbered
houses are hidden in small back lanes off
the High Street, itself an impressive wide
road sweeping down the centre of the town.
Overall effect is Georgian, but there are a
number of periods manifest here.

TOURIST INFORMATION CENTRE
George Lane Car Park, Marlborough SN18 1EE
Tel: (01672) 513989

ATTRACTION
ALEXANDER KEILLER MUSEUM (NT)
Avebury, Nr. Marlborough SN8 1RF
Tel: (01672) 539250   Fax: (01672) 539388
Museum is a site museum for Avebury
Monuments, situated 250m from the stone
circle on the western side of Avebury
Manor farmyard. New museum gallery in
C17th thatched barn in farmyard designed
with access. Avebury Manor, just behind
the Museum is not accessible.

SD ⬧ CP ⬧ E ⬧ RF ⬧ S ⬧ WC ⬧

SALISBURY
Built on the junction of the rivers Avon
and Nadder, the city's history dates back to
C13th when the bishop's see was moved
from old Sarum and the famous
cathedral's foundations were laid here in
1220. It has been a market town since its
inception. There is much of interest in the
streets, flanked by gabled houses and in
buildings of all periods set in comfortable
juxtaposition. See C16th facade of Joiner's
Hall in St. Ann Street; C17th Shoemaker's
Guildhall: C15th Poultry Cross in Silver
Street, etc.

TOURIST INFORMATION CENTRES
Fish Row, Salisbury SP1 1EJ
Tel: (01722) 234956   Fax: (01722) 422059
Also at Salisbury Station (summer
months).
SALISBURY DISTRICT COUNCIL
Bourne Hill, Salisbury SP1 3UZ
Tel: (01722) 434373

SALISBURY INFORMATION AROUND DISABILITY (SID)
3 Priory Square, The Maltings, Salisbury SP1 1BD
Tel: (01722) 416189
General information on all aspects of
disability, very helpful.

BUSES
Wilts and Dorset: Tel: (01722) 336855
Some low-floor buses
Wiltshire County Council Bus line:
Tel: (0345) 090899

TAXIS
Value Cars: Tel: (01722) 505050
Seven adapted vehicles.

TRAINS
South West Trains: Special Needs:
Tel: (0845) 6050440
Minicom: (0845) 6050441
web: www.swtrains.co.uk
Wales & West: Special Needs:
Tel: (0845) 3003005
Minicom: (0845) 585469

CAR PARKS
2 hours free parking in city council-owned
car parks, free unlimited orange badge
spaces. If staying with a resident, a free
parking permit may be obtained.
Tel: (01722) 713000

SHOPMOBILITY
The Maltings Car Park, Malthouse Lane,
Salisbury.
Tel/Fax: (01722) 328068

HOTEL
GRASMERE HOUSE HOTEL
70 Harnham Road, Salisbury SP2 8JN
Tel: (01722) 338388   Fax: (01722) 333710
No. of Accessible Rooms: 4. Bath
Accessible Facilities: Lounge, Restaurant,

Garden. Victorian family residence, set in 1.5 acres of mature gardens laid largely to lawn, with towering beech trees and small woodland fir copse. Built in 1896 of red brick with attractive pointed filials on the roof gables. Converted and extended with ambience of comfortable Victorian home.

ROSE & CROWN
Harnham Road, Salisbury SP2 8JQ
Tel: (01722) 399955 Fax: (01722) 339816
No. of Accessible Rooms: 3. Bath
Accessible Facilities: Lounge, Restaurant.
Charming hotel located by the River.

BED AND BREAKFAST
WEBSTERS
11 Hartington Road, Salisbury SP2 7LG
Tel/Fax: (01722) 339779
e-mail: websters.salis@eclipse.co.uk
No. of Accessible Rooms: 1. Roll-in Shower
Accessible Facilities: Lounge, Dining Room
1996 Holiday Care Service Award winner.
Situated in cul-de-sac on end of colourful Victorian terrace.

ATTRACTION
SALISBURY CATHEDRAL
33 The Close, Salisbury SP1 2EJ
Tel: (01722) 555120 Fax: (01722) 555716
e-mail: headvisits@aol.com
Built between 1220 and 1258, a medieval masterpiece of Early English Gothic architecture with an elegant spire, the tallest in England at 123m. Artefacts include one of the original Magna Carta documents and probably the oldest working clock in the world, c.1386.
Accessibility leaflet available.
WARNING: ENTRANCE RAMPED AT 1:8.
THE BUILDING HAS BEEN INCLUDED BECAUSE OF ITS IMPORTANCE.

SD ☐ CP ☐ E n/a C ☐ S ☐ WC ☐

SALISBURY AND SOUTH WILTSHIRE MUSEUM
The King's House, 65 the Close, Salisbury SP1 2EN
Tel: (01722) 332151 Fax: (01722) 325611
e-mail:
museum@salisburymuseum.freeserve.co.uk
One of several beautiful buildings in Cathedral Close, with fascinating displays including galleries on Stonehenge, Early Man, History of Salisbury, Pitt Rivers

collection, ceramics and Wedgwood room. Good summer exhibitions.

SD ☐ CP ☐ E ☐ RF ☐ C ☐ S ☐ WC ☐ RFE ☐

WILTON HOUSE
The Estate Office, Wilton, Salisbury SP2 0BJ
Tel: (01722) 746720 Fax: (01722) 744447
e-mail: Tourism@Wiltonhouse.com
web: www.wiltonhouse.com
Set in 21 acres of landscaped parkland, Wilton House is the famous family home of the 17th Earl of Pembroke and considered one of the premier houses of England. The Palladian-style house contains a fine art collection, Victorian laundry and Tudor kitchen. Setting for scenes from Sense and Sensibility and Mrs. Brown. Video in Visitor Centre provides introduction to house and family. Grounds include Palladian bridge, Woodland Walk and Old English Rose Garden.

SD ☐ CP ☐ E ☐ RF ☐ C ☐ S ☐ WC ☐ RFE ☐

WARMINSTER
Situated 130m. above sea-level, above the valley of the Wylye, the town grew rich from the manufacture of cloth and the sale of wheat. There are Georgian houses and cottages and some lovely inns in this rather graceful town.

TOURIST INFORMATION CENTRE
Central Car Park, Warminster BA12 9BT
Tel: (01985) 218548 Fax: (01985) 846154

ATTRACTION
STOURTON HOUSE FLOWER GARDEN
Stourton, Zeals, Warminster BA12 6QF
Tel: (01747) 840417
4-acre plant lovers' garden lies hidden just before the car park of Stourhead House (NT). Grassy paths lead through the 12 Apostles walk, through hedged borders, ponds, and varied vistas of colourful shrubs, trees and unusual plants.

SD ☐ CP ☐ E ☐ RF ☐ C ☐ S ☐ WC ☐ RFE ☐

YORKSHIRE

YORKSHIRE – NORTH AND EAST

YORKSHIRE TOURIST BOARD
312 Tadcaster Road, York YO2 2HF
Tel: (01904) 707961   Fax: (01904) 701414
E-mail: mkt@yorkshire-tourist-board.org.uk

EAST RIDING OF YORKSHIRE TOURISM
County Hall, Beverley HU17 9BA
Tel: (01482) 885035   Fax: (01482) 884851

WHEELCHAIR HIRE
ABLE LIVING CENTRE
3 Enterprise Complex, Walmgate, York
Tel: (0500) 432158
Manual and powered wheelchairs available
for hire.

NORTH YORK MOORS NATIONAL PARK
North York Moors National Park,
The Old Vicarage, Bondgate,
Helmsley YO6 5BP
Tel: (01439) 770657   Fax: (01439) 770691
Bleak, but glorious wide open spaces and
panoramic views across the heather
moorland and out to sea. Wheelchair hire.

Pickering Tourist Information Centre
Eastgate Car Park. Tel: (01751) 473791

Flintoft Ironmongers
22 Hungate. Tel: 01751 472202

Park and View
Cowhouse Bank. 3 miles north of
Helmsley on Bransdale Road. No
restroom.
Newgate Bank. 6 miles north-west of
Helmsley on B1257. No adaptive
restroom.
Clay Bank. 3 miles north of Chop Gate on
B1257. Refreshments, no restroom.
Sheepwash. 2 miles north of Osmotherley
on Swainby Road.
Hazel Heads. 3 miles north-west of
Helmsley on Osmotherly Road. No
restroom.
Peak Scar. 3 miles north of Sutton Bank.
No restroom.

Helmsley Bank. 4.5 miles north of
Helmsley on road to Baxtons. No
restroom.
Thimbley Moor and **Chequers.** Both are
on the road to Osmotherly from Hawnby.
Carlton Bank. 1 mile south-east of
Carlton-in-Cleveland on the road to Chop
Gate. Café.
Rudland Rigg. 6 miles north-north-west of
Kirkbymoorside. On road to Bransdale
from Kirkby there are several viewing
places.
Gillamoor, Surprise View. In Gillamoor
village, 3 miles north of Kirkbymoorside,
by the side of the church.
Saltergate Bank. 7/5 miles north-east of
Pickering on A169. No restroom.
Blue Bank. 1 mile south of Sleights on
A169. No restrooms.
Bell Heads. Nr. Hackness at top of steep
hill on road to Silpho. No restroom.
Highwood Brow. Forest Enterprise car
park. No restroom.
Scaling Dam. 7 miles west of Sandsend on
A1717 at Scaling Reservoir. Facilities for
angling for the disabled. Enquiries, call
01287 640214. Restroom.
Ravenscar. Roadside lay-by. Restroom.
Sandsend. Car park at foot of Lythe Bank,
fronting onto sea. Ramp access to sandy
beach.
Runswick Bay. Car park in village with sea
views.
Whitby. Abbey Plains car park. Follow
signs from Whitby to the abbey.

Public restrooms with disabled facilities:
Farndale, Hutton-le-Hole, Goathland,
Grosmont Station, Kildale, Thornton-le-
Dale, Low Dalby, Staindale Lake (Dalby
Forest), Kirkbymoorside, Pickering
(Ropery and Eastgate Car Parks), Coxwold,
Newton-under-Roseberry, Ravenscar,
Danby Moors Centre, Sutton Bank,
Swainby, Scaling Dam, Helmsley
(Cleveland Way Car Park and Borogate).

Accessible Trails and Paths
Farndale. Daffodil path suitable from Low
Mill car park. Able-bodied companion
recommended.
Mulgrave Woods, Sandsend. Parking at
East Row Car Park, walk borders two steep

ravines reaching almost to the sea. Mixed woodland, meadow and beckside glade.
Cawthorn Roman Camps, Nr. Cropton. Only short part of archaeological trail is accessible, but possible to see earth ramparts of the most westerly of the camps.

Cleveland Way National Trail
110 miles long, running from Helmsley around the North York Moors to Saltburn and along the coast to Filey. The accessible routes below spread throughout the length of the walk. These routes have compact hard surface or are fairly smooth with compact earth/short even grass and a gradient of not more than 1/20. Remember to take your RADAR key with you.
Sutton Bank, Nr. Thirsk. From Thirsk take A170 towards Scarborough. Visitor Centre is at the top of Sutton Bank on the left, about 7 miles beyond Thirsk. Go south for 1.5 miles towards the Kilburn White Horse, or north for 0.5 mile to overlook Lake Gormire. Both walks start from Visitor Centre (accessible restroom) car park. For walk south, follow stone path towards Bank and cross road. Walk follows escarpment edge along smooth stone surface to finish at White Horse. Going north, head for escarpment and turn right. Path remains flat and smooth as far as views over Lake.
Hambleton Drove Road, Nr. Kepwick. Kepwick is north-east of Thirsk. Turn off A19 at Knayton, 3 miles north of Thirsk. Follow signs to Kepwick, and carry straight on up steep and climbing hill, ignoring sign saying no motor vehicles. There are 2 gates along this road that must be opened before reaching start of walk. Park beyond top gate on reaching the moor and head downhill on gentle grass slope. This is a linear moor land walk of 0.65 mile, there and back. You will reach the ruins of Limekiln House after 0.33 mile.

BEDALE
An important meeting point since Saxon times, Bedale flourished as a thriving country town, particularly at the height of the coaching era. With its long, curving High Street, flanked by Georgian buildings

and a market cross at its centre, Bedale forms the gateway to the Yorkshire Dales.

TOURIST INFORMATION CENTRE
(Open Easter-end September)
Bedale Hall, North End, Bedale DL8 1AA
Tel: (01677) 424604   Fax: (01677) 427146

SELF-CATERING ACCOMMODATION
ELMSFIELD HOUSE COTTAGES
Arrathorne, Bedale DL8 1NE
Tel: (01677) 450558   Fax: (01677) 450557
No. of Accessible Units: 2. Roll-in Shower
No. of Beds per Unit: 3
Accessible Facilities: Open plan Kitchen, Dining Room, Lounge.
Cottages adjacent to country guest house.

ATTRACTION
BEDALE MUSEUM
Beadale Hall, Bedale DL8 1AA
Tel/Fax: (01677) 422037
Building of C17th with famous exhibit of 1742 fire engine. Artefacts give interesting account of the lives of ordinary people.
SD   CP   E   RF

BROUGH
A coaching town in the last century. Brough is at the foot of the long ascent over Stainmore, with a castle dating from C11th. The National Trust has a protected area to the north, Musgrave Fell, which is a limestone pavement.

BED AND BREAKFAST
RUDSTONE WALK
South Cave, Brough HU15 2AH
Tel: (01430) 422230   Fax: (01430) 424552
e-mail: office@rudstone-walk.co.uk
web: www.rudstone-walk.co.uk
No. of Accessible Rooms: 3. Roll-in Shower/Bath. Accessible Facilities: 400-year-old farmhouse forms the heart of this property, with cottages, including adapted Woodland Cottage, converted from the farm buildings adjacent to the house, where meals are served. Set in its own grounds and wooded hills, overlooking the Vale of York. Located a few miles from historic Beverley, and 1.5 miles from the village of South Cave.

DARLINGTON

Busy town, renowned for locomotives and known as the cradle of railways although locomotive engineering shops were closed in 1966.

TOURIST INFORMATION CENTRE
13 Horsemarket, Darlington DL1 5PW
Tel: (01325) 388666

TRAINS
Great North Eastern Railway: Special Needs:
Tel: (0845) 7225444
Mincom: (0191) 2330173
Virgin Trains: Special Needs:
Tel: (0845) 7443366
Minicom: (0845) 7443367

HOTEL ACCOMMODATION
ST. GEORGE AIRPORT HOTEL
Teesside Airport, Darlington DL2 1RH
Tel: (01325) 332631
Fax: (01325) 333851
No. of Accessible Rooms: 1
Accessible Facilities: Restaurant, Lounge/Bar. Originally the officer's mess on site of WWII bomber airfield of Middleton St. George, now converted into a modern hotel.

BED AND BREAKFAST
CLOW-BECK HOUSE
Monkend Farm, Crofton-on-tees, Darlington DL2 2SW
Tel: (01325) 721075
Fax: (01325) 720419
e-mail: ifanet@cityscape.co.uk
web: www.clowbeckhouse.co.uk
No. of Accessible Rooms: 1
Accessible Facilities: Lounge (1 step), Dining Room. Charming country residence, set in rolling countryside and deriving its name from the Beck, winding its way through the farm to the River Tees. Dinner also available.

GRASSINGTON

This Wharfedale village is very appealing: its buildings crowd around a small market place paved with cobblestones and along irregular passages. The river is crossed by a stone bridge of 1603. There are numerous prehistoric sites here.

SELF-CATERING
THE BARN
21A Broughton Fold, Grassington BD23 5AL
Tel: (01756) 753037
To book: Call Mrs. Evans on
(01274) 561546
No. of Accessible Units: 1. Bath,
No. of Beds per Unit: 1D/1S
Accessible Facilities: Lounge/Dining Room, Kitchen, Garden, secluded, south facing with patio.
Ground floor cottage forming part of converted Dales barn, situated in quiet private part of the village square.

HARROGATE

A stately and genteel town in a high and airy location with spacious parks, an abundance of trees and lavish flower beds. Famous for fine shopping and rich teas, Edwardian and Victorian buildings in its centre and its annual flower show that is a social must.

TOURIST INFORMATION CENTRE
Royal Baths Assembley Rooms, Crescent Road, Harrogate HG1 2RR
Tel: (01423) 537537
Fax: (01423) 537305

BUSES
Local bus and rail information:
Tel: (0113) 2457676
Harrogate District Travel:
Tel: (01423) 507227

TAXIS
Blueline Cars: Tel: (01423) 530830
Eight adapted vehicles.
Central Radio Cabs: Tel: (01423) 505050
Five adapted vehicles, two minibuses.

TRAINS
Northern Spirit: Special Needs:
Tel: (0845) 6008008

CAR PARKS
Free unlimited orange badge parking, either in car parks or off-street.

SHOPMOBILITY
10th floor, Victoria Car Park, Harrogate
Tel: (01423) 500666

HOTEL
HARROGATE MOAT HOUSE   🚶
Kings Road, Harrogate HK1 1XX
Tel: (01423) 849988   Fax: (01423) 524435
No. of accessible Rooms: 1. Bath
Accessible Facilities: Lounge, Restaurant.
Quality town-centre hotel.

SELF-CATERING
HELM PASTURE COTTAGES   🚶
Hartwith Bank, Summerbridge,
Harrogate HG3 4DR
Tel: (01423) 780279   Fax: (01423) 780994
No. of Accessible Units: 6. Bath
No. of Beds per Unit: 2 - 10
Accessible Facilities: Open plan
Lounge/Dining Room/Kitchen
Scandinavian lodges in woodland
overlooking the Nidd Valley.

ATTRACTION
HARLOW CARR BOTANICAL GARDENS
Crag Lane, Harrogate HG3 1QB
Tel: (01423) 565418   Fax: (01423) 530663
68 fine acres of ornamental and woodland
gardens with craft weekends throughout
the summer.

SD ♿   CP ♿   E ♿   RF ♿   C ♿
S n/a   WC 🚶   RFE ♿

RIPLEY CASTLE
Ripley, Harrogate HG3 3AY
Tel: (01423) 770152   Fax: (01423) 771745
e-mail: ripleyestate@ripley castle.co.uk
Home of the Ingilby family, dating from
1320s in extensive Capability Brown
designed estate. Fine paintings, furnishings
and Civil War memorabilia. Home to the
National Hyacinth collection.

SD ♿   CP ♿   E ♿   RF ♿
C ♿   S 🚶   WC ♿   RFE - Gardens 🚶

HELMSLEY
Helmsley lies in a hollow of the River Rye,
an excellent gateway to Ryedale and the
North Yorkshire Moors. The view dropping
into it from the south takes in the red-
roofed house, spacious market square,
pinnacled church tower and the gaunt
shell of Helmsley Castle.

TOURIST INFORMATION CENTRE
Town Hall, Market Place, Helmsley YO6 5DL
Tel: (01439) 770173
web: www.ryedale.gov.uk

SELF-CATERING
ANGEL COTTAGE   🚶
Wheatfield, Newton Grange,
Oswaldkirk YO62 5YE
Tel/Fax: (01439) 788493
No. of Accessible Units: 1. Roll-in Shower
No. of Beds per Unit: 4
Accessible Facilities: Lounge,
Kitchen/Diner
Holiday cottage 3 miles from Helmsley.

ATTRACTION
NUNNINGTON HALL (NT)
Nunnington, Nr. Helmsley YO62 5UY
Tel: (01439) 748283   Fax: (01439) 748284
C16th. country manor house with panelled
rooms and a superb staircase, plus display of
the Carlisle collection of miniature rooms.

SD ♿   CP 🚶   E ♿   RF 🚶   C 🚶
S 🚶   WC 🚶   RFE 🚶

RIEVAULX TERRACE AND TEMPLES (NT)
Rievaulx, Helmsley YO61 5LJ
Tel: (01439) 748283   Fax: (01439) 748284
Firm gravel path through woodland or
wheelchair route straight onto Terrace.
Picnic along elegant half-mile created over
300 years ago. Superb views of Rievaulx
Abbey and landscape of Hambleton Hills.
Two C18th. classical temples, neither
accessible inside, but well worth a look.
Pre- book Battericar or wheelchair.

SD ♿   CP ♿   E ♿   S ♿

INGLETON
At the north-west extreme of Yorkshire,
with hills and moors above the village
showing weathered limestone outcrops so
typical of the area. There are 5 pubs and 3
cafes with reasonable access.

TOURIST INFORMATION CENTRE
Community Centre Car Park, Ingleton LA6 3HG
Tel: (015242) 41049

BED AND BREAKFAST
RIVERSIDE LODGE
24 Main Street,
Ingleton, via Carnforth LA6 3HJ
Tel: (015242) 41359
No. of Accessible Rooms: 2. Shower
Accessible Facilities: Lounge, Restaurant,
Country guesthouse with conservatory
with beautiful views, level access to top
garden, sauna, games room (the latter two
on lower ground floor, accessible from
outside with 1 step, then 3 steps).

KINGSTON-UPON-HULL
Severely damaged during WWII, with
modern, rather unexciting buildings
combining with the lawns, flower-beds and
pools of Queens Gardens. Third largest
port in UK, its docks run for
seven miles along the north bank of the
Humber, and the country's largest
fishing operation.

HULL TOURISM
1 Paragon Street, Kingston-upon-Hull HU1 3NA
Tel: (01482) 223559
web: www.hull700.co.uk

HOTEL
QUALITY ROYAL HOTEL
170 Ferensway, Hull HU1 3UF
Tel: (01482) 325087   Fax: (01482) 323172
No. of Accessible Rooms: 2. Bath
Accessible Facilities: Lounge, Restaurant
Located in city centre.

ATTRACTION
BURTON CONSTABLE HALL
Burton Constable, Sproatley, Nr. Hull HU11 4LN
Tel: (01964) 562400 Fax: (01964) 563229
Lovely Elizabethan house built in 1570
with fine reception rooms and Tudor long
gallery and much Chippendale furniture.
200-acre park designed by Capability
Brown. Located a few miles NW of Hull.

SD   CP   E   RF   L
C   S   WC   RFE

KIRBYMOORSIDE
Just off the Pickering-Helmsley road, its
main street climbs steeply toward the hills.

On the Vivers hill behind the church are
the sketchy remains of a Norman castle.
Fine Georgian houses in its broad main
street and a cobbled market square.

BED AND BREAKFAST
THE CORNMILL
Kirby Mills, Kirbymoorside, York YO62 6NP
Tel: (01751) 432000   Fax: (01751) 432300
e-mail: cornmill@kirbymills.demon.co.uk
web: www.kirbymills.demon.co.uk
No. of Accessible Rooms: 1. Roll-in Shower
Accessible Facilities: Lounge/Bar, Dining
Room. Renovated C18th watermill and
farmhouse with glass-floored dining room
over millrace. Accommodation in annexed
Victorian farmhouse.

LEYBURN
A broad mile-long terrace shaded with
evergreens, oaks and sycamores allows fine
views over Wensleydale. Among other landmarks are Bolton and Middleham castles.

TOURIST INFORMATION CENTRE
4 Central Chambers, Railway Street,
Leyburn DL8 5BB
Tel: (01969) 623069 Fax: (01969) 622833

HOTEL ACCOMMODATION
EASTFIELD LODGE
1 St. Matthews Terrace, Leyburn DL8 5EL
Tel: (01969) 623196
No. of Accessible Rooms: 1. Bath
Accessible Facilities: Lounge, Restaurant.
Private hotel, built in mid-1800s, in lovely
Wensleydale with attractive south-facing
public rooms and garden.

GOLDEN LION HOTEL
Market Place, Leyburn DL8 5AS
Tel: (01969) 622161   Fax: (01969) 623836
No. of Accessible Rooms: Several (via
accessible lift)
Accessible Facilities: Dining Room (1 step),
Bar. Dating from 1765, a traditional family
hotel of 15 rooms. Ideal base for exploring
Yorkshire Dales.

MALTON
Historic centre of Ryedale since Roman

times. North of Roman fort site at Orchard Fields is the original town of Old Malton, in the centre of which stands a fragment of St. Mary's the only Gilbertine Priory in use in England. Traditional agricultural town, holding thrice-weekly cattle market.

MALTON TOURIST INFORMATION CENTRE
58 Market Place, Malton YO17 7LW
Tel: (0800) 137233

RYEDALE TOURISM NORTH YORKSHIRE
Rydedale District Council, Rydedale House, Malton YO17 0HH
Tel: (01653) 600666   Fax: (01653) 696801
web: www.fyedale.gov.uk

ATTRACTION
EDEN CAMP MODERN HISTORY THEME MUSEUM
Malton YO17 6RT
Tel: (01653) 697777   Fax: (01653) 698243
e-mail: admin@edencamp.co.uk
The People's War, a fascinating range of WWII exhibits on the Home Guard, Street at War, U-Boat Menace, Prisoners of War, Civil Defence, The Blitz etc. Also six new exhibitions on military and political events complementing the civilian story.

| SD | CP | E | RF |
| C | S | WC | RFE |

MALTON MUSEUM
Town Hall, Market Place, Malton YO17 0LT
Tel: (01653) 695136
Well known for its rich archaeological collection, there are depictions of the famous Roman settlements in the area, particularly of the Roman fort at Derventio.

| SD | CP | E | RF | S |

MIDDLESBROUGH
Large town, administrative centre of Teesside with several museums and galleries.

TOURIST INFORMATION CENTRE
(Open April-end October)
High Green Car Park, Great Ayton, Middlesbrough TS9 6BJ
Tel: (01642) 722835

ATTRACTIONS
CAPTAIN COOK BIRTHPLACE MUSEUM

Stewart Park, Marton, Middlesbrough TS7 6AS
Tel: (01642) 311211   Fax: (01642) 813781
Unique perspective on the life and times of Captain James Cook through this superb museum with films, special effects, inter-active hands-on exhibits about Cook's three great voyages. Discover the creaking timbers, the perils of the ocean and the recordings of artists and scientists among the strange plants and animals of the South Seas and the Americas. Superb in content and access. Not to be missed. NB. Entrance is through The Grove, not the main car park.

| SD n/a | CP | E | RF | C |
| S | WC | L | | |

ORMESBY HALL (NT)
Church Lane, Ormesby, Middlesbrough TS7 9AS
Tel: (01642) 324188
Fax: (01642) 300937
e-mail: yorkor@smep-ntrust.org.uk
C18th. Palladian mansion, noted for plasterwork and carved wood decoration.

| SD | CP | E | RF |
| C | S | WC | RFE |

NORTHALLERTON
Set in the rich farmland of the Vale of Mowbray, Northallerton is the county town with elegant redbrick buildings. It has a long history and a town trail points out sites and buildings with historical connections. The Church of All Saints at the north end of the High Street dates from 1120 and just outside the town a memorial stone marks the site of the Battle of the Standard.

TOURIST INFORMATION CENTRE
Applegarth, Northallerton DL7 8LZ
Tel/Fax: (01609) 776864

HERRIOT COUNTRY TOURISM
Hambleton District Council, Civic Centre, Stone Cross, Northallerton, DL6 2UU
Tel: (01609) 767110   Fax: (01609) 780017

BED AND BREAKFAST
LOVESOME HILL FARM
Lovesome Hill, Northallerton DL6 2PB

Tel: (01609) 772311
No. of Accessible Rooms: 1. Shower
Accessible Facilities: Dining Room.
Dinner is available. 165-acre working farm
four miles north of Northallerton with
accommodation in granary conversion,
Granary Mill is accessible. Fine touring
base being between Yorkshire Dales and
North Yorkshire Moors.

PICKERING
Reputed to be one of the oldest towns in
the area dating back to 270BC. Skyline
dominated by fine spire of the Church of
St. Peter and St. Paul. Hidden high above
the town are the ruins of Pickering Castle.
Narrow streets lead off in all directions,
the market place straggling along the hilly
main street.

TOURIST INFORMATION CENTRE
Eastgate Car Park, Eastgate, Pickering YO18 7DB
Tel: (01751) 473791

SELF-CATERING
MOONPENNY COTTAGE   ♿
Levisham, Pickering YO18 7NL
Tel: (01751) 460311
No. of Accessible Units: 1. Shower
No. of Beds per Unit: 2
Accessible Facilities: Lounge, Dining Room,
Kitchen, Patio, Garden. Tourist board
award-winning renovation of a Grade II
listed C18th farm, preserving its historic
character. The village is full of stone-built
houses and wide grass verges along a main
street, surrounded by moorland and forest.

CLOTH FAIR COTTAGE   ♿
Rawcliffe House Farm, Stape,
Nr. Pickering YO18 8JA
Tel: (01751) 473292 Fax: (01751) 473766
e-mail: sheilarh@yahoo.com
No. of Accessible Units: 1. Roll-in Shower
No. of Beds per Unit: 2
Accessible Facilities: Kitchen, Lounge,
Dining Room. The farm is set in 42 acres
of rolling pasture and wild flower meadows
in heart of North York Moors National
Park. Three cottages converted from old
stone barns are arranged around stone
courtyard.

BYRE COTTAGE AND DAIRY HOUSE   ✠
Manor Farm, Newton upon Rawcliffe,
Pickering YO18 8QA
Tel: (01751) 472601
No. of Accessible Units: 2. Bath
No. of Beds per Unit: Byre - 3: Dairy - 6
Accessible Facilities: Byre – Kitchen,
Lounge/Diner: Dairy – Kitchen/Diner,
Lounge. Stone-built cottages in small,
unspoilt village cluster of stone farms
around village green and duckpond. Much
of interest within easy reach.

ATTRACTION
RYEDALE FOLK MUSEUM
Hutton-le-Hole, Nr. Pickering YO6 6UA
Tel/Fax: (01751) 417367
Open air museum with 13 historic buildings
showing the lives of ordinary people from
earliest times to tnow. Roman artefacts.
Saxon stone crosses, medieval crofter's
cottage and an Elizabethan manor house
combine with C18th Stangend, a Victorian
Cottage and a C20th Edwardian studio.

SD ♿	CP n/a	E ♿	RF ♿
S ♿	WC ♿	RFE ♿	

REDCAR
Holiday resort for Teesside with 3 beaches
and long rocky reefs running out to sea that
are left bare, but for seaweed at low tides.

TOURIST INFORMATION CENTRE
West Terrace, Esplanade, Redcar TS10 3AE
Tel: (01642) 471921

SPORTING VENUE
REDCAR RACECOURSE
Redcar TS10 2BG
Admin & Booking-Box Office: (01642) 484068
Fax: (01642) 488272
Open venue with large open concourse
served by tarmac walkways and areas
providing free movement to facilities.
CP ♿   RE ♿   ED ♿ (No door entrance,
through gates adjoining Main entrance)
INT ♿   L ♿
WC ♿ (3 sites at centre of course, behind Tattersalls and
in Members' Paddock Rooms)
SS ♿ (1 space in viewing area)
B/R - Ground floor facilities have level access: first floor
accessed by manned lift.

RICHMOND

Set dramatically at the entrance to steep-sided Swaledale. Striking ruined Norman fortress on its sheer rock. Large, cobbled market place surrounded by an easy blend of Georgian and Victorian stone buildings.

TOURIST INFORMATION CENTRE
Friary Gardens, Victoria Road,
Richmond DL104AJ
Tel: (01748) 850252

BED AND BREAKFAST
MOUNT PLEASANT FARM ⬚🚶
Whashton, Richmond DL11 7JP
Tel: (01748) 822784
No. of Accessible Rooms: 1. Shower
Accessible Facilities: Lounge, Dining Room. The accessible Piggery Room is one of several cottage style rooms in a converted stable on a working farm of sheep and beef cattle. The stone farmhouse of 1850 is situated in rolling countryside 3 miles from Richmond and just outside peaceful Whashton, with fine views of Vale of York.

SPORTING VENUE
CATTERICK RACECOURSE
Catterick Bridge, Richmond
Admin & Booking-Box Office: (01748) 811478
Fax: (01748) 811082
Complies with Part M, Building Regulations Open venue with open concourses served by tarmac walkways providing free movement to enclosures and facilities.

CO ♿   RE ♿   ED ♿ (except manual door)
INT ♿   L ♿
WC ♿ (1 site in Gods Solution Bar)
SS ♿ (1 space only in viewing area, no seating in stands)
B/R ♿

RIPON

Small market town with great cathedral and rectangular market place.

TOURIST INFORMATION CENTRE
Minster Road, Ripon HG41LT
Tel: (01765) 604625 (Seasonal)

SELF-CATERING
MULBERRY LODGE ♿🚶
Book through holidays for You & Me.

Lacon Hall, Sawley, Nr. Ripon HG4 3EE
Tel: (01765) 620658
No. of Accessible Units: 1. Roll-in Shower
No. of Beds per Unit: 1,D.
Accessible Facilities: Open plan Lounge/Diner/Kitchen
Lacon Hall dating from c1600, is in lovely countryside. Mulberry Lodge is a charming stone cottage within the old courtyard.

SWALLOW COTTAGE 🚶
Moor End Farm, Knaresborough Road,
Littlethorpe, Ripon HG4 3LU
Tel: (01765) 677419
No. of Accessible Units: 1. Shower
No. of Beds per Unit: 2
Accessible Facilities: Lounge/Diner, Kitchen. Detached cottage recently converted from an old byre, retaining old trusses and beams, located on small working sheep farm. Set in its own courtyard adjacent to main farmhouse. Three miles from Ripon.

ATTRACTION
BLACK SHEEP BREWERY VISITOR CENTRE
Wellgarth, Mashon, Ripon HG4 4EN
Tel: (01765) 689227   Fax: (01765) 689746
e-mail: visitor.centre@blacksheep.co.uk
The brewhouse and fermenting rooms included in the Brewery Tour, make the whole tour inaccessible, but wheelchair users can see a video of the brewing process, a and history explained by a tour guide. Ingredients are shown and tasted by visitors, smell the hops and taste the malts. Good photographic display of the whole process.

SD ♿   CP ♿🚶   E ♿   RF ♿
C ♿   S ♿   WC 🚶

THE NIDDERDALE MUSEUM
King Street, Pately Bridge, Nr. Ripon HG3 5LE
Tel: (01423) 711225
10 rooms illustrating past local life including Victorian sitting room and kitchen, schoolroom and cobblers' shop.

SD ♿   CP 🚶   E ♿   RF ♿
L-Stair lift from ground floor entrance to first floor.
WC ♿🚶   RFE-See lift
Wheelchair available on first floor to tour museum all on one level

285

SCARBOROUGH

Big, breezy North Sea resort that combines castle ruins, a fishing village, working port, luxury hotels, boarding houses, sands, terraced gardens, long wave-swept promenades, views and carnival-style amusements. Scarborough is built below and on top of a cliff with steep steps, footpaths and lifts connecting the parts.

SCARBOROUGH AND DISTRICT DISABLEMENT ACTION GROUP
Allatt House, 5/6 West Parade,
Scarborough YO12 5ED
Tel/Fax and Minicom: (01723) 379397
e-mail: scardag@onyxnet.co.uk
scardag@onyxnet.co.uk
Produces Travelling Around. Very helpful.

TOURIST INFORMATION CENTRE
Unit 3, Pavilion House, Valley Bridge Road,
Scarborough YO11 2UZ
Tel: (01723) 373333   Fax: (01723) 363785

SCARBOROUGH, WHITBY AND FILEY TOURISM
Londesborough Lodge, The Crescent
Scarborough, YO11 2PW
Tel: (01723) 369151   Fax: (01723) 376941

SCARBOROUGH MOBILITY CENTRE
8/9 Hanover Road, Scarborough
Tel: (01723) 500045
Manual wheelchairs available for hire.

WHEELCHAIR HIRE
St. Mary's Hospital, Dean Road
Scarborough.
Tel: (01723) 353177
Manual wheelchairs available for hire.

Quality Life Mobility: Tel: (01482) 506030

BUSES
East Yorkshire Motor Services:
Tel: (01482) 327142
Some low-floor buses.

TAXIS
Station Taxis: Tel: (01723) 366366
Eight adapted vehicles.

TRAINS
Northern Spirit: Special Needs:
Tel: (0845) 6008008

CAR PARKS
Three-hour free parking in the city centre, free unlimited further hour. Council-owned car parks charge.
Tel: (01723) 373333

HOTEL
THE GRAINARY HOTEL   ♿
Keasbeck Hill Farm, Harwood Dale,
Scarborough YO13 9DT
Tel/Fax (01723) 870026
No. of Accessible Rooms: 4. Roll-in Shower
Accessible Facilities: Lounge, Restaurant
Family run hotel on 200-acre mixed farm in the heart of the National Park. Located midway between Scarborough and Whitby.

THEATRE
STEPHEN JOSEPH THEATRE
Westborough, Scarborough YO11 1JW
Admin: (01723) 370540
Booking-Box Office: (01723) 370541
Minicom: (01723) 370555
Fax: (01723) 360506
Complies with Part M, Building Regulations.
CP ♿   RE ♿   ED ♿ (except Manual Door)
INT ♿   L ♿
WC ♿ (2 sites on 1st floor, 1 on 2nd floor)

SETTLE

Narrow streets, tiny courtyards and fine Georgian houses contribute to an interesting townscape in this picturesque centre for touring in an area of great limestone hills and crags, across the Ribble from Giggleswick.

TOURIST INFORMATION CENTRE
Town Hall, Cheapside, Settle BD24 9EJ
Tel: (01729) 825192

ATTRACTION
YORKSHIRE DALES FALCONRY AND CONSERVATION CENTRE
Crows Nest, Nr. Giggleswick, Settle LA2 8AS
Tel: (01729) 822832 Fax: (01729) 823160
Privately owned falconry centre with many species of birds of prey from around the

world: eagles, vultures, hawks, falcons and owls in natural habitats. Regular free-flying demonstrations, the star attraction being an Andean Condor, the largest bird in the world. Children's Area, Hawk Walk, bird feeding and educational talks.

| SD [♿] | CP [♿] | E [♿] | RF [♿] |
| C [♿] | S [♿] | WC [♿] | RFE [♿] |

SKIPTON

A good gateway to Wharfedale, the town has charming old houses and courtyards, an old toll-booth and stocks in Sheep Street. Very lively market four times a week, a medieval church and a beautiful castle.

TOURIST INFORMATION CENTRE
The Old Town Hall, 9 Sheep Street, Skipton BD23 1JH
Tel: (01756) 792809

HOTEL
CRAVEN HEIFER INN [♿]
Grassington Road, Skipton BD23 3LA
Tel: (01756) 792521 Fax: (01756) 794442
e-mail: philandlynn@cravenheifer.co.uk web: www.cravenheifer.co.uk
No. of Accessible Rooms: 1. Shower
Accessible Facilities: Lounge, Restaurant. Traditional dales country inn serving ales and home cooked food with adjoining barn converted to a selection of rooms.

BED AND BREAKFAST
HIGH FOLD [♿]
Kettlewell, Skipton BD23 5RJ
Tel: (01756) 760390
No. of Accessible Rooms: 2. Roll-in Shower
Accessible Facilities: Lounge, Dining Room.

SELF-CATERING
THE GHYLL COTTAGES [♿]
Dalegarth, Buckden, Skipton BD32 5JU
Tel/Fax: (01756) 760877
e-mail: dalegarth@aol.com
web:www.yorkshirenet.co.uk/acgde/dalegarth
No. of Accessible Units: 3. Roll-in Shower
No. of Beds per Unit: 4 - 6
Accessible Facilities: Lounge, Dining Room, Kitchen, Spa Bath, Indoor Pool with ramped entrance, assistance required with steps. National award-winning cottages

offering tranquillity with wonderful views of Dales National Park.

CAWDER HALL COTTAGES [♿]
Cawder Lane, Skipton BD23 2QQ
Tel: (01756) 791579 Fax: (01756) 797036
No. of Accessible Units: 1. Shower or Bath
No. of Beds per Unit: 4-5
Accessible Facilities: Living Room, Kitchen. The Smithy is 1 of 5 traditional farm buildings now converted. Peaceful rural setting, surrounded by fields and moorland. A mile from Skipton

ATTRACTION
BOLTON ABBEY GARDENS
Bolton Abbey, Skipton BD23 6EX
Tel: (01756) 710533 Fax: (01756) 710535
e-mail: boltonabbey@dalesweb.co.uk
Bolton Abbey Estate has been in the family of the Dukes of Devonshire since 1754, providing 75 miles of footpaths through wonderful scenery of moorland, woodland and riverside with walks for all ages and abilities. There are three car parks, we have selected the most accessible:

BOLTON ABBEY VILLAGE CAR PARK:
From the village green head north along the main road (no pavement), Turn down drive marked No Cars. On reaching the priory door proceed around the north side to avoid obstacles. Firm path. No steps into church.

| SD [♿] | CP [♿] | E [♿] | RF [♿] |
| S [♿] | WC [♿] | RF [♿] | |

STRID WOOD CAR PARK:
The Cumberland Trail is accessible, it winds through the wood with resting places and viewing platform overlooking Barden Beck. Fully accessible bird hide.

| SD [♿] | CP [♿] | S [♿] | WC [♿] | TRAIL [♿] |

THIRSK

Small market town, prosperous in medieval times as evidenced by a large, cobbled market place, and also in Georgian times, with many houses still standing on Kirkgate. Known to many as James Herriot's town, Thirsk is closely associated with this famous author vet, and the surgery where the real Mr. Herriot worked can be seen in Kirgate. Horse racing has been popular here since C18th. Sutton Bank, housing the National Park Visitor Centre, is reached via the A170 with a 1:4 incline as it climbs 170m, to offer incredible views across the Vale of York to the Pennines.

TOURIST INFORMATION CENTRE
14 Kirkgate, Thirsk YO7 1PQ
Tel: (01845) 522755   Fax: (01845) 526230
(Seasonal)

SUTTON BANK VISITOR CENTRE
Sutton Bank, Thirsk YO7 2EK
Tel: (01845) 597426

BED AND BREAKFAST
DOXFORD HOUSE
73 Front Street, Sowerby, Thirsk YO7 1JP
Tel/Fax: (01845) 523238
No. of Accessible Rooms: 1. Bath
Accessible Facilities: Lounge, Dining Room. Comfortable Georgian guest house overlooking village greens.

ATTRACTION
FALCONRY UK
Sion Hill Hall, Kirby Wiske,
Nr. Thirsk YO7 4EU
Tel: (01845) 587522   Fax: (01845) 523735
web: www.falconry.co.uk
Birds of prey centre where eagles, hawks and owls swoop and dive around you in a lovely English garden. Skilled handlers explain all there is to know. The flying displays and information on breeding and training programmes is fascinating.

SD 🔵   CP 🔵   E 🔵   RF 🔵
C 🔵   S 🔵   WC 🔵   RFE 🔵

WHITBY
Charming town on the coast,with the Esk emptying into the sea. It divides the town, connected by a swing bridge. Associated with seagulls, the smell of fish, the sight of red roofs up the steep banks from the quay, and above the ruin of the C7th. Abbey on the cliff. Captain Cook served an apprenticeship here in 1746.

WHITBY AND DISTRICT DISABLEMENT ACTION GROUP
Church House, Flowergate, Whitby YO21 3BA
Tel: (01947) 821991
TOURIST INFORMATION CENTRE
Langbourne Road, Whitby TO21 1YN
Tel: (01947) 602674

SELF-CATERING
THE BYRE
Millinder House, Westerdale, Whitby YO21 2DE
Tel: (01287) 660053
No. of Accessible Units: 1. Roll-in Shower
No. of Beds per Unit: 5
Accessible Facilities: Lounge/Diner, Kitchen. Cottage in courtyard

CAPTAIN COOK'S HAVEN
Larpool Lane, Whitby UO22 4JE
Tel: (01947) 601396   Fax: (01947) 893573
No. of Accessible Units: 1. Roll-in Shower
No. of Beds per Unit: 4
Accessible Facilities: Open plan Lounge/Kitchen
Resolution Bungalow is in a modern cottage complex located on the Esk, a mile from Whitby.

YORK
Normans, Saxons and Danes preceded our own Plantagenets for whom York became the commercial capital of the north. Although much restored, the city's fine walls are mainly C14th, though fragments of Norman work still survive. Medieval York is everywhere, not least in the web of narrow streets. The city contains England's greatest concentration of medieval stained glass, mainly in York Minster, Britain's largest Gothic building. Start a city tour here, visit the Shambles or walk around the walls to Exhibition Square and Museum Street and then the Jorvik Centre.

YORK TOURISM BUREAU
20 George Hudson Street, York YO1 6WR
Tel: (01904) 554488   Fax: (01904) 554460
e-mail: yt@york-tourism.co.uk
web: www.york-tourism.co.uk

TOURIST INFORMATION CENTRES
The de Grey Rooms, Exhibition Square,

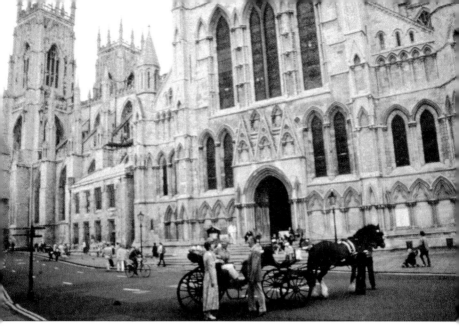

Masterful York Minster seems almost bigger inside.

York YO1 2HB
Tel: (01904) 621756

Railway Station, Outer Concourse,
York YO2 2AY
Tel: (01904) 621756

TIC Travel Office, 6 Rougier Street,
York YO2 1JA
Tel: (01904) 620557

YORK DISABILITY RIGHTS
Tel: (01904) 638467

BUSES
General Enquiries: Tel: (01904) 551400
Also includes train information.

TAXIS
Station Taxis: Tel: (01904) 554455
Five adapted vehicles.
K Jibb: Tel: (01904) 654500
Two adapted vehicles.
A & P Transport: Tel: (01904) 471300
Seven adapted minibuses.

TRAINS
Great North Eastern Railway: Special Needs:
Tel: (0845) 7225444

Minicom: (0191) 2330173
Northern Spirit : Special Needs:
Tel: (0845) 6008008
Virgin Trains: Special Needs:
Tel: (0845) 7443366
Minicom: (0845) 7443367
York and Selby Line (York-Leeds):
Tel: (0345) 484950
See also under BUSES.
York Station has disabled parking bays,
disabled WCs, underpass tunnel to far
platform. Also accessible via lifts,
Minicom telephones available, automatic
doors into ticket office/travel
information.

CAR PARKING
Limited orange badge parking for 3 hours.
Much of York is pedestrianised.
Tel: (01904) 613161

SHOPMOBILITY
2nd Floor, Piccadilly Car Park, the
Coppergate Centre, Piccadilly, York
Tel/Fax: (01904) 679222

WHEELCHAIR HIRE
Able Living, Unit 3, Enterprise Complex,
Walmgate, York
Tel: (01904) 611516

HOTELS

SWALLOW HOTEL YORK
Tadcaster Road, Dringhouses, York YO2 2QQ
Tel: (01904) 701000   Fax: (01904) 702308
No. of Accessible Rooms: 2. Bath
Accessible Facilities: Lounge, Restaurant, Lift, Beauty Salon. Quality hotel near the racecourse.

NOVOTEL YORK
Fishergate, York YO1 4AD
Tel: (01904) 611660   Fax: (01904) 610925
No. of Accessible Rooms: 4
Accessible Facilities: Lounge, Restaurant, Pool. Modern hotel a mile from city centre.

CLIFTON BRIDGE HOTEL
Water End, Clifton, York YO30 6LL
Tel: (01904) 610510   Fax: (01904) 640208
No. of Accessible Rooms: 3. Bath
Accessible Facilities: Lounge, Restaurant
Private hotel opposite Homestead Park and beside the river. 0.5 mile from city centre.

JARVIS INTERNATIONAL HOTEL
Shipton Road, Skelton, York YO3 6XW
Tel: (01904) 670222   Fax: (01904) 670311
web: www.jarvis.co.uk

No. of Accessible Rooms: 2. Bath
Accessible Facilities: Lounge, Restaurant
Very spacious Georgian country house, modernised, but retaining many original features, in six acres of grounds. All public areas easily accessed. Located close to A19 York ring road and A1. 2.5 miles from York city centre.

HEWORTH COURT HOTEL
76 - 78 Heworth Green, York YO3 7TQ
Tel: (01904) 425156   Fax: (01904) 415290
e-mail: hotel@heworth.co.uk
web: www.heworth.co.uk
No. of Accessible Rooms: 2, in courtyard, ground floor.
Accessible Facilities: Restaurant, Bar
Charming family run hotel within 1 mile of city centre. Located off A1036 Malton Road

SAVAGES HOTEL
St. Peter's Grove, Clifton, York YO3 6AQ
Tel: (01904) 610818
No. of Accessible Rooms: 1. Bath
Accessible Facilities: Lounge, Restaurant
Victorian hotel in peaceful tree-lined street close to city centre and attractions.

STAKIS YORK HOTEL
1 Tower Street, York YO1 1SB
Tel: (01904) 648111
No. of Accessible Rooms: 3. Bath
Accessible Facilities: Lounge, Restaurant. Well situated within city walls, close to the Minster, the Shambles and main attractions.

SELF-CATERING
YORK LAKESIDE LODGES
Moor Lane, York YO24 2QU
Tel: (01904) 702346   Fax: (01904) 701631
Mobile: (01831) 885824
No. of Accessible Units: Several
No. of Beds per Unit: Willow - 6/8:
Beech - 4/6
Accessible Facilities: Willow Lodge (Cat.2) has Roll-in Shower. Lounge/Diner Kitchenette. Beech Lodges. Some are Cat.3 with Lounge/Diner, Kitchenette.
Family owned and run, these attractive

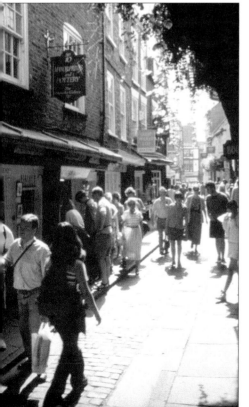

Early shopping mall –the Shambles.

lodges are situated along one side of a 10-acre lake, facing south with fine views over the water. Reached via south outer ring road (A64), close to Tesco and Park & Ride.

ATTRACTIONS

JORVIK VIKING CENTRE
Coppergate, York YO1 9WT
Tel: (01904) 643211   Fax: (01904) 627097
e-mail: jorvik@jvcyork.demon.co.uk
web: www.jorvik-viking-centre
Jorvik was the Viking name for York and the centre takes you on a journey from audio-visual introduction, on time-cars (one is accessible for wheelchairs) from WWII back to Norman times and then a full-scale reconstruction of the C10th. Coppergate where remarkable discoveries were made, and the dig of the 1970s. Voices speak in old Norse language and the smells and sounds give an authentic air. NOT TO BE MISSED.
NB. Although the centre does not have parking facilities, there are disabled spaces at Piccadilly car park within easy reach of the centre and with its own Shop Mobility department. Piccadilly is at a right angle to Coppergate. Free orange badge parking.

SD n/a   CP n/a   E 🦽   RF 🦽   L 🦽
C 🦽   S 🦽   WC 🚹   RFE 🦽

MERCHANT ADVENTURERS' HALL
Fossgate, York YO1 9RD
Tel/Fax: (01904) 654818
e-mail: The.Clerk@mahall-york.demon.uk
Medieval, mid C14th guild hall where merchants carried out business with early furniture, paintings and other artefacts. Also an Undercroft (ramped) where the poor were cared for.

SD 🦽   CP n/a   E 🚹   RF 🚹
WC 🚹   RFE 🚹

NATIONAL RAILWAY MUSEUM
Leeman Road, York YO26 4XJ
Tel: (01904) 621261   Fax: (01904) 631319
e-mail: nrm@nmsi.ac.uk
web: www.nmsi.ac.uk/nrm
The story of the train. From Stephenson's rocket and giant steam trains to Eurostar and miniature railways, rail is brought to life with interactive displays and exhibitions.

SD 🦽   CP 🦽   E 🦽   RF 🦽   L 🦽

C 🦽   S 🦽   WC 🚹

THE ORIGINAL GHOST WALK OF YORK
C/o King's Arms Pub, Ouse Bridge, York
Tel/Fax: (01759) 373090
e-mail: york@talk21.com
This is a guided tour around the city, i.e. outdoors, leaving the pub at 22.00 every night. The walk aims to be accurate and authentic, exploring a world of folklore, legend and dreams. Guides will amend the route to avoid steps.

SD 🦽   CP n/a (street parking adjacent to pub)

YORK CITY ART GALLERY
Exhibition Square, York YO1 2EW
Tel: (01904) 551861   Fax: (01904) 551866
e-mail: art.gallery@york.gov.uk
600 years of superb paintings represented here by Bellotto, Lowry and Nash, plus a fine pottery collection. Stairlift to upper collections of Victorian and modern paintings and modern stoneware pottery.

SD 🦽   CP n/a Nearest CP in Marygate   E 🦽
RF 🦽   L 🦽   S 🦽   WC 🚹

YORK MINSTER
Deangate, York YO1 7HH
Tel: (01904) 557216   Fax: (01904) 557218
The minster was built between 1220 and 1472, although parts of a previous Norman church survive in the building. It is the largest medieval church north of the Alps, and renowned for its original stained glass. The main area of the minster is on one level. There is a ramped facility into the choir area, but crypt is not accessible to wheelchairs that are available on loan. NB. Call in advance.

SD 🦽   CP 🚹 (NE side of the Minster)
E 🦽 (Chapter House Yard)
RF 🚹   S 🚹   WC 🚹

BURNBY HALL GARDENS
The Balk, Pocklington, York YO42 2QF
Tel: (01759) 302068
Age Concern award winner. 7 wonderful acres of park and garden with fine varieties of trees and shrubs, a picnic area and lakes. National collection of water lilies is here. 14 miles east of York.

SD 🦽   CP 🦽   E 🦽   RF 🦽
C 🦽   S 🦽   WC 🦽

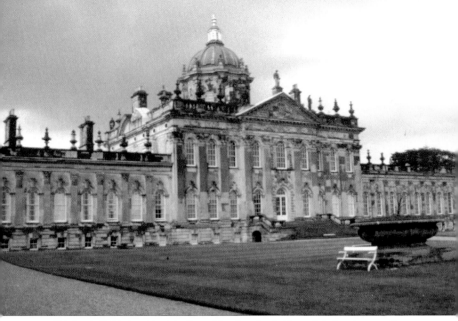

TV classic 'Brideshead Revisited' was filmed at Castle Howard during the seventies.

CASTLE HOWARD

Castle Howard Estate Office, York YO60 7DA
Tel: (01653) 648444   Fax: (01653) 648501
e-mail: admin@castlehoward.demon.co.uk

C18 palace designed by Vanbrugh, with 2 original Vanburgh rooms. He later created Blenheim Palace. Built for the 3rd Earl of Carlisle, Charles Howard, his descendants still call it home. An immense painted and gilded dome tops the facade and the interior contains richly furnished rooms and a superb family chapel that is not accessible. 1,000 acres of gardens.

Near Malton, 15 miles from York off A 64. Stable courtyard entrance adjacent to car park with 4 shops, cafeteria and WC. Land train, ramped with 2 wheelchair places, transports visitors to the house that is 300m from the courtyard along a difficult gravel path. Surrounded by grass it should be fine in summer, but could be difficult in winter. If in doubt, take the land train. Main area also has cafeteria, a shop and WC. Main floor of house accessed through the shop, round to main staircase and up by Stannah Chairlift, staff member always on duty to assist. Once on main floor, surfaces flat, wooden or tiled.

SD   CP   E   RF   C [♿]
S [♿]   WC [♿]   G [♿]

SPORTING VENUE
YORK RACECOURSE

The Knavesmire, York YO23 1EX
Admin & Booking-Box Office: (01904) 620911
Fax: (01904) 611071

CP [♿] (D2 Car park outside Stands Enclosure near Paddock Gates)   RE [♿]
WC [♿] (4 sites at Course Enclosure, Silver Ring, County and Melrose Stands)
SS - Silver Ring [♿]. Raised race viewing platform
Tattersalls - Access to Stand and Parade Ring. Raised viewing platform
County Stand - Raised viewing platform
Parade Ring - raised viewing platform

THEATRE
YORK THEATRE ROYAL

St. Leonard's Place, York YO1 2HD
Admin: (01904) 658162
Fax: (01904) 611534
Booking-Box Office: (01904) 623568

SD [♿]
CP [♿] Public CP-Marygate. Taxi Rank-around corner.
RE [♿]   ED [♿]   INT [♿]
WC [♿] (ground floor). AUD [♿]
B/R [♿] accessed via disabled lift..
Add. Notes: access straight through front doors to Stall doors, 1.5m from doors to spaces.

YORKSHIRE – SOUTH AND WEST

KIRKLESS FEDERATION OF DISABLED PEOPLE
Zetland Street, Huddersfield HD1 2RA
Tel: (01484) 435838 Fax: (01484) 450739

METROLINE
Tel: (0113) 2457676
Minicom: (0113) 2428888
web: www.ukbus.u-net.co.uk
Bus and trains times in West Yorks.

BARNSLEY
Positioned in the exact centre of the
Yorkshire coalfield. A huge market that
started in 1249 is still held weekly on the
original town centre site.

SPORTING VENUE
BARNSLEY FOOTBALL CLUB
Oakwell Stadium, Barnsley S71 1ET
Admin & Booking-Box Office: (01226) 211211
Fax: (01226) 211444
e-mail: thereds@barnsleyfc.co.uk
web: www.barnsleyfc.co.uk
Complies with Part M, Building Regulations.
CP 🦽   RE 🦽   ED 🦽   INT 🧍
WC 🦽 (4 units, close to disabled seating areas)
SS 🦽 Route via Entrance 1 to Welcome and Ora Stands,
via Entrance 33, turn right to Ora Stand
B/R 🧍 (Access via lift)

BATLEY
ATTRACTION
BAGSHAW MUSEUM
Wilton Park, Batley WF17 0AS
Tel: (01924) 326155 Fax: (01924) 326164
Victorian Gothic mansion in wooded park.
Collections include Life and death in Egypt
in the Kingdom of Osiris.
SD 🦽   CP 🧍   E 🧍   RF 🦽
WC 🦽   RFE 🧍

OAKWELL HALL GARDEN
Nutter Lane, Birstall, Batley WF17 9LG
Tel: (01924) 326240 Fax: (01924) 326249
The hall is not accessible, but the country
park with a wildlife garden is.
SD n/a   CP 🧍   RF 🦽   S 🦽
WC 🧍   RF 🦽

BRADFORD
In its prime, the town was the world's
largest producer of worsted cloth and
much of the town looks confidently
Victorian, but there is considerable new
building. Bradford was the first town to
have a variety of educational services, such
as school meals and a nursery school, plus
a municipal hospital.

TOURIST INFORMATION CENTRE
Central Library, Prince's Way,
Bradford BD1 1NN
Tel: (01274) 753678

HOTEL
NOVOTEL BRADFORD   🧍
Merrydale Road, Bradford BD4 6SA
Tel: (01274) 683683   Fax: (01274) 651342
No. of Accessible Rooms: 2. Bath
Accessible Facilities: Open plan
Lounge/Bar, Restaurant.
One of first Novotels to be built in Britain,
recently undergoing refurbishment: three
miles from the city centre.

ATTRACTION
THE COLOUR MUSEUM
Perkin House, 1 Providence Street,
Bradford BD1 2PW
Tel: (01274) 390955 Fax: (01274) 392888
e-mail: museum@sdc.org.uk
Britain's only Museum of Colour with 2
galleries full of exhibits on the effects of
light and colour-optical illusions and the
story of dyeing and textile printing.
There is no setting down point nor car
park, all else is varyingly accessible.
SD n/a   CP n/a   E 🧍   RF 🦽
L 🦽   S 🦽   WC 🦽   FRE 🦽

DONCASTER
Modern town, transformed from an
agricultural to an industrial centre by the
arrival of the railway in 1848. Ringed by
mining villages, it now manufactures
agricultural equipment and the famous
butterscotch.

TOURIST INFORMATION CENTRE
Central Library, Waterdale, Doncaster DN1 3JE
Tel: (01302) 734309

HOTELS

DONCASTER MOAT HOUSE 🚶
Warmsworth, Doncaster DN4 9UX
Tel: (01302) 799988   Fax: (01302) 310197
No. of Accessible Rooms: 3. Roll-in Shower.
Accessible Facilities: Lounge, Restaurant
Near A1M (J36), close to Earth Centre and
several cultural/art/industrial sites.

MOUNT PLEASANT HOTEL 🚶
Great North Road, Rossington,
Doncaster DN11 0HP
Tel: (01302) 868696   Fax: (01302) 875130
No. of Accessible Rooms: 14. Bath.
Accessible Facilities: Lounge, Restaurant
Former estate house for Rossington Hall.
This family-owned, Georgian house stands
in 100 acres of private wooded parkland.

ATTRACTION

DONCASTER MUSEUM AND ART GALLERY
Chequer Road, Doncaster DN1 2AE
Tel: (01302) 734293   Fax: (01302) 735409
Home to collections of the Kings Own
Yorkshire Infantry and a wide variety of
decorative art and sculpture.

| SD ♿ | CP 🚐♿ | E ♿ | L ♿ |
| S ♿ | WC ♿ | | |

SPORTING VENUE

DONCASTER RACECOURSE
The Grandstand, Leger Way, Doncaster DN2 6BB
Admin & Booking-Box Office:
(01303) 320066   Fax: (01302) 323271

CP 🚐♿	RE ♿	ED ♿	L 🚶
WC 🚶 (10 units)			
SS ♿ (Disabled stand position by winning post)			
B/R 🚐♿			

HALIFAX

Built on the cloth trade from C13th. The
town is set in the Pennine foothills, rising
on steep hills from Hebble Brook, and is
largely C19th in appearance.

TOURIST INFORMATION CENTRE
Piece Hall, Halifax HX1 1RE
Tel: (01422) 368725

ACCESS FOR ALL IN CALDERDALE
Calderdale Borough Council,
Tourist Information Centre,

1 Bridge Gate, Hebden Bridge HX7 8EX
Tel: (01422) 843831
web: www.calderdale.gov.uk
Information on access to public buildings
in Halifax, Brighouse, Elland, Hebden
Bridge, Sowerbybridge and Todmorden.

ATTRACTION

EUREKA! THE MUSEUM FOR CHILDREN
Discovery Road, Halifax HX1 2NE
Tel: (01422) 330069   Fax: (01422) 330275
e-mail: Eureka-Museum@compuserve.com
First hands-on museum in Britain
designed for children up to 12. Touch,
listen, smell and look at four main areas -
Me and My Body, Living and Working
Together, Invent, Create, Communicate
and Things.

SD ♿	CP 🚐♿	E ♿	RF ♿
L ♿	C ♿	S ♿	
WC ♿ (hinged support rail 30cm from seat centre)			
RFE ♿			

HAWORTH

Home to the Bronte family, the village is
all grey-stone houses, slate roofs and
smoking chimney pots. The main street,
paved with stones, and requiring a strong
pusher, struggles up a very steep bank. Near
the top the street widens into a little square
with the Black Bull Hotel, where Branwell
Bronte drank. At the top is the parsonage, the
Bronte's home, behind lies moorland and a
hint of the windswept isolation recalled from
the Bronte sisters' writings. The parsonage is
not accessible, and the village a tourist spot,
but it is very evocative and not to be missed.

TOURIST INFORMATION CENTRE
2-4 West Lane, Haworth BD22 8EF
Tel: (01535) 642329

BRONTE COUNTRY TOURISM – See Keighley.

SELF-CATERING

STABLE COTTAGE 🚐♿
West Field Farm, Tim Lane, Haworth BD22 7SA
Tel: (01535) 644568   Fax: (01535) 646686
e-mail: c.p.pickles@bradford.ac.uk
web: www.webscape.co.uk/farmaccom/
england/Yorkshire_dales/westfield/
No. of Accessible Units: 1. Roll-in Shower

No. of Beds per Unit 2. One of 5 cottages converted from old farm buildings in an elevated south position near the village. Stunning views. NB: Steep hill to village centre, requires powered wheelchair or car.

HUDDERSFIELD

Extremely hilly town covering a spectacular site in the Colne Valley on the edge of the Pennines. Huddersfield has been the centre of textile production for centuries, and the town is still famous for worsted, and more recently, music.

TOURIST INFORMATION CENTRE
3-5 Albion Street, Huddersfield HD1 2NW
Tel: (01484) 223200

ATTRACTION
KIRKLEES LIGHT RAILWAY
Park Mill Way, Clayton West, Nr. Huddersfield HD8 8SX
Tel/Fax: (01484) 865999
3 steam locomotives operating on narrow 37cm gauge railway running through gently rolling farmland for 4 miles. Picnic facilities provided at both ends.
CARRIAGES CANNOT TAKE WHEELCHAIRS
From platform to carriages there is one step, approx. 200m high.

| SD ♿ | CP 🚶 | E ♿ | RF ♿ |
| C 🚶 | S 🚶 | WC 🚶 | RFE 🚶 |

TOLSON MEMORIAL MUSEUM
Ravensknowle Park, Wakefield Road, Huddersfield HD5 8DJ
Tel: (01484) 223830   Fax: (01484) 223843
Discover Huddersfield's past from the tools of earliest settlers to modern collections from local people. Ground floor galleries on one level or shallow ramp. First floor has 2 short flights of steps (3 steps) and a Stannah stairlift.

| SD ♿ | CP ♿ | E-(REAR) 🚶 | RF 🚶 |
| C 🚶 | S 🚶 | WC 🚶 | |

KEIGHLEY
BRONTE COUNTRY TOURISM
Cedar House, Aire Valley Business Centre, Lawkholme Lane, Keighley BD21 3DD
Tel: (01535) 670700   Fax: (01535) 671373

e-mail: espencer@brontecountry.co.uk
web: www.brontecountry.co.uk

ATTRACTIONS
CLIFFE CASTLE MUSEUM AND PARK
Spring Gardens Lane, Keighley BD20 6LH
Tel: (01535) 618231   Fax: (01535) 610536
Completed in 1833 in Elizabethan style, the owner re-constructed the castle and grounds from a wide range of medieval architectural styles in 1875. Permanent displays on the local area including its natural history, minerals and domestic, social, agricultural and industrial bygones.

| SD ♿ | CP ♿ | E ♿ | RF ♿ |
| C 🚶 | S 🚶 | WC 🚶 | RFE 🚶 |

VINTAGE RAILWAY CARRIAGE MUSEUM
Ingrow Railway Centre, Keighley BD22 8NJ
Tel: (01535) 680425   Fax: (01535) 646472
e-mail: vct@mwdjcope.demon.co.uk
web: www.neotek.demon.co.uk/vct/
Unique display of historic railway carriages with sound presentations bringing the story to life. Railway memorabilia available in large shop.

| SD ♿ | CP 🚶 | E ♿ | RF ♿ |
| S ♿ | WC 🚶 | RFE ♿ | |

LEEDS

Spread over a large, hilly area, the town centres on Victoria Square. The Town Hall is a successful example of classic revival architecture. Briggate Street offers examples of the typical Leeds arcades, with delightful glass-roofed passages lined with shops.

GATEWAY YORKSHIRE REGIONAL TOURIST INFORMATION CENTRE
The Arcade, Leeds City Station, Leeds LS1 1PL
Tel: (0800) 808050
web: www.leeds.gov.uk

BUSES
Black Prince Coaches: Tel: (0113) 2532305
Some low-floor buses.
First Leeds: Tel: (0113) 2451602
Some low-floor buses.
Metroline: Tel: (0013) 2457676
Minicom: (0113) 2428888
web: www.ukbus.u-net.co.uk
All information on buses and trains.

TAXIS

Streamline: Tel: (0113) 2443322
40 adapted vehicles.
Telecabs: Tel: (0113) 2792222
20 adapted vehicles.
City Cabs: Tel: (0113) 2469999
5 adapted vehicles.

TRAINS

Midland Mainline: Special Needs:
Tel: (0114) 2537654
Minicom: (0845) 7078051
Northern Spirit: Special Needs:
Tel: (0845) 6008008
Great North Eastern Railway: Special Needs:
Tel: (0845) 7225444
Minicom: (0191) 2330173
Virgin Trains: Special Needs:
Tel: (0845) 7443366
Minicom: (0845) 7443367

CAR PARKS

Free unlimited orange badge parking in all
council car parks, 4 free hours in marked
bays, some on-street parking
Tel: (0113) 2477500

SHOPMOBILITY

White Rose Shopping Centre, Dewsbury Road,
Leeds LS11 8LU
Tel: (0113) 2773636   Fax: (0113) 2291122

61 Vicar Lane, Leeds LS1 6BA
Tel/Minicom: (0113) 2460125

HOTEL

HILTON NATIONAL LEEDS CITY
Neville Street, Leeds LS1 4BX
Tel: (0113) 2442000   Fax: (0113) 2433577
No. of Accessible Rooms: 1
Accessible Facilities: Restaurant, Lounge
(3rd Floor), Lift. Bright, modern hotel
adjacent to railway station.

CROWNE PLAZA HOTEL
Wellington Street, Leeds LS1 4DL
Tel: (0113) 244 2200 Fax: (0113) 2440460
Web: www.crowneplaza.com
No. of Accessible Rooms: 4
Accessible Facilities: Restaurant,
Lounge/Bar (first floor via accessible lift).
Quality hotel located in city centre.

ATTRACTION

LOTHERTON HALL
Rangers Office, Stable Courtyard,
Lotherton Hall Estate, Towton Road,
Nr. Aberford, Leeds LS25 3EB.
Tel/Fax: (0113) 2813068
Rebuilt in present form during Victorian
and Edwardian times, Lotherton was
owned by the Gasgoigne family until given
to Leeds City Council in 1968. The hall,
despite its rich collection, retains a family
ambience – the type of home we would all
love to live in. Beyond delightful bird and
formal gardens, the estate offers lovely
countryside walks. The hall is accessed by 3
steps. The ground-floor flat and wide
corridors, formal gardens, paths and
countryside walks and bird garden.

SD ♿	CP ♿	RF ♿	C ♿
S ♿	WC ♿	Hall ♿	G ♿

MIDDLETON RAILWAY
The Station, Moor Road, Hunslet,
Leeds LS10 2JQ
Tel: (0113) 2710230
e-mail: howill@globalnet.co.uk
World's oldest working railway, established
by the first British Railway Act of Parliament
in 1758. Built to carry coal from the mines
of Middleton to Leeds Bridge. Steam trains
run each weekend in the season.

SD ♿	CP ♿	E ♿	RF ♿
C ♿	S ♿	WC ♿	RFE ♿

ROYAL ARMOURIES
Armouries Drive, Leeds LS10 1LT
Tel: (0113) 2201890   Fax: (0113) 2201955
e-mail: enquiries@armouries.org.uk
web: www.armouries.org.uk
Experience 3,000 years of history through
this famous collection of arms and armour.
Live interpretations, fine displays and
exhibits.

SD ♿	CP ♿	E ♿	RF ♿
L ♿	C ♿	S ♿	WC ♿

THACKRAY MEDICAL MUSEUM
Beckett Street, Leeds LS9 7LN
Tel: (0113) 244 4343   Fax: (0133) 247 0219
e-mail: medical_museum@msn.com
The story of health care and medicine told
through audio-visual displays,
reconstructions, and hands-on exhibits

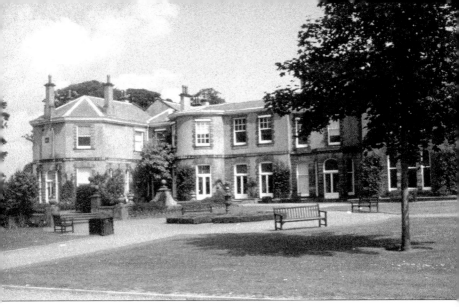

The imposing Lotherton Hall.

showing how developments and improvements have transformed our lives.

SD 🦽　CP 🦽　E 🦽　RF 🦽
L 🦽　C 🚶　S 🦽　WC 🦽

THWAITE MILLS MUSEUM
Thwaite Lane, Stourton, Leeds LS10 1RP
Tel: (0113) 249 6453 Fax: (0133) 2776737
Water-powered mill whose enormous cogs crushed stone for putty and paint during C19th. The Georgian mill-owner's house has been restored, displays tell the mill's history.

SD 🦽　CP 🚶　E 🦽　RF 🦽
S 🚶　WC 🚶

THEATRE
WEST YORKSHIRE PLAYHOUSE
Playhouse Square, Quarry Hill, Leeds LS2 7UP
Tel: (0113) 2137800 Fax: (0113) 2137250
Web: www.wyp.com
Box Office: Tel: (0113) 2137700. Minicom: (0113) 2137299 Fax: (0113) 2137210
Complies Part M, Building Regulations.

CP 🚶　RE 🚶　ED 🦽 (except Manual Door)
INT 🦽　L 🦽　WC 🚶
AUD 🚶　Quarry – lift (in foyer) to level 1, access to Row H via disabled entrance. Courtyard - as above but accessed through main theatre doors.
B/R 🦽　all accessed by lift, low level counters in restaurant and low-level tables.

SPORTING VENUE
LEEDS UNITED FOOTBALL CLUB
Elland Road. Leeds LS11 0ES
Admin & Booking-Box Office: (0113) 2266000

CP 🦽　RE 🦽　ED 🦽 (except Manual Door)
INT 🦽　L 🦽　WC 🦽　SS 🦽 (West Stand Paddock 40 spaces & helper seating and 80 ambulant spaces: North Stand 25 spaces & helper seating and 58 ambulant spaces: South West Corner 26 spaces & helper seating and 40 ambulant spaces: Family Stand 10 spaces & helper seating. Route through either NW tunnel or up low gradient ramp in SW corner)　B/R 🦽　DISABLED LOUNGE open 1.5 hours prior to kick off, tea/coffee at subsidised rate.

PONTEFRACT
There are some fine C18th and C19th buildings and the town is famous for the liquorice in its Pontefract Cakes.

SPORTING VENUE
PONTEFRACT RACECOURSE
Administration: 33 Ropergate, Pontefract WF8 1LE
Admin & Booking-Box Office: (01977) 703224 Fax: (01977) 600577
Booking: As above
Complies with Part M, Building Regulations
CP 🦽　RE 🦽　Gate adjacent Paddock Ent.
Second Enclosure not accessible, Third Enclosure open to

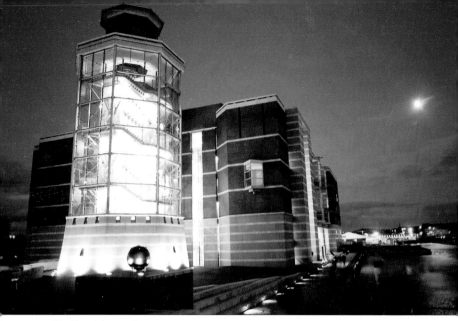

The Royal Armouries.

cars at a charge.   ED ⬛♿

INT ⬛♿ Access along back of both Main Stands which connect all Enclosures.

WC ⬛🚶 (2 sites, in Club and in Paddock by Main Stairs).

SS ⬛♿ No. special viewing area. Enclosures pronounced slope provides good all-round visibility but some obstacles for those with mobility problems.

B/R ⬛♿

ROTHERHAM

Coal mines, iron, steel, brass and glass works dominate its situation in the Don Valley. There has been much rebuilding in recent years, but some of the medieval street plan remains.

TOURIST INFORMATION CENTRE
Central Library, 65 Walker Place, Rotherham S65 1JH
Tel: (01709) 823611

HOTEL
HELLABY HALL HOTEL   ⬛♿
Old Hellaby Lane, Hellaby, Rotherham S66 8SN
Tel: (01709) 702701   Fax: (01709) 700979
No. of Accessible Rooms: 2. Bath
Accessible Facilities: Lounge, Restaurant, Pool, Sauna, Whirlpool

Unique C17th building, Flemish in style with baronial reception rooms.

ATTRACTION
ROTHERHAM ART GALLERY/YORKS AND LANCASTER REGIMENTAL MUSEUM
Rotherham Arts Centre, Walker Place, Rotherham S65 1JH
Tel: (01709) 823635   Fax: (01709) 823631
web: www.rma.org.uk
Regularly changing exhibitions of contemporary and fine art.

SD ⬛♿   CP ⬛♿   E ⬛♿   RF ⬛♿
L ⬛♿   C ⬛♿   WC ⬛🚶

SHEFFIELD

England's fourth largest city, still famous for its steel, cutlery, engineering and toolmaking industries, but the city centre is being transformed as work begins on the Heart of the City Millennium project.

TOURIST INFORMATION CENTRE
Peace Gardens, Sheffield S1 2HH
Tel: (0114) 2734571

TRAVELINE
Tel: (01709) 515151
Information on buses, trams and trains

BUSES
First Mainline: Tel: (01709) 566000

TAXIS
Central Cabs: Tel: (0114) 2769869
30 adapted vehicles.
Shefftax: Tel: (0114) 2720000
30 adapted vehicles

TRAMS
Accessible to wheelchairs.

TRAINS
First North Western: Special Needs:
Tel: (0845) 6040231
Midland Mainline: Special Needs:
(0114) 2537654
Minicom: (0845) 7078051
Virgin Trains: Special Needs: (0845) 7443366
Minicom: (0845) 7443367
Sheffield Station has some lifts, but lots of
stairs and no subways.

CAR PARKING
Free unlimited orange badge parking in
council-owned car parks, some on-street
parking also.

SHOPMOBILITY
Bank Street, Sheffield
Tel: (0114) 2812278   Fax: (0114) 2787173

HOTEL
SHEFFIELD MOAT HOUSE   [人]
Chesterfield Road South,
Sheffield S8 8BW
Tel: (0114) 2829988   Fax: (0114) 2378140
No. of Accessible Rooms: 4. Bath
Accessible Facilities: Lounge, Restaurant,
Bar, Pool. Located near M1 motorway
south of the city.

SPORTING VENUE
SHEFFIELD WEDNESDAY FOOTBALL CLUB
Hillsborough,
Sheffield S6 1SW
Admin: (0114) 2212121 Fax: (0114) 2212122
Booking: Tel: (0114) 2212400
Fax: (0114) 2212401
Complies with part M, Building
Regulations.
CP [人&] (request in advance)   RE [人&]
ED [&] (except Manual Door)

WC [人&] (Located on North Stand)
SS [&] (Westfield Enclosure with ramp access in north
Stand — 56 spaces and helper seating: West Lower
Disabled Enclosure — 32 spaces and helper seating)
B/R [人&] (Ramped/Lift access to some)

WAKEFIELD
City centre is the Bull Ring, redeveloped
with modern shops, but some good
Georgian houses remain on the South and
West parades.

TOURIST INFORMATION CENTRE
Town Hall, Wood Street,
Wakefield WF1 2HQ
Tel: (01924) 305000

ATTRACTIONS
NATIONAL COAL MINING MUSEUM FOR
ENGLAND
New Road, Overton, Wakefield WF4 4RH
Tel: (01924) 848806
Award-winning museum offering visitors
the working world of mining. See the
conditions in a 75cm. seam and meet
genuine pit ponies, now in retirement.
New visitor centre with access.
Underground tour available for wheelchair
users. Contact in advance for details.
SD [&]   CP [人&]   E [&]   RF [&]
C [人]   S [&]   WC [人]

YORKSHIRE SCULPTURE PARK
Bretton Hall, West Bretton,
Wakefield WF4 4LG
Tel: (01924) 830579 Fax: (01924) 830044
e-mail: FES @ysp.co.uk
web: www.ysp.co.uk
Over 200 acres of C18th parkland are used
to display some of the best sculpture in the
country produced by artists worldwide.
Alongside changing exhibitions permanent
features include C19th bronzes by Rodin,
contemporary sculptures and Henry Moore
bronzes in the adjacent 100-acre Bretton
country park. The blend of landscape and
sculpture is extraordinary: the soothing
peace of the countryside arrested and
stimulated by the sight of a single piece of
work alongside sheep, the park's natural
inhabitants. But it works. Not to be
missed! Four scooters and one powerchair

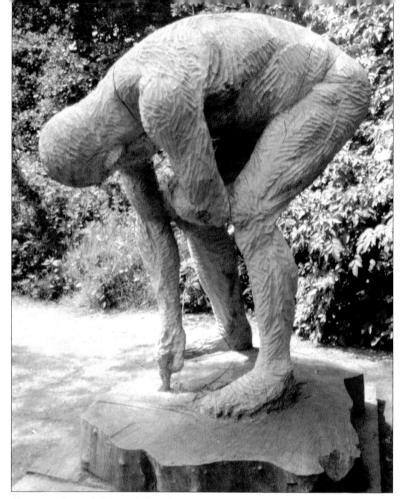

Famous artists and their works have brought monumental acclaim to Wakefield.

for use in the park free of charge from the Information Centre. The main entrance is to be moved early in 2001, to facilitate more disabled parking spaces.

SD [♿]   CP [♿]   C [♿]

E [♿] (Information Centre at Car Park)

S [♿] (Information Centre)

[♿] (Pavilion Gallery Bookshop)

[🚶] (Bothy Shop)   WC - Several [🚶]

RFE [♿] (Access Sculpture Trail)

[♿] Lakeside, Hillside, Driveside, Bothy Garden, Bretton Country Park.

Formal Garden (can be viewed from terrace)

WETHERBY
TOURIST INFORMATION CENTRE
24 Westergate, Wetherby LS22 6NL
Tel: (0113) 247 7251

SPORTING VENUE
WETHERBY RACECOURSE
York Road, Wetherby LS22 5ET
Admin & Booking-Box Office:
(01937) 582035
Fax: (01937) 580565

Complies with Part M, Building Regulations. Open venue with large viewing concourses served by tarmac paths/walkways providing freedom of movement to all enclosures and facilities.

CP [♿]   RE [♿]

ED [♿] through main gate onto centre of course

INT [♿]   L [♿]

WC [♿] (2 sites, rear of Tattersalls Stand and Weighing Room. Further 4 under construction in new members stand)

SS [♿]   B/R [♿]

SCOTLAND

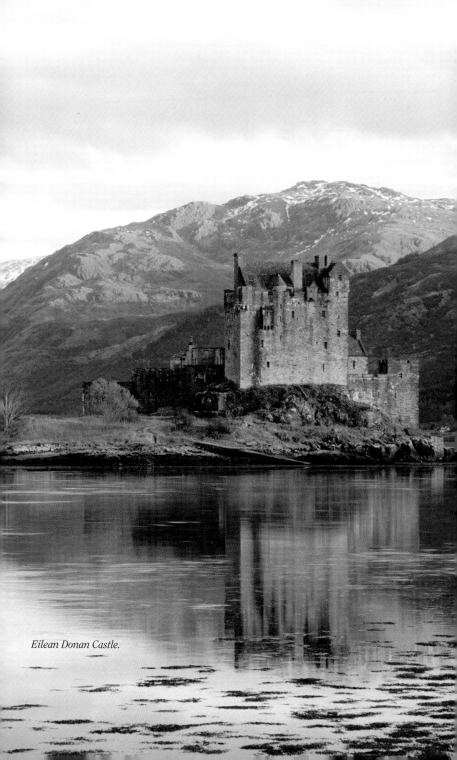

Eilean Donan Castle.

Apart from the Central Information Department, Scotland is now divided into eight areas, some with several tourist boards within each of these regions.

SCOTTISH TOURIST BOARD CENTRAL INFORMATION DEPARTMENT

23 Ravelston Terrace, Edinburgh EH4 3TP
Tel: (0131) 3322433   Fax: (0131) 3431513
web: www.holiday.scotland.net

REGION 1
SOUTH OF SCOTLAND

DUMFRIES and GALLOWAY TOURIST BOARD
64 Whitesands, Dumfries DG1 2RS
Tel: (01387) 245550   Fax: (01387) 245551
e-mail: infor@dgtb.demon.co.uk
web: www.galloway.co.uk

AYRSHIRE and ARRAN TOURIST BOARD
Burns House, Burns Statue Square, Ayr KA7 1UP
Tel/fax: (01292) 262555
Fax: (01292) 288686
e-mail: ayr@ayrshire-arran.com
web: www.ayrshire-arran.com

SCOTTISH BORDERS TOURIST BOARD
Tourist Information Centre, Murray's Green, Jedburgh TD8 6BE
Tel: (01835) 863435/863688
Fax: (01835) 864099
e-mail: info@scot-borders.co.uk

REGION 2
EDINBURGH AND LOTHIANS

EDINBURGH and LOTHIANS TOURIST BOARD
4 Rothesay Terrace, Edinburgh EH3 7RY
Tel: (0131) 4733600   Fax: (0131) 4733626
e-mail: esic@eltb.org
web: www.edinburgh.org

REGION 3
GREATER GLASGOW AND CLYDE VALLEY

GREATER GLASGOW and CLYDE VALLEY TOURIST BOARD

11 George Square, Glasgow G2 1DY
Tel: (0141) 2044400   Fax: (0141) 2213524
e-mail: tourismglasgow@ggcvtb.org.uk
web: www.seeglasgow.com

REGION 4
ARGYLL, THE ISLES, LOCH LOMOND, STIRLING AND TROSSACHS TOURIST BOARD

Dept. SOS, 7 Alexandra Parade, Dunoon, Argyll PA23 8AB
Tel: (01369) 701000   Fax: (01369) 706085
e-mail: infor@scottish.heartlands.org.uk

REGION 5
PERTHSHIRE, ANGUS AND DUNDEE AND THE KINGDOM OF FIFE

ANGUS and CITY OF DUNDEE TOURIST BOARD
7-12 Castle Street, Dundee DD1 3AF
Tel: (01382) 527527   Fax: (01382) 527550
e-mail: arbroath@sol.co.uk
web: www.angusanddundee.co.uk

KINGDOM OF FIFE TOURIST BOARD
70 Market Street, St. Andrews KY16 9NU
Tel: (01334) 472021   Fax: (01334) 478422
web: www.standrews.co.uk

PERTHSHIRE TOURIST BOARD
Lower City Mills, West Mill Street, Perth PH1 5QP
Tel: (01738) 627958   Fax: (01738) 630416
e-mail: perthtouristb@perthshire.co.uk
web: www.perthshire.co.uk

REGION 6
GRAMPIAN HIGHLANDS, ABERDEEN AND THE NORTH EAST COAST

ABERDEEN and GRAMPIAN TOURIST BOARD
27 Albyn Place, Aberdeen AB10 1YL
Tel: (01224) 632727   Fax: (01224) 581367
e-mail: tourism@agtb.org
web: www.agtb.org

REGION 7
THE HIGHLANDS AND SKYE

HIGHLANDS OF SCOTLAND TOURIST BOARD
Peffery House, Strathpeffer, Ross-shire IV14 9HA
Tel: (01997) 423019   Fax: (01997) 421168
e-mail: info@host.co.uk
web: www.host.co.uk

ISLES OF SKY TOURIST BOARD
Bayfield House, Bayfield Road, Portree IV51 9EL
Tel: (014768) 612137   Fax: 901478) 612141

REGION 8
OUTER ISLANDS

WESTERN ISLES TOURIST BOARD
Head Office, 4 South Beach, Stornoway,
Isle of Lewis HS1 2XY
Tel: (0185)1 703088   Fax: (01851) 705244
e-mail: witb@sol.co.uk
web: www.witb.co.uk

ORKNEY TOURIST BOARD
6 Broad Street, Kirkwall, Orkney KW15 1NX
Tel: (01856) 872856   Fax: (01856) 875056
e-mail: orkneytb@csi.com
web: www.orkneyislands.com

SHETLAND ISLANDS TOURISM
Market Cross, Lerwick, Shetland ZE1 0LU
Tel: (01595) 693434   Fax: (01595) 695807
e-mail: shetland.tourism@zetnet.co.uk
web: www.shetland-tourism.co.uk

USEFUL ORGANISATIONS
HISTORIC SCOTLAND
Longmore House, Salisbury Place,
Edinburgh EH9 1SH
Tel: (0131) 6688800   Fax: (0131) 6688888
web: www.historic-scotland.gov.uk

NATIONAL MUSEUMS OF SCOTLAND
Chambers Street, Edinburgh EH1 1JF
Tel; (0131) 2257534   Fax: (0131) 2204819
web: www.nms.ac.uk

SCOTTISH AIRPORTS LTD
St. Andrew's Drive, GLASGOW Airport, Paisley,
Renfrewshire PA3 2SW
Tel: (0141) 8484441

Fax: (0141) 8421412
web: www.baa.co.uk

THE NATIONAL TRUST FOR SCOTLAND
28 Charlotte Square, Edinburgh EH2 4ET
Tel: (0131) 2265922   Fax: (0131) 2439302
e-mail: information@nts.org.uk
web: www.nts.org.uk

DISABILITY ORGANISATIONS
DIAL SCOTLAND
Braid House, Labrador Avenue, Mowden, West
Lothian EH54 6DU
Tel: (01506) 433468   Fax: (01506) 431201
Information service for disabled people.

DISABILITY RESOURCE CENTRE
130 Langton Road, Pollock, Glasgow G53
Tel: (0141) 8832997

DISABILITY SCOTLAND
Princes House, 5 Shandwick Place,
Edinburgh EH2 4RG
Tel: (0131) 2298632   Fax: (0131) 2295168
Information on all aspects of disability.

MULTIPLE SCLEROSIS IN SCOTLAND
2a North Charlotte Street, Edinburgh,
Lothian EH2 4HR
Tel: (0131) 2253600   Fax: (0131) 2205188

PHAB SCOTLAND
Princes House, 5A Warriston Road,
Edinburgh EH3 5LQ
Tel: (0131) 5589912

**SCOTTISH SPORTS ASSOCIATION FOR THE
DISABLED**
Fife Institute PRE, Viewfield Road,
Glenrothes KY6 2RA
Tel: (01592) 771700   Fax: (01592) 415710

SCOTRAIL RAILWAYS
Caledonian Chambers, 87 Union Street,
Glasgow G1 3TA

SPINAL INJURIES SCOTLAND (SIS)
The Festival Business Centre, 150 Brand street,
Glasgow G51 1DH
Tel: (0141) 3140056
Equivalent of SIA in Scotland.

303

SOUTH OF SCOTLAND

DUMFRIES & GALLOWAY

CASTLE DOUGLAS

Laid out in the C18th by local lad, William Douglas, this is a planned village, which Douglas hoped would become a major commercial and industrial centre - but it didn't happen.

SELF-CATERING
BARNCROSH LEISURE CO.
Barncrosh, Castle Douglas DG7 1TX
Tel: (01556) 680216   Fax: (01556) 680442
No. of Accessible Units: 4
No. of Beds per Unit: 2 - 9
Accessible Facilities: Lounge, Kitchen. Comfortable cottages on working farm with access to seashore, hills, forests and botanical gardens.

ATTRACTION
THREAVE GARDEN (NT for S)
Castle Douglas DG7 1RX
Tel: (01556) 502575   Fax: (01556) 502683
64 acres with fine springtime displays of daffodils, colourful summer herbaceous borders and trees and heathers in autumn.

SD ♿	CP ♿	E ♿	RF ♿
C ♿	S ♿	WC ♿	RFE ♿

DALBEATTIE

Forms the meeting point of A710 and A711 around north coast of Solway Firth. Good day's tour from Dumfries, driving through Dalbeattie Forest and hamlets of Kippord and Colvend.

HOTELS
AUCHENSKEOCH LODGE ♿
By Dalbeattie, DG5 4PG
Tel/Fax: (01387) 780277
No. of Accessible Rooms: 1. Roll-in Shower
Accessible Facilities: Lounge, Restaurant. Formerly a Victorian shooting lodge,

Auchenskeoch is set in 20 acres of grounds in a quiet and unspoilt corner of SW Scotland. 5 miles from Dalbeattie and 3 from the coast. Traditional furnishings, log fires and lots of books.

CLONYARD HOUSE ♿
Colvend, Dalbeattie, DG5 4QW
Tel: (01556) 630372   Fax: (01556) 630422
No. of Accessible Rooms: 1. Shower
Accessible Facilities: Lounge Bar, Restaurant. The Garden Wing houses the room for disabled guests, modern, ground floor with own small patio overlooking quiet area of the gardens. Small, family run hotel situated in 7 acres of woodland in secluded position on Solway Coast between Rockliffe and Kippord. This is Scotland's waiting-to-be-discovered south west corner with high cliffs, sheltered creeks, lochs and forest clad hills.

DUMFRIES

Known as Queen of the South, Dumfries was a seaport in the middle ages. Regularly invaded by the English, this red sandstone town beside river Nirth is still important as a focus for the area's agricultural prosperity.

TOURIST INFORMATION CENTRE
64 Whitesands, Dumfries DG1 2RS
Tel: (01387) 245550

SOCIAL WORKS DEPARTMENT
8 Gordon Street, Dumfries DG1 1EG
Tel: (01387) 261234

BUSES
Stagecoach/Western Buses:
Tel: (01387) 253496
5 low-floor buses each taking 1 wheelchair.

TAXIS
Beehive Taxis: Tel: (01387) 263103
Only firm with wheelchair facilities.

TRAINS
GNER – Special Needs Tel: (0145) 7225444
Minicom: (0191) 2330173
Wheelchair space in both first and standard class. Dumfries Station offers assistance when booked in advance.

SHOPMOBILITY
Holywood Trust Building, Old Assembly Close, Dumfries.
Tel: (0345) 090904   Fax: (0345) 269026

HOTEL
HETLAND HALL HOTEL
Carrutherstown, Dumfries DG1 4JX
Tel: (01387) 840201   Fax: (01387) 840211
No. of Accessible Rooms: 1
Accessible Facilities: Lounge, Restaurant, Pool, Sauna. Charming hotel in countryside location, situated by main A75, 8 miles from Dumfries

BED AND BREAKFAST
ORCHARD HOUSE
298 Annan Road, Dumfries DG1 3JE
Tel: (01387) 255099
No. of Accessible Rooms: 1
Accessible Facilities: Dining Room
Converted farm stead with one acre of garden, overlooking open country to the back with sheep pastures next to the main area. Located 1.5 miles from Dumfries centre.

SELF-CATERING
CAIRNYARD HOLIDAY LODGES
Cairnyard House, Beeswing, Dumfries DG2 8JE
Tel: (01387) 730218
No. of Accessible Units: 4
No. of Beds per Unit: 2 sleeping 2, 2 sleeping 4.
Accessible Facilities: Unit for 2. Open plan kitchen/Dining/Lounge, verandah. Unit for 4 – kitchen/diner, Lounge. Located 5 miles from Dumfries, in the former orchard of a large Victorian house set in mature grounds and surrounded by countryside.

ATTRACTION
DUMFRIES MUSEUM
The Observatory, Dumfries DG2 7SW
Tel: (01387) 253374   Fax: (01387) 265081
e-mail: info@dumfriesmuseum.demon.co.uk
Largest museum in southwest Scotland, with 150 years' worth of collections and exhibits on the history and landscape of the region.
SD [&] CP E [&] RF [&]
L S [&] WC [人]

ROBERT BURNS CENTRE
Mill Road, Dumfries DG2 7BE
Tel: (01387) 264808

Situated in the town's C18th watermill on west bank of river Nith. Tells the story of Burns' last years in Dumfries in the 1790s. Exhibition illuminated by original documents and personal relics, plus scale model of Dumfries at the time and AV presentation.
SD [&] CP [&] E [&] RF [&]
C [&] (Stannah Stairlift) S [人] WC [&]

NEWTON STEWART
Typical Galloway town on banks of river Cree, where gamefishing is popular.

BED AND BREAKFAST
ROWANTREE GUEST HOUSE
38 Main Street, Glenluce,
Newton Stewart DG8 0PS
Tel: (01581) 300244
No. of Accessible Rooms: 1
Accessible Facilities: Lounge, Dining Room. C19th guest house, formerly the shoe shop, in peaceful village midway between Stranraer and Newton Stewart.

ATTRACTION
CREETOWN GEM ROCK MUSEUM
Chain Road, Creetown DG8 7HJ
Tel: (01671) 820357   Fax: (01671) 820554
e-mail: gen.rock@bt.internet.com
Fine privately owned collection of gemstones, crystals, minerals, gemstone objects d'art and fossils. Almost every known gemstone and mineral is represented plus recent additions of a fossilised dinosaur egg and dung along with meteorites from outer space. Located 19km from Newton Stewart.
SD [&] CP [&] E [&] RF [&]
C [&] S [&] WC [人] RFE [&]

PORTPATRICK
Harbour town and holiday resort with charming streets and cottages and a calm harbour backed by low cliffs.

HOTEL
FERNHILL HOTEL
Heugh Road, Portpatrick DG9 8TD
Tel: (01776) 810220   Fax: (01776) 810596
No. of Accessible Rooms: 3
Accessible Facilities: Lounge, Restaurant
High above the village, fine harbour views.

305

WANLOCKHEAD
Scotland's highest village at 421m, and the centre of the metal mining industry.

ATTRACTION
THE MUSEUM OF LEAD MINING
Wanlockhead, by Biggar ML12 6UT
Tel: (01659) 74387   Fax: (01659) 74481
Guided tour of Lochnell Lead Mine plus Visitor Centre, housing a collection of rare minerals. There are hands-on displays, mineral collecting areas and a 1.5 mile walkway to C18th lead mine and miners cottages. Gold panning tuition available at Gold Panning Centre. Fascinating museum.

| SD 🦽 | CP 🦽 | E 🦽 | RF 🦽 |
| C 🚶 | S 🚶 | WC 🚶 | RFE 🚶 |

AYRSHIRE & ISLE OF ARRAN

ALLOWAY
Robert Burns was born here in 1759, his cottage standing on Monument Road, and much of the village is associated with his poetry, particularly the Burns National Heritage Park,

ATTRACTION
BURNS COTTAGE
Alloway KA7 4PY
Tel: (01292) 441215
Home for his first 7 years of the most famous Scottish poet, born in Alloway in January 1759. Interpretative presentation, including audio/visual, offers an interesting experience of how cottage looked when the Burns family lived here.

| SD 🦽 | CP 🦽 | E 🦽 | RF 🦽 |
| C 🦽 | S 🦽 | WC 🚶 | RFE 🚶 |

ISLE OF ARRAN
Two ferry services to the island. Caledonian McBrayne all year round from Ardrossan (rail link to Glasgow) – 55-minute crossing by modern roll-on roll-off ferry with facilities for the disabled. Smaller ferry between Lochranza and Kintyre during the summer. Passengers may remain in their cars. 20 miles long and about 57 miles around, Arran has mountainous peaks,

dense forests and ever-changing shoreline. Lying across the path of the gulf stream, Arran enjoys sub-tropical conditions, palm trees grow well and basking sharks and dolphins can be seen from the shore.

BRODICK
The main village on Arran, busy but unspoilt, with a wide beach stretching around Brodick Bay.

HOTEL
AUCHRANNIE COUNTRY HOUSE HOTEL 🦽
Brodick, Arran KA27 8BZ
Tel: (01770) 302234
Fax: (01770) 302812
No. of Accessible Rooms: 1
Accessible Facilities: Lounge, Restaurant, Pool, Sauna, Spa, Fitness Suite, Snooker Room, Hairdressing Salon, Aromatherapy Room.

BED AND BREAKFAST
STRATHWHILLIAN HOUSE 🦽
Brodick, Aran KA27 8BQ
Tel: (01770) 302331
No. of Accessible Rooms: 8
Accessible Facilities: Lounge Dining Room, Gardens. Privately owned, the original house is over 150 years old, carefully renovated with a new wing. It lies in lovely grounds of courtyards, lawns and flower beds with views over Brodick Bay to the castle and mountains beyond. Situated 0.5 mile from Brodick, with shore and ferry terminal within 200m.

LAMLASH
3 miles south of Brodick, a secluded village with some jolly pubs. Coming down into Lamlash there are fine views across the golf course and bay to Holy Island.

LILYBANK HOTEL 🚶
Shire Road, Lamlash, Arran KA27 8LS
Tel: (01770) 600230
No. of Accessible Rooms: 1. Shower
Accessible Facilities: Lounge, Restaurant. Hotel on the seafront.

MAYBOLE
Robert Burns' parents were said to have met close to a clock tower in the high street.

306

SELF-CATERING
ROYAL ARTILLERY COTTAGE

Culzean Castle, Maybole KA19 8LE
Tel: (01655) 760274   Fax: (01655) 760615
No. of Accessible Units: 1
No. of Beds per Unit: 4
Accessible Facilities: Lounge, Kitchen.
Owned by the National Trust for Scotland.

ATTRACTION
CULZEAN CASTLE AND COUNTRY PARK (NT for S)
Maybole KA19 8LE
Tel: (01655) 884400   Fax: (01655) 884522
Built on clifftop 50m above the sea, this is
one of Scotland's finest castles. Built in
C18th, designed by Robert Adam for 10th
Earl of Cassillis. Noted for oval staircase,
circular drawing room and plasterwork.
Country park of 560 acres with walled and
terraced gardens. All castle rooms on display
accessible (lift to first floor). Ground floor of
Visitor Centre only. Firm gravel and grass
paths with ramps in Walled Garden. Access
to Fountain Court Garden via graded path
down side of Viaduct. Dropping off point
below Viaduct for easier access. Woodland
area not very accessible, but hide at Swan
Pond accessible by ramp. Wheelchairs and
batricars available at Castle, Visitor Centre
and kiosk. Batricars should be booked in
advance.

SD ⌣ CP ⚹ E ⌣ RF ⌣
L ⌣ C ⌣ S ⌣ WC ⚹

WHITING BAY
Peaceful, but cosmopolitan atmosphere,
views of the bays and palm-fringed gardens.

HOTEL
GRANGE HOUSE HOTEL

Whiting Bay, Arran KA27 8QH
Tel/Fax: (01770) 700263
No. of Accessible Rooms: 1
Accessible Facilities: Lounge, Restaurant.
Located in the south of the island with
wonderful views to Holy Island and the
Ayrshire coast.

AYR
Important seaport and commercial
centre. A popular resort in Victorian
times, the beach still is so. Ayr racecourse

is the most prestigious in Scotland.

HOTEL
MONKTON LODGE TRAVEL INN
Kilmarnock Road, Monkton,
Nr. Ayr KA29 2RJ
Tel: (01292) 678262
Fax: (01292) 678248
No. of Accessible Rooms: check.
Accessible Facilities: check.
Situated on A77/A78 roundabout by
Prestwick Airport, north of Ayr.

DISABLED FORUM
Ground Floor, Burns House, Burns Statue
Square, Ayr KA7 1UP
Tel: (01292) 616261

BUSES
Stagecoach/Western Buses: Tel: (01292)
613700/613500
12 low-floor buses, limited wheelchair
space.

TAXIS
All Black Cabs fully equipped
Tel: (01292) 284545

TRAINS
Scotrail: Special Needs Tel: (0845) 6057021

Ayr Station offers wheelchair unassisted
access and ramps.

SHOPMOBILITY
33 Carrick Street, Ayr KA7 1NS
Tel: (01292) 618086

GIRVAN
Traditional family resort with a lovely
harbour, once a major landing site for
herring catch.

ATTRACTION
BARGANY GARDEN
Bargany Estate, by Girvan KA26 9PF
Tel: (01465) 871249   Fax: (01465) 871282
Woodland gardens free of charge. Main
area with rhododendrons and azaleas and
a pond. Flat Walled garden with slightly
inclined approach.

SD   CP   E   RF

GALSTON

East of Kilmarnock, off the A71

ATTRACTION

LOUDOUN CASTLE THEME PARK
Galston KA4 8PE
Tel: (01563) 822296   Fax: (01563) 822408
e-mail: loudouncastle@btinternet.com
Scotland biggest theme park surrounding
Loudoun Castle, the whole park is steeped
in history. The Museum and Visitor Centre
tells the story of the Earl of Loudon who
inhabited the castle c1714. 500 acres of
entertainment including rides, gentle
countryside walks and children's farm.

| SD ♿ | CP ♿ | E ♿ | RF ♿ |
| C ♿ | S ♿ | WC 🚶 | RFE ♿ |

IRVINE

Originally a maritime settlement, some
remains visible around the harbour. Centre
of town is cobbled.

HOTEL

THE THISTLE IRVINE   ♿
46 Annick Road, Irvine KA11 4LD
Tel: (01294) 274272   Fax: (01294) 277287
No. of Accessible Rooms: 1
Accessible Facilities: Lounge, Restaurant,
Pool, Jacuzzi. Quality hotel designed in
Moroccan style.

TURNBERRY

Along the south-west Ayrshire coast, 40
minutes from Glasgow. Renowned as home
of one of the great hotels.

HOTEL ACCOMMODATION

TURNBERRY HOTEL   ♿
Ayrshire KA26 9LT
Tel: (01655) 331000   Fax: (01655) 331706
No. of Accessible Rooms: 1
Accessible Facilities: Lounge, Restaurant.
Luxury hotel, created at the turn of the
century by the Marquess of Ailsa who built
a private golf course on his estate in 1902.
Turnberry is about golf, but also about the
Edwardian love of ease and luxury which is
reflected in the antiques, paintings and
oriental art.

WEST KILBRIDE

HUNTERSTON VISITOR CENTRE
West Kilbride KA23 9QJ
Tel: (0800) 838557   Fax: (01294) 826008
Advanced gas-cooled reactor type of nuclear
power station. Purpose-built centre with
exhibits, inter-active models and videos.

| SD ♿ | CP ♿ | E ♿ | RF ♿ |
| S ♿ | WC ♿ | RFE ♿ | |

SCOTTISH BORDERS

COLDSTREAM

Known as the birthplace of the
Coldstream Guards, the regiment's
history is featured in the local museum.
August sees the ride to Flodden Field to
honour the dead in battle in 1513.

TOURIST INFORMATION CENTRE

Town Hall, High Street, Coldstream TD12 4DH
Tel: (01890) 882607

ATTRACTIONS

COLDSTREAM MUSEUM
12 Market Square, Coldstream TD12 4BD
Tel: (01890) 882630   Fax: None
Displays explore the history of Coldstream
and its people with a special section on the
Coldstream Guards.

| SD n/a | CP ♿ | E ♿ | RF ♿ | C n/a |
| S ♿ | WC 🚶 | RFE ♿ | Outside Courtyard | |

HIRSEL COUNTRY PARK

Hirsel Estate Office, Coldstream TD12 4LP
Tel/Fax: (01890) 882834
Museum of Estates, past and present, arts
and crafts centre, picnic area and
playground.

| SD ♿ | CP 🚶 | E ♿ | RF 🚶 |
| C 🚶 | S 🚶 | WC 🚶 | |

EYEMOUTH

Historic town lying 5m. north of the
border where the mouth of the River Eye
provides a natural harbour and sandy
beaches. People have fished here since
C13th and the harbour is still busy.

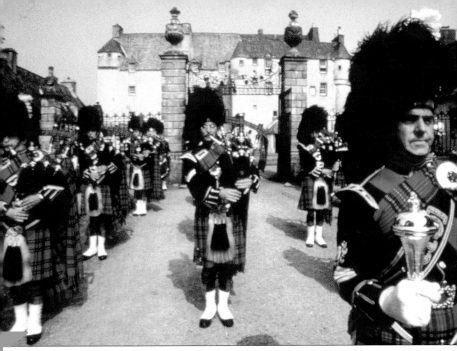

The pipes! The pipes! Coldstream, birthplace of the famous Coldstream Guards.

x

TOURIST INFORMATION CENTRE

Auld Kirk, Market Place, Eyemouth TD14 5HE
Tel: (01890) 750678

BED AND BREAKFAST

WESTWOOD GUEST HOUSE

Houndwood, Eyemouth TD14 5TP
Tel: (01361) 850232   Fax: (01361) 850333
e-mail: westwood@zetnet.co.uk
web: www.users.zetnet.co.uk/westwood/

No. of Accessible Rooms: 1
Accessible Facilities: Lounge, Dining Room,
Tea Room, Garden. Mary Queen of Scots
hunted with her hounds in the woods here,
hence the name. Originally an C18th
coaching inn, the property retains much
character and is set in over an acre of
landscaped gardens with ducks and rare
chickens roaming around.

HAWICK

Famous for wool production, located on the
banks of the river Teviot.

TOURIST INFORMATION CENTRE

Drumlanrig's Tower, Tower Knowe,
Hawick TD9 9EN
Tel: (01450) 372547   Fax: (01450) 373993

right

right

right

SELF-CATERING

CHERRY COTTAGE

right

309

Blacklee Square, Bonchester Bridge,
Hawick TD9 9TD
Tel/Fax: (01450) 850678
e-mail: kate@blacklee.demon.co.uk
web: www.aboutscotland.co.uk/quince/
cherry.html

No. of Accessible Units: 1
No. of Beds per Unit: 6
Accessible Facilities: Sun Lounge, Dining
Room, Kitchen, ramped access to Garden.
Originally tradesmen's workshops for local
estate, Blacklee Square comprises 4 stone
built cottages in traditional courtyard
setting with unspoilt countryside of hills,
forests, woods and rivers.

INNERLEITHEN

Tweedsdale village, famous in C19th for its
spa. A pump room was built by the owners
in Traquair House.

ATTRACTIONS

TRAQUAIR HOUSE

Innerleithen EH44 6PW. Tel: (01896) 830 323
Fax: (01896) 830 639
The oldest inhabited house in Scotland.

Once a pleasure ground for Scottish kings, a refuge for catholic priests in times of terror, the Stuarts of Traquair supported Mary Queen of Scots and the Jacobite cause. Imprisoned, fined and isolated for their beliefs, their home, untouched by time, reflects the tranquillity of their family life. Secret stairs, spooky cellars, books, embroideries, modern Scottish art in the gallery. Search for the centre of the maze.

SD 🅿   CP ♿   E 🅿   RF 🅿
C 🚹   S ♿   WC 🚹

ROBERT SMAIL'S PRINTING WORKS
7-9 High Street, Innerleithen EH44 6HA
Tel: (01896) 830206

This museum contains a Victorian office, paper store, composing and press rooms. Machinery is in full working order and visitors can see the printer at work and try their hands at typesetting. All bottom levels can be reached by various routes, top area is not accessible but staff will bring items downstairs for visitors.

SD 🅿   CP n/a   E 🅿   S 🚹

MELROSE
Quiet small hamlet set around a square. Ruins of Melrose Abbey has very limited disabled access.

TOURIST INFORMATION CENTRE
Abbey House, Abbey Street, Melrose TD5 7HE
Tel: (01896) 822555

SELF-CATERING
EILDON HOLIDAY COTTAGES   🅿
Dingleton Mains, Melrose TD6 9HS
Tel/Fax: (01896) 823258
web: www.aboutscotland.co.uk/eildon/
cottages.html
No. of Accessible Units: 5
No. of Beds per Unit: 2 - 6 (Showers in Hamiltons, Langrig and The Croft.)
Accessible Facilities: various room combinations. Converted C18th farm steading with fine views of the Tweed Valley to the Lammermuir and Moorfoot Hills. 4 miles from Abbotsford (see below). Able-bodied and disabled visitors can holiday here without differentiation. Alternatively disabled people can holiday

with their carers. Electric hoists are fitted with continuous ceiling track to transport from bed to bath (Single Tree) and bed to shower (Langrig). Portable hoist available for use in other cottages.

ATTRACTIONS
ABBOTSFORD
Melrose TD6 9BQ
Tel: (01896) 752043   Fax: (01896) 752916

Set on the River Tweed, this was the lovely home of Sir Walter Scott, which he built and lived in from 1812 until his death in 1832. A passionate collector of historic relics, there is a fine collection of armour and weapons, including Rob Roy's gun. There are also extensive gardens.

SD 🅿   CP 🚹   E 🚹   RF ♿
S 🅿   WC 🚹   RFE 🅿

DRYBURGH ABBEY
Dryburgh, St. Boswells, Melrose TD6 0RG
Tel/Fax: (01835) 822381

Remarkably complete ruins, much of which are of C12th and C13th origin. Sir Walter Scott and Field Marshall Earl Haig are both buried here. Flat approach to the Abbey, mostly accessible, apart from cloisters.

CP 🅿   E 🅿   WC 🚹

PRIORWOOD DRIED FLOWER GARDEN (NT FOR SC)
Abbey Street, Melrose TA6 9PX
Tel/Fax: (01896) 822493

Walled garden and orchard specialising in flowers for drying and historic apple varieties. Picnic area.

SD 🚹   CP 🚹   E 🅿   RF 🚹   S 🚹

PEEBLES
Large town with country shops lining the high street. Famous for the annual display of local horse power in *Common Riding of the Marches*.

TOURIST INFORMATION CENTRE
High Street, Peebles EH45 8AG
Tel: (01721) 720138
Fax: (01721) 724401

HOTEL
HORSESHOE INN

Eddleston, Peebles EH45 8QP
Tel: (01721) 730223   Fax: (01721) 730268
e-mail: horshoe.inn@virgin.net
web: www.horseshoeinn.com
No. of Accessible Rooms: 1
Accessible Facilities: Lounge, Restaurant (2
steps). The inn was originally a forge on the
stagecoach route Edinburgh/London, now
an oak-beamed traditional inn, with
bedrooms in separate building, once the old
village school. 30 minutes from Edinburgh.

SELKIRK
Standing above Ettrick and Yarrow valleys
and known for waterpowered textile mills
in C19th. Cashmere, tweed and tartan are
still produced here, plus Selkirk Glass.
Statue of Sir Walter Scott at one end of the
town with Battle of Flodden memorial at
the other end. And the main A7 goes
through the town centre,

TOURIST INFORMATION CENTRE
Halliwell's House, Selkirk TD7 4BL
Tel: (01750) 20054

ACCESSIBLE ATTRACTIONS
BOWHILL HOUSE and COUNTRY PARK
Bowhill, Selkirk TD7 5ET
Tel/Fax: (01750) 22204
Home of the Duke of Buccleuch and
Queensberry, with superb collection of
paintings by Van Dyck, Gainsborough and
Canaletto and others. Also porcelain and
furniture. Lovely wooded grounds.

SD ⑂   CP ⑂   E ⑂   R ⑂
C ⑂   S ⑂   WC ⑂

SELKIRK GLASS VISITORS CENTRE
Selkirk TD7 5EF
Tel: (01750) 20954   Fax: (01750) 22883
Watch skilled craftsmen at work creating
art glass paperweights, candlesticks and
visit the showroom to take advantage of
reduced factory prices.

SD ⑂   CP ⑂   E ⑂   C ⑂
S ⑂   WC ⑂

REGION 2:
EDINBURGH AND LOTHIANS

LOTHIAN COALITION OF DISABLED PEOPLE
Norton Park, 57 Albion Road, Edinburgh EH7
5QY
Tel/Minicom: (0131) 4752360
Fax: (0131) 4752392
Full information service and publishers of
excellent Guide to Access in Lothian.

ABERLADY
Aberlady Bay was the first area in Britain to
be called a Local Nature Reserve in 1952 and
there is much wildlife here in this charming
pantile-roofed village.

HOTEL
KILSPINDIE HOUSE HOTEL
High Street, Aberlady, East Lothian EH32 0RE
Tel: (01875) 870682   Fax: (01875) 870304
No. of Accessible Rooms: 3. Bath
Accessible Facilities: Lounge, Restaurant.
Coastal hotel Northeast of Edinburgh.

ATTRACTION
MYRETON MOTOR MUSEUM
Aberlady, East Lothian EH32 0PZ
Tel: (01875) 870288
Dating from 1896, a large collection of cars,
motor cycles, commercials and WWII
vehicles military vehicles, plus collection of
period advertising, posters and enamel signs.

SD ⑂   CP ⑂   E ⑂   RF ⑂   WC ⑂

EAST FORTUNE

ATTRACTION
MUSEUM OF FLIGHT
East Fortune Airfield, East Fortune,
Midlothian EH39 5LF
Tel: (01620) 880308   Fax: (01620) 880355
e-mail: aes@nms.ac.uk
Housed in former airship base with exhibit
of airship 34 which flew to New York in
1919. Aircraft on display include Hawker
Sea Hawk and Spitfire MK 16.

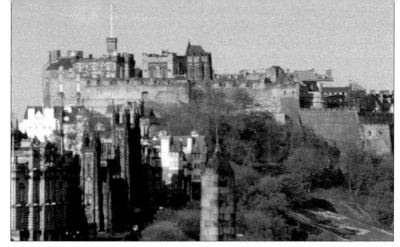

Edinburgh Castle dominates the city skyline.

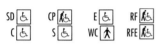

SD 🖰 CP 🖰 E 🖰 RF 🖰
C 🖰 S 🖰 WC 🖰 RFE 🖰

EDINBURGH

Capital of Scotland whose Castle Rock, overlooking the Firth of Forth, has been a stronghold since 1,000BC. Holyrood Palace, a mile to the east, was built by James IV in 1498. The town growing along this route became known as The Royal Mile which offers a wealth of historic sights, including the house of John Knox and the seat of Scotland's new Parliament. Overcrowding in this part of the city led to a Georgian New Town to the north in the 1700s. The city is divided in half by Princes Street, the principal shopping street with the Royal Mile to its south and New Town to its north. It is a compact city and easy to get around, although the centre is best avoided by car.

TOURIST INFORMATION CENTRE
3 Princes Street, Edinburgh EH2
Tel: (0131) 4733800

LOTHIAN COMMUNITY TRANSPORT SERVICES
129b Willowbrae Road,
Edinburgh EH8 7HL
Tel: (0131) 2298632

BRITISH RED CROSS
Beaverhall House, 27 Beaverhall Road,
Edinburgh EH7 4JH
Tel: (0131) 557 9898

ARTSLINE (see London)
Produce excellent Reel Guide to cinemas in Edinburgh.

TRAVEL LINE
2 Cockburn Street, Edinburgh EH1 1BL
Tel: (0800) 232323/ (0131) 2253858

TAXIS
Central Radio Taxis: Tel: (0131) 2292468
Capital Castle: (0131) 22825555
City Taxis: (0131) 2281211
Festival City/Waverley Taxis:
Tel: (0131) 2203160/55217777
Radiocabs: Tel: (0131) 2259000/2256736

HANDICABS
58 Canaan Lane, Edinburgh EH10 4SG
Tel: (0131) 4479949

Dial a Ride: Tel: (0131) 4479949
7 days a week.
Dial a Bus: Tel: (0131) 4471718
Monday to Friday.

TRAINS
Scotrail: Tel: for disabled assistance:
(0845) 6057021
Tel: for booking in advance for assistance:
(0131) 5502301
Tel: for any other facilities: (0131) 5502263

LOTHIAN SHOPMOBILITY
King's Stables Yard, King's Stables Road,
Edinburgh EH1 2YJ
Tel: (0131) 2259559

Unit 42D, The Gyle Shopping Centre, South Gyle, Broadway, Edinburgh West EH12 9JY
Tel: (0131) 3171460

HOTELS IN CITY CENTRE AND WEST END
SIMPSONS HOTEL   ♿
79 Lauriston Place, Edinburgh EH3 9HZ
Tel: (0131) 622 7979   Fax: (0131) 622 7900
e-mail: reception@simpsons-hotel.demon.co.uk
web: hotel.demon.co.uk
No. of Accessible Rooms: 3
Accessible Facilities: Lounge, Lift
NB. No restaurant but many close by.
Continental breakfast is served in guests' rooms. Opened in 1998, close to Princes Street and the castle.

SHERATON GRAND   ♿
1 Festival Square, Edinburgh EH3 9SR
Tel: (0131) 2299131   Fax: (0131) 2284510
No. of Accessible Rooms: 2
Accessible Facilities: Lounge, Restaurants (2). Luxury modern property in the centre of West End of city with imposing public areas.

THISTLE EDINBURGH   ♿
St. James Centre, Edinburgh EH1 3SW
Tel: (0131) 5560111   Fax: (0131) 5575333
No. of Accessible Rooms: 1
Accessible Facilities: Lounge, Restaurant
Modern hotel in good location just off Princes Street.

THE CALEDONIAN   ♿
Princes Street, Edinburgh EH1 2AB
Tel: (0131) 4599988   Fax: (0131) 2256632
No. of Accessible Rooms: 2
Accessible Facilities: Lounge, Restaurants (2), Pool, Sauna, Spa. Renowned hotel of Victorian splendour in heart of the city, with good views of the castle.

HOLIDAY INN GARDEN COURT   ♿
107 Queensferry Road, Edinburgh EH4 3HL
Tel: (0131) 3322442   Fax: (0131) 332 3408
No. of Accessible Rooms: 1
Accessible Facilities: Lounge, Restaurant
Modern hotel on western side of city with panoramic views.

HOTEL IBIS   ♿
Hunter Square, Edinburgh EH11 1QR
Tel: (0131) 2407000   Fax: (0131) 2407007

No. of Accessible Rooms: Check
Accessible Facilities: Open plan Lounge/Bar, Restaurant. Located in City Centre, close to Royal Mile with modern accommodation converted from old warehouses.

STAKIS EDINBURGH GROSVENOR   ♿
7-21 Grosvenor Street, Edinburgh EH12 7BJ
Tel: (0131) 2266001   Fax: (0131) 2202387
No. of Accessible Rooms: 3. Bath
Accessible Facilities: Lounge, restaurant. city-centre elegant Victorian building, well refurbished.

BARNTON HOTEL   🚶
Queensferry Road, Barnton, Edinburgh EH4 6AS
Tel: (0131)339 1144   Fax: (0131) 339 5521
No. of Accessible Rooms: 1
Accessible Facilities: Lounge, Restaurant.
Located on A90, 4m. from city centre, Forth road bridge and airport. Comfortable public areas.

EDINBURGH CAPITAL MOAT HOUSE   🚶
187 Clermiston Road, Edinburgh EH12 6UG
Tel: (0131) 5359988   Fax: (0131) 3349712
No. of Accessible Rooms: 4
Accessible Facilities: Restaurant, Bar.
Modern hotel located close to Corstorphine Park, 3 miles from airport and city centre.

KING'S MANOR HOTEL   🚶
100 Milton Road East, Edinburgh EH15 2NP
Tel: (0131) 6690444   Fax: (0131) 6696650
No. of Accessible Rooms: 2
Accessible Facilities: Lounge, Dining room, Bar. Former Laird's home, now family owned and managed hotel in east end of the city, close to by-pass.

BED AND BREAKFAST
ARDGARTH GUEST HOUSE   ♿
1 St. Mary's Place, Portobello, Edinburgh EH15 2QF
Tel: (0131) 6693021   Fax: (0131) 4681221
e-mail: enquiries@ardgarth.demon.co.uk
No. of Accessible Rooms: 2
Accessible Facilities: Dining Room.
Lounge has 2 steps. Evening meals can be provided. Special diets catered for. Owners hold RADAR WC keys for guests. Adapted from large Victorian home with well proportioned rooms in a wide, quiet street

close to the beach and 3.5 miles east of Princes Street, Edinburgh. Portobello is on the south shore of the Firth of Forth with a beach and promenade.

TREFOIL HOUSE
Gogarbank EH12 9DA
Tel: (0131) 339 3148   Fax: (0131) 317 7271
e-mail: info@trefoil.org.uk
No. of Accessible Rooms: 12
Accessible Facilities:
Lounge, Dining Room, Pool, Library, Games Room, Shop, Bar, Minibus with tail lift, Woodland Walk, Nature Trail, Roundabout and Swings. Manor house set in lovely countryside, a few miles from city centre and totally adapted holiday centre for both groups and individuals.

LINDSAY GUEST HOUSE
108 Polwarth Terrace, Edinburgh EH11 1NN
Tel: (0131) 3371580   Fax: (0131) 3379174
No. of Accessible Rooms: 1. Roll-in Shower
Accessible Facilities: Dining Room.
a listed building of red sandstone, situated in quiet residential area, close to city centre.

ATTRACTIONS
CITY ART CENTRE
2 Market Street, Edinburgh EH1 1DE
Tel: (0131) 5293993   Fax: (0131) 5293957
e-mail: enquiries@city-art-centre.demon.co.uk
Home to Edinburgh's permanent fine art collection and temporary world-wide exhibitions on 6 floors of display galleries (lift).

SD ⬤   E ⬤   L ⬤   C ⬤
S ⬤   WC ⬤

EDINBURGH CASTLE
Castle Rock, Edinburgh
Tel: (0131) 2259846   Fax: (0131) 2204733
The castle stands of the precipitous crag of Castle Rock. In 1018 King Malcolm defeated the English at the Battle of Carham and a royal castle at Edinburgh emerges at the end of that century, of which only the C11th chapel of Queen Margaret remains. The last siege here was in 1745. Shortly after the esplanade was built, it became the site of the Military Tattoo. Apartments of Mary Queen of Scots can be seen. The Scottish crown is displayed in the crown room.

Route to features includes vehicle available from esplanade to top of the castle - Cat 1: to Crown Jewels - Cat. 3. The guided tour includes 26 areas of most interest.

The Lower Ward:
1-Gatehouse,
2-Old Guardhouse
3-Inner Barrier all accessible:
4-Portcullis- Cat. 3
The Middle Ward:
5-Lang Stairs,
6-Argyle Battery - n/a:
7-Cartshed (restaurant) accessible:
8-Governor's House,
9-New Barracks-n/a:
The Upper Ward:
10-Foog's Gate - vehicle passes through
11-St. Margaret's Chapel
12-Dog Cemetery -not inside, but good view of both from platform
13- Argyle Tower - n/a
14-Forwall Battery
15 -Fore Well
16-Half-Moon Battery - all accessible
Buildings in Crown Square:
17-Palace - Crown Room via lift accessible:
18-Great Hall - via ramp:
19-Queen Anne Building - via rear entrance:
20-Scottish National War Memorial - accessible. Off the beaten track
21-Castle Vaults - majority accessible:
22-Military Prison
23-Dury's Battery-n/a
24-Ordnance Storehouse
25-Hospital
26 -Back Well - all accessible.

S ⬤   CP ⬤   E ⬤   RF ⬤
L ⬤ Stair Climber.   C ⬤   S ⬤
WC ⬤ ⬤ -   RFE ⬤ ⬤

PALACE OF HOLYROOD HOUSE
Edinburgh EH8 8DX
Tel: (0131) 5567371   Fax: (0131) 5575256
e-mail: hh@royalcollections.org.uk
The Queen's Scottish residence at the end of the Royal Mile. Founded in 1128, Holyrood evolved from a fortress into a palace. Home to the court of Mary Queen of Scots 1561/67. C17th state rooms and picture galleries are open when the Queen is not in residence.

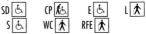
SD ⬤   CP ⬤   E ⬤   L ⬤
S ⬤   WC ⬤   RFE ⬤

NATIONAL GALLERY OF SCOTLAND
The Mound, Edinburgh EH2 2EL
Tel: (0131) 6246200   Fax: (0131) 3433250
Scotland's greatest collection of European paintings and sculpture from renaissance to post-impressionist, including Raphael, Constable, Velasquez, Gaugin and Van Gogh. The collection of Scottish paintings is particularly extensive.

SD [&]   E [&]   L [人]
S [&]   WC [人]

MUSEUM OF SCOTLAND
Chambers Street, Edinburgh EH1 1JF
Tel: (0131) 2474422   Fax: (0131) 2204819
Minicom: (0131) 2474027
e-mail (to Disability Officer): clt@nms.ac.uk
webs: www.nms.ac.uk
Stand adjacent to Royal Museum and together Present the World to Scotland and Scotland to the World. Chronological history of Scotland from 900AD to C20th. through rich national collections and colour-coded themes. NB: No car park but 2 designated spaces in layby near entrance. Otherwise main street metered parking.

SD [&]   CP n/a   E [&]   RF [&]   C [&]
S [&]   WC [&]   L [&]

ROYAL MUSEUM
Chambers Street, Edinburgh EH1 1JF
Tel: (0131) 2474219   Fax: (0131) 2204819
e-mail/web: as above

Palace of Holyrood House.

Victorian building housing fine international collections of decorative arts, science and industry, archaeology and the natural world. NB. Single yellow line parking adjacent or meters in Chamber Street or at rear in Lothian Street. Level entry through the Museum of Scotland is available.

SD [&]   P n/a   E [&]   RF [&]
C [&]   S [&]   WC [&]   L [&]

ROYAL SCOTTISH ACADEMY
5/1 Fettes Rise, Edinburgh EH2 2EL
Tel: (0131) 2256671   Fax: (0131) 2252349
Fine collection of Old Scottish Masters, plus 2 main exhibitions of fine art, the Annual Exhibition during the summer and the Edinburgh Festival Exhibition.

SD [&]   CP n/a   E [&]   RF [&]   L [&]
C n/a   S n/a   WC [人]

THE ROYAL YACHT BRITANNIA
Ocean Drive, Leith, Edinburgh EH6 6JJ
Tel: (0131) 5555566   Fax: (0131) 5558835
e-mail: enquiry @try-britannia.co.uk
Full wheelchair accessibility in both Visitor Centre and for the whole tour on board (4 decks, accessible via Lift Cat. 2).

SD [&]   CP [&]   E [&]   RF [&]
L [&]   C [&]   S [&]   WC [人]

SCOTCH WHISKY HERITAGE CENTRE
354 Castlehill, the Royal Mile, Edinburgh EH1 2NE
Tel: (0131) 2200441   Fax: (0131) 2206288

315

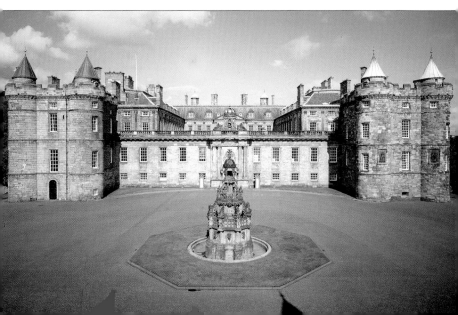

e-mail: enquiry@whisky-heritage.co.uk
web: www.whisky-heritage.co.uk
Travel through time exploring the history
of this famous export. Meet the Ghostly
Blender and enjoy the sights, sounds, smells
and the secrets of whisky making.

SD ♿   CP n/a   E 🚶   RF ♿   L ♿
C 🚶   S ♿   WC 🚶   RFE 🚶

SCOTTISH NATIONAL PORTRAIT GALLERY
1 Queen Street, Edinburgh EH2 1JD
Tel: (0131) 6246200 Fax: (0131) 3433250
Portraits of prominent people who shaped
Scotland's history, including Mary Queen of
Scots and Sir Walter Scott. All the portraits
are of Scots, but not all are by Scots, with
works by Van Dyck, Gainsborough, Copley
and Rodin.

SD 🚶   E ♿   RF ♿   C ♿
S ♿   WC 🚶

SCOTTISH NATIONAL GALLERY OF MODERN ART
73 Bedford Road, Edinburgh EH4 3DK
Tel: (0131) 6246200 Fax: (0131) 3433250
Home to Scotland's finest collection of C20th
paintings including works by Picasso,
Matisse, Sickert and Hockney. Also Scottish
modern art and important Dada and
Surrealist collection with masterpieces by
Dali, Magritte and Ernst. Extensive grounds
are home to sculptures by Moore, Hepworth,
Paolozzi and others.

SD ♿   CP ♿   E ♿   RF ♿
C ♿   S ♿   WC 🚶

CRAIGMILLAR CASTLE (HS)
Craigmillar Castle Road, Edinburgh EH16 4SY
Tel/Fax: (0131) 6614445
Fifteenth century stronghold where the plot
to murder Darnley, the second husband of
Mary Queen of Scots, was hatched. C16th
and C17th apartments.

SD ♿   CP ♿   E ♿   RF ♿
C 🚶   S 🚶   WC 🚶

EDINBURGH BUTTERFLY AND INSECT WORLD.
Dobbies Garden World, Lasswade,
Midlothian EH18 1AZ
Tel: (0131) 6634932 Fax: (0131) 6542774
e-mail: ebiw@compuserve.com
web: www.edinburgh-butterfly-world.co.uk
Exotic rainforest, splashing waterfalls and
pools provide a setting for watching

hundreds of the world's spectacular and
colourful butterflies flying all around you.
Ten minutes from Edinburgh city centre.

SD ♿   CP ♿   E ♿   C ♿
S ♿   WC 🚶   RFE ♿

EAST LINTON
East Lothian was one of the foremost grain-
growing areas in Scotland when techno-
logical changes in the C18th led to a rapid
increase in grain production. East Linton's
Preston Mill has always been of major
importance in this riverside setting with the
sea and Lammermuir hills only a short
distance away.

ATTRACTION
PRESTON MILL (NT for S)
Preston Road, East Linton, East Lothian EH40 3DS
Tel: (01620) 860426
Oldest water-driven mill in Scotland, last
used commercially in 1957. Old mill pond
with ducks. No access to upper floor of mill
or kiln. Excellent brochure for information
and history.

CP 🚶   E ♿   RF ♿   S ♿
WC 🚶   RFE ♿

LINLITHGOW
Lively town centre surrounded by dismal
1960s concrete blocks. St. Michael's Parish
church dedicated in C12th, was rebuilt in
C16th. A modern spire was added in 1946.

ATTRACTION
HOUSE OF THE BINNS (NT for S)
Linlithgow EH49 7NA
Tel: (01506) 834255
Historic home of the Dalyell family, General
Tam Dalyell raised the Royal Scots Greys
here in 1681. Originally a fortified
stronghold when built in 1612 it gradually
became a large mansion. Notable particularly
for fine C17th moulded plaster ceilings.

SD ♿   CP 🚶   E ♿
RF ♿   C n/a   S n/a   WC 🚶
No. shop or catering facility on site.

LIVINGSTON
Medium-sized community west of

Edinburgh off the M8

HOTEL
HILTON NATIONAL LIVINGSTON
Almondview, Livingston, West Lothian EH54 6QB
Tel: (01506) 431222   Fax: (01506) 434666
No. of Accessible Rooms: 4
Accessible Facilities: Lounge, Restaurant,
Pool, Sauna, Spa. Situated between
Edinburgh and Glasgow on the M8.

ATTRACTION
ALMOND VALLEY HERITAGE CENTRE
Millfield, Livingston Village, Livingston, West
Lothian EH54 7AR
Tel: (01506) 414957   Fax: (01506) 497771
e-mail: almondheritage@cableinet.co.uk
20-acre site exploring history of the local
environment with animals on Mill Farm,
vintage farm machinery in Livingstone Mill
and a shale oil museum. Lovely family day out.

SD 🚾   CP 🚶   E 🚾   RF 🚾
C 🚶   S 🚶   WC 🚶

NEWTOWNGRANGE
Located south of Bonnyrigg, that is SE of
Edinburgh off the A72.

ATTRACTION
SCOTTISH MINING MUSEUM
Lady Victoria Colliery, Newtowngrange,
Midlothian EH22 4QN
Tel: (0131) 6637519   Fax: (0131) 6541618
At 800 years old, this is the oldest
documented coal mining site in Britain. See
the Cornish beam engine plus several
relevant sites and exhibitions: Cutting the
Coal; A Race Apart; Pithead; Smithy;
Interactive and audio visual areas; Coal
Roadway; At the Coal Face Exhibition; and
Old Washer.

SD 🚾   CP 🚾   E 🚾   RF 🚾
L 🚾   C 🚾   S 🚾   WC 🚾

UPHALL
11 miles from Edinburgh, this is a good base
for touring central Scotland. Within a few
miles of the M8, M9 and M90, the principal
motorways for the central area. In the
immediate locale there are good recreational
facilities and restaurants.

BED AND BREAKFAST
COILLE-MHOR 🚾
20 Houston Mains, Uphall, West Lothian EH52 6PA
Tel: (01506) 854044   Fax: (01506) 855118
No. of Accessible Rooms: 6
Accessible Facilities: Lounge, Dining Room,
Family run guest house with a house
speciality of good porridge laced with a
liqueur, giving the day a kick!

SOUTH QUEENSFERRY
Small village on the bank of the river Forth,
10 miles west of Edinburgh. Famous for its
Forth Bridge, below which the old ferry is
still used for pleasure craft.

ATTRACTION
DALMENY HOUSE
South Queensferry, West Lothian EH30 9TQ
Tel: (0131) 3311888   Fax: (0131) 3311788
Built in 1815 in Tudor Gothic style, and
home to the Earl and Countess of Rosebery,
with collections of French and early
Scottish furniture, tapestries and china
from the Rothschild Mentmore Collection.
Situated on the Firth of Forth.

SD 🚾   CP n/a   E 🚶   RF 🚶   WC 🚶

WEST CALDER
Located on north side of the Pentland Hills,
18 miles west of Edinburgh city centre. Less
than an hour's drive away are palaces,
castles, stately homes and many other
attractions.

SELF-CATERING
CROSSWOODHILL FARM 🚾
By West Calder, West Lothian EH55 8LP
Tel: (01501) 785205   Fax: (01501) 785308
No. of Accessible Units: 1
No. of Beds per Unit: 6
Accessible Facilities: Lounge/Dining Room.
NB Kitchen too narrow for a wheelchair.
1,700-acre livestock farm. Steading Cottage
is for those happy to be at the heart of the
farm. Set back from the road with a small
garden, it nestles right beside the farm
buildings and a field. Despite thick walls
and double glazing you may hear tractors,
cattle or perhaps smell the odd farm whiff
outside!

REGION 3:
GREATER GLASGOW AND CLYDE VALLEY

STRATHCLYDE PASSENGER TRANSPORT DIAL-A-BUS
Tel: (0141) 3333252
Mon/Sat: easy and flexible door-to-door service. Sunday service in SE Glasgow, Renfrew and Kilmarnock and Thursday evening service in NW Glasgow, Hamilton, East Kilbridge, Cumbernauld and Monklands.

GLASGOW
Occupied by the Romans 2,000 years ago, Glasgow's modern city grew wealthy from the British Empire and the Industrial Revolution to become the UK City of Architecture in 1999. In 1991 it was European City of Culture. The streets run on a grid system on the north bank of the River Clyde, which includes rail stations and main shopping facilities. Outside the centre is the West End with bars and restaurants. A vibrant and exciting city to visit.

TOURIST INFORMATION CENTRE
11 George Square, Glasgow G2 1DY
Tel: (0141) 2044400

CENTRE OF INDEPENDENT LIVING
117-127 Brook Street, Bridgeton, Glasgow G40 3AP
Tel: (0141) 5504455   Fax: (0141) 5504858

GLASGOW CITY COUNCIL
Cultural and Leisure Services
37 High Street, Glasgow G1 1LX
Tel: (0141) 2875064   Fax: (0141) 2875918
Contact for general queries pertaining to museums, theatres etc.

TAXIS
Taxis Owner's Association
Radio Systems Ltd. 6a Lynedoch Street, Glasgow G3
Tel: (0141) 3327070

Wheelchair accessible metro and facility cabs
Taxi Cab Association: Tel: (0141) 3326666
If you require portable ramps, request the facility car when booking.

TRAINS
Scotrail, Caledonian Chambers, 87 Union Street, Glasgow G1 3TA
Tel: (0141) 3354590
Tel: Disabled Users: (0845) 6057021

National Rail Travel
Passenger Enquiries: (0345) 484950

Glasgow Station offers unassisted wheelchair access and ramps. 24 hours' notice is advisable.

CAR PARK
Charing Cross Car Park, Embankment Crescent, Glasgow.
Tel: (0141) 2219320
Orange badge parking available.

SHOPMOBILITY
Sauchiehall Centre, 179 Sauchiehall Street, Glasgow G2 3ER
Tel: (0141) 3326486

HOTELS
GLASGOW HILTON ♿
1 William Street, Glasgow G3 8HT
Tel: (0141) 2045555   Fax: (0141) 2045552
No. of Accessible Rooms: 4
Accessible Facilities: Lift, Lounge, Restaurant, Pool, Sauna, Spa.
Located 0.5 miles from the city centre.

GLASGOW MOAT HOUSE ♿
Congress Road, Glasgow G3 8QT
Tel: (0141) 3069988   Fax: (0141) 2212022
No. of Accessible Rooms: 2
Accessible Facilities: Lounge, Restaurant, Pool, Sauna, Spa. Impressive hotel overlooking the Clyde is located beside the SECC and Armadillo Conference Centre, a mile from the railway station.

THE SHAWLANDS HOTEL AND TRAVEL LODGE ♿
Ayr Road, Larkhall, Nr. Hamilton ML9 2TZ
Tel: (01698) 791111   Fax: (01698) 792001
No. of Accessible Rooms: 2
Accessible Facilities: Lounge, Restaurant.

Privately owned with accessible accommodation in Lodge. Located south of Glasgow.

STAKIS EAST KILBRIGE 🚹
Stewartfield Way, East Kilbride G74 5LA
Tel: (01355) 236300   Fax: (01355) 233552
No. of Accessible Rooms: 2
Accessible Facilities: Lounge, 2 Restaurants, Cafe, Bar, Pool, Sauna, Whirlpool.
Located on the southern outskirts of Glasgow, this is a modern hotel with a Living Well healthclub.

BED AND BREAKFAST
GLASGOW GUEST HOUSE ♿
56 Dumbreck Road, Glasgow GA1 5NP
Tel/Fax: (0141) 4270129
No. of Accessible Rooms: 2
Accessible Facilities: Lounge, Dining Room.

ATTRACTIONS
THE BURRELL COLLECTION
Pollock Country Park, Glasgow G43 1AT
Tel: (0141) 2872550   Fax: (0141) 2872597
Superb collection of art works ranging from Chinese ceramics, European medieval art, stained glass and British silverwork to paintings and sculptures from C15th to the early C20th with works by Rembrandt, Degas and Cezanne. An absolute must, this really needs two visits!

SD n/a   CP ♿   E ♿   RF ♿
L 🚹   C 🚹   S ♿   WC 🚹

GLASGOW ART GALLERY AND MUSEUM
Kelvingrove, Glasgow G3 8AG
Tel: (0141) 2872699
Fine collection of French Impressionists, Post-Impressionists and Scottish artists from C17th onward, plus works by Rembrandt and Giorgione. The Glasgow style represented by Charles Rennie Mackintosh furniture is now as well known for silver jewellery design.

SD ♿   CP ♿   E ♿   L ♿
C ♿   S ♿   WC 🚹

GALLERY OF MODERN ART
Queen Street, Glasgow G1 3AZ
Tel: (0141) 2291996   Fax: (0141) 2045316
Opened in 1996 and set in a marvellous refurbished neo-classical building in the city centre. Houses post-war art and design,

themed to reflect natural elements of earth, water, fire and air. International and Scottish artists. All six levels are accessible via either of the two lifts, and each gallery is accessible.

SD ♿   CP n/a   E ♿   RF ♿
L ♿   C ♿   S ♿   WC ♿

GLASGOW BOTANIC GARDENS
730 Great Western Road, Glasgow G12 OUE
Tel: (0141) 3342422   Fax: (0141) 339 6964
Dedicated to education, conservation and research there are 10 main points of interest of which the riverwalk and sorbus and birch areas of arboretum are not accessible. The main range Glasshouse and the area around Kibble Palace are particularly fine. Many of the plants represent temperate geographical regions: Mediterranean, Australasian, South American and temperate Asian. All paths around the gardens are tarmac, mostly level or slightly sloping.

SD ♿   CP 🚹   E ♿   RF ♿
C ♿   WC 🚹   RFE ♿

Glasgow Art Gallery.

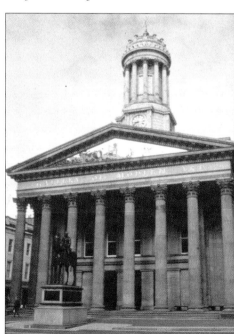

McLELLAN GALLERIES
270 Sauchiehall Street, Glasgow G2 3EH
Tel: (0141) 3311854   Fax: (0141) 3329957
Range of major and changing international exhibitions.
SD 🦽   CP n/a   E 🚶   L 🦽   WC 🚶

PEOPLE'S PALACE
Glasgow Green, Glasgow G40 1AT
Tel: (0141) 554 0223   Fax: (0141) 5500892
Victorian building purpose-built in 1898 as a cultural museum, which houses a wide range of exhibits on the city's social history from the C12th to the C20th. A fine conservatory at the rear of building contains a winter garden and tropical plants and birds.
SD 🦽   CP 🚶   E 🦽
L 🦽   S 🦽   WC 🦽

UNIVERSITY OF GLASGOW VISITOR CENTRE
University of Glasgow, University Avenue, Glasgow G12 8QQ
Tel: (0141) 3305511   Fax: (0141) 3305225
e-mail: visitorcentre@gla.ac.uk
Starting point for guided tours of the university's many attractions.
SD 🦽   CP 🦽   E 🚶   RF 🦽
C 🚶   S 🦽   WC 🚶   RFE 🚶

THEATRE
THE KING'S THEATRE
297 Bath Street, Glasgow
Admin: (0141) 2875006   Fax: (0141) 2483361
Booking-Box Office: (0141) 2875511
Fax: (0141) 2875016
CP 🚶   RE (accessible entrance in Elmbank Street.)
ED 🦽   INT 🦽
WC 🦽 (except inward opening door)
AUD 🦽 (5 spaces).   B/R 🦽

GREENOCK
Developed through industrial growth on the Clyde. Good new leisure development on Inverclyde's waterfront.

HOTEL
JAMES WATT COLLEGE   🦽
Halls of Residence, Custom House Way, Greenock PA15 1EN
Tel: (01475) 731360   Fax: (01475) 730877

No. of Accessible Rooms: 16
Accessible Facilities: Lounge, Restaurant.
Located 0.25 mile from the town centre.

LANGBANK
30 minutes west of Glasgow, between Glasgow and Greenock,

ATTRACTION
FINLAYSTONE COUNTRY ESTATE
Langbank
Tel: (01475) 590505   Fax: (01475) 540265
e-mail: info@finlaystone.co.uk
web: www.finlaystone.co.uk
Delightful Victoriana exhibition in the house, but the grounds are particularly splendid with formal and walled gardens, including a scented garden, and woodland walks.
SD 🦽   CP 🦽   E 🦽   RF 🦽
C 🦽   S 🦽   WC 🦽   RFE 🦽

NEW LANARK
The village, founded in 1785 as a completely new industrial settlement, is now A World Heritage Village and restored as a living and working community. New Lanark is the gateway to the Scottish Wildlife Trust's Falls of the Clyde Wildlife Reserve (limited access for wheelchairs) and there is a Wildlife Centre in the village, together with shops, craft workshops and various exhibitions, all advised as accessible.

TOURIST INFORMATION CENTRE
Horsemarket, Ladyacre Road, Lanark ML11 7LQ
Tel: (01555) 661661   Fax: (01555) 666143

HOTEL
NEW LANARK MILL HOTEL   🦽
Mill One, New Lanark ML11 9DB
Tel: (01555) 667200   Fax: (01555) 667222
e-mail: hotel@newlanark.org
web: www.newlanark.org
No. of Accessible Rooms: 5. Roll-in Shower
Accessible Facilities: Lounge, Restaurant.
Set on the upper reaches of the River Clyde in unique surroundings of restored C18th mill village.

REGION 4
WEST HIGHLANDS AND ISLANDS, ARGYLL, LOCH LOMOND, STIRLING AND TROSSACHS

ALLOA

Industrial town of coalmining, textiles and glass-making, close to the north bank of the River Forth.

ATTRACTION
ALLOA TOWER (NT for S)
Alloa FK10 1PP
Tel/Fax: (01259) 211701

A C15th medieval tower house, now restored, is all that remains of the ancestral home of the Earls of Mar. It has rare medieval features, particularly the timber roof. Flat access to ground floor, wide shallow stairs to first floor. Other floors are inaccessible because of a turnpike staircase.

SD   CP   E
RF   S   WC

ABERFOYLE

ATTRACTION
QUEEN ELIZABETH FOREST PARK
Visitor Centre, Aberfoyle
Tel: (01877) 382258

30 miles from Glasgow, the park takes in east Loch Lomond and the Trossachs with breath-taking scenery. Wheelchair loan scheme operates from the Visitor Centre. Woodlands walks and trails.

APPIN

Between Ballahulish and Oban

SELF-CATERING
APPIN HOUSE APARTMENTS AND LODGES
Appin House, Appin PA38 4BN
Tel: (01631) 730207   Fax: (01631) 730567

Shuna Apartment
No. of Accessible Units: 1
No. of Beds per Unit: 2
Accessible Facilities: Open plan Lounge/Dining/Kitchen

Pine Lodge
No. of Accessible Units: 1
No. of Beds per Unit: 4
Accessible Facilities: Lounge, Dining room
Both the above are in landscaped gardens of five acres in an elevated position overlooking Loch Linnhe with the hills of Mull in the background and the mountains of Morven to the west.

Oak Tree Cottage
No. of Accessible Units: 1
No. of Beds per Unit: 10
Accessible Facilities: Lounge, Dining room. Located in Duror, five miles north of Appin House, and under the same ownership. Standing on its own at the head of a peaceful glen, overlooked by Bheinn Beithir, it is five minutes from the local shop and restaurant/pub with Cuil Bay beach and Glencoe very close.

BALLOCH

At the southern tip of Loch Lomond and a starting point for loch cruises. Fine view of loch can be had at Duncryne, a small hill three miles NE of Balloch.

ATTRACTION
BALLOCH CASTLE COUNTRY PARK
Balloch G83 8LX
Tel: (01389) 758216   Fax: (01389) 720922

At the southern end of Loch Lomond, the castle, built in 1808, has a visitor centre with an introduction to local history and wildlife. It overlooks the park that offers trails, a walled garden and lawns for picnics.

SD    CP   E   RF
C   S   WC   RFE

CALLANDER

Capital of the Trossachs region, can be very busy as a popular base for exploring

Trossachs. Known as Tannochbrae of *Dr. Finlay's Casebook* in the 1960s.

HOTEL
ROMAN CAMP COUNTRY HOUSE HOTEL
off Main Street, Callander FK17 8BG
Tel: (01877) 330003   Fax: (01877) 331533
e-mail: mail@roman-camp-hotel.co.uk
No. of Accessible Rooms: 1
Accessible Facilities: Lounge (1 step),
Restaurant. Built in 1625 in 20 acres of
secluded gardens by the river Teith.

BED AND BREAKFAST
AIRLIE HOUSE
Main Street, Strathyre, Callander FK18 8NA
Tel: (01877) 384247   Fax: (01877) 384305
No. of Accessible Rooms: 1
Accessible Facilities: Lounge, Dining Room
Victorian house built in late 1800s. Being
converted into a guesthouse with 4
bedrooms, one specially adapted. Tourist
Board assistance on access compliance
requirements. Check when booking.

DALMALLY
Quiet village with good access to Western
Isles, located on A85 from Perth and Crieff
heading west toward Oban.

BED AND BREAKFAST
CRUACHAN
Dalmally PA33 1AA
Tel: (01838) 200496   Fax: (01838) 200650
No. of Accessible Rooms: 2. Roll-in Shower
Accessible Facilities: Lounge, Dining room,
Garden. Traditional villa with lovely scenery.

ATTRACTION
CRUACHAN THE HOLLOW MOUNTAIN POWER STATION
Dalmally PA33 1AN
Tel: (01866) 822618   Fax: (01866) 922509
e-mail: VISIT.cruachan@scottishpower.plc.uk
Free exhibition contains touch-screen
information on the vast cavern hidden
inside Ben Cruachan, containing 400,000-
kilowatt hydro-electric power station. Access
to the surface exhibition only. Buses going
inside the mountain cannot take wheelchairs.
Visitors with their own diesel transport can
be taken in by prior arrangement.

SD ☐ CP   E ☐ RF
C ☐ S   WC ☐

DRYMEN
Located north-west of Glasgow, almost at
the south-western tip of Loch Lomond.

ATTRACTION
LOCH LOMOND PARK CENTRE
Balmaha, by Drymen
Tel: (01360) 870479   Fax: (01360) 870471
The main exhibition explores the geography
of Loch Lomond landscapes. The centre is
the focal point for the Millennium Trail
with boat yard, pier, car park and shops all
set round a lovely bay below Conic Hill.

SD ☐ CP ☐ E ☐ RF ☐
S ☐ WC ☐ RFE ☐

DUNOON
Popular Victorian holiday resort, which
once had a strong US influence from the
submarine base at Holy Loch now reduced
since the base closed. Disabled riding
facilities five miles.

BED AND BREAKFAST
MONCRIEFF
133 Alexandra Parade, Dunoon PA23 8AN
Tel/Fax: (01369) 707945
e-mail: willypeel@aol.com
No. of Accessible Rooms: 1
Accessible Facilities: Lounge, Dining Room.
Guesthouse by the seafront.

FALKIRK
This thriving industrial town of the C18th
and C19th, maintains a busy shopping
centre. Five miles away at Rough Castle are
remains of the Antonine Wall, built by the
Romans in AD142.

BED AND BREAKFAST
ASHBANK GUEST HOUSE
105 Main Street, Redding, Falkirk FK2 9UQ
Tel: (01324) 716649   Fax: (01324) 712431
e-mail: house.freeserve.co.uk
No. of Accessible Rooms: 1
Accessible Facilities: Dining Room, Garden
Detached stone house situated on the east

side of the town with gardens on all sides and views over the Forth Valley. Falkirk is 10 minutes' drive away, Stirling 20 minutes, and Edinburgh 30 minutes.

ATTRACTION
CALLENDAR HOUSE
Callendar Park, Falkirk FK1 1YR
Tel: (01324) 503770   Fax: (01324) 503771
900 years of history demonstrated in the Story of Callendar House exhibition. Costumed interpreters explain local C19th life.

SD   CP  E   RF   L
C [人] S [人] WC [人] RFE [♿]

HELENSBURGH
Holiday town, home of John Logie Baird who invented the TV in 1926, and of the designer Charles Rennie MacKintosh.

HOTELS
ARDENCAPLE HOTEL   [♿]
Shore Road, Rhu, Nr. Helensburgh G84 8LA
Tel: (01436) 820200   Fax: (01436) 821099
No. of Accessible Rooms: 1
Accessible Facilities: Lounge, Restaurant.

ROSSLEA HALL HOTEL   [♿]
Ferry Road, Rhu, Helensburgh G84 8NF
Tel: (01436) 439955   Fax: (01436) 820897
No. of Accessible Rooms: 2
Accessible Facilities: Lounge, Restaurant
Country house hotel.

ISLE OF ISLAY
Most southerly of Western Isles, home to fine Highland heavily peated malt whiskies with much to see of historical and archaeological interest.

ATTRACTION
LOCH GRUINART NATURE RESERVE (RSPB)
Bushmill Cottages, Gruinart, Bridgend,
Islay PA44 7PP
Tel: (01496) 850505   Fax: (01496) 850575
e-mail: loch.gruinart@interramp.co.uk
Super beaches on Islay support a variety of bird life at the reserve. Hide is accessible with wheelchair viewing window. NB: Visitor Centre is ramped at 1:8 and is not accessible.

SD n/a   CP   RF-(WC)
WC [人]   RFE [♿]

ISLE OF MULL
Largest of the Inner Hebrides with most roads following an irregular coastline backed by mountains. Tobermory, the capital in the north, has colourful houses and a sheltered harbour. Several mountain peaks are over 2,000feet, Ben More is the highest at 3,169. Some lovely beaches.

HOTEL
THE TOBERMORY HOTEL   [人]
53 Main Street, Tobermory,
Isle of Mull PA75 6NT
Tel: (01688) 302091   Fax: (01688) 302254
No. of Accessible Rooms: 2. Roll-in Shower
Accessible Facilities: Lounge, Restaurant (both with 1 step). Family hotel situated in the lovely Tobermory Bay.

ATTRACTIONS
MULL AND WEST HIGHLANDS NARROW GAUGE RAILWAY CO.
Craignure, Isle of Mull PA65 6AY
Tel: (01680) 812474
Steam and diesel trains run from Torosay Castle to Craignure, 1.5 miles, with woodland and mountain scenery.

SD [♿] CP [人] E [♿]  RF [♿]
S [♿]   WC [人]

TOROSAY CASTLE
Craignure, Isle of Mull PA65 6AY
Tel: (01680) 812421   Fax: (01680) 812470
Victorian castle of Scottish baronial architecture with a fascinating variety of interior displays. Edwardian library and archive rooms. Italian terraced gardens include statue walk and water gardens

SD [♿] CP [♿] E [♿] RF [♿]
C [人] S [♿] WC [人] G [♿]

LOCHGILPHEAD
A market town and hub for smaller communities with bank, supermarket etc. A good base for a tour of the Kintyre Peninsula.

BED AND BREAKFAST
EMPIRE TRAVEL LODGE
Union Street, Lochgilphead PA31 8JS
Tel: (01546) 602381
No. of Accessible Rooms: 1

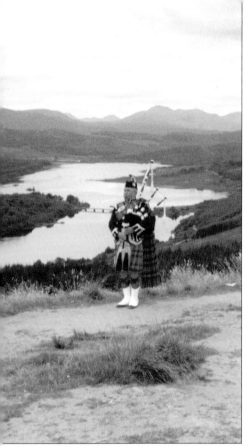

More pipes! Well that's what Scotland's all about.

Trails and Hides – two trails (Dubbs Water and Aird Meadow) and three bird-watching hides are all accessible to wheelchair users. Open water is a most obvious feature of the reserve with many species – great crested grebes being a summer favourite. Trails follow marsh and meadow and also a small woodland.

SD n/a CP ♿ E ♿ RF ♿
C 🚶 WC ♿ RFE ♿

LUSS

Attractive C19th estate village where many cottages were erected to house factory workers. Now restored, Luss is a Conservation Village, famous for the roses around the doors. Set at the foot of the glen, on the shores of Loch Lomond, where the Luss runs into the loch.

ATTRACTION
LOCH LOMOND PARK CENTRE
Luss Village
Tel: (01436) 860601
The main exhibit provides an insight into landscape, wildlife and the cultural history of Loch Lomond.

SD ♿ CP ♿ E ♿ RF ♿
S ♿ WC 🚶

OBAN

Known as the Gateway to the Isles, this is a busy port on the Firth of Lorne with good views of the Argyll coast, and an attractive sea-front shopping area with fresh fish for sale on the pier. The town is dominated by McCraig's Tower (1800). August attracts yachtsmen for West Highland Week.

SELF-CATERING
MELFORT PIER AND HARBOUR ♿
Kimelford, by Oban PA34 4XD
Tel: (01852) 200333   Fax: (01852) 200329
e-mail: melharbour@aol.com
No. of Accessible Units: 4
No. of Beds per Unit: 2 - 6
Accessible Facilities: Lounge/Diner, Kitchen, Balcony. Self-contained harbour houses in superb and unique location right on the shores of Loch Melfort, protected on seaward side by uninhabited islands and

Accessible Facilities: Breakfast served in bedrooms. there are five steps to the breakfast room. Built originally as a cinema, now fully refurbished to create mid-Argyll's only purpose-built travel lodge.

LOCHWINNOCH
ATTRACTION
RSPB LOCHWINNOCH NATURE RESERVE
Larges Road, Lochwinnoch PA12 4JE
Tel: (01505) 842663   Fax: (01505) 813026
e-mail: HYPERLINK
mailto:Lochwinnoch@interramp.co.uk
Lochwinnoch@interramp.co.uk
Useful information sheet for people with disabilities visiting the Reserve.
Visitor Centre shop/reception and visitor's area accessible. The observation tower is not accessible. A wheelchair is available free of charge.

sheltered by the hills of Melfort to the North.

ELERAIG HIGHLAND CHALETS
Kilninver, by Oban PA34 4UX
Tel/Fax: (01852) 200225
web: www.Scotland2000.com/eleraig
No. of Accessible Units: 1. Bath
No. of Beds per Unit: 6
Accessible Facilities: Open plan Lounge/
dining/kitchenette.
One of seven Norwegian chalets in a private
glen with wonderful scenery and close to
Loch Tralaig, 1.5 miles long.

ATTRACTION
ARDUAINE GARDENS (NT for S)
Arduaine, Oban PA34 4XQ
Tel/Fax: (01852) 200366
C18th garden planted on a hillside beside
the sea, notable for rhododendrons and
azaleas, with variable terrain. Two
wheelchair-friendly waymarked routes
around the garden. Wheelchair on site.

SD 　　CP 　　E
RF 　　WC

OBAN SEAL AND MARINE CENTRE
Barcaldine, Oban PA37 1SE
Tel: (01631) 720386　Fax: (01631) 720529
Set among pine trees on the shore of Loch
Creran, this is Scotland's leading marine
animal rescue centre. Crystal clear waters
allow exploration of over 30 natural marine
habitats and dramatic loch-side wildlife trails,
seal sanctuary and multi-level viewing
enhance this fascinating attraction.

SD | CP | E | RF
C | S | WC

STIRLING
The town grew up around its castle, one of
the most important fortresses in Scotland,
built in C15th and C16th. Beneath the
castle, the Old Town is protected by original
C16th walls and is well preserved with a fine
medieval church of the Holy Rude, guild
hall, tolbooth and wide market place. North
of the city is the Bridge of Allan, established
as a Victorian spa town and now home to
the University of Stirling with landscaped
wooded grounds which are worth visiting.

BED AND BREAKFAST
UPPER GARTINSTARRY
Buchlyvie, Nr. Stirling FK8 3PD
Tel/Fax: (01360) 850309
e-mail: goldings@bigfoot.com
No. of Accessible Rooms: 2
Accessible Facilities: Lounge, Dining Room
Country guesthouse a few miles west of
Stirling.

ATTRACTIONS
OLD TOWN JAIL
St. John Street, Stirling FK8 1EA
Tel: (01786) 450050　Fax: (01786) 471301
Built in 1847, this Victorian architectural
gem offers a living history performance
about the daily life of its prisoners. The lift
accesses the rooftop with panoramic views
of Stirling and beyond. Guided tour takes
place in a level, wide corridor.

SD n/a　　CP 　　E　　RF
L 　　S　　WC

STIRLING CASTLE
Stirling FK8 1EJ
Tel: (01786) 450000　Fax: (01786) 464678
Strategically built on the Firth of Forth,
much remaining from C15th and C16th.
James II was born here in 1430: Mary
Queen of Scots spent time here. All
apartments are accessible apart from the
museum of Argyll and Sutherland
Highlanders. The lower level of Queen Anne
Gardens is also accessible. Only medieval
kitchens and Elphinstone Tower are not
accessible.

SD | CP | E | RF
C | S | WC

SMITH ART GALLERY AND MUSEUM
Dumbarton Road, Stirling
Tel: (01786) 471917　Fax: (01786) 449523
e-mail: museum@smithartgallery.demon.co.uk
Located beneath Stirling Castle, with a fine
collection of Scottish painting, and an
important and little-known history
collection, including the Stirling Jug
(1457), the oldest dated curling stone in the
world (1511) and ancient tartans.

SD | CP | E (not main entrance)
RF | L | C
S | WC | RFE

REGION 5:

PERTHSHIRE, ANGUS AND DUNDEE, KINGDOM OF FIFE

ANGUS & DUNDEE

ARBROATH

Fishing and holiday town famous for red stonework, C12th, and Arbroath Smokies, smoked haddock. Many fishmongers gather on the seafront where visitors can watch the smoking process and enjoy a treat in one of the wonderful fish and chip shops.

ATTRACTION
ARBROATH ABBEY (HS)
Abbey Street, Arbroath
Tel/Fax: (01241) 878756
Robert the Bruce was declared king in this C12th abbey in 1320. A rose garden along the south wall of the abbey church is accessible. The sacristy not accessible.

SD 🔽 CP 🧍 E ♿ RF 🔽
C 🧍 WC 🧍 (50m from Abbey)

CARNOUSTIE

Pleasant seaside town best known for its championship golf course.

HOTEL
CARLOGIE HOUSE HOTEL 🔽
Carlogie Road, Carnoustie DD7 6LD
Tel: (01241) 853185 Fax: (01241) 856528
No. of Accessible Rooms: 4
Accessible Facilities: Lounge, Restaurant. Set in secluded grounds and close to over 50 golf courses. Situated just off the A92 road from Dundee to Arbroath, the latter five miles away.

DUNDEE

Major shipbuilding centre in C18th and C19th and the country's fourth largest city.

Good views over the River Tay to Fife from its riverfront, where at Victoria Dock lies HM Frigate Unicorn, the oldest British-built warship still afloat (1824). Several historic relics include the Howff, an old burial ground and Old Steeple, C15th tower fragment of the largest medieval church in Scotland.

TOURIST INFORMATION CENTRE
4 City Square, Dundee DD1 3AA
Tel: (01382) 434664

BUSES
Strathtay Scottish: Tel: (01382) 228345
Thistle Coaches: Tel: (01382) 87212
16-seater vehicles with ramps, straps and private hire if required.

TAXIS
Blackcabs:
Discovery Taxis: Tel: (01382) 732111/731222
Findhorn: Tel: (01382) 504040
Four adapted vehicles.
Handytaxis: Tel: (01382) 225825
Two adapted vehicles.

Peter Fraser-Minibuses: Tel: (0385) 266845
One adapted vehicle, taking two wheelchairs.

TRAINS
Dundee Scotrail: Tel: (0345) 484950
No. for disabled passengers: (0845) 6057021
Ramps and staff assistance available with 24 hours' notice.
GNER – Special Needs: Tel: (0845) 225444
Minicom: (0191) 2330173
Wheelchair space in first and standard class. Assistance available at stations when booked in advance.

HOTEL
STAKIS DUNDEE HOTEL 🧍
Earl Grey Place, Dundee DD1 4DE
Tel: (01382) 229271 Fax: (01382) 200072
No. of Accessible Rooms: 3. 1 room has a shower, 2 have baths. Accessible Facilities: Lounge, Restaurant. Quality hotel set on the banks of the River Tay, five minutes' drive from the A90.

SWALLOW HOTEL 🧍
Kingsway West, Invergowrie, Dundee DD2 5JT

Tel: (01382) 541122   Fax: (01382) 568340
No. of Accessible Rooms: 3
Accessible Facilities: Lounge, Restaurant,
Pool, Sauna, Spa. Victorian mansion in
delightful gardens, located off the by-pass,
10 minutes' drive from the city centre.

BED AND BREAKFAST
ALCORN GUEST HOUSE
5 Hyndford Street, Dundee, Angus DD2 3DY
Tel: (01382(668433
No. of Accessible Rooms: 1. Bath
Accessible Facilities: Lounge, Dining Room

SELF-CATERING
KINGENNIE LODGES
The Kingennie Fishings, Kingennie,
Broughtyferry, Dundee DD5 3RD
Tel: (01382) 350777   Fax: (01382) 350400
e-mail: kingennie@easynet.co.uk
No. of Accessible Units: 1
No. of Beds per Unit: 3
Accessible Facilities: Lounge, Kitchen/Diner,
Trout Fishing. Luxury self-catering lodges of
which Glenclova is fully accessible. Situated
in woodland overlooking trout lakes and old
boathouse of 1855. Located five miles north
of Dundee. Some areas of the lake are
wheelchair accessible.

ATTRACTION
DISCOVERY POINT
Discovery Quay, Dundee DD1 4XA
Tel: (01782) 201245   Fax: (01382) 225891
e-mail: dundeeheritage@sd.co.uk
Home of Captain Scott's Antarctic ship RRS
Discovery. There are eight exhibition areas
with lighting, special effects and graphics
telling the Discovery story. A must.

SD | CP | E | RF
C | S | WC | RFE

FORFAR
Market town, once a jute and flax milling
centre, now producing man-made fabrics
and agricultural products.

ATTRACTION
GLAMIS CASTLE GROUNDS
by Forfar DD8 1RJ
Tel: (01307) 840393   Fax: (01307) 840733
e-mail: glamis@great-houses-scotland.co.uk

Unfortunately this wonderful turreted and
battlemented castle is not accessible, but
worth viewing from outside. Home of the
Bowes-Lyon family since C14th, The
Queen Mother was born here. The
grounds are lovely, details below.

SD | CP | E | RF
C | S | WC

KIRRIEMUIR
Typical Angus town with red sandstone
buildings, agricultural and textile works
and famous as birthplace of J. M. Barrie, a
little cottage at 9 Brechin Road. Statue of
Peter Pan in town square.

ATTRACTION
LOCH OF KINNORDY RSPB RESERVE
The Flat, Kinnordy Home Farm,
Kirriemuir DD85ER
Tel/Fax: (01250) 881496
3 bird-watching hides, two are accessible.
SD n/a   CP   E

MONTROSE
A wealthy town accumulated through rich
agricultural land and more recently oil
revenues. Situated at the mouth of river,
South Esk is an important area for
wintering geese, many thousands roost
here. There is a medieval market square
and the seafront offers a fine beach.

HOTEL
THE LINKS HOTEL
Mid Links, Montrose, Angus DD10 8RL
Tel: (01674) 671000   Fax: (01674) 672698
No. of Accessible Rooms: 1
Accessible Facilities: Lounge, Restaurant.
Small hotel situated in the Links in the
centre of Montrose.

KINGDOM OF FIFE
For all information regarding accessible
transport throughout Fife, contact Anne
Cowan, Transport Department, Fife
House, Glenrothes.
Tel: (01592) 414141

ANSTRUTHER

Once the home of Scotland's main fishing fleet, now leisure boats fill the harbour.

ATTRACTION
SCOTTISH FISHERIES MUSEUM
Harbourhead, Anstruther KY10 3AB
Tel: (01333) 310628
Both real and model boats and fisherman's cottages are housed in various C16th and C19th buildings.

SD 🚻 CP 🚻 E 🚻 RF 🚹
C 🚻   S 🚻   WC 🚹

DUNFERMLINE

Capital of Scotland in 1603, dominated by the ruins of the C12th abbey. The abbey church contains the tombs of 22 Scottish kings and queens including Robert the Bruce.

HOTEL
PITBAUCHLIE HOUSE HOTEL   🚹
Aberdour Road, Dunfermline KY11 4PB
Tel: (01383) 722282   Fax: (01383) 620738
No. of Accessible Rooms: 1
Accessible Facilities: Lounge, Restaurant. Family-run hotel on the south side of town set in wooded, landscaped grounds with modern public rooms.

SELF-CATERING
BENARTY HOLIDAY COTTAGES   🚹
Benarty House, Kelty, Nr. Dunfermline KY4 0HT
Tel/Fax: (01383) 830235
No. of Accessible Units: 1. Bath
No. of Beds per Unit: 6
Accessible Facilities: Living/Dining Room, Kitchen. The Steading is 1 of 2 cottages situated on a working farm in woodland adjacent to Lochore Meadows Country Park and over the hill from Loch Leven. Located 4 miles north of Dunfermline.

ATTRACTION
ABBOT HOUSE
Maygate, Dunfermline KY12 7NE
Tel: (01383) 733266   Fax: (01383) 624908
Journey through 1,000 years of history in this medieval house which has born witness to the intrigues of church and state.

SD 🚻 CP 🚻 E 🚻 RF 🚻
C 🚻   S 🚻   WC 🚹

GLENROTHES

Planned town of 1950s built to house Fife's colliery workers, it is full of 60s architecture. Transport details for Kirkcaldy, a few miles south, are also given.

DIAL A RIDE
Rothesay House, Glenrothes DY7 5LT
Tel: (01592) 413434
Useful for information on Taxicard.

SHOPMOBILITY
Multi Storey Car Park, Kingdom Centre, Glenrothes. Tel: (01592) 414199

HOTEL
BALBIRNIE HOUSE HOTEL   🚻
Balbirnie Park, Markinch,
by Glenrothes KY7 6NE
Tel: (01592) 610066   Fax: (01592) 610529
e-mail: balbirnie@btinternet.com
web: www.balbirnie.co.uk
No. of Accessible Rooms: 4
Accessible Facilities: Lounge, Restaurant. Listed Grade A Georgian mansion set in 416 acre estate with trees and rhododendrons. Restored with open fires and antiques, providing a wonderful ambience. 30 minutes from Edinburgh and St. Andrews.

KIRKCALDY TRANSPORT
PUBLIC TRANSPORT INFORMATION HELPLINE
Tel: (01592) 416060

BUSES
First Fife Bus: limited bus service, One throughout Fife with low-floor access but no restraints.

TAXIS
VoBus: Tel: (01592) 758978
One adapted 12-seater minibus takes two wheelchairs.
Derek Tapp Taxis: Tel: (0836) 717225
One adapted taxicab, takes one wheelchair.
Glenrothes Mini Coaches: Tel: (01592) 754004
One adapted 8-seater minibus takes three wheelchairs.
Bernards Minibuses: Tel: (01592) 640404
One adapted 6-seater minibus, takes two wheelchairs.

Ellis Taxis: Tel: (01592) 654100
One adapted 4-seater vehicle takes one
wheelchair.
Forth Taxis: Tel: (01592) 646464
One adapted 5-seater vehicle takes one
wheelchair.

TRAINS
Scotrail, Platform 14, Edinburgh Waverley Station.
Super-Sprinter and Class 158 trains, wheelchair
spaces.
Train Enquiries for Disabled Users:
Tel: (0141) 3354652
Staff Assistance: Tel: (0845) 6057021
Passenger Superintendent: Tel: (01383) 730346

SHOPMOBILITY
Mercat Centre Car Park, Tolbooth Street,
Kirkcaldy KY1 1NJ
Tel: (01592) 412199/414199

NORTH QUEENSFERRY
Important originally as a north terminal for
ferry crossing to carry pilgrims to nearby
Dunfermline. Ferry lasted 800 years until
road bridge opened in 1964.

ATTRACTION
DEEP SEA WORLD
North Queensferry KY11 1JR
Tel: (01383) 411880   Fax: (01383) 410514
e-mail: deepsea@sol.co.uk
Amazing underwater world viewed from
moving walkway travelling along viewing
tunnel through the sea bed. Come face to
face with sharks, giant rays and conger eels.

SD	CP	E	RF
C	S	WC	RFE

PITTENWEEM
Home of the Fife fishing fleet with bustling
early morning harbour. Overlooking harbour
is St. Fillan's Cave, a refuge in the C17th for
a Christian missionary. Pittenweem means
place of the cave in Pict dialect.

ATTRACTION
KELLIE CASTLE GARDENS (NTS)
Pittenweem KY10 2RF
Tel: (01333) 720271   Fax: (01333) 720326
The castle is not accessible, but smooth

paths run round the lovely Victorian walled
garden where plants and shrubs are grown
organically.

SD	CP	E	RF
C	S	WC n/a	

ST. ANDREWS
Scotland's oldest university town and one
time ecclesiastical capital, now synonymous
with golf. Charming crooked housefronts in
streets and alleyways, medieval churches
and C12th cathedral.

TOURIST INFORMATION CENTRE
70 Market Street, St. Andrews KY16 9NU
Tel: (01334) 472021

HOTEL
RUFFLETS COUNTRY HOUSE
Strathkinness Low Road, St. Andrews KY16 9TX
Tel: (01334) 472594   Fax: (01334) 478703
No. of Accessible Rooms: 1. Roll-in Shower
Accessible Facilities: Unknown
Lovely country house set in 10-acre gardens,
1.5 miles from the famous golf course. Close
to several visitor attractions.

SELF-CATERING
CAULSIDE FARMHOUSE
Easter Kincaple, St. Andrews   KY16 9SG
Tel: (01334) 473224   Fax: (01334) 472457
No. of Accessible Units: 1
No. of Beds per Unit: 8.
Accessible Facilities: 2 Lounges, Large
Kitchen/Diner. Large attractive house facing
south, with Swilken Burn running a few feet
away. Two miles west of St. Andrews.

ST. ANDREW'S COUNTRY COTTAGES
Mountquhanie Estate, Cupar,
Nr. St. Andrews KY15 4QJ
Tel: (01382) 330252   Fax: (01382) 330480
e-mail: enquiries@standrews-cottages.com
web: www.standrews-cottages.com
No. of Accessible Units: 1
No. of Beds per Unit: 6
Accessible Facilities: Lounge, Kitchen/Diner
One of several charming, secluded cottages
and farmhouses on Nydie Mains Farm, three
miles west of St. Andrews. Formerly two
traditional farm cottages, it has its own
enclosed garden. It overlooks the valley of

the river Eden with panoramic views towards the Tay and the foothills of the Grampians.

ATTRACTION
ST. ANDREWS CASTLE
The Scores, St. Andrews KY16 9AR
Tel: (01334) 477196 Fax: (01334) 475068
C13th defence with visitor centre showing multi-media exhibition describing castle's history and that of St. Andrews Cathedral.

| SD | [symbol] | E | [symbol] | RF | [symbol] |
| S | [symbol] | WC | [symbol] | RFE | [symbol] |

PERTHSHIRE

ABERFELDY
Popular, but less touristy than its neighbours though busy in summer with some cafes and shops. Close to the town centre is the 1733 Wades Bridge, and the water mill – powered by Moness Burn that runs through the town centre – has been restored to a working mill again.

TOURIST INFORMATION CENTRE
The Square, Aberfeldy PH15 2DD
Tel: (01887) 820276 Fax: (01887) 829495

SELF-CATERING
LOCH TAY LODGES
Remony, Aberfeldy PH15 2HR
Tel: (01887) 830209 Fax: (01887) 830802
e-mail: remony@btinternet.com
No. of Accessible Units: 1
No. of Beds per Unit: 6
Accessible Facilities: Lounge, Dining Room, Kitchen. Laggan Lodge is one of six lodges, originally constructed by the Earl of Breadalbane in the mid 1800s as estate workers cottages, now rebuilt. Situated on the eastern side of the small village of Acharn, close to Loch Tay in tranquil countryside of hill farms and sporting estates. Fine views in all directions.

BLAIRGOWRIE
Main centre for skiing in Glen Shee Ski area, 39km to the north. Famous as major

raspberry growing area since 1898. Woollen mill, shops and cafes add to a pleasant ambience.

TOURIST INFORMATION CENTRE
26 Wellmeadow, Blairgowrie PH10 6AS
Tel: (01250) 872960 Fax: (01250) 873701

HOTEL AAIRLIE MOUNTMANSION HOUSE
2 Albert Street, Alyth, Nr. Blairgowrie
Tel: (01828) 632986 Fax: (01828) 632563
No. of Accessible Rooms: 1
Accessible Facilities: Lounge, Dining Room
Family run Victorian mansion house set within mature gardens, specialising in accommodation for elderly or disabled people. Many historic sights within an hour's drive.

KINLOCH HOUSE HOTEL
By Blairgowrie PH10 6SG
Tel: (01250) 884237 Fax: (01250) 884333
No. of Accessible Rooms: 4
Accessible Facilities: Lounge, Restaurant.
Country house hotel in 25 acres of woods, parkland and highland cattle.

CRIEFF
Located on the cultural and physical border between the Highlands and Lowlands, Once a famous cattle market town, Crieff sits on the southern slope of the Knock, a large hill with woods.

TOURIST INFORMATION CENTRE
Town Hall, High Street, Crieff PH7 3HU
Tel: (01764) 652578 Fax: (01764) 655422

HOTEL
CRIEFF HYDRO HOTEL
Ferntower Road, Crieff PH7 3LQ
Tel: (01764) 655555 Fax: (01764) 653087
No. of Accessible Rooms: 2
Accessible Facilities: Lift (Cat.1), Lounge, Restaurant, Pool, Sauna, Spa, Cinema, Disabled Riding School, Victorian Garden, Beauty Salon, Boutique, Coffee Shop, Ballroom. Well-known, quality hotel on northern edge of the town combining traditional values and all modern conveniences, plus enormous range of sporting and leisure facilities.

ATTRACTION
GLENTURRET DISTILLERY
The Hosh, Crieff PH7 4HA
Tel: (01764) 656565   Fax: (01764) 654366
web: www.glenturret.com

Oldest distillery in Scotland, dating back to 1775, uses water from the Turret Burn to make award-winning whiskies.

SD   CP   E    RF
C [♿]   S [♿]   WC [♿]

DUNKELD
Situated by river Tay and almost destroyed in the Battle of Dunkeld in 1689. The little houses lining Cathedral Street were the first to be rebuilt. Ruins of a C14th. cathedral can be seen.

TOURIST INFORMATION CENTRE
The Cross, Dunkeld PH8 0AN
Tel/Fax: (01350) 727688

ATTRACTION
THE HERMITAGE (NT for S)
11 The Cross, Dunkeld PH8 0AN
Tel: (01350) 728641

A designed landscape with a woodland walk leading to St. Ossian's Hall, an C18th folly overlooking the dramatic Falls of Braan. Orange badge holders park at Ossian's Hall by going from the car park through an unlocked barrier behind the main notice board and following the track for 0.25 mile.

CP [🚶]

FORGANDENNY
Located in the River Earn valley, a few miles from Perth, lying within a short distance of an ancient Roman road connecting a string of outposts, forts and camps along the valley.

BED AND BREAKFAST
BATTLEDOWN BED AND BREAKFAST   [♿]
Battledown, Forgandenny PH2 9EL
Tel/Fax: (01738) 812471
e-mail: ian@battledown34-freesave.co.uk

No. of Accessible Rooms: 1
Accessible Facilities: Lounge, Dining Room. Late C18th cottage that once belonged to the village baker. Set in a mature garden with trees and shrubs, including rare

rowans. Secluded and sheltered in an old part of Forgandenny village that was on the stage route from Perth until early this century.

KILLIN
Charming little village dominated by Ben Lawers. The river Dochart runs through the centre with much photographed scenic falls.

HOTEL
DALL LODGE COUNTRY HOUSE HOTEL   [♿]
Main Street, Killin FK21 8TN
Tel: (01567) 820217   Fax: (01567) 820726
e-mail: wilson@dalllodgehotel.co.uk
web: www.dalllodgehotel.co.uk

No. of Accessible Rooms: 1. Bath
Accessible Facilities: Lounge, Restaurant. Country house hotel at the head of Loch Tay.

SELF-CATERING
THE SHIELING   [🚶]
Aberfeldy Road, Killin FK21 8TX
Tel/Fax: (01567) 820334

No. of Accessible Units: 3. Bath
No. of Beds per Unit: 1-4
Accessible Facilities: Lounge, Kitchen, Verandah with patio furniture, barbecue. Log cabins and chalets (accessible) situated adjacent to woodland and overlooks rolling hills at west end of Loch Tay. Located on the north (A827) side of Loch Tay, close to Killin Golf Course.

KINROSS
Located at the south entrance to Tayside, with fine C17th tolbooth.

HEART OF SCOTLAND TOURIST INFORMATION CENTRE
Service Area, J.6, M90 Kinross
Tel: (01577) 863680   Fax: (01577) 863370

HOTELS
LOMOND COUNTRY INN   [♿]
Main Street, Kinnesswood, Kinross KY13 7HN
Tel: (01592) 840253   Fax: (01592) 840 693
e-mail: the.lomond@dial.pipex.com

No. of Accessible Rooms: 1
Accessible Facilities: Lounge, Restaurant

Charming, small hotel lying in the slopes of the Lomond Hills, overlooking Loch Lomond in a small village, with wonderful Loch views. Good base for touring.

WINDLESTRAE HOTEL [🚶]
The Muirs, Kinross KY13 7AS
Tel: (01577) 863217   Fax: (01577) 864233
No. of Accessible Rooms: 3. Bath
Accessible Facilities: Lounge, Restaurant (3 steps). Attractive hacienda style frontage leads into this rather cosy 45-roomed property, located close to M90 (J6).

ATTRACTION
KINROSS HOUSE GARDENS
Kinross KY13 8ET
Tel: (01577) 862900
C17th house, not open to the public, but lovely formal gardens with yew, roses and herbaceous borders to view.
SD [♿]   CP [🚶]   E [🚶]   RFE [🚶]

PERTH

Once the capital of medieval Scotland with wonderful historic buildings remaining – the Fair Maid's House c1600, on North Park, is the oldest in town. The River Tay runs through the centre. John Knott preached his fiery sermons here in the Church of St. John in 1559.

TOURIST INFORMATION CENTRE
Lower City Mills, West Mill Street, Perth PH1 5QP
Tel: (01738) 627958   Fax: (01738) 630416
PUBLIC TRANSPORT LINE
Tel: (0845) 3011130

PERTH AND KINROSS COUNCIL
Recreation/Outdoor Divisions
3-5 High Street, Perth PH1 5JS
Tel: (01738) 475200   Fax: (01738) 441690

Arts and Heritage Division
George Street, Perth , PH1 5LB
Tel: (01738) 632488   Fax: (01738) 443505

BUSES

(ask for Traffic Manager).
Service 1 and 2 are wheelchair accessible

and run every 12 minutes.

TAXIS
A & M King Taxis: Tel: (01738) 622255
Fully equipped but advisable to book.
TRAINS
Scotrail: Tel: for special assistance
(0845) 6057021

GNER: Special Needs Tel: (0845) 7225444
Wheelchair spaces in first and standard class trains, advisable to book. One space in each with straps. Perth station has no wheelchair unassisted access but there are ramps and staff assistance when notified 24 hours in advance.

HOTEL
SUNBANK HOUSE HOTEL [🚶]
50 Dundee Road, Perth PH2 7BA
Tel: (01738) 624882   Fax: (01738) 442515
No. of Accessible Rooms: 3
Accessible Facilities: Lounge, Restaurant.
Small hotel close to city centre

SPORTING VENUE
THE PERTH HUNT
Perth Racecourse, Scone Palace Park, Perth
Tel: (01738) 551597   Fax: (01738) 553021
Complies with Part M, Building Regulations.
CP [♿]   RE [♿]   ED [♿]   INT [♿]
WC [♿] (2 adapted WC's on ground level of public enclosure)
SS [♿] Route from main entrance around paddock to racecourse on rails – good viewing. 6 spaces
B [🚶] (ground floor)

PITLOCHRY

One of Queen Victoria's favourite European resorts, the town is surrounded by the pine-covered hills of the central Highlands. A busy town with good shops and restaurants along its main street.

TOURIST INFORMATION CENTRE
22 Atholl Road, Pitlochry PH16 5BX
Tel: (01796) 472215   Fax: (01796) 474046

HOTELS
CRAIGVRACK HOTEL [🚶]
38 West Moulin Road, Pitlochry PH16 5EQ
Tel: (01796) 472399   Fax: (01796) 473990

No. of Accessible Rooms: 1
Accessible Facilities: Lounge, Restaurant
Comfortable holiday hotel, with elevation
located beside Braemar Road and fine views
over surrounding wooded hills.

BED AND BREAKFAST
BALLINDUIN BOTH   🦽
Strathtay, by Pitlochry PH9 0LP
Tel/Fax: (01887) 840460
No. of Accessible Rooms: 3
Accessible Facilities: Lounge, Dining Room,
Garden. Converted farm buildings, quiet,
with lovely views of wildlife and birds.

ATTRACTIONS
BLAIR ATHOLL DISTILLERY VISITOR CENTRE
Perth Road, Pitlochry PH16 5LY
Tel: (01796) 482003   Fax: (01796) 482001
By 1579 whisky making took so much barley
that food supplies were threatened. Sadly,
much of the actual tour of this Bells-owned
distillery is inaccessible, but join in
beneath the stills room and continue to the
bonded warehouse with rolling stock of 15
million litres. Oak casks of a minimum
three years, usually eight, and eight casks of
1968. These, with 50% evaporation, will
make the intended dram a wee pricey!

SD 🦽	CP 🚶	E 🦽	RF 🦽
C 🚶	S 🦽	WC 🚶	

BLAIR CASTLE
Blair Atholl, Pitlochry PH18 5TL
Tel: (01796) 481207   Fax: (01796) 431487
e-mail: scotland.co.uk
Scotland's most visited privately owned
home of the Dukes of Atholl with 32 fully
furnished rooms of beautiful furniture, a
fine collection of paintings, armour, china,
lace and embroidery displays. Extensive
parklands, deer park, highland cattle,
picnic area and nature trail in the grounds.

SD 🦽	CP 🦽	E 🦽	RF 🦽
C 🚶	S 🚶	WC 🚶	RFE 🦽

EDRADOUR DISTILLERY
Pitlochry PH16 5JP
Tel: (01796) 472095   Fax: (01796) 472002
Scotland's smallest distillery producing a
handmade malt in limited quantity. Enjoy
a wee dram in the Malt Barn where the
history and whisky maker's art will be
revealed, and then tour the distillery.

SD 🦽	CP 🚶	E 🦽	C n/a
RF 🦽	S 🦽	WC 🚶	RFE 🚶

333

Pitlochry boat station.

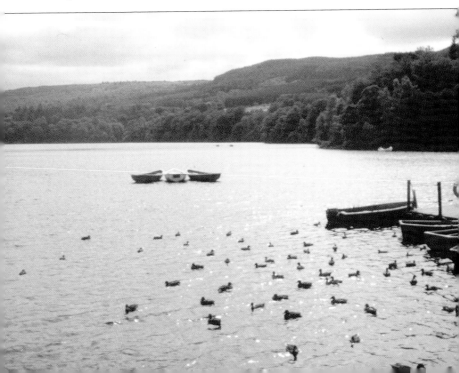

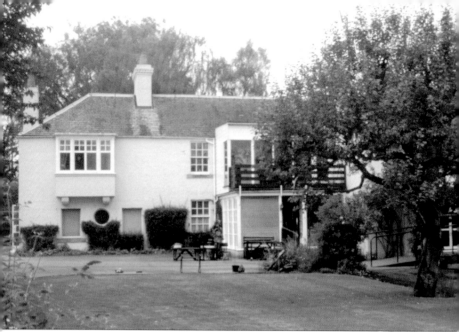

Wildwood House.

GLENGOULANDIE DEER PARK
Glengoulandie, Foss, by Pitlochry PH15 5NL
Tel/Fax: (01887) 830261

Drive-through park with herds of red deer and cattle and numerous native birds and animals in natural surroundings.

S 🚶 WC 🚶

PITLOCHRY ANGLING CLUB
Sunnknowe, 7 Nursing Home Brae, Pitlochry PH16 5HP
Tel: (01796) 472 484

Fly fishing for trout and grayling on Loch Kindardochy. Information and permits available in local tackle shops. Parking 50m up the slope from the lochside. There is provision on one loch for a boat with an accessible seat for boat fishing. Booking is necessary.

PITLOCHRY BOATING STATION
Loch Faskally, Cluniebridge Road, Pitlochry
Tel: (01796) 472919

Charming spot on lovely loch with coffee shop and picnic facilities, boats and ducks.

CP ♿   E ♿   RF ♿
C ♿   S ♿   EC ♿

STANLEY

River Tay runs close to the village of Stanley that is close to Perth, Dunkeld, Blairgowrie and Pitlochry.

HOTEL
WILDWOOD HOUSE   ♿
Stanley, Perthshire PH1 4PX
Tel: (01738) 828932

No. of Accessible Rooms: 4
Accessible Facilities: Lounge, Dining Room, Gardens. One room on ground floor, others on first floor accessed by four-person professional lift. One room has a Closomat WC that washes and dries: another has an hydraulic adjustable washbasin: two have roll-in showers. Mattresses of various heights and lounge chairs of various heights with adjustable arms. Small, secluded country house in lovely gardens run by a delightful, caring couple who cater for elderly and disabled guests.

BALLATHIE HOUSE HOTEL   🚶
Kinclaven, by Stanley PH1 4QN
Tel: (01250) 883268   Fax: (01250) 883396

No. of Accessible Rooms: 2, 1 being a suite.
Twin-shower: Suite-Spa bath.
Accessible Facilities: Lounge, Restaurant
Lovely country house in a delightful location overlooking River Tay.

REGION 6

GRAMPIAN HIGHLANDS, ABERDEEN AND NORTH EAST COAST

ABERDEEN

Maritime city and one-time royal burgh, the sea is the essence of this city, where gas and oil, rather than fish, are now paramount. It has a distinctive townscape formed by the many buildings of locally quarried silver granite used since the C18th to shape the town, hence it is known as the granite city. There are many shopping malls, and continuous floral displays in the gardens of Duthies Park and other city parks. The university was founded here in 1494. 3km of sands between the mouths of the rivers Dee and Donn maintain its seaside town appeal.

TOURIST INFORMATION CENTRE
St. Nicholas House, Broad Street,
Aberdeen AB10 1DE
Tel: (01224) 632727

ABERDEEN CITY COUNCIL
Woodhill House, Westburn Road,
Aberdeen AB1 5GB
Tel: (01224) 664580

BUSES
Freepark Community Service: Tel: (01224) 680100.
4 minibuses with straps and ramps.
(Ronnie Devlin-Transport).
J.W.Coaches: Tel: (01330) 823300

TAXICARD OPERATORS LIST
Tel: (01224) 665566
Bluebird: Tel: (01224) 212266
Campbell Cars: Tel: (01224) 625444
Dennis Davidson: Tel: (01224) 590406
Duncans Large Cabs: Tel: (01224) 744263
Fyvie Taxis: Tel: (01224) 890937
Falcon Taxis: Tel: (01224) 697569

DJ Grayson: Tel: (01224) 208478
Brian L Hay: Tel: (01224) 693235
Mairs-City: Tel: (01224) 494949
Eric McDermid: Tel: (07990) 840521
Phoenix Taxis: Tel: (01224) 698869
T0.D.A.: Tel: (01224) 648648

TRAINS
Scotrail: Telephone for disabled Assistance:
(0845) 6057021

GNER - Telephone for Special Needs:
(08457) 225444
Minicom: (0191) 2330173
Wheelchair space in first and standard class. Assistance at station when booked in advance. Aberdeen Station offers staff assistance and ramps available.

SHOPMOBILITY
Flourmill Lane Car Park, Flour Mill Lane,
Aberdeen AB10 1AG
Tel/Minicom: (01224) 630009
Fax: (01224) 640741

HOTELS
MARCLIFFE at PITFODELS ♿
North Deeside Road, Aberdeen AB15 9YA
Tel: (01224) 861000   Fax: (01224) 868860
e-mail: reservations@marcliffe.com
No. of Accessible Rooms: 1
Accessible Facilities: Lounge, Restaurant. Country hotel in the city, 20 minutes from airport. Dining room under glass.

SPEEDBIRD INNS ♿
Aberdeen Airport, Argyll Road, Dyce, Aberdeen AB21 0AF
Tel: (01224) 772884   Fax: (01224) 772560
No. of Accessible Rooms: 3
Accessible Facilities: Lounge, Restaurant. Comfortable, modern airport hotel.

THISTLE ABERDEEN AIRPORT ♿
Argyll Road, Dyce, Aberdeen AB21 7DU
Tel: (01224) 725252   Fax: (01224) 723745
No. of Accessible Rooms: 1
Accessible Facilities: Lounge, Restaurant, Outdoor Pool. Quality hotel located adjacent to the airport, just off the A96 with rail station. Nine miles, 15 minutes' drive, to the city centre.

THISTLE ABERDEEN ALTENS ♿
Souterhead Road, Aberdeen AB12 3LF
Tel: (01224) 877000 Fax: (01224) 896964
No. of Accessible Rooms: 1.
Accessible Facilities; Lounge, Restaurant
Located in the south of the city close to the
Altens Industrial Estate, popular with
visiting businessmen.

BRITANNIA HOTEL ABERDEEN 🚶
Malcolm Road, Bucksburn, Aberdeen AB21 9LN
Tel: (01224) 409988 Fax: (01224) 714020
No. of Accessible Rooms: 1.
Accessible Facilities: Restaurant, Bar.
Modern business hotel in north-west suburb.

ATTRACTIONS
ABERDEEN MARITIME MUSEUM
Shiprow, Aberdeen AB11 5BY
Tel: (01224) 337700 Fax: (01224) 213066
Housed in the city's oldest building (1593)
explore the history of the North Sea with
exciting exhibitions and multi-media
displays about the offshore oil industry,
shipbuilding, fishing and the story of
Aberdeen harbour. Centrepiece is the 8.5m
high model of the Murchison oil platform.

SD ♿ CP n/a E ♿ L ♿
C ♿ S ♿ WC ♿

CRUIKSHANK BOTANIC GARDENS
University of Aberdeen, Dept. of Plant and Soil
Sciences, St. Machar Drive, Aberdeen AB24 3UU
Tel: (01224) 272704 Fax: (01224) 272703
The majority of the garden is level,
although some areas are grass and will
present some difficulty. 11 acres of rock
gardens, rose garden, herbaceous borders,
arboretum and patio garden.

CP ♿ (call in advance) E ♿ RF n/a
C n/a S n/a WC n/a

GORDON HIGHLANDERS MUSEUM
St. Lukes, Viewfield Road, Aberdeen AB15 7XH
Tel: (01224) 311200 Fax: (01224) 319323
e-mail: museum@gordonhighlanders.com
Story of this famous regiment which spans
200 years of world history, with interactive
displays, a unique collection of regimental
treasures, an AV theatre and detailed life-
size and scale reproductions of some of the
regiment's finest moments in battle.

SD n/a CP ♿ E ♿ RF ♿
C ♿ S ♿ WC 🚶

SATROSPHERE
19 Justice Hill Lane, Aberdeen AB11 6EQ
Tel: (01224) 213232 Fax: (01224) 211685
e-mail: satrosphere@ssphere.ifb.co.uk
web: www.ifb.co.uk/-ssphere/
Science and technology come alive through
hands-on exhibits. Find out about energy,
communications, growing plants, weather,
the earth and the world around us.

SD ♿ CP ♿
E 🚶 (side entrance for wheelchairs, ramped at 1:10)
C ♿ S 🚶 WC 🚶 RFE ♿

BALLATER
Queen Victoria purchased Balmoral Estate
in 1852 and the it has been the summer
home of Royal Family ever since. Ballater is
an old Deeside railway town, almost 250m
above sea level with an impressive backdrop
of forest and mountain. Many of the shops
have royal warrants. It developed in the
C19th as a spa town, its waters reputedly
good for curing tuberculosis.

BALLATER ROYAL DEESIDE TOURISM
36 Golf Road, Ballater AB35 5RS
Tel: (013397) 55467 Fax: (013397) 55283
e-mail: royaldeeside@compuserve.com
web: www.royal-deeside.org.uk/brd.htm

TOURIST INFORMATION CENTRE
Albert Hall, Station Square, Ballater.
Tel: (013397) 55306

HOTEL
DARROCH LEARGE HOTEL ♿
Braemar Road, Ballater AB35 5UX
Tel: (013397) 55443 Fax: (013397) 55252
e-mail: nigel@darroch-learg.demon.co.uk
No. of Accessible Rooms: 1
Accessible Facilities: Lounge, Restaurant
Family run hotel built in 1888 as a
comfortable residence in Royal Deeside. It
became a hotel about 50 years ago. It is set
in four acres of wooded grounds on the
slopes of Craigendarroch. Located high
above Ballater with fine views of the
Grampians across the Dee Valley.

ATTRACTION
BALMORAL ESTATES
The Estate Office, Balmoral, Ballater AB35 5TBA

Tel: (013397) 42334   Fax: (013397) 42271
e-mail: info@balmoral/castle.co.uk
web: www.balmoral-castle.co.uk

The castle is closed to the public, except for the ballroom. Carriage hall exhibitions are accessible with exhibitions of carriages, commemorative china, plus wildlife display in natural habitat. The three-acre gardens contain a range of glasshouses and a conservatory, plus a large kitchen garden and a water garden created by the Duke of Edinburgh. The garden cottage, where Queen Victoria used to write her diaries that was rebuilt in 1895, is not open to the public, but one can peek through the windows to view the unchanged interior.

SD n/a   CP 🧑‍🦽   E ♿   RF ♿
C ♿   S 🧑‍🦽   WC 🚹   RFE ♿

BALLINDALLOCH

Situated on a spur of the Speyside Way where the Glenlivet Estate is part of the Crown Estate.

SELF-CATERING
TORVUE COTTAGE   🚹
Achnascraw Farm, Braes of Glenlivet,
Ballindalloch AB37 9JT
Tel: (01807) 590256

No. of Accessible Units: 1. Bath
No. of Beds per Unit: 5
Accessible Facilities: Lounge, Kitchen.
Step from outside into porch and porch into kitchen. Modern bungalow with expansive views onto surrounding hills in peaceful, scenic countryside of secluded Braes of Glenlivet. 6 miles from Tomintoul.

ATTRACTION
GLENLIVET DISTILLERY VISITOR CENTRE
Glenlivet, Ballindalloch AB37 9DBA
Tel: (01542) 783220   Fax: (01542) 783218

200 years ago, whisky was closely bound up in the lives of every family in the glen of the Livet. This whisky, favoured by aristocracy and royalty, can be made only in this single spot. An audio-visual programme explores the turbulent history of whisky smugglers, teaches the intriguing mysteries of distilling and of course you must sample this true spirit of Scotland.

SD ♿   CP ♿   E ♿   RF ♿   L ♿
C ♿   S ♿   WC 🚹   RFE ♿

BANCHORY

Holiday town of elegant buildings with excellent salmon fishing on river Dee and trout on river Fengh.

TOURIST INFORMATION CENTRE
Bridge Street, Banchory
Tel: (01330) 822000

ATTRACTION
CRATHES CASTLE AND GARDENS
Banchory AB31 5QJ
Tel: (01330) 844525   Fax: (01330) 844797

Impressive C16th castle not accessible. Walled garden of three acres with unusual plants, and seven other gardens, extensive grounds and a disabled nature trail. Lower level of gardens only is accessible.

SD ♿   CP 🚹   RF ♿   C 🚹
S 🚹   WC 🚹   G 🧑‍🦽

BUCKIE

One of the largest of the Moray towns, extending along three miles of coastline, its principal industry is fishing. The Fish Market operates daily with harbour particularly full of boats on Friday nights. Good bird watching along shore.

ATTRACTION
THE BUCKIE DRIFTER MARITIME HERITAGE CENTRE
Freuchny Road, Buckie AB56 1TT
Tel: (01542) 834646   Fax: (01542) 835995

History of the herring-boom years in the Moray area during the 1890s and 1930s. Active participation includes finding out how to catch herring and packing fish in a barrel, plus hands-on displays and changing exhibits.

SD ♿   CP 🧑‍🦽   E ♿   L ♿
C ♿   S ♿   WC 🚹   RFE ♿

DUFFTOWN

On the malt whisky trail.

TOURIST INFORMATION CENTRE
The Clock Tower, The Square, Dufftown
Tel: (01340) 820501

ATTRACTION
THE GLENFIDDICH DISTILLERY

William Grant & Sons Ltd.,
Dufftown AB55 4DH
Tel: (01340) 820373 Fax: (01340) 820805
Founded in 1887 by William Grant this
remains a family firm. View the stages of
the whisky-making process and sample the
finished product! Audio-visual display of
the history and manufacture of whisky,
and a visit to the Scotch whisky museum.

| SD ♿ | CP ⚠ | E ♿ | RF ♿ |
| C ⚠ | S ♿ | WC ⚠ | RFE ♿ |

ELGIN

Major town of Moray, famous as Scotland's
malt whisky country. Retains its medieval
layout with a cobbled market place and
narrow lanes and the ruins of a C13th.
cathedral. There are some C18th buildings
with original arched facades.

TOURIST BOARD
17 High Street, Elgin IV30 1EG
Tel: (01343) 543388 Fax: (01343) 552982

SELF-CATERING
CARDEN SELF-CATERING   ♿
The Old Steading, Carden, Alves, Elgin,
Moray IV30 8UP
Tel: (01343) 850222 Fax: (01343) 850626
e-mail: carden@enterprise.net
web: www.carden.co.uk
No. of Accessible Units: 2, Bothy and
Stables, both with Roll-in Showers.
No. of Beds per Unit: 2
Accessible Facilities: Open plan
Lounge/Diner/Kitchen, Courtyard patio.
Two of six courtyard cottages created from
the original C18th farm steading.
Open views of surrounding countryside
with the hills of distant Sutherland visible
over the Moray Firth to the north and
farmland views to the south.

ATTRACTION
PLUSCARDEN ABBEY
Elgin IV30 3UA
Tel: (01343) 890257 Fax: (01343) 890258
Monastery founded in 1230, burnt down
and restored in C14th and C19th. Once
more it is a religious community. All
services are open to the public, with
Gregorian chant. Beeswax polish and

natural apiary remedies can be purchased.

| SD ♿ | CP ♿ | E ♿ | RF ♿ |
| S ⚠ | WC ♿ | RFE ♿ | |

FORRES

There has been a settlement here for at
least 2,000 years. See the topiary gardens
in Grant Park, and Nelson's Tower that
overlooks the town. It was built in 1806 to
celebrate victory at Trafalgar.

TOURIST INFORMATION CENTRE
116 High Street, Forres
Tel: (01309) 672938

ATTRACTION
BRODIE CASTLE (NT for S)
Brodie, Forres
Tel: (01309) 641371
Owned and lived in by the Brodie family
since 1160, this gabled castle offers fine
furniture and a collection of C17th Dutch
art, C19th English watercolours and
French impressionists. Lovely grounds.
Wheelchairs to loan, and a wheelchair lift
to the first floor.

| SD ♿ | CP ⚠ | E ⚠ | C ⚠ | S ⚠ |

INVERURIE

Thriving market town and centre of castle
country with easy access to the whisky
trail. Progressive agricultural centre with
auctions daily.

TOURIST INFORMATION CENTRE
18 High Street, Inverurie AB51 3XQ
Tel: (01467) 625800

HOTEL
STRATHBURN HOTEL   ⚠
Burghmuir Drive, Inverurie AB51 4GY
Tel: (01467) 624422 Fax: (01467) 625133
No. of Accessible Rooms: 2
Accessible Facilities: Lounge, Restaurant.
Built by the present owners in 1985, and
gradually extended to 25 rooms, this
pleasant property is located just off the
main A96 Aberdeen/Inverness road
overlooking Strathburn Park. 10 miles
from Aberdeen Airport.

KEITH

Fine 1830 catholic church and Auld Brig.
Built in 1609, it is among the oldest
bridges in Scotland.

SELF-CATERING
PARKHEAD COTTAGES ♿
Drummuir, Keith, Banffshire AB55 5PQ
Tel/fax: (01542) 810365
e-mail: LinCollins@tesco.net
No. of Accessible Units: 1. Roll-in Shower
No. of Beds per Unit: 6
Accessible Facilities: Open-plan living,
Dining, kitchen. Specially designed for
both disabled and able-bodied
holidaymakers, Parkhead Croft is a single
storey detached stone house set in well
planted gardens in a secluded valley in the
Grampian mountains midway between
Dufftown and Keith. The owners are now
restoring a second cottage, Garden
Cottage, situated at Forgie overlooking
Spey Forests and the Hills of Strathspey.
Due for completion during 2000.
Telephone to check.

MACDUFF

Former spa town and still a busy fishing
and boat-building centre, looking out
across the Moray Firth.

ATTRACTION
MACDUFF MARINE AQUARIUM
11 High Shore, Macduff AB44 2SL
Tel: (01261) 833369   Fax: (01261) 831052
e-mail:
macduffaquarium.ed@aberdeenshire.gov.uk.
web: www.marine-aquarium.com
Offers a unique centrepiece display tank
open to the sky in which a Moray firth kelp
reef thrives, complete with kelp and other
seaweeds and a whole community of fish –
don't miss the divers feeding the fish.

SD ♿   CP ♿   E ♿   RF ♿
S ♿   WC 🚹   RFE ♿

PETERHEAD

Famous for its harbour, fish-market and
prison, it is the busiest whitefish port in
Europe, its harbour is full of trawlers.

ATTRACTION
ABERDEENSHIRE FARMING MUSEUM
Aden Country Park, Mintlaw, Peterhead AB42 5FR
Tel: (01771) 622906   Fax: (01771) 622884
e-mail: heritage@aberdeenshire.gov.uk
Unique semi-circular steading surrounded
by the beautiful woodlands of Aden Country
Park, bringing alive the story of this region's
farming history. There are three related
interpretive themes: the Aden Estate
Story: Well Worked Ground, farming from
1780s to present day: and thirdly a video on
the newly reconstructed Hareshowe
Working Farm.

SD ♿   CP 🚹   E ♿   RF 🚹
C ♿   S 🚹   WC 🚹

PETERHEAD MARITIME HERITAGE
The Lido, South Road, Peterhead AB42 2YP
Tel/Fax: (01779) 473000
e-mail: itstrachan.er@aberdeenshire.gov.uk
The story of Peterhead's seafaring history
told through an AV presentation, touch-
screen computers and other displays,
including period kitchen and tableaux of
shipbuilding. Set by the shore of the
Harbour of Refuge on south side of town,
this is a fascinating visit.

SD ♿   CP ♿   E ♿   RF ♿
C ♿   S ♿   WC 🚹

STONEHAVEN

Holiday resort with lovely pebble and sand
beach reached from the central Allardice
Street. Oldest part of town is the charming
little harbour, where Tolbooth Museum is to
be found.

TOURIST INFORMATION CENTRE
66 Allardice Street, Stonehaven
Tel: (01569) 762806

ATTRACTION
TOLBOOTH MUSEUM
Old Pier, Stonehaven, Kincardineshire
Tel: (01771) 622906   Fax: (01771) 622884
e-mail: heritage@aberdeenshire.gov.uk
Stonehaven's oldest building – the Earl
Marischal's C16th storehouse – served as
the County Tolbooth from 1600-1767.
Episcopal priests imprisoned here in 1748.

SD ♿   CP 🚹   E ♿   S ♿

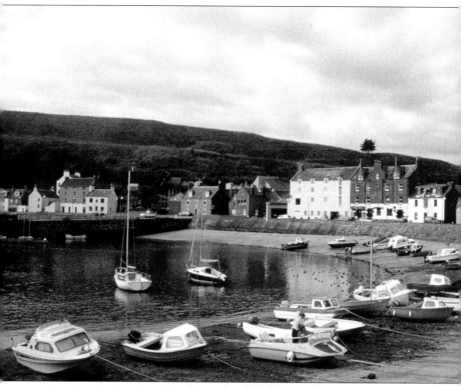

Stonehaven harbour has all the charm of an old Ealing comedy.

TOMINTOUL

On the Glenlivet Estate, one of the highest villages in Britain and the highest north of the Highland line. Planned and laid out by the 4th Duke of Gordon in 1776.

**TOURIST INFORMATION CENTRE and
TOMINTOUL and GLENLIVET HIGHLAND
HOLIDAYS**
The Square, Tomintoul AB37 9ET
Tel: (01309) 580285/580770

ATTRACTION
TOMINTOUL MUSEUM
The Square, Tomintoul AB37 9ET
Tel: (01309) 673701   Fax: (01309) 675863
e-mail: kris.sangster@techleis.moray.gov.uk
Displays on local wildlife, history of the town and local skiing industry with reconstructed crofters kitchen and smithy.
SD   CP   E   S

TURRIFF

Historic town situated at confluence of the Idoch Water and River Deveron, and once a capital of the Picts. The Old Church was built in C11th and in 1179 the Knights Templar were given land here. One of the main centres of the Covenanter Rebellion of mid C17th. Today Turriff is a thriving community and a main shopping centre for surrounding farmlands.

SELF-CATERING
ELMWOOD
Delgatie Castle Estates Trust, Delgatie Castle, Turriff AB53 8ED
Tel/Fax: (01888) 563479
No. of Accessible Units: 1
No. of Beds per Unit: 4 - 7
Accessible Facilities: Lounge, Dining Room, Kitchen. North wing in C11th castle, One of five houses in the grounds.
Delgatie was a private home and has fine painted ceilings, paintings, and furniture in a parkland setting.

THE HIGHLANDS AND SKYE

ACHNASHEEN

Located just east of Loch a'Chroisg on the road to Torridon.

HOTELS
LOCH TORRIDON HOTEL   🚾
By Achnasheen IV22 2EY
Tel: (01445) 791242 Fax: (01445) 791296
e-mail: david@lochtorridonhotel?????
web: www.s/h.com
No. of Accessible Rooms: 20
Accessible Facilities: Lounge, Restaurant
Former shooting lodge at the foot of the Torridon Mountains, on the shores of Loch Torridon.

LOCH MAREE HOTEL   🚶
Talladale, Loch Maree, by Achnasheen IV22 2HN
Tel: (01445) 760288 Fax: (01445) 760241
No. of Accessible Rooms: 1
Accessible Facilities: Lounge, Restaurant, Bar. Built in 1872 in superb scenery on Loch Maree, its restaurant is supplied daily by the fishing fleet of Gairloch.

AVIEMORE

Originally a small village, now the region's commercial centre. Its location in the foothills of the Cairngorm mountains means many concrete blocks accommodate tourists, particularly in the ski season, when buses transport visitors to ski area 13km away.

TOURIST INFORMATION CENTRE
Grampian Road, Aviemore PH22 1OO
Tel: (01479) 810363 Fax: (01479) 811063

SELF-CATERING
SILVERGLADES HOLIDAY HOMES   🚾
Dalnaby, Aviemore PH22 1TD
Tel: (01479) 810165 Fax: (01479) 811246
No. of Accessible Units: 1
No. of Beds per Unit: 1 - 8
Accessible Facilities: Lounge/Diner, Room, Kitchen. The Macdui unit is one of six chalet-style units here, situated at the foot of the Cairngorms, surrounded by glorious scenery.

PINE BANK CHALETS   🚶
Shieling Apartment,
Dalfaber Road, Aviemore PH22 1PX
Tel: (01479) 810000 Fax: (01479) 811469
e-mail: Pinebank@enterprise.net
web: www.aviemore.co.uk/pinebank.html
No. of Accessible Units: 1
No. of Beds per Unit: 5
Accessible Facilities: Lounge, Kitchen
Chalets and apartments in lovely riverside location close to Aviemore village.
Craigellachie Hill and nature reserve behind and Cairngorm Mountains in front.

BALLACHULISH

Located on Loch Linnhe, very close to Glencoe with fantastic scenery surrounding the Loch.

TOURIST INFORMATION CENTRE
Albert Road, Ballachulish PA39 4JR
Tel: (01855) 811296 Fax: (01855) 811720

HOTELS
**THE ISLES OF GLENCOE HOTEL and
LEISURE CENTRE**   🚾
Ballachulish PA39 4HL
Tel: (01855) 811602 Fax: (01855) 811770
No. of Accessible Rooms: 2
Accessible Facilities: Lounge, Restaurant.
Located 250m from the village centre on Loch Leven, one is almost afloat! Set on an highland estate with two harbours and 3kms of water frontage and spectacular views.

BALLACHULISH HOTEL   🚾
Ballachulish PA38 4YJ
Tel: (01855) 821582 Fax: (01855) 821463
e-mail: reservations@mysteryworld . co.uk
web: www.freedomglen.co.uk
No. of Accessible Rooms: 1
Accessible Facilities: Lounge, Restaurant
One of Scotland's oldest and best known hotels in fine lochside location.

BED AND BREAKFAST
CRAIGLINNHE GUEST HOUSE   🚶
Ballachulish PA39 4JX

Tel/Fax: (01855) 811270
e-mail: craiglinnhe@ballchulish.almac.co.uk
web: www.milford.co.uk/scotland/accom
No. of Accessible Rooms: 1. Shower
Accessible Facilities: Lounge, Dining
Room.
Lovely C19th villa in lochside setting.

BEAULY

Charming village with good range of
shops, restaurants, hotels, pubs, a craft
centre and ruins of C13th priory.
Established centre for salmon and brown
trout fishing and for Campbells world
famous wool shop.

SELF-CATERING
DUNSMORE LODGES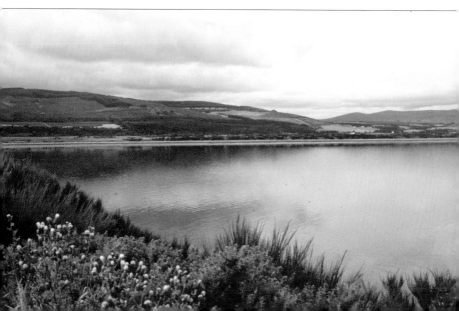
Farley, by Beauly IV4 7EY
Tel: (01463) 782424   Fax: (01463) 782839
e-mail: inghammar@cali.co.uk
web: www.cali.co.uk/dunsmore
No. of Accessible Units: 1
No. of Beds per Unit: 3
Accessible Facilities: Open Plan
Lounge/Kitchen/Diner
Scandinavian lodges, with Dornie being
accessible. Situated on two wooded hillside
sites, 0.25 mile apart, 100-300m. above the
Beauly river with great views of hills and
mountains. Four miles from Beauly.

BRORA

Rather charming small town with lovely
beaches around Kintradwell Bay and salmon
and trout fishing on River Brora. A good
base for touring this part of the north east.

BED AND BREAKFAST
GLENARVERON
Golf Road, Brora, Sutherland KW9 6QS
Tel/Fax: (01408) 621601
No. of Accessible Rooms: 1. Shower (slight ramp).
Accessible Facilities: Lounge, Dining Room,
Gardens. Absolutely charming old stone
house built in 1904 in mature gardens. Very
spacious interior with warm ambience, pine
and oak furnishings and a family atmosphere.
One of our most impressive visits.

CULLODEN

Desolate stretch of moorland, 6km east of
Inverness, looking as it did in April 1746.

ATTRACTION
CULLODEN BATTLEFIELD (NT for S)
Culloden Moor Visitor Centre, Culloden Moor,
Inverness IV2 5EN
Tel: (01463) 790607   Fax: (01463) 794294
Site of the last battle fought on mainland
Britain on 16 April 1746 when Bonny
Prince Charles Edward Stuart's army was
routed by the Duke Butcher of Cumberland.

The coastline around Brora is magical.

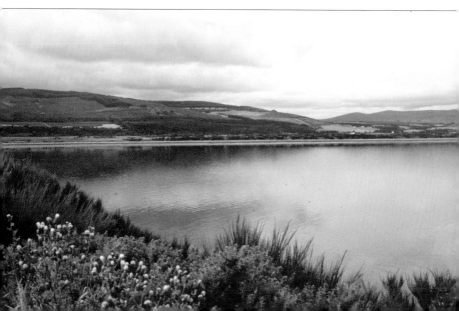

The battlefield has been restored to its state on that day. Visitor Centre with Jacobite exhibition and audio-visual show. Rough nature of the site and its size means that those in wheelchairs and the less-able may find it tiring to go round the whole site.

| SD 🦽 | CP ♿ | E 🦽 | RF 🦽 |
| C 🦽 | WC 🦽 | RFE 🚶 | |

DINGWALL

Established by Victorian penchant for the Highlands, Dingwall is the main centre for the region, and birthplace of Macbeth.

HOTEL
KINKELL HOUSE HOTEL 🚶
Easter Kinkell, Conon Bridge,
By Dingwall IV7 8HY
Tel: (01349) 861270   Fax: (01349) 865902
No. of accessible Rooms: 1
Accessible Facilities: Lounge, Restaurant
Small country house hotel in own grounds surrounded by trees and pasture land. Situated 10 miles north of Inverness on the Black Isle with fine view of the Cromarty Firth and West Ross hills.

DRUMNADROCHIT

Third of the way down Loch Ness with thriving monster mania through Monster Exhibition Centre, shops and crafts. 3km away is Urquart Castle offering good photographic access to the Loch.

HOTELS
CLUNEBEG LODGE ♿
Clunebeg Estate, Drumnadrochit IV3 6UU
Tel: (01456) 450387   Fax: (01456) 450854
web: www.host.co .
No. of Accessible Rooms: 6
Accessible Facilities: Lounge, Restaurant.
Comfortable modern lodge, set on quiet farm, overlooking the town by Loch Ness.

DRUMNADROCHIT HOTEL 🚶
Drumnadrochit IV3 6TU
Tel: (01456) 450202   Fax: (01456) 450793
e-mail: drumhotel@lochness.demon.co.uk
web: www.host.co.uk
No. of Accessible Rooms: *check*
Accessible Facilities: *check*

Award=winning hotel at Loch Ness with Travel Inn style rooms.

SELF-CATERING
LOCHLETTER LODGES 🦽
Balnain, Drumnadrochit, Glenurquhart IV3 6TJ
Tel: (01456) 476313   Fax: (01456) 476301
No. of Accessible Units: 1
No. of Beds per Unit: 4 – 6
Accessible Facilities: Lounge, Kitchen, Full Disability equipment available free of charge. Glomach Lodge is one of four pine lodges situated in Glenurquhart which stretches from Loch Ness to Glen Affrice, well placed for highland touring. Located in mature birchwood with own access road.

DUNBEATH

Between Wick and Brora on the north-east coast.

ATTRACTION
LAIDHAY CROFT MUSEUM
Dunbeath KW6 6EH
Tel: (01593) 731244
Housed in a 200-year-old thatched Caithness longhouse, furnished as of 100 years ago. Also a collection of early farm tools and machinery.

| SD 🦽 | CP 🚶 | E 🚶 | RF 🚶 |
| WC 🚶 | RFE 🚶 | | |

FORT GEORGE
Aerdersier, by Inverness IV1 2TD
Tel: (01667) 46277
Although there has been a royal stronghold and military garrison at Inverness since C12th, Fort George dates back to 1725 when it was rebuilt and extended. It is one of the outstanding military fortifications in Europe and still an active army barracks. Within the Fort is the Regimental Museum of the Queen's own Highlanders (see below).
Many grassed areas that can be soft, but a wide path runs throughout. Battlements are not accessible.

| CP ♿ (although 200m from entrance, surface is good and slightly sloped) | E ♿ | RFE ♿ |
| S ♿ | WC 🚶 | |

343

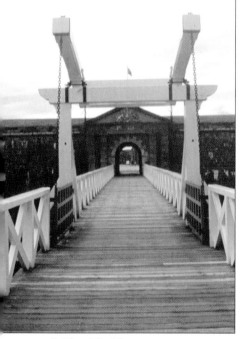

Brtidge at Fort George

REGIMENTAL MUSEUM

Collection of the Queen's Own Highlanders (Cameron and Seaforth) located in the house of the former Lieutenant Governor. Fascinating displays of uniforms, medals, pictures and weaponry on three floors. Ground floor and first floor (stairlift) accessible. The second floor, dedicated to WWII, is not accessible.

FORT WILLIAM

Known for its location at the foot of Ben Nevis, this has always been a good base for touring this area of the Highlands. Stores for climbers, skiers and sightseers line the main street. Can get very busy in summer.

TOURIST INFORMATION CENTRE
Cameron Centre, Cameron Square,
Fort William PH33 6AJ
Tel: (01397) 703781   Fax: (01397) 705184

HOTELS
LODGE ON THE LOCH
Onich, by Fort William PH33 6RY
Tel: (01855) 821237
Fax: (01855) 821463
No. of Accessible Rooms: 1. Shower
Accessible Facilities: Lounge (Side entrance), Restaurant.
Delightful country house hotel facing south across a mile-wide bay off Loch Linnhe, the sea loch at the south-western end of the Great Glen. 10 miles south of Fort William.

OLD PINES RESTAURANT WITH ROOMS
Spean Bridge, by Fort William PH34 4EGA
Tel: (01397) 712324   Fax: (01397) 712433
e-mail: goodfood.at.oldpines@lineone.net
No. of Accessible Rooms: 5
Accessible Facilities: Lounge, Restaurant
Warm family home built 20 years ago in Scandinavian style with recent stone and wood additions. Situated above the village of Spean Bridge, it is set among mature Scots Pines in 30 acres of ground with good views across the Great Glen and Glen Spean to Ben Nevis. Winner of 1994 Holiday Car Service Award for best small (under 20 rooms) hotel in Great Britain. Legendary Restaurant. Disabled British downhill ski champion has been a guest here. Good base for exploring West Highlands and Islands. 10 miles from Fort William.

BED AND BREAKFAST
LOCHAN COTTAGE GUEST HOUSE
Lochyside, Fort William PH33 7NX
Tel: (01397) 702695
web: www.host.co.uk
No. of Accessible Rooms: 1
Accessible Facilities: Lounge, Dining Room.
Situated in lovely gardens with panoramic views over Ben Nevis.

SELF-CATERING
MOSSFIELD APARTMENTS
Lochyside, Fort William,
Invernesshire PH33 7NY
Tel/Fax: (01397) 703087
No. of Accessible Units: 1. Shower
No. of Beds per Unit: 2
Accessible Facilities: Lounge/Diner. Kitchen
One of a group of seven holiday flats, three miles from Fort William.

ATTRACTION
THE WEST HIGHLAND MUSEUM
Cameron Square, Fort William PH33 6AJ
Tel/Fax: (01397) 702169

Displays on traditional Highland life, with Jacobite artefacts, including the famous secret portrait of Bonnie Prince Charlie, that looks like splash of paint but is indeed a portrait when reflected in a metal cylinder.

SD [♿] E [♿] RF [♿]
S [♿] (Sales point at entrance) WC [♿]

GAIRLOCH
Traditional coastal crofting town and holiday village, now rather tourist conscious. The road through the village leads to a campsite with good views of the Torridon range and lovely beaches.

TOURIST INFORMATION CENTRE
Achtercairn, Gairloch IV22 2DN
Tel: (01445) 712130   Fax: (01445) 712071

SELF-CATERING
WILLOW CROFT   [♿]
Big Sand, Gairloch, Wester Ross
Tel: (01445) 712448

No. of Accessible Units: 1
No. of Beds per Unit: 6
Accessible Facilities: Lounge, Dining room, Kitchen, Sauna. Five miles from the village.

GLENCOE
Awesome scenery combines with a savage history here with steep cliffs, craggy peaks and the river Coe. Famous for the Massacre of Glencoe in 1692 in which the Glencoe Macdonalds were betrayed and killed by soldiers of William III.

ATTRACTION
GLENCOE AND NORTH LORN FOLK MUSEUM
Glencoe PA39 4HS
Tel: (01855) 811664

2 heather-thatched cottages with exhibits on the Macdonald and the Jacobite uprisings, plus local artefacts.

SD [♿] CP [♿] E [♿] RF [♿]
S [♿] WC [♿] (0.25 miles from museum)

GRANTOWN-ON-SPEY
Victorian resort offering a peaceful highland holiday with fishing and golf popular.

TOURIST INFORMATION CENTRE
54 High Street, Grantown on Spey PH26 3EH
Tel/Fax: (01479) 872773

BED AND BREAKFAST
DUNALLAN HOUSE   [♿]
Woodside Avenue, Grantown-on-Spey PH26 3JN
Tel/Fax: (01479) 872140
e-mail: dunallan@mcmail.com
web: www.dunallan.mcmail.com

No. of Accessible Rooms: 1.Bath
Accessible Facilities: Lounge, Dining Room. Lovely, traditional seven-bedroomed Victorian villa.

KINROSS HOUSE   [♿]
Woodside Avenue, Grantown-on-Spey, Morayshire PH26 3JR
Tel: (01479) 872042   Fax: (01479) 873504
web: www.kinrosshouse.freeserve.co.uk

No. of Accessible Rooms: 1
Accessible Facilities: Lounge, Dining Room, Sauna. Attractive Victorian villa, with warm ambience, on the wooded southside of Grantown, a good base for exploring this part of the Highlands.

ATTRACTION
SPEYSIDE HEATHER GARDEN AND VISITOR CENTRE
Skye of Curr, Dulnain Bridge, by Grantown on Spey PH26 3PA
Tel: (01479) 851359   Fax: (01479) 851396
e-mail: enquiries@heathercentre.com

Heather Heritage Exhibition, gallery/antique shop and show gardens

SD [♿] CP [♿] E [♿] RF [♿]
C [♿] S [♿] WC [♿]

HELMSDALE
Famous as holiday home destination of authoress Barbara Cartland, the town is set on craggy headland with small harbour in north east Highlands.

TOURIST INFORMATION CENTRE
Coupar Park, Helmsdale KW8 6HH
Tel/Fax: (01431) 821640

HOTEL
NAVIDALE HOUSE HOTEL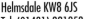
Helmsdale KW8 6JS
Tel: (01431) 821258   Fax: (01431) 821531
web: www.host.co.uk
No. of Accessible Rooms: 6
Accessible Facilities: Lounge, Restaurant.
Comfortable country house in lovely clifftop
location,

ATTRACTION
TIMESPAN
Dunrobin Street, Helmsdale KW8 6JX
Tel: (01431) 821327
History of the Highlands from the Picts and
Vikings to the Highland clearances and the
oil industry. Re-creations with life-size sets,
sound effects and audio-visual material.

SD 🔲   CP 🔲   E 🔲   L 🔲
C 🔲   S 🔲   WC 🔲   RFE 🔲

INVERNESS
Highland capital, compact and easily
accessible centre, with unattractive modern
architecture softened by lovely floral displays
in summer. River Ness flows through centre
of the town, which is dominated by
Inverness Castle, a Victorian red sandstone
building, now the court house.

TOURIST INFORMATION CENTRE
Castle Wynd, Inverness IV2 3BJ
Tel: (01463) 234353   Fax: (01463) 710609

BUSES
Scots City Link: Tel: (0990) 505050
2 journeys per day for local buses with
ramps and straps.

TAXIS
Serving Inverness and Fort William.
**Ace Taxis, Tom Na Faire, North Road, Fort
William PH33 6TQ**
Tel: (01397) 704000
Several adapted taxis and metrocabs, fully
equipped for wheelchairs.

TRAINS
Scotrail: Disabled passengers no:
Tel: (0845) 6057021
Wheelchair unassisted access and ramps
available, with 24 hours' notice.

GNER – Special Needs: Tel: (0845) 7225444
Minicom: (0191) 2330173
Wheelchair space in first and standard
class. Assistance available at stations if
booked in advance.

SHOPMOBILITY
Eastgate Pedestrian Precinct, Inverness
Tel: (01463) 717624

HOTELS
KINGSMILLS HOTEL 🔲
Culcabock Road, Inverness IV2 3LP
Tel: (01463) 237166   Fax: (01463) 225208
No. of Accessible Rooms: 2. Bath.
Accessible Facilities: Lounges, Restaurant.
(Conservatory has 4 steps). Delightful
property set in 4 acres of gardens, a mile
south of Inverness.

GLEN MHOR HOTEL and RESTAURANTS 🔲
9-12 Ness Bank, Inverness IV2 4SG
Tel: (01463) 234308   Fax: (01463) 713170
No. of Accessible Rooms: 2
Accessible Facilities: Lounge, 2
Restaurants.
Lovely quiet central riverside location near
the historic sites.

ATTRACTIONS
CLANLAND
Foulis Ferry Point, Easter Ross, Invernesshire
IV16 9UX
Tel/Fax: (01349) 830000
e-mail: clanland@cali.uk
web: www.clanland.com
Opened in summer 1998, this excellent
attraction, set on the shore of the
Cromarty Firth, offers a fascinating history
of the fully restored Girnal, which houses a
series of entertaining and educational
history and wildlife exhibitions. Unravel
secrets of 7 centuries of land and people
brought to life in Rogues Gallery theatre.
Learn about the Munro Clanlands history
and heritage. Fascinating Sealpoint
exhibition. Outside are traditional fishing
cobbles and picnic area. Located 20
minutes north of Inverness on main A9.

CP 🔲   E 🔲   RF 🔲   C 🔲
S 🔲   WC 🔲   RFE 🔲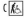

346

KINGUSSIE

Originally a weaving and spinning centre, the arrival of the railway in 1890 encouraged building of lovely Victorian homes for English families travelling to the Highlands by train. River Spey runs through the town.

TOURIST INFORMATION CENTRE
c/o Highland Folk Museum, Duke Street, Kingussie PH21 1JG
Tel: (01540) 661297

HOTEL
AVONDALE GUEST HOUSE
Newtonmore Road, Kingussie PH21 1HF
Tel: (01540) 661731
No. of Accessible Rooms: 1
Accessible Facilities: Lounge, Dining Room
Edwardian property, 5 minutes' walk from the town centre.

ATTRACTION
HIGHLAND WILDLIFE PARK
Kincraig, Kingussie PH21 1NL
Tel: (01540) 651270   Fax: (01540) 651236
260-acre site with an amazing variety of native Scottish wildlife, visit the new Wolf Territory, herds of red deer, secretive roe deer, Highland cattle, bison, ancient breeds of sheep and Przewalski's horses, one of the world's rarest mammals. Clear driving route, although exploration on foot to themed habitats also available .

SD 🔥	CP 🔥	E 🔥	RF 🔥
C 🔥	S 🔥	WC 🔥	

HIGHLAND FOLK MUSEUM
Duke Street, Kingussie PH21 1JG
Tel: (01540) 661307   Fax: (01540) 661631
Touch, feel and smell the World of the Highlander as you walk through material remains of 400 years of Highland life from clansman to crofter. Unique collection of everyday domestic artefacts, plus countryside furniture, machinery and implements

CP 🔥	E 🔥	RF 🔥
S 🔥	WC 🔥	RFE 🔥

KINLOCHLEVEN

One of the first industrial towns in the Highlands, where Scots and Irish workers constructed the Blackwater Dam. Situated at the head of Loch Leven at the foot of the Mamore Hills, with the West Highland way passing through the town.

HOTEL
TIGH-na-CHEO
Kinlochleven PA40 4SE
Tel: (01855) 831434 Fax: (01855) 831441
e-mail: napier@tigh-na-cheo.demon.co.uk
web: www.scottish-highlands.com
No. of Accessible Rooms: 1
Accessible Facilities: Lounge, Restaurant, Sauna. Family run delightful small hotel located between Fort William and Oban, close to Glencoe.

KINLOCHEWE

Village lying at foot of Glen Docherty, the road west from here leading into startling mountain scenery of Torridon Hills, Beinn Eighe National Nature Reserve bordered by Loch Maree and Loch Torridom, 50 miles W. of Inverness

BED AND BREAKFAST
CROMASAIG
Torridon Road, Kinlochewe IV22 2PE
Tel: (01445) 760234 Fax: (01445) 760333
e-mail: cromasaig@email.msn.com
web: mountains.com/cromasaig
No. of Accessible Rooms: 1
Accessible Facilities: Lounge, Dining Room
Small family run accommodation surrounded by fine mountain scenery.

ISLE OF RAASAY

In his Hebridean Journals, Samuel Johnson recounts great tales of a stay on Raasay. Raasay is a small, close knit crofting community, who welcome visitors. With breathtaking views of Torridon peaks to the east and Cuillins of Skye to the west, Raasay is a treasure-trove for nature lovers. Wildlife, plants and archaeology are on the menu with wonderful walks for those who both wish and are able to do so.

ISLE OF RAASAY HOTEL
Raasay, by Kyle of Lochalsh,
Inverness-shire IV40 8PD
Tel/Fax: (01478) 660222

No. of Accessible Rooms: 6. Bath.
Accessible Facilities: Lounge, Restaurant.
Small, family-run hotel with a blend of old
and new. Modern wings have been added to
the renovated old stone mansion house, with
views across the glittering Narrows of Raasay
to Skye. Lovely gardens. To get to Raasay,
first you must get to Skye, and then by road
to Sconser and from this village on Loch
Sligachan you sail to Raasay. Several daily
sailings (except Sundays) in each direction,
duration of 15 minutes. NB No petrol on
Raasay, so fill up in Broadford (Skye).

LAIDE

Situated above the shoreline of Gruinard
Bay, between outflows of Little Gruinard
and Inverianvie rivers.

SELF-CATERING
ROCKLEA
Little Gruinard, Laide, Wester Ross IV22 2NG
BOOK THROUGH: Mr/Mrs Gilchrist, Grassvalley
Cottage, 12 Woodhall Road, Colinton,
Edinburgh EH13 0X
Tel: (0131) 441 6053   Fax: (0131) 441 4849
e-mail: aandagilchrist@cwcom.net
No. of Accessible Units: 1
No. of Beds per Unit: 5
Accessible Facilities: Lounge, Dining room,
Kitchen. Log constructions standing in own
grounds of about 5 acres. Uninterrupted
outlook across bay towards Gruinard Island
and beyond.

NAIRN

Refined Victorian holiday town on the
shores of the Moray Firth with long sandy
beaches.

TOURIST INFORMATION CENTRE
62 King Street, Nairn IV12 4DN
Tel/Fax: (01667) 452753

HOTEL
CLAYMORE HOUSE HOTEL
Seabank Road, Nairn IV12 4EY
Tel: (01667) 453731   Fax: (01667) 455290
e-mail:
ClaymoreNairnbScotland@compuserve.com

No. of Accessible Rooms: 1. Roll-in Shower
Accessible Facilities: Lounge, Restaurant
Quality hotel located in the centre of Nairn.

BED AND BREAKFAST
GREENLAWNS
13 Seafield Street, Nairn IV12 4HG
Tel/Fax: (01667) 452738
e-mail: greenlawns@fsbdial.co.uk
No. of Accessible Rooms: 3
Accessible Facilities: Lounge, Dining Room,
Bar. Will do packed lunch and dinner by
arrangement. Large 100-year-old house
restored to original Victorian past. Set in
own grounds at the western end of town.

SELF-CATERING
BURNSIDE AND MILL LODGES
Raitloan, Geddes, Nairn IV12 5SA
Tel: (01667) 454635
No. of Accessible Units: 2
No. of Beds per Unit: 6
Accessible Facilities: Open plan
Lounge/Diner/Kitchen, Patio (Burnside),
Timber Deck (Mill).
Lovely situation in quiet wooded setting,
3 miles from Nairn.

LAIKENBUIE
Grantown Road, Nairn IV12 5QN
Tel: (01667) 454630
e-mail: musbus@bigfoot.com
No. of Accessible Units: 2
No. of Beds per Unit: 6
Accessible Facilities: Open plan Lounge,
Dining Room, Kitchen.

NETHYBRIDGE

Lovely Highland village between Grantown-
on-Spey and Boat of Garten.

SELF-CATERING
FHUARAIN FOREST COTTAGES
Badanfhuarain, Nethybridge,
Nr. Grantown-on-Spey PH25 3ED
Tel/Fax: (01479) 821642
e-mail: dv.dean@virgin.net
web: freespace.virgin.net/dv.dean/
Owner is Chairperson of Badenoch and
Strathspey Disabled Access Panel.
Flox and Badanfhuarain Cottages:

No. of Accessible Units: 2. Badanfhuarain -
Roll-in shower,
Flox - Bath.
No. of Beds per Unit: 5
Accessible Facilities:
Flox: Kitchen/Dining/Living
Badanfhuarain: Kitchen, Dining/Living
Quite delightful C19th forest cottages with
fenced gardens. Four miles from
Grantown-on-Spey.

CREGGAN COTTAGE

Causer, Nethybridge.
Bookings: Speyside Holiday Cottages,
1 Chapelton Place, Forres, Moray IV36 2NL
Tel/Fax: (01309) 672505
e-mail: speyside@enterprise.net
No. of Accessible Units: 1. Bath
No. of Beds per Unit: 6
Accessible Facilities: Open plan Living
room/Kitchen
Comfortable cottage in lovely Highland
village close to river and forest, with
private fenced gardens.

ATTRACTION
RSPB LOCH GARTEN OSPREY CENTRE

Forest Lodge, Abernethy Forest Reserve,
Nethbridge PH25 3EF
Tel: (01479) 821409   Fax: (01479) 821069
Once widespread in the UK, egg-collectors
and hunters almost wiped out the fish-
eating osprey. Now, from a single pair in
1959, ospreys have returned to nest here,
in trees, on the Loch and surroundings.
The centre enables one to watch these
superb birds of prey at close quarters.
Centre located 400m from car park, use the
set-down facility. Centre overlooks famous
nesting ospreys with viewing slots at
various heights, including low level ones
for visitors in wheelchairs.

| SD 🚲 | CP n/a | E 🚲 | RF ♿ |
| S 🚲 | WC ♿ | RFE 🚲 | |

NEWTOWNMORE

Situated in the heart of the Highlands,
close to Kingussie and the facilities of
Aviemore. A delightful village dominated
by Creag Dubh and close to the River Spey,
with secluded glens such as Glen Banchor
less than a mile from the village centre.

HOTEL
BALAVIL SPORT HOTEL

Main Street, Newtonmore PH20 1DL
Tel: (01540) 673220   Fax: (01540) 673773
web: www.host.co.uk
No. of Accessible Rooms: 10 (ground floor)
and 9 (via lift) Accessible Facilities: Lounge,
restaurant. Family owned hotel in
Newtonmore.

SELF-CATERING
CRUBENBEG FARM STEADING

Newtonmore PH20 1BE
Tel: (01540) 673566   Fax: (01540 673509
e-mail: enquiries@crubenbeg.netlineuk/net
No. of accessible Units: 1. Roll-in Shower
No. of Beds per Unit: 2
Accessible Facilities: Lounge, Kitchen, Trout
fishing from disabled platform.
Original derelict farm buildings converted
into seven holiday cottages of which one is
accessible. Situated on a wooded hillside at
the foot of Crubenbeg Hill above the River
Trium as it tumbles toward the River Spey.
Located 5 miles south of the village.

BALVATIN HOLIDAY COTTAGES

Perth Road, Newtonmore PH20 1BB
Tel: (01540) 673433   Fax: (01540) 673303
e-mail: gm.ferrer@virgin.net
web: business.virgin.net/gm.ferrier/index.htm
No. of Accessible Units: 1
No. of Beds per Unit: 4S, 1D.
Accessible Facilities: Lounge, Dining Room,
Kitchen. Small complex of 9 properties with
lovely gardens and pine trees.

ATTRACTION
WALTZING WATERS (SCOTLAND)

Balavil Brae, Newtownmore PH20 1DR
Tel/Fax: (015406) 673752
Elaborate water, light and music production
with thousands of dazzling patterns of
moving water synchronised with music.

| SD n/a | CP ♿ | E 🚲 | RF 🚲 |
| S 🚲 | WC 🚶 | RFE 🚲 | |

POOLEWE

Located between Loch Ewe and Loch
Gairloch, 6 miles from Gairloch. Famous for
the popular Inverewe Gardens (some parts
difficult for wheelchairs).

SELF-CATERING
AN BOTHAN
8 Naast, Poolewe IV22 2LL
Tel/Fax: (01445) 781360
e-mail: highlands.dreams@virgin.net
web: freespace.virgin.net/nicola.taylor/
highlands-dreams.htm
No. of Accessible Units: 1.Bath
No. of Beds per Unit: 5
Accessible Facilities: Lounge,
Kitchen/Diner, Garden (shared with
owner's bungalow)
Absolutely charming former croft house in
crofting community with just 8 houses on
the western shore of Loch Ewe, 3 miles
north of Poolewe. Fine views across Loch
Ewe to mountains by Loch Maree and those
beyond Ullapool up to Sutherland. Nearest
shop is in Inverasadale, 1 mile north of
cottage. Safe sandy beach at Firemore
Beach, two miles north of Naast.

INNES-MAREE BUNGALOWS
Poolewe IV22 2JU
Tel/Fax: (01445) 781454
e-mail: maree@lineone.net
web: www.destinations-scotland.com/innes/
No. of Accessible Units: 1. Shower
No. of Beds per Unit: 6.
Accessible Facilities: Lounge, open plan
kitchen/dinette. One of 6 modern purpose-
built bungalows in lovely village. Area
around Poolewe offers mountain and forest,
loch and glen and safe sandy beaches. The
bungalows are a few minuets from
Inverewe Gardens.

SHIELBRIDGE
Tiny community just off the main A87 Kyle
of Lochalsh road.

BED AND BREAKFAST
TIGH UR
MacInnes Park, Ratagan, Glenshiel, Ross-shire
IV40 8HR
Tel: (01599) 511292
e-mail: TIGHUR88@aol.com
No. of Accessible Rooms: 2. Roll-in shower.
Twin room -pneumatic height adjusting
bed and manual ARGO sling lift. Double
has monkey pull.
Accessible Facilities: Lounge, Dining

Room. Evening Meal available. Spacious,
unpretentious bungalow owned by
charming couple, she in a wheelchair, who
create a homely ambience. Superb
location in hamlet of Ratagan, metres
from, and with views of, the lovely Loch
Duich, in the foothills of Kintail. From
A87, Ratagan is 1.5 miles from
Shielbridge. Good location for touring
Skye and Western Highlands.

ISLAND OF SKYE
Largest of Inner Hebrides and reached by
bridge linking Kyle of Lochalsh on
mainland with Kyleakin. Varied dramatic
scenery, divided by sea lochs, inland area
never more than 8km from sea. Volcanic
plateau in the north, grasslands in the
south. Historically known for association
with Bonnie Prince Charlie.

BUSES
Highland County Buses: Tel: (01463) 222244
Regular service with ramps and straps.
Citylink: Tel: (0900) 505050
National Express: Tel: (0990) 808080

TAXIS
Waterloo Taxis: (01471) 822630
Regular service with ramps and straps.

TRAINS
Scotrail: Tel: 90345 550033

SELF-CATERING
BROADFORD, SKYE
Second largest town on Skye in south-
east.

TOURIST INFORMATION CENTRE
The Car Park, Broadford IV49 9AB
Tel: (01471) 822361   Fax: (01471) 822141

CORREIGORM BEAG
Bayview Crescent, Broadford, Isle of Skye
IV49 9AB
Tel: (01471) 822575   Fax: (01471) 822860
No. of Accessible Units: 1
No. of Beds per Unit: 1
Accessible Facilities: Lounge, Kitchen.

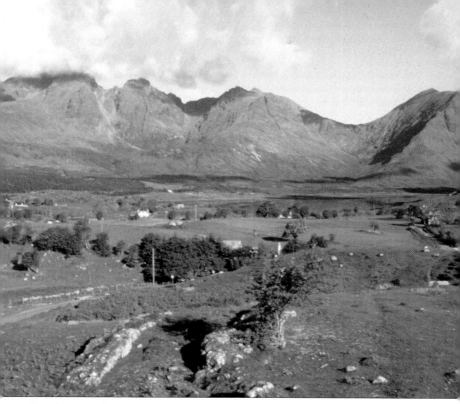

Over the sea to Skye. You can go by bridge now. It's well worth the effort.

DUNVEGAN, SKYE

On Durinish Peninsula on western shores of island.

TOURIST INFORMATION CENTRE
2 Lochside, Dunvegan IV55 8WB
Tel: (01470) 521581   Fax: (01470) 521582

HOTEL/RESTAURANT
THE THREE CHIMNEYS
Colbost, Dunvegan IV55 8ZT
Tel: (01470) 511258   Fax: (01470) 511358
e-mail: eatandstay@threechimneys.co.uk
web: www.threechimneys.co.uk
No. of Accessible Rooms: 1.
Accessible Facilities: Restaurant.
A famous award-winning Restaurant with 6 luxurious rooms in the House Over-By, completed in 1999.Located in small village just SW of Dunvegan, 5 miles from Dunvegan Castle.

KILMUIR, SKYE

BED & BREAKFAST
WHITEWAVE ACTIVITIES
No. 19 Linicro, Kilmuir IV51 9YN
Tel: (01470) 542414   Fax: (01470) 542443
e-mail: activities@whiteact.demon.co.uk
web: www.whiteact.demon.co.uk
No. of Accessible Rooms: check
Accessible Facilities: check
A cross between an outdoor centre, a ceilidh place and a family home with accessible activities of all kinds.

PORTREE, SKYE

TOURIST INFORMATION CENTRE
Bayfield House, Bayfield Road,
Portree IV51 9EL
Tel: (01478) 612137   Fax: (01478) 612141

BED & BREAKFAST
AUCHENDINNY GUEST HOUSE
Treaslane, by Portree IV51 9NX
Tel/Fax: (01470) 532470

web: www.host.co.uk
No. of Accessible Rooms: 1. Bath
Accessible Facilities: Lounge, Dining Room
House in 2 acres of gardens with lawns and
wooded areas, overlooking Loch Treaslane,
a sea loch 70m. away. Located just off the
Portree/Dunvegan road (A850).

SLEAT, SKYE

Adjacent to Armadale, with an active pier
and ruins of Armadale Castle, built in 1815,
adjoining the Clan Donald Centre.

ATTRACTION
CLAN DONALD VISITOR CENTRE
Armadale, Sleat IV45 8RS
Tel: (01471) 844305   Fax: (01471) 844275
e-mail: cland.demon.co.uk
Clan Donald's history dates back 1300
years, a history of fighting, diplomacy,
governing, clearances, triumph and defeat.
Video on bygone days shown in a restored
part of Armadale Castle. 40 acres of
woodland gardens surround the castle.

| SD ♿ | CP ♿ | E ♿ | RF ♿ |
| C ♿ | S ♿ | WC 🚻 | RFE ♿ |

WATERNISH, SKYE

SELF-CATERING
GREENBANK ♿
4 Halistra, Waternish IV55 8GL
Tel/Fax; (01470) 592369
No. of Accessible Units: 1.Roll-in Shower
No. of Beds per Unit: 4
Accessible Facilities: Purpose built bungalow
for wheelchair users. Spectacular loch and
sea views.

STRATHCARRON

Located at southern end of Loch Torridon.

BED AND BREAKFAST
INNIS MHOR ♿
Ardheslaig, Shieldaig, Strathcarron IV54 8XH
Tel/Fax: (01520) 755 339
e-mail: cjsermon@primex.co.uk
No. of Accessible Rooms: 2
Accessible Facilities: Lounge, Dining Room.
Country guest house.

STRATHPEFFER

Located west of Dingwall, a popular spa
town and health resort in C19th and now a
quiet town with lots of huge hotels as
residue. Sample the water at the Water
Tasting Pavilion in the town centre.

TOURIST INFORMATION CENTRE
The Square, Strathpeffer IV14 9DW
Tel: (01997) 421415   Fax: (01997) 421460

HOTEL
ACHILTY HOTEL ♿
Contin, by Strathpeffer IV14 9EG
Tel: (01997) 421355   Fax: (01997) 421923
No. of Accessible Rooms: 4
Accessible Facilities: Lounge, Restaurant.
Renovated C18th coaching inn west of
Contin. Owner-managed.

ATTRACTION
HIGHLAND MUSEUM OF CHILDHOOD
The Old Station, Strathpeffer IV14 9DH
Tel: (01997) 421031
e-mail: info@freeserve.co.uk
Located in Victorian railway station of
1885, alongside various craft shops.

| SD ♿ | CP ♿ | E ♿ | RF ♿ |
| C ♿ | S 🚻 | WC 🚻 | RFE ♿ |

STROMFERRY

Close to Kyle of Lochalsh.

SELF-CATERING
GLENVIEW ♿
Birchwood, Achmore, Stromeferry IV5 8UT
Tel: (01599) 577211
e-mail: dennis@achmore-freeserve.co.uk
web:members.netscapeonline.co.uk/dfife577211
No. of Accessible Units: 1
No. of Beds per Unit: 4
Accessible Facilities: Lounge/Kitchen,
Dining Room. Modern bungalow within
grounds of owner's house in rural location.
Nearest facilities at Balmacara .

TALMINE

Three miles north of Tongue and off the
main tourist route between John O'Groats
and Cape Wrath. Seals, otter, deer and a
variety of bird life can be observed here.

SELF-CATERING
CLOISTERS
Church Holme, Talmine IV27 4YP
Tel/Fax: (01847) 601286
No. of Accessible Rooms: 1
Accessible Facilities:
Lounge, Breakfast Room
Newly built in traditional style to harmonise
with owners' home, an existing C19th
church, the property is set in an acre of wild
coastal scenery with views over Rabbit
Islands to the Orkneys.

THURSO
Located 32km west of John O'Groats, a well
organised little town with shops and hotels
leading off a main central square. Surfing
and windsurfing are popular off local
beaches. One can catch the ferry here from
Scrabster to Stromness on Orkney. Close by
is the gigantic white dome of Dounreay
nuclear reprocessing plant, no longer open.

TOURIST INFORMATION CENTRE
Riverside, Thurso KW14 8BU
Tel: (01847) 892371   Fax: (01847) 893155

HOTEL
CASTLE ARMS HOTEL
Mey, by Thurso KW14 8XH
Tel/Fax: (018457) 851244
No. of Accessible Rooms: 1
Accessible Facilities: Lounge, Restaurant,
Wheelie fishing boat on nearby loch (trout)
Small country hotel.

FORSS COUNTRY HOUSE HOTEL
Forss, by Thurso KW14 7XY
Tel: (01847) 861201   Fax: (01847) 861301
web: www.host.co.uk
No. of Accessible Rooms: 6
Accessible Facilities: Lounge, Restaurant.
Lovely country house set in 25 acres of
woodlands by River Forss with an
abundance of wildlife.

SELF-CATERING
CURLEW COTTAGE
Hilliclay Mains, Weydale, Thurso KW14 8YN
Tel: (01847) 895638
No. of Accessible Units: 1
No. of Beds per Unit: 3

Accessible facilities: Lounge, Dining Room
(includes a piano), Kitchen, Garden
Set amid high farmland, 4 miles from
Thurso with grand views across Caithness to
the distant mountains.
Good base for touring Caithness and
Northern Sutherland with two-mile stretch
of Dunnet Sands, other secluded beaches
and fine coastal scenery within a short drive.

ULLAPOOL
Very pretty village with palm trees and
white-washed houses on the west coast,
planned and built as a fishing community in
1788, it juts into Loch Broom. Embarkation
point for ferry to Stornoway on Isle of Lewis.

TOURIST INFORMATION CENTRE
Argyle Street, Ullapool IV26 2UB
Tel: (01854) 612135   Fax: (01854) 613031

BED AND BREAKFAST
DROMNAN GUEST HOUSE
Garve Road, Ullapool IV26 2SX
Tel: (01854) 612333   Fax: (01854) 613364
e-mail: dromnan@msn.com
web: www.destination-scotland.com/dromnan
No. of accessible Rooms: 1. Shower
Accessible Facilities: Lounge, Dining Room
Family-run guest house in peaceful location
overlooking Lochbroom.

WICK
The community grew on Wick as it became
the busiest herring port in Europe, it is still
a busy town.

TOURIST INFORMATION CENTRE
Whitechapel Road, Wick KW1 4EA
Tel: (01955) 602596   Fax: (01955) 604940

BED AND BREAKFAST
24 LINDSAY DRIVE
Wick KW1 4PG
Tel: (01955) 603001
web: www.host.co.uk
No. of Accessible Rooms: 1
Accessible Facilities: Lounge, Dining Room
Bungalow in quiet cul-de-sac on route to
Sinclair and Girnigoe Castle. Good
overnight stay for Orkneys.

REGION 8
OUTER ISLANDS

ORKNEY

Seventy flat, undulating islands, twenty inhabited, two hours' sailing time from Scrabster. Spectacular coastline with famous landmark of 150m Old Man of Hoy. The islands are well known for the most dense concentration of archaeological sites in Britain, evidence of more than 5,000 years of settlements here. Notable are Skara Brae Prehistoric village, and many Iron Age brochs all along the coast. There also are traces of Vikings everywhere. Farming and fishing remain very important to the Orcadians.

ORKNEY DISABILITY FORUM
Anchor Buildings, Bridge Street,
Kirkwall, Orkney KW15 1HR
Tel/Fax: (01856) 870340
Publishes very useful book: *Holiday Accommodation for People with Disabilities.*

DIAL A BUS and SHOPMOBILITY KIRKWALL
Tel: (01856) 871515
You can join this on a temporary basis as a visitor.

BUSES
Highland Scott Omnibus/City Link
Tel: (01463) 233371

BIRSAY

Located on the north-west corner of the mainland, once an important Viking settlement. See the ruins of the C16th earl's palace.

BED AND BREAKFAST
PRIMROSE COTTAGE
Birsay KW17 2NB
Tel: (01856) 721384
No. of Accessible Rooms: 3
Accessible Facilities: Lounge, Dining Room
Single storey house.

DOUNBY
Located north-east of Kirkwall on the mainland.

SELF-CATERING
LOCHLAND CHALETS
Dounby KW17 2HR
Tel: (01856) 771340
No. of Accessible Units: 1
No. of Beds per Unit: 4
Accessible Facilities: Open plan Lounge/Kitchen.
Bird Hide on site.

EVIE
Located 10 minutes from Kirkwall and Stromness.

BED AND BREAKFAST
WOODWICK HOUSE
Evie, Orkney KW17 2PQ
Tel: (01856) 751330   Fax: (01856) 751383
No. of Accessible Rooms: 2. Bath. Shower
Accessible Facilities: Lounge, Dining Room, Gardens. Delightful house surrounded by trees, secluded corners, lawns and wonderful views overlooking the island of Gairsay and beyond.

KIRKWALL
Main town, dominated by St. Magnus Cathedral, c1140, yellow and red stone church. Flag-stoned streets and a small, busy harbour.

ATTRACTION
THE ORKNEY MUSEUM
Broad Street, Kirkwall KW15 2DH
Tel: (01856) 873191   Fax: (01856) 871560
C16th building, 'A' listed, with exhibits on Orkney's history and archaeology.

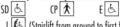

SD ⬚   CP ⬚   E ⬚   RF ⬚
L ⬚ (Stairlift from ground to first floor and another to extension area).   S ⬚   WC ⬚

NORTH RONALDSAY
Remote island lying at the north eastern extremity of Orkney with open sea beyond towards Shetland and Norway. Farming and kelp sustain the island's economy.

BED AND BREAKFAST
NORTH RONALDSAY BIRD OBSERVATORY
North Ronaldsay KW17 2BE
Tel: (01857) 633200   Fax: (01857) 633207
e-mail: alison@nrbo.prestel.co.uk
No. of Accessible Rooms: 1
Accessible Facilities: Lounge, Dining Room.
Established in 1987, the bird observatory
provides comfortable, inexpensive
accommodation with special opportunities
for visitors interested in birds and natural
history. Set on the crofts of Twingness and
Lurand, its 30 acres follow traditional
farming practice. Rich grassland and
remnant coastal heath are combined with
bere barley and a flock of sheep.

SHETLAND
Over 100 cliff-edged islands, (15
inhabited), closer to Norway than
mainland Scotland and nowhere more
than 5km from the sea. Fishing and
salmon fishing are still important while
North Sea oil has had a great impact on
the economy. Fine beaches and a striking
coastline.

DISABILITY SHETLAND
Harbour House, Esplanade, Lerwick,
Shetland ZE1 0LL
Tel/fax: (01595) 692196
Free and independent advice on holidays,
aid, equipment.

SOCIAL WORK DEPARTMENT
92 St. Olaf's Street, Lerwick, Shetland ZE1 0ES
Tel: (01595) 744400/744872
Provide temporary orange badges for car
parks.

BUSES
John Leask and Son, Lerwick:
Tel: (01595) 693162
Wheelchair accessibility on route betwen
Lerwick Town Centre – North and South
Sandwick – Sumburgh Airport.
Shalder Coaches, Scalloway:
Tel: (01595) 880217
Wheelchair accessibility on route Walls-
Lerwick Walls.

LERWICK
Mainland Shetland's major town with flagstones narrow lanes, grey stone buildings

HOTEL
SHETLAND HOTEL
Holmsgarth Road, Lerwick ZE1 0PW
Tel: (01595) 695515   Fax: (01595) 695828
No. of Accessible Rooms: 1. Roll-in Shower
Accessible Facilities: Lounge, Restaurant
Modern purpose-built hotel located
opposite main ferry terminal at northern
end of the town.

BED AND BREAKFAST
WHINRIG
12 Burgh Road, Lerwick ZE1 0LB
Tel: (01595) 693554
No. of Accessible Rooms: 1
Accessible Facilities: Dining Room
Attractive house, centrally located, but in a
quiet area.

SELF-CATERING
THE CHALETS
Gord, Cunningsburgh, Nr. Lerwick
Booking: Lyjastan, Tow,
Cunningsburgh ZE2 9HB.
Tel: (01950) 477384
No. of Accessible Units: 2
No. of Beds per Unit: 4, 6. Bath
Accessible Facilities: Lounge, Kitchen.
Working farm, 10 miles from Lerwick.

1 CHALET
Laebrak, Gulberwick
Booking: Mrs. Leask, Garth Lodge, Asta,
Scalloway ZE1 0UQ
Tel: (01595) 880231
No. of Accessible Units: 1
No. of Beds per Unit: 3
Accessible Facilities: check
In peaceful location just outside Lerwick,
overlooking lovely Gulberwick Bay. Near
sandy beach.

SUMBURGH HEAD
Located at southern tip of the mainland,
famous for seabird colonies. RSPB have a
site here. Within three miles of Jarlshof
archaeological site.

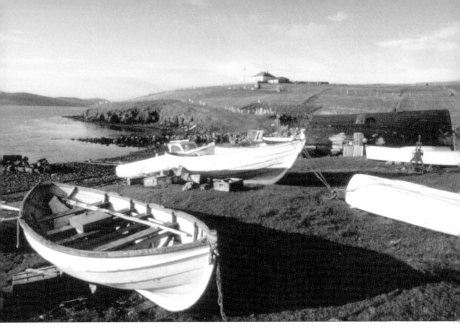

Typical Shetland shoreline.

SELF-CATERING

PRINCIPAL LIGHTHOUSE-KEEPER'S HOUSE 🚶
Sumburgh Head Lighthouse, Sumburgh Head.
Bookings: c/o T. Johnson-Ferguson,
Solwaybank, Canonbie, Dumfries-shire DG14 0XS.
Tel: (013873) 72240

No. of Accessible Units: 1. Bath
No. of Accessible Beds: 6
Accessible Facilities: Lounge/Diner,
Kitchen.

Fascinating property, 1 of 4 lighthouse
keepers' cottages in spectacular clifftop
location, along with fields and land enclosed
within drystone walls. In summer puffins
and fulmars come within a few metres of
the dining/sitting room. Within three miles
are wonderful white sandy beaches, the
RSPB site and the Pool of Virkie (for birds).

ATTRACTION

RSPB SUMBURGH HEAD SEABIRD VIEWPOINT

About 13,000 guillemots breed here, laying
their single egg directly onto the cliff
ledges. Razorbills, shags and gannets can
also be seen. In the seas around there are
harbour porpoises and white-beaked
dolphins, orcas (killer whales), minke and
humpback whales can sometimes be seen.
Lighthouse compound separated from cliffs
by high dry-stone dykes: at one point the
dykes are low enough for wheelchair users
to see over the top and view the birds on the
cliffs. This low section of dyke is adjacent to
where a car may be parked. The reserve is
not ideal for wheelchair users, but with
some assistance, certain areas of the reserve
can be enjoyed.

SD n/a

CP Use small car park near the lighthouse.　　E

UPPER SCALLOWAY

Second town to Lerwick. Standing over an
attractive bay looking out to the Atlantic.
Large catches of cod and haddock brought
in daily. The town is dominated by ruins of
C7th Scalloway Castle.

BED AND BREAKFAST

HILDASAY GUESTHOUSE ♿
Upper Scalloway ZE1 0UP
Tel: (01595) 880822

No. of Accessible Rooms: 4
Accessible Facilities: Lounge, Dining Room.
Family owned and managed Scandinavian
designed property, standing in own grounds
with fine views overlooking sea and
surrounding countryside. 10-minute drive
from Lerwick.

WALLS

Main village in the western area of the mainland. With attractive shoreline both here and nearby at Sandness that has views of the island of Papa Stour.

HOTEL
BURRASTOW HOUSE ♿
Walls, Shetland ZE2 9PD
Tel: (01595) 809307   Fax: (01595) 809213
No. of Accessible Rooms: 1
Accessible Facilities: Lounge, Restaurant.
C18th house on a promontory facing the island of Vaila. Otters and seals can be seen from the windows and wild orchids flourish in the grounds. Peat fires and a library complete the country house ambience.

ISLAND OF FETLAR

SELF-CATERING
2 CHALETS 🚶
Tigh Sith, Fetlar
Tel/Fax: (01957) 733303
Bookings: Society of our Lady of the Isles, Aithness, Fetlar ZE2 9DJ
No. of Accessible Units: 1
No. of Beds per Unit: 2
Set on the headland of Aithness, ideal for a peaceful break and for an opportunity of living alongside and worshipping with the community.

ISLAND OF UNST

Britain's most northerly inhabited island is one of the most spectacular, varied and interesting in Europe. Just 12 miles long by five miles wide there are stupendous cliffs, jagged sea stacks, sheltered inlets, golden beaches, heathery hills, freshwater lochs, peat bogs and fertile farmland. Rich variety of wildlife include Shetland ponies and seabirds. Lying north of the 60 degree parallel, Unst experiences perpetual daylight at midsummer. Modern roads and frequent roll-on/roll-off vehicle ferries link Shetland mainland to Unst via neighbouring island of Yell. From Lerwick it is a 45-minute drive north on main A970 to Toft ferry terminal: crossing to Yell takes 20 minutes, then follow main road to Gutcher ferry terminal

(30-minute drive) for 10-minute crossing to Unst. It is always advisable to book well in advance for ferries, particularly in summer. Ferry Booking Office – Ulsta, Yell Tel: (01957) 722259/722268.

HOTEL
BALTASOUND HOTEL ♿
Baltasound, Central Unst, Shetlands ZE2 9DS
Tel: (01957) 711334   Fax: (01957) 711358
e-mail: balta.hotel@zetnet.co.uk
No. of Accessible Rooms: 3
Accessible Facilities: Lounge, Restaurant.
Britain's most northerly hotel, an old stone house and pine log chalets in the garden, with great views over Baltasound. Village has shops, post office, marina and leisure centre. The Keen of Hamar nature reserve with its abundance of rare plants, is very close.

ATTRACTION
UNST HERITAGE CENTRE-BOAT HAVEN
Haroldswick, Shetland ZE2 9ED
Tel: (01957) 711528
Preserves fine examples of traditional Shetland working boats, together with artefacts and photographs, capturing a glimpse of Shetlands' fishing history.
SD ♿   CP 🚶   E ♿   RF ♿   WC 🚶

WESTERN ISLES

Comprising Lewis, Harris, North Uist, South Uist, Benbecula and Barra. Stornaway, on Lewis, is the only town in the islands and is the main administrative and shopping centre. Ullapool ferry sails into Stornaway and the airport has regular flights to and from Glasgow and Inverness.

WESTERN ISLES TOURIST BOARD
26 Cromwell Street, Stornoway,
Isle of Lewis HS1 2DD
Tel: (01851) 703088

LOCAL AUTHORITY TRANSPORT DEPARTMENT
Tel: (01851) 703773

MINIBUSES
Neil MacNeil: Tel: (01851) 703840
8-seater taxi bus with wheelchair facilities and ramp.

Graham Minibus Hire: Tel: (01851) 705716
8-seater minibus with wheelchair facilities
and ramp.

ISLE OF HARRIS

Separated from Lewis by two sea lochs,
Harris has a craggy east coast dominated by
An Clisham, the highest mountain in the
outer islands. Rocky landscape can be rather
desolate, but there are superb sandy beaches.

TOURIST INFORMATION CENTRE
Pier Road, Tarbert
Tel: (01859) 502011 (Seasonal)

SELF-CATERING
CABHALAN COTTAGE
Quidinish, Harris HS3 3JQ
Tel/Fax: (01463) 712661.
BOOK THROUGH: Mr/Mrs Luty, 35 Telford
Road, Inverness IV3 8JA on the same number.
No. of Accessible Units: 1
No. of Beds per Unit: 6
Accessible Facilities: Lounge, Dining Room,
Kitchen. Very secluded stone cottage
overlooking the sea.

LEWIS

Largest in 130-mile long chain of islands,
this is low lying with moors and meadows.
The capital, Stornaway, hosts many Gaelic
events. Don't miss the broch at Carloway
and the bronze age Standing Stones at
Callanish.

ATTRACTION
COLL POTTERY
Back, Isle of Lewis, Western Isles HS2 0JP
Tel: (01851) 820219   Fax: (01851) 820565
e-mail: collpot@sol.co.uk
Manufacture of widest range of ceramics in
Scotland made in crofting town of Coll.
Famous for earthenware figurines reflecting
Hebridean life and marbled ware
representing lands, sea and sky of locale.
Stunning domestic and artistic pieces.

SD   CP   E   RF
C [⚹]   S [⚹]   WC [⚹]

NORTH UIST

Linked to South Uist by a causeway through
Benbecula, the main centre here is
Lochmaddy, a good touring base. The island
is dominated by sea lochs birds, there are
also standing stones, chambered caves and
stone circles, all worth viewing.

TOURIST INFORMATION CENTRE
Pier Road, Lochmaddy
Tel: (01876) 500321 (Seasonal)

ATTRACTION
UIST ANIMAL VISITORS CENTRE
Kyle Road, Bayhead, North Uist, Outer Hebrides
Tel: (01876) 510706   Fax: (01876) 510223
Meet some exotic animals, pot-bellied pigs,
llama which children can pet and feed, rare
poultry and game breeds with much of the
centre undercover.

CP   E   C [⚹]
S [♿]   WC [⚹]

SOUTH UIST

Hill island with a mountainous spine
running down the eastern side. Many
historical and archaeological sites, wonderful
beaches, abundance of wild life, including
many rare breeding birds and rich variety of
plant life. Worth visiting village of Howmore.

TOURIST INFORMATION CENTRE
Pier Road, Lochboisdale
Tel: (01878) 700286 (Seasonal)

HOTEL
ORASAY INN
Lochcarnan, South Uist HS8 5PD
Tel: (01870) 610298   Fax: (01870) 610390
e-mail: orasayinn@btinternet.com
No. of Accessible Rooms: check
Accessible Facilities: Lounge, Dining Room
Small, privately owned hotel, with views
across the Minch in an area of outstanding
natural beauty.

BED & BREAKFAST
CROSS ROADS
Stoneybridge, South Uist HS8 5SD
Tel: (01870) 620321
No. of Accessible Rooms: 2
Accessible Facilities: Dining Room.

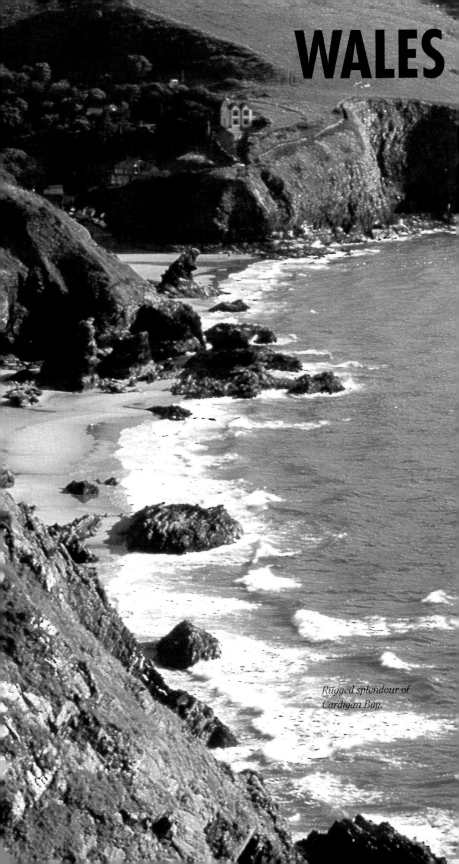

WALES

*Rugged splendour of
Cardigan Bay.*

WALES TOURIST BOARD
Brunel House, 2 Fitzaland Road,
Cardiff CF2 1UY
Tel: 01222 499909   Fax: 01222 485031
e-mail: info@tourism.wales.gov.uk
web: www.visitwales.com

REGIONAL WALES TOURIST BOARDS
THE ISLE OF ANGLESEY
Llangefni LL77 7TW
Tel: (01248) 752411   Fax: (01248) 752192
e-mail: bkxpl@anglesey.gov.uk

LLANDUDNO, COLWYN BAY
Tourism & Leisure Dept. Civic Offices
Colwyn Bay LL29 8AR
Tel: (01492) 575387   Fax: (01492) 513664
e-mail: gwen.roberts@conwy.gov.uk

RHYL & PRESTATYN
Coastal Tourism Unit, West Promenade
Rhyl LL18 1HZ
Tel: (01745) 344515   Fax: (01745) 342255

NORTH WALES BORDERLANDS
Flintshire County Council, County Offices,
St. David's Park, Ewloe,
Deeside CH5 3ZQ
Tel/Fax: (01352) 702468
e-mail: David_P_Evans@flintshire.gov.uk

SNOWDONIA MOUNTAINS & COAST
Gwynedd Council, Cae Penarlag
Dolgellau LL40 2YB
Tel: (01341) 423558   Fax: (01342) 424440
e-mail: tourism@gwyness.gov.uk
web: www.gwynedd.gov.uk

MID WALES LAKES & MOUNTAINS
Powys Tourism, Neuadd Maldwyn,
Severn Road, Welshpool SY21 7AS
Tel: (01938) 551255
e-mail: tourism@powys.gov.uk

MID WALES TOURISM
The Station, Machynlleth SY20 8TG
Tel: Freephone: (0800) 273747
Fax: (01654) 703855
e-mail: info@brilliantbreaks.demon.co.uk

CEREDIGION-CARDIGAN BAY
Section VW2K, Ceredigion Tourism,
Lisburn House, Terrace Road,

Aberystwyth SY23 2AG
Tel: (01970) 612125   Fax: (01970) 626566
e-mail: econ@ceredigion.gov.uk

PEMBROKESHIRE
PO Box 103, Pembroke Dock SA72 6TQ
Tel: (01646) 682278   Fax: (01646) 682281
e-mail: tourism@pembrokeshire.gov.uk

CARMARTHENSHIRE-COAST &
COUNTRYSIDE IN WEST WALES
Carmarthenshire County Council
Ty'r Nant, Trostre Business Park,
Llanelli SA14 9UT
Tel: (01554) 747508   Fax: (01554) 747501
e-mail: dgodbeer@carmarthenshire/gov.uk

SWANSEA BAY
Swansea Tourist Information Centre,
Plymouth Street, Swansea SA1 3Q
Tel: (01729) 468321   Fax: (01729) 464602
e-mail: swantrsm@cableol.co.uk

NORTH WALES TOURISM
77 Conway Road, Colwyn Bay LL29 7LN
Tel: (01492) 531731   Fax: (01492) 530059
e-mail: croeso@nwt.co.uk
web: www.nwt.co.uk

VALLEY OF SOUTH WALES
Valley Breaks, Tourism S & W Wales
Charter Court, Enterprise Park,
Swansea SA7 9DBA
Tel: (01792) 781212   Fax: (01792) 781300
e-mail: valleys@tsww.com

GLAMORGAN HERITAGE COAST
& COUNTRYSIDE
Tourism Unit, Vale of Glamorgan Council,
Dock Office, Barry CF6 4RT
Tel: (01446) 709328   Fax: (01446) 704612
e-mail: tourism@valeofglamorgan.gov.uk
web: valeofglamorgan.gov.uk

WYE VALLEY & VALE OF USK
Tourism Section, Monmouthshire County Council
County Hall, Cwmbran NP44 2XH
Tel: (01633) 644842   Fax: (01633) 644800
e-mail: tourism@monmouthshire.gov.uk

DISABILITY ORGANISATIONS
ACCESSMATTERS
Gorslwyd Farm, Tanygroes, Cardigan,
Ceredigion SA43 2HZ
Tel: (01239) 810593
Researches and publishes *Discovering
Accessible Wales*, an extremely
comprehensive guide to tourist
information, attractions and
accommodation throughout the country.

ARTS FOR DISABLED PEOPLE IN WALES
Channel View. Jim Driscoll Way, The Marl,
Grangetown, Cardiff CF1 7NF
Tel: (029) 20 377885

DISABILITY WALES
Llys For, Crescent Road, Caerphilly,
Glamorgan CF8 1XL
Tel: (029) 20 887325
Freephone: (0800) 731 6282
All Wales disability information and
campaigning organisation.

DISABILITY HELPLINE WALES
3 Links Court, Business Park, St. Mellons,
Cardiff CF3 0SP
Tel: (029) 20 798633
Information and advice for disabled people.

TRAVEL FREEDOM WALES
Unit 2b. St. David's Industrial Estate,
Pengam NP2 1SW
Tel: (01443) 831000   Fax: (01443) 839800
Provides detailed information on aspects of
travel, transport, accommodation and
services for disabled visitors.

TRANSPORT

RAIL
WALES AND WEST PASSENGER TRAINS
Brunel House, 2 Fitzalan Road, Cardiff CF2 1SU
Special Needs: Tel: (0845) 300 3005
Minicom: (0845) 758 5469

CARDIFF
Welsh capital with fusion of ancient
heritage and successful modernity.
Dominated by a splendid Norman castle,
converted in mid C19th to present medieval
appearance. Cardiff Bay is a striking
combination of old dock buildings and
spectacular new developments. Barrage
across the rivers Taff and Ely has created a
huge 500-acre lake. Other major
developments include the demise of the
much-loved Cardiff Arms Park Stadium and
its re-birth as the Millennium Stadium,
built for the Rugby World Cup in 1999.
Shopping here is fun in eight delightful
Victorian and Edwardian arcades and a
Victorian market. A thriving city. Not to be
missed.

TOURIST INFORMATION CENTRE
16 Wood Street, Cardiff CF10 1ES
Tel: (029) 20 227281   Fax: (029) 20
239162

CARDIFF BAY VISITOR CENTRE
Harbour Drive, Cardiff Bay, Cardiff
Tel: (029) 20 463833

PUBLIC TRANSPORT INFORMATION
Tel: (029) 20 873252

BUSES
Cardiff Bus: Tel: (029) 20 396521

TAXIS
Black Cabs: Tel: (029) 20 345345
Some adapted vehicles.

TRAINS
First Great Western: Special Needs:
Tel: (0845) 7413775
Valley Line: Special Needs:
Tel: (029) 20 449944
Virgin Trains: Special Needs:
Tel: (0845) 7443366
Minicom: (0845) 7443367
Wales and West: Special Needs:
Tel: (0845) 3003005
Minicom: (0845) 7585469

CAR PARKS
Free unlimited orange badge parking.
Tel: (029) 20 872000

SHOPMOBILITY
Oxford Arcade Car Park, Bridge Street,
Cardiff CF2 2EB
Tel: (029) 20 399355

HOTELS
COPTHORNE CARDIFF
Copthorne Way, Culverhouse Cross,
Cardiff CF5 6DH
Tel: (029) 20 599100   Fax: (029) 20 599080
No. of Accessible Rooms: 2
Accessible Facilities: Lounge, Restaurant.
Quality hotel in picturesque lakeside
setting four miles from the city centre.

CARDIFF MARRIOTT HOTEL
Mill Lane, Cardiff CF1 1EZ
Tel: (029) 20 399944   Fax: (029) 20 395578
Web: www.marriott.com/marriott/cwldt
No. of Accessible Rooms: 2
Accessible Facilities: Lounge, Restaurant,
bar, disabled changing rooms in leisure
club. Quality hotel located in the heart of
the city opposite colourful café quarter.

CARDIFF WEST TRAVELODGE
Granada Service Area, M4 Junction 33,
Pontyclun, Cardiff CF72 8SA
Tel: (029) 20 891141   Fax: (029) 20 892497
No. of Accessible Rooms: 2
Accessible Facilities: Restaurant.
Located 11 miles from Cardiff city centre.

CARDIFF MOAT HOUSE
Circle Way East, Llanederyn, Cardiff CF3 7XF
Tel: (029) 20 589988   Fax: (029) 20 549092
No. of Accessible Rooms: 2
Accessible Facilities: Lounge, Restaurant,
Bar. Conveniently located for M4 also
with easy access to the city centre.

SELF-CATERING
PARC-COED-MACHEN COUNTRY COTTAGES
St. Brides super-Ely, Nr. Cardiff CF5 6EZ
Tel: (01446) 760684
Fax: (01446) 760289
No. of Accessible Units: 2
No. of Beds per Unit: 3
Accessible Facilities: Lounge, Dining
Room, Kitchen, Patio with garden
furniture. Situated in the north-east of
the Vale, this is a working organic stock
farm with cottages around a central
courtyard of original farm buildings.

ATTRACTIONS
CARDIFF BAY VISITOR CENTRE
Harbour Drive, Cardiff Bay
Tel: (029) 20 463833   Fax: (029) 20 486650
e-mail: viscen@cardiff-bay.co.uk
web: www.cardiff-bay.co.uk
Known locally as The Tube, the visitor
centre was designed by avant-garde
architect William Alsop, creating a
futuristic giant telescope offering
panoramic views of the bay. Also a large-
scale model of Cardiff Bay, the largest
architectural model in the UK.

SD	CP	E	RF
S	WC	RFE	

DYFFRYN GARDENS
St. Nicholas, Nr. Cardiff CF5 6SU
Tel: (029) 20 593328   Fax: (029) 20 598254
A superb landscaped garden of 55 acres,
with small themed gardens, kitchen
garden, arboretum and glass house.

SD	CP	E	RF
C	S	WC	RFE

NATIONAL MUSEUM AND GALLERY
Cathays Park, Cardiff CF1 3NP
Tel: (029) 20 397951
Fax: (029) 20 577010 (Marketing Dept.)
Neo-classic building, a treasure house,
with extensive range of art and science
displays. Art Galleries – works by famous
artists, including the Impressionists in
the fine Davies collection. Evolution of
Wales exhibition traces the country's
development from 4,600 million years
ago. Also the Natural History of Wales
exhibition as well as displays of bronze
age gold, Christian monuments and Celtic
treasures.

SD	CP	E	RF
L	C	S	WC

TECHNIQUEST
Stuart Street, Cardiff CF1 6BW
Tel: (029) 20 475475   Fax: (029) 20 482517
e-mail: gen@tquest.org.uk
UK's leading Science Discovery Centre,
located in waterfront site in the heart of

Cardiff Bay. Over 160 hands-on exhibits: freeze your own shadow, launch a hot-air balloon or even film your own animation. 1996 award for most accessible building for disabled visitors in Cardiff.

    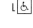

THEATRE
THE SHERMAN THEATRE
Sendhennydd Road, Cathays, Cardiff CF2 4YE
Admin: (029) 20 646901
Fax: (029) 20 646902
Booking-Box Office: (029) 20 646900
Minicom: (029) 20 646909
SD
CP Public CP-Humphries Place, 5-10 minutes walk
Taxi Rank -Outside main entrance. RE ED
INT WC (main foyer)
AUD – Main Theatre studio – n/a
B/R forms part of Foyer

SPORTS VENUE
THE MILLENNIUM STADIUM
CARDIFF ARMS PARK
A Millennium Project
1st Floor St. David's House, Wood Street, Cardiff CF1 1ES
Tel: (029) 20 232661
Fax: (029) 20 232678
e-mail: info@cardiff-stadium.co.uk
web: www.cardiff-stadium.co.uk
Produces comprehensive leaflet on access for disabled visitors. 20 designated spaces in basement car park, access across level plazas with no ramp steeper than 1:20. Entrances from north along riverwalk to Gate 1. From east across Westgate Plaza to Gate 3: from south across Millennium Plaza to Gates 6 and 7: Wheelchair-accessible terraces at level 3 (324 spaces + 206 companion spaces): Level 4 (28 spaces + 24 companion spaces): Level 6 (28 spaces + 24 companion spaces). Lifts access spaces on upper levels (lift size unknown). Adapted WCs available on Levels 3, 4, 6, plus private boxes level 5 (boxes and WCs adapted). NB. Quality of adaptation not known. Catering close to accessible viewing areas at all levels. 10 wheelchairs available for loan.

CARMARTHENSHIRE
web: www.carmarthenshire.gov.uk

CARMARTHEN
Centre of West Wales' agricultural community with flourishing cattle market and excellent covered market; pork butchers a speciality. Built cAD74 around the Roman fortress of Maridunum, the town was an important administration centre in Roman Britain. Reputed to be the birthplace of Merlin, the wizard of Arthurian folklore.

TOURIST INFORMATION CENTRE
Lammas Street SA31 3AQ
Tel: (01267) 231557   Fax: (01267) 221901

PUBLIC TRANSPORT INFORMATION
Tel: (01267) 231817

BUSES
First Cymru: Tel: (01792) 580580

TAXIS
Chris Cars: Tel: (01267) 234438
2 adapted vehicles.

TRAINS
Wales and West: Special Needs:
Tel: (0845) 3003005
Minicom: (0845) 7585469

CAR PARKS
Free unlimited orange badge parking:
Tel: (01267) 231557

WHEELCHAIR HIRE
British Red Cross. Tel: (01686) 626663

HOTEL
CWMTWRCH HOTEL
Nantgaredig, Nr. Carmarthen SA32 7NY
Tel: (01267) 290238 Fax: (01267) 290808
No. of Accessible Rooms: 3
Accessible Facilities: Restaurant, Garden, Indoor Pool. Set in 30 acres off the beaten track in lovely countryside. Nantgaredig is between Carmarthen and Llandeilo.

BED AND BREAKFAST
ALLT-Y-GOLAU UCHAF

Felingwm Uchaf, Nantgaredig,
Nr. Carmarthen SA32 7BB
Tel: (01267) 290455
No. of Accessible Rooms:1
Accessible Facilities: Dining Room
Georgian stone-walled farmhouse built in
1812 with many original features.
Panoramic views over Tywi Valley and
beyond to Black Mountains.

GOLDEN GROVE
Located in the lovely Towy valley, overlooked
by Dinefwr Castle, close to Llandeilo.

SELF-CATERING
HAMDDEN LLETY MEIRI C
Golden Grove SA32 8NL
Tel/Fax: (01558) 823059
e-mail: mcloughlin.patrick@virgin.net
No. of Accessible Units: 3
No. of Beds per Unit: 4
Accessible Facilities: Lounge/ Kitchen/Diner,
Games room, Fitness room, Laundry,
Gardens, fishing from specially constructed
platforms. Located in lovely countryside in
the Towy Valley, 3 cottages, all accessible,
built of traditional Welsh stone, set around a
central courtyard next to a large orchard.

KIDWELLY
Historic town with a magnificent C11th.
Norman castle, one of the best preserved in
Wales. Nine miles south of Carmarthen.
Also lovely river walks.

ATTRACTION
KIDWELLY CASTLE
5 Castle Road, Kidwelly SA17 5BQ
Tel: (01554) 890104
Fine example of late C13th design with
defensive system of walls within walls. Later
additions, including chapel from about
1400. Approach to castle entrance gently
sloping, with slightly steeper stretch on
approach to drawbridge.

SD   CP   E
RF   from car park   S   WC

KIDWELLY INDUSTRIAL MUSEUM
Broadford, Kidwelly SA17 4LW
Tel: (01554) 891078

Established in 1980 on the site of the
second oldest tinplate works in Britain to
preserve and interpret the nation's sole
surviving pack mill. Tinplate production
started here in 1737, the works closing in
1941. Fascinating displays include Engine
House and Coal Museum, Brynlliw Locomotive and Bessie, a steam-powered crane.

SD   CP   E   RF
C   S

LLANDEILO
The former capital of West Wales retains its
old world atmosphere with narrow streets
and historic buildings. Many reflect the
agricultural prosperity of the C18th and early
C19th. Charming market on the last Saturday
of every month. Best enjoyed from the south
across the many-arched bridge of 1848.

TOURIST INFORMATION CENTRE
Municipal Car Park, Crescent Road,
Llandeilo SA19 6HN
Tel/Fax: (01558) 824226
Seasonal, in winter contact Carmarthen.

HOTEL
THE PLOUGH INN AT RHOSMAEN
Rhosmaen, Llandeilo SA19 6NP
Tel: (01558) 823431   Fax: (01558) 823969
e-mail: ploughinn@rhosmaen.demon.co.uk
No. of Accessible Rooms: 1
Accessible Facilities: Restaurant, End of
Towy Lounge (1 step).
Situated on the A40, a mile north of
Llandeilo and within the heart of the Towy
Valley. Wonderful views of the Black
Mountains.

SELF-CATERING
THE STABLE
Book through Holidays for You & Me.
Maerdy Cottages, Taliaris, Nr. Llandeilo SA19 7BD
Tel: (01550) 777448   Fax: (01550) 777067
No. of Accessible Units: 2. Shower
No. of Beds per Unit: 6
Accessible Facilities: Open plan
Kitchen/Diner, Lounge, level to wide
Garden terrace, Ramped to Garden,
Barbecue, Catering available.
The Maerdy was the home farm of the historic
Robert Peel Estate and the 300-year-old

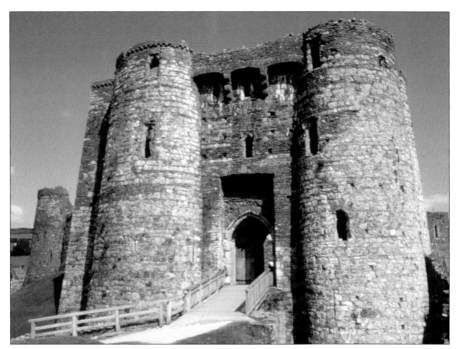

Kidwelly Castle, built to keep the natives in their place.

farmhouse and its original stone buildings have now been converted into six cottages, two accessible. A tranquil setting among mature and wooded gardens with a stream. Midway between Llandovery and Carmarthen.

LLANDOVERY

Small grey-stone town that had a Roman fort, fragments of bricks are still visible in the walls of the site now covered by St. Mary's Church. Cattle drovers stopped here en route from the grazing area in the west to Smithfield Market in London. Located in north-west corner of Brecon Beacons National Park.

TOURIST INFORMATION CENTRE
Kings Road, Llandovery SA20 0AW
Tel/Fax: (01550) 720693

HOTEL
LLANERCHINDDA FARM   🚶
Cynghordy, Llandovery SA20 0NB
Tel: (01550) 750274   Fax: (01550) 750300
e-mail: nick@cambrianway.com
web: www.cambrianway.com
No. of Accessible Rooms: Several. Roll-in

Showers. Accessible Facilities: Lounge, Library Dining Room. West wing of old farmhouse in tranquil location on working sheep farm at 200m on southern slopes of Cambrian Mountains foothills. Fine views. Awarded Best B & B in Wales in 1997.

ATTRACTION
LLANDOVERY HERITAGE CENTRE/TOURIST INFORMATION CENTRE/BRECON BEACONS NATIONAL PARK
Tyllwyd, Kings Road, Llandovery SA20 0AW
Tel/Fax: 01550 720693
SD ♿   CP ♿   E ♿   WC 🚶
Heritage Centre – 1 Wheelchair/stair lift to upper floor.

LLANELLI

Originally the tinplate capital of the world although coal from the Amman Valley and copper are equally important industries now. Its rapid industrial growth in the C19th meant much of the town was based on the Victorian terraced house. The town centre and market are pedestrianised.

TOURIST INFORMATION CENTRE
The Central Library, Vaughan Street,

Llanelli SA15 3AS
Tel: (01554) 772020   Fax: (01554) 750125
Seasonal, in winter contact Carmarthen.

ATTRACTION
THE WILDFOWL AND WETLANDS TRUST
Llanelli Centre, Penclacwydd, Lewynhandy,
Llanelli SA14 9SH
Tel/Fax: (01554) 741087
Excellent visitor centre with fine views to
Gower Peninsula.

SD ♿   CP ♿   E ♿   RF ♿
C ♿   S 🚶   WC 🚶   RFE ♿

WHITLAND
Market town with remains of C12th Abbey.

SELF-CATERING
HOMELEIGH COUNTRY COTTAGES   ♿
Red Roses, Whitland SA34 0PN
Tel: (01834) 831765
No. of Accessible Units: 3.
No. of Beds per Unit: 4, 5, 7
Accessible Facilities: Lounge, Dining
Room, Kitchen.
Small friendly complex designed around
ease and accessibility of wheelchair users
and their families. Set in picturesque village
amid many farm animals. Located on the
edge of the Pembrokeshire National Park.

CEREDIGION
TOURIST INFORMATION
e-mail: econ@ceredigion.gov.uk
web: www.cerdigion.gov.uk/

ABERAERON
Striking harbour and neat Georgian layout,
purpose-built in early 1800s. Poor beach.

TOURIST INFORMATION CENTRE
The Quay, Aberaeron SA46 0BT
Tel: (01545) 570602 Fax: (01970) 626566
e-mail: aberaeron.tic@ceredigion.gov.uk

ATTRACTION
SEA AQUARIUM/COASTAL VOYAGES
2 Quay Parade, Aberaeron SA46 0BT
Tel: (01545) 570142 Fax: (01545) 570160
Insight into marine life in coastal waters of

Cardigan Bay with various tanks stocked
with local fish and shellfish, plus own small
lobster and fish hatcheries. Large screen
AV presentation describes a fisherman's
working life, past and present. Wheelchair
users are welcome on Sea Leopard, a rigid
inflatable boat, on 1 and 2-hour trips
around the bay to see many sea birds and
mammals such as puffin and dolphin.

SD ♿   CP n/a   E ♿   RF ♿
C n/a   S n/a   WC 🚶

ABERPORTH
Small seaside village, traditionally
depending on farming and fishing, but
now a delightful holiday base for some of
the finest scenery on Ceredigion's Heritage
Coast with its award-winning beaches.

BED AND BREAKFAST
FFYNONWEN COUNTRY GUEST HOUSE   ♿
Aberporth SA43 2HT
Tel: (01239) 810312
No. of Accessible Rooms: 1
Accessible Facilities: Lounge/Bar, Dining
Room, Tarmac area with close access to
farm animals and views over small lakes.
Farmhouse, about 300 years old, set in 20
acres with unspoiled coastline.

ABERYSTWYTH
A favourite traditional seaside resort with
many visitor attractions and easy access to
the open hills, coastline and beaches.

TOURIST INFORMATION CENTRE
Terrace Road, Aberystwyth SY23 2AG
Tel: (01970) 612125   Fax: (01970) 626566
e-mail: aberystwyth.tic@ceredigion.gov.uk
Will hire out Red Cross wheelchairs.

PUBLIC TRANSPORT INFORMATION
Tel: (01545) 572504

BUSES
Arriva Cymru: Tel: (01970) 617951

TRAINS
Central Trains: Assistance:
Tel: (0845) 7056027
web: www.centraltrains.co.uk

CAR PARKS
Some free unlimited orange badge parking on-street and in car parks.
Tel: (01545) 572413/572440

HOTEL
GWEST MARINE HOTEL
Marine Terrace, The Promenade,
Aberystwyth SY23 2BX
Tel: (01970) 612444   Fax: (01970) 617435
No. of Accessible Rooms: 1.
Accessible Facilities: Restaurant, Bar.
Large seafront hotel with disabled entrance.

ATTRACTIONS
BWLCH NANT YR ARIAN
Ponterwyd, Aberystwyth SY24 5DF
Tel: (01970) 890500   Fax: (01970) 890340
Forest enterprise.
SD ☒ CP ☒ E ☒ RF ☒
C ☒ S ☒ WC ☒

NATIONAL LIBRARY OF WALES
Aberwystyth SY23 3BU
Tel: (01970) 632800   Fax: (01970) 615709
e-mail: mgm@llgc.org.uk
Huge library, one of Britain's six copyright libraries, specialising in Welsh and Celtic literature. There are maps, manuscripts and drawings plus books and a permanent exhibition on A Nation's Heritage.
SD n/a CP ☒ E ☒ RF ☒ L ☒
C ☒ S ☒ WC ☒ RFE ☒

RHEIDOL POWER STATION
Cwm Rheidol, Aberwystwyth SY23 3NF
Tel: (01970) 880667   Fax: (01970) 880670
Power station lying in a secluded valley with a visitor centre. Also fish farm, forest trails and lakeside picnic area.
SD ☒ CP ☒ E ☒ RF ☒
C ☒ WC ☒ RFE ☒

BORTH
Popular holiday village with lovely firm sandy beach. Fine views from Ynyslas dunes to the north across the Dovey Estuary. Lies to the north of Aberystwyth on a scenic coastline.

TOURIST INFORMATION CENTRE
Cambrian Terrace, Borth SY24 5HU
Tel: (01970) 871174   Fax: (01970) 626566
e-mail: borth.tic@ ceredigion.gov.uk
Seasonal, winter contact Aberystwyth.

SELF-CATERING
ABERLERI FARM COTTAGES
Dept.C. Cambrian Coast Park, Borth SY24 5JU
Tel: (01970) 871233   Fax: (01970) 871124
No. of Accessible Units: 2
No. of Beds per Unit:6
Accessible Facilities: Lounge, Kitchen
Complex of farmhouse and 4 cottages adjoining quality holiday park facilities. Close to sandy beach.

CARDIGAN
Second largest town in the county where in 1176, the very first National Eisteddford was held. Handsome C18th bridge, ruined castle on its mound and long, curving Victorian High Street.

TOURIST INFORMATION CENTRE
Theatr Mwldan, Bath House Road,
Cardigan SA43 2YJ
Tel: (01239) 613230   Fax: (01970) 626566
e-mail: cardigantic@ceredigion.gov.uk

HOTEL
PENBONTBREN FARM HOTEL
Glynarthen, Nr. Cardigan SA44 6PE
Tel: (01239) 810248   Fax: (01239) 811129
No. of Accessible Rooms: 2
Accessible Facilities: Lounge, Restaurant
Old farm buildings now a hotel in the secluded valley of the river Dulais. Victorian farmhouse overlooks the complex. 90 acres of livestock-raising farmland within three miles of sandy beaches.

SELF-CATERING
GORSLWYD FARM
Tanygroes, Cardigan SA43 2HZ
Tel: (01239) 810593 Fax: (01239) 811569
e-mail: bob.donaldson@virgin.net
No. of Accessible Units: 8
No. of Beds per Unit: 6
Accessible Facilities: Lounge, Games Room, Laundry Facilities, Adventure play area, Gardens, Nature Trail, Barbecue, Farm Animals. Comfortable cottages in attractive gardens, 7 miles from Cardigan and close to

sandy beaches. THE OWNER IS A WHEELCHAIR USER AND AN ACCESS CONSULTANT TO THE WALES TOURIST BOARD. HOME OF ACCESSMATTERS, WHO HAVE RESEARCHED AND PUBLISHED *DISCOVERING ACCESSIBLE WALES*, WHICH IS SUPERB.

CANLLEFAES GANOL COTTAGES
Penparc, Cardigan SA43 1SG
Tel/Fax: (01239) 613712
e-Mail: Canllefaes@clara.co.uk
No. of Accessible Units: 1
No. of Beds per Unit: 2 – 8, + cot
Accessible Facilities: Lounge, Dining Room, Kitchen, Outdoor Pool (2 steps).

CROFT FARM AND CELTIC COTTAGES
Croft Farm, Nr. Cardigan SA43 3NT
Tel: (01239) 615179   Fax: (01239) 615179
No. of Accessible Units: 4
No. of Beds. Per Unit: 1
Accessible Facilities: Lounge, Kitchen Comfortable accommodation in unspoilt countryside.

ATTRACTION
FELINWYNT RAINFOREST & BUTTERFLY CENTRE
Felinwynt, Cardigan SA43 1RT
Tel/Fax: (01239) 810882
Wander among free-flying exotic butterflies, observe their life history and how they use both tropical and native plants for breeding and feeding. Waterfall, ponds and streams provide humidity. Accompanied by recorded sounds of the Peruvian Amazon.

| SD ♿ | CP ♿ | E ♿ | RF ♿ |
| C 🚶 | S ♿ | WC 🚶 | RFE ♿ |

LAMPETER
Situated on River Teifi amid rolling farmland, Lampeter is both a university and a market town. The centre of St. David's College is a single Tudor-style quadrangle in attractive grounds. Mostly Georgian and Victorian in character with a large livestock market held on Tuesdays generally.

BED AND BREAKFAST
BRYNCASTELL FARMHOUSE
Llanfair Road, Lampeter SA48 8JY
Tel: (01570) 422447
No. of Accessible Rooms: 2
Accessible Facilities: Lounge, Dining Room. Join this traditional bilingual Welsh farming family on their 140-acre riverside farm overlooking the Teifi valley. Located a mile from Lampeter.

SELF-CATERING
GAER COTTAGES
Cribyn, Lampeter SA48 7LZ
Tel/Fax: (01570) 470275
No. of Accessible Units: 1 (Shippon)
No. of Beds per Unit: 4
Accessible Facilities: Open plan Lounge/diner, kitchen. Pool with Oxford dipper hoist. 1 accessible of 9 attractive cottages set among established lawns, each with a private patio. Beamed ceilings and stone walls and pine furniture. Smallholding 10 miles from the coast, with fine views of surrounding countryside.

TY GLYN DAVIS TRUST
1 Dolfor, Cilia Aeron, Lampeter SA48 8DE
Tel: (01570) 470947
No. of Accessible Units: 1
No. of Beds per Unit: 18
Accessible Facilities: Lounge, Dining Room, Kitchen, Wild Life Garden. Purpose-built centre for young people with disabilities just outside the seaside town of Aberaeron. Situated in woodlands on the banks of the River Aeron.

LLANDYSUL
Teifi-side village in historic textile-producing area where woollen mills still exist. Salmon fishing is popular here.

ATTRACTION
MUSEUM OF THE WELSH WOOLLEN INDUSTRY
Drefach Felindre, Llandysul SA44 5UP
Tel: (01559) 370929   Fax: (01559) 371592
Exhibits tracing history of the woollen industry include C19th textile machinery with demonstrations of fleece to fabric.

| SD ♿ | CP | E ♿ | RF |
| C 🚶 | S ♿ | WC | |

CONWY

ABERGELE

A historic market town, now popular with families for its award-winning beach. Located between Colwyn Bay and Rhyl.

BED AND BREAKFAST
DOLHYFRYD LODGE
Rhuddlan Road, Abergele LL22 7HL
Tel: (01745) 826505 Fax: (01745) 827402
No. of Accessible Rooms: 1
Accessible Facilities: Lounge, Restaurant. Pub and Italian restaurant just down road.

BETWS-Y-COED

Nestling among the forested slopes of Snowdonia, the town's glorious mountain backdrop draws many ramblers and rock-climbers. Full of rather severe slate-roofed houses in local stone, rather like a Victorian mountain resort. It lies jut within the eastern boundary of Snowdonia National Park and is an excellent centre from which to explore.

TOURIST INFORMATION CENTRE
Snowdonia National Park, Royal Oak Stables LL24 0AH
Tel: (01690) 710426 Fax: (01690) 710665

SELF-CATERING
GLANY-Y-BORTH APARTMENT
Book through Holidays for You & Me. Glay-y-Borth Holiday Village, Betws Road, Llanwrst, Nr. Betws-y-Coed LL26 0HB
Tel: (01492) 641543
No. of Accessible Units: 1. Roll-in Shower
No. of Beds per Unit: 4. 1D/1T
Accessible Facilities: Open plan Lounge/Diner, Kitchenette. Ramped landscaped gardens, large barbecue area on the bank of the River Conwy.

ATTRACTION
CONWY VALLEY RAILWAY MUSEUM
The old Goods Yard, Betws-y-Coed LL24 0AL
Tel: (01690) 710568 Fax: (01690) 710132
Two large museum buildings with displays on North Wales railways, including stock and other memorabilia. Working model railway layouts, steam-powered 4-acre miniature railway in the grounds and tramway to the woods.

| SD 🚾 | CP 🚾 | E 🚾 | RF 🚾 |
| C 🚾 | S 🚾 | WC 🚶 | RFE 🚾 |

COLWYN BAY / RHOS-ON-SEA

Late-Victorian and Edwardian seaside resort with beautiful sands and curving promenade running three miles from Rhos-on-Sea in the north to the village of Old Colwyn in the east. Rhos has a mixture of red brick villas and hotels with some older cottages, producing the ambience of an old fishing village.

CB.TOURIST INFORMATION CENTRE
Imperial Buildings, Station Square, Princes Drive, Colwyn Bay LL29 8LA
Tel: (01492) 530478 Fax: (01492) 534789

RHOS. TOURIST INFORMATION CENTRE
The Promenade, Rhos on Sea LL28 4EP
Tel: (01492) 548778
Seasonal, in winter contact Colwyn Bay.

SHOPMOBILITY
44 Sea View Road, Colwyn Bay LL29 8DG
Tel: (01492) 533822 Fax: (01492) 535372
Small collection/delivery charge and small daily charge.

HOTELS
NORTHWOOD HOTEL
47 Rhose Road, Rhos-on-Sea, Colwyn Bay LL28 4RS
Tel: (01492) 549931
No. of Accessible Rooms: 1
Accessible Facilities: Lounge, Dining Room, Bar. Small family-run hotel in the centre of Rhos-on-Sea, 175m from shops and Promenade. Rhos is a charming resort at the western end of Colwyn, but retains a quiet atmosphere with a backcloth of the Pwllcrochan Woods and Clwydian Hills.

SELF-CATERING
BAY COURT
105 Rhos Promenade, Rhos-on-Sea, Colwyn Bay LL28 4NG
Tel: (01492) 549365
No. of Accessible Units: 1

No. of Beds per Unit: 1
Accessible Facilities: Lounge, Kitchen
Seafront holiday apartments opposite
harbour and sandy beach.

BEACHMOUNT
67 Colwyn Avenue, Rhos-on-Sea,
Colwyn Bay LL28 4NN
Tel: (01492) 549314
e-mail: Hhalewood:aol.com
No. of Accessible Units: 2
No. of Beds per Unit: 2-4
Accessible Facilities: Lounge/Diner,
Kitchen. Delightful Victorian residence
50m from sea front in pleasant quiet
avenue with award-winning garden. Five
minutes' level walk to the village centre.

CONWY

A World Heritage Site, Conwy has a C13th
castle, complete town walls and many
historic buildings including a C14th
merchant's house, a fine Elizabethan town
house, the smallest house in Britain. There
is also a charming harbour full of yachts
and fishing boats.

TOURIST INFORMATION CENTRE
Cadw Visitor Centre, Castle Entrance,
Conwy LL32 8LD
Tel: (01492) 592248
Can supply Conwy Public Transport
Information booklet which gives all
information on buses and trains.

BUSES
Tel: (01492) 575412
Some low-floor buses on some routes.

TAXIS
Castle Cabs: Tel: (01492) 593398
3 adapted vehicles.

TRAINS
First North Western: Special Needs:
Tel: (0845) 6040231

CAR PARKS
Free unlimited orange badge spaces
Tel: (01492) 592248

SHOPMOBILITY
44 Sea View Road, Colwyn Bay,
Conwy LL29 8DG
Tel: (01492) 533822   Fax: (01492)
535372
Small collection/delivery charge and
small daily charge.

HOTEL
THE LODGE HOTEL
Tal-y-Bont, Conwy LL32 8YX
Tel: (01492) 6600766
Fax: (01492) 660534
e-mail: b.baldon@lodgehotel.co.uk
Number of Accessible Rooms: 6. Bath
Accessible Facilities: Lounge, Restaurant,
Bar. Built in 1974 on the site of a
smallholding and well converted into a
charming small hotel, with 3.5 acres of
gardens. Located on the B5106 six miles
south of Conwy. Tal-y-Bont is a peaceful
rural village in the heart of the lovely
Conwy Valley, on the edge of Snowdonia
National Park. The hotel is framed by the
Cardeddau mountains.

ATTRACTION
THE SMALLEST HOUSE IN GREAT BRITAIN
The Quay, Conway LL32 8BB
Tel/Fax: (01492) 593484
Occupied until 1900, this house is only 72
inches (180cm) wide and 122 inches
(305cm) high. There is a tiny fireplace
where cooking was done: a settle with a lift-
up seat that doubled as a coal bunker, a
small round table, a water tap hidden
behind the stairs and a minute bedroom
with a long single bed. WC used to be at the
back. The last occupant was a mussel
fisherman standing 6ft 3in. (187.5cm).
Access to downstairs room only.

SD   CP   E

LLANDUDNO

Wales' largest resort, located between the
Great and Little Ormes, with the award-
winning North Shore beach and the quiet
sand-duned West Shore beach. Although
full of modern attractions, Llandudno
retains much Victorian and Edwardian
elegance.

TOURIST INFORMATION CENTRE
1/2 Chapel Street, Llandudno LL30 2SY
Tel: (01492) 876413   Fax: (01492) 872722

HOTEL
THE WEST SHORE HOTEL
Grooms Holidays.
West Parade, Llandudno LL30 2BB
Tel: (01492) 876833   Fax: (01492) 875461
No. of Accessible Rooms: All
Accessible Facilities: Lounge, Dining Room,
Bar. Situated at the foot of the magnificent
Great Orme and a short walk from the
ornate Victorian Pier and Promenade.

BEDFORD HOTEL
The Promenade, Craig-y-Don,
Llandudno LL30 1BN
Tel: (01492) 876647   Fax: (01492) 860185
No. of Accessible Rooms: 2. Bath
Accessible Facilities: Lounge, Restaurant.
On the promenade, many rooms enjoy fine
views of the sweeping bay.

BELMONT HOTEL
21 North Parade, Llandudno LL30 2LP
Tel: (01492) 877770
No. of Accessible Rooms: 6
Accessible Facilities: Lounge, Restaurant.
Hotel owned by Henshaw's Society for the

Blind close to the beach (100m) and 300m
from the town centre.

EPPERSTONE HOTEL
15 Abbey Road, Llandudno LL30 2EE
Tel: (01492) 878746   Fax: (01492) 871223
No. of Accessible Rooms: 1
Accessible Facilities: Lounge, Restaurant.
Small quiet detached hotel retaining some
fine Edwardian features. 600m from town
centre and 800m from the beach.

THE ROYAL HOTEL
Church Walks, Llandudno LL30 2HN
Tel: (01492) 876476   Fax: (01492) 870210
No. of Accessible Rooms: 6. Bath
Accessible Facilities: Lounge, Restaurant.
Established in 1857, this is the oldest hotel
in Llandudno, retaining an air of Victorian
elegance. Situated at the foot of the Great
Orme within easy distance of both North
and West shores and the town centre.
Large, secluded gardens.

SELF-CATERING
BEAVER LODGE
4 Old Road, Llandudno LL30 2QQ
Tel: (01492) 877443
No. of Accessible Units: 1
No. of Beds per Unit: 2
Accessible Facilities: Lounge, Kitchen

371

Llandudno bay from Great Orme.

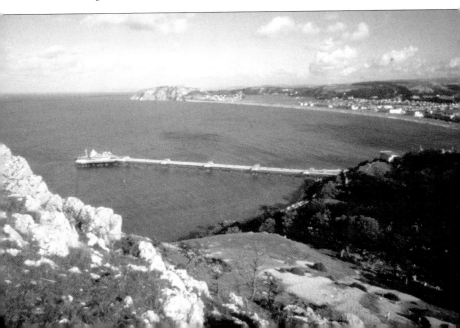

DENBIGHSHIRE

DENBIGH

Pretty walled and old market town dominated by the scanty remains of a huge castle begun in 1282. There are narrow streets, piazza and historic buildings, plus C16th. hall now housing a good museum. Denbigh was once the centre of glove-making in Wales. Famous as the birthplace of Henry Morton Stanley who uttered the immortal words "Dr. Livingstone, I presume."

HOTEL
BRYN GLAS HOTEL
St. Asaph Road, Trefnant,
Nr. Denbigh LL16 5UD
Tel: (01745) 730868   Fax: (01745) 730590
No. of Accessible Rooms: 8
Accessible Facilities: Lounge, Restaurant, Bar, Lawn, Grounds. Privately owned hotel purpose built in 1988, previously the site of an old farm. The proprietor's son is a spinal injured person and the hotel is staffed by the family who are very familiar with special requirements.

CORWEN

Market town in Vale of Edeyrnion with regular livestock market. Located 12 miles from Llangollen, it is a good centre for Snowdonia.

ATTRACTION
LLYN BRENIG VISITOR CENTRE
Cerrigdrudion, Corwen LL21 9TT
Tel: (01490) 420463   Fax: (01490) 420694
A 1,800 acre estate with archaeological and nature trails. Specially adapted fishing boat for disabled anglers, the centre has an exhibition on geology, archaeology, history and natural history of the region.

EWLOE

Located 10 miles west of Chester with a castle that is proudly Welsh, built by native princes in a wooded hollow to attack the English.

HOTEL
ST. DAVID'S PARK HOTEL
St. David's Park, Ewloe,
Nr. Chester CH5 3YB
Tel: (01244) 520800   Fax: (01244) 520930
e-mail: reservations@st.davids-park-hotel.co.uk
web: www.st.davids-park-hotel.co.uk
No. of Accessible Rooms: 6
Accessible Facilities: Bar, Restaurant
Quality hotel in delightful grounds, with nearby Northrop Country Park Golf Club.

HOLYWELL

Associated with a virtuous virgin of C7th. St. Winefride was restored to life after her head had been chopped off by the holy water of the Holywell stream. The buildings associated with the spring are set into a steep hillside and there is a well and chapel in her name.

ATTRACTION
GREENFIELD VALLEY COUNTRY PARK MUSEUM AND FARM
Administration Centre, Basingwerk House,
Greenfield, Holywell CH8 7QB
Tel: (01354) 714172
Fax: (01352) 714791
web: www.mksite.co.uk/greenfeild/
Set in 50 acres of woodland, within the Abbey Farm complex is a museum complete with machinery, equipment and animals, restored cottages depicting a way of life long gone and a Victorian school. Explore further for ruined mills, good picnic spots and silent pools.

LLANGOLLEN

Situated on the banks of the River Dee, this lovely town is famous for its steam railway and horse-drawn canal boats. In the town, a C14th bridge spans the river, and there are many historical buildings.

TOURIST INFORMATION CENTRE
Town Hall, Castle Street, Llangollen LL20 5PD
Tel: (01978) 860828
Fax: (01978) 861563

PUBLIC TRANSPORT INFORMATION
Tel: (01824) 706968

BUSES
Arriva Cymru: Tel: (01970) 617951
Some low-floor buses.

TRAINS
Nearest station is Ruabon, Central Trains.

CAR PARKS
Orange badge spaces available in off-street car park, but chargeable at normal rate. 3-hour free parking on-street.

WHEELCHAIR HIRE
Red Cross North Wales
Tel: (01492) 877886

HOTEL
BRYN HOWEL HOTEL AND RESTAURANT
Llangollen LL20 7UW
Tel: (01978) 860331
Fax: (01978) 860119
e-mail: hotel@brynhowel.demon.co.uk
No. of Accessible Rooms: 1
Accessible Facilities: Lounge Bar, Restaurant. Built in 1896 as a private home, a lovely red brick property family owned and managed. Good location for exploring Vale of Llangollen.

ATTRACTION
LLANGOLLEN WHARF CANAL MUSEUM AND HORSEDRAWN BOATS
Wharf Hill, Llangollen LL20 8TA
Tel (01978) 860702
The museum offers imaginative displays on canal life in its heyday. New horse-drawn boats accessible via ramp in order to take full advantage of a 45-minute boat trip along the lovely Llangollen valley.

SD 🦽	CP 🚹	E 🦽	RF 🦽
C 🦽	S 🦽	WC 🚹	RFE 🦽

PRESTATYN
Seaside resort on which vast amounts of money have been spent to make the town an oasis of family fun, so there is much to do. Don't miss Offa's Dyke trail, stretching from the town to Chepstow. The poet Philip Larkin wrote a poem Sunny

Prestatyn that captures the flavour of the resort.

TOURIST INFORMATION CENTRE
Offa's Dyke Centre, Central Beach, Prestatyn LL19 7EY
Tel: (01745) 889092
Seasonal, in winter contact Conwy.

HOTEL
TRAETH GANOL HOTEL 🚹
41 Beach Road West, Prestatyn LL19 7LL
Tel: (01745) 853594
Fax: (01745) 886687
No. of Accessible rooms: 3
Accessible Facilities: Lounge, Restaurant, Bar. Located opposite the sea at Central Beach with Promenade access by the Nova Leisure Centre 100m. away. Small and personal family-owned hotel.

373

Llangollen canal Pontcysyllte aquaduct.

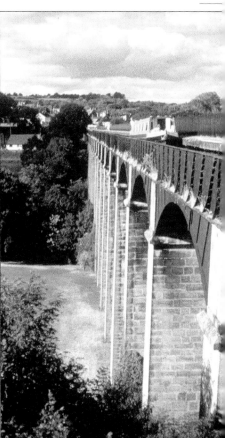

GWYNEDD

ABERSOCH

Popular small resort, calling itself the Welsh Riviera. There are two sandy bays full of dinghies and windsurfers, and offshore are St. Tudwal's Islands with seals and seabirds.

TOURIST INFORMATION CENTRE
Abersoch LL53 7EA
Tel/Fax: (01758) 712929

SELF-CATERING
RHYDOLION
Llangian, Abersoch, LL53 7LR
Tel/Fax: (01758) 712342
No. of Accessible Units: 1
No. of Beds per Unit: 6
Accessible Facilities: Lounge/Diner, Kitchen.
Cottage on working farm.

BALA

Market town on the edge of Snowdonia with a single street lined with trees. In the deep valley to the SW of the town is Bala Lake, the largest natural body of water in Wales. Originally founded as an English borough in 1310, the back lanes running parallel to the High Street show the limits of the original burbage plots.

TOURIST INFORMATION CENTRE
Pensarn Road, Bala LL23 7NH
Tel/Fax: (01678) 521 021
e-mail: bala.tic@gwynedd.gov.uk

ATTRACTION
BALA LAKE RAILWAY
The Station, Llanuwchllyn, Bala LL23 7DD
Tel/Fax: (01678) 540666
Narrow gauge train running along the shores of Wales' largest natural lake. Lovely nine-mile return journey through Snowdonia national park with fine views of the lake and surrounding pastoral and woodland scenery and nearby mountains.

SD		CP		E	RF
C		S		WC	

RFE Platform – Direct Access at Llanuwchllyn, but NOT AT BALA. Train- Ramped Access

BANGOR

Cathedral and university city overlooking the scenic Menai Strait. A wide variety of architectural styles, a Victorian pier and its cathedral, founded in AD525, said to be the oldest in Britain. The city began to grow at the end of the C18th when Penrhyn slate was exported. The university arrived in 1884 and Bangor is now a small metropolis.

TOURIST INFORMATION CENTRE
Town Hall, Deiniol Road, Bangor LL57 7RE
Tel: (01248) 352786   Fax: (01248) 362701
e-mail: bangor.tic@gwynedd.gov.uk

PUBLIC TRANSPORT INFORMATION
Tel: (01286) 679535

BUSES
Arriva Cymru: Tel: (01248) 351879/750444
Some low-floor buses.

TRAINS
First North Western: Special Needs:
Tel: (0845) 6040231
Virgin Trains: Special Needs:
Tel: (0845) 7443366
Minicom: (0845) 7443367

WHEELCHAIR HIRE
Mantell Gwynedd (Caernarfon)
Tel: (01286) 672626
Red Cross (Llandudno): Tel: (01492) 877886

HOTEL
THE BRITISH HOTEL
High Street, Bangor LL57 1NP
Tel: (01248) 364911   Fax: (01248) 370569
e-mail: BritishHotelBangor@compuserve.com
web: www.S-H-Systems.co.uk/Hotels/Brit,Html
No. of Accessible Rooms: 40 (via lift)
Accessible Facilities: Lounge, Restaurant, Buttery and Cocktail Bar. Purpose-built property close to university halls, main shopping and entertainment areas.

ATTRACTION
PENRHYN CASTLE (NT)
Bangor LL57 4HN
Tel: (01248) 353084   Fax: (01248) 371281
Neo-Norman castle with towers and battlements commissioned in 1827 as a sumptuous family home. Notable rooms

include the Great Hall, Library and Dining Room with a fine collection of paintings. Also an industrial railway museum in the Stableyard, and Victorian terraced walled garden in the 40-acre grounds. Ground floor rooms only are accessible. Wheelchairs available and volunteer-driven 3-passenger vehicles to assist in viewing the grounds.

SD ♿ CP ♿ E ♿ RF ♿
C ♿ S ♿ New – in Stable block
WC ♿ RFE ♿

THE GREENWOOD CENTRE
Y Felinheli, Nr. Bangor LL56 4QN
Tel: (01248) 671493   Fax: (01248) 670069
e-mail: trees@greenwood-centre.demon.co.uk
Set up to provide an insight into the extraordinary world of trees, with conservation a priority. Forest and Adventure Park with herb garden, sculpture trail, tree world in the great hall, adventureland, Welsh crafts and animals. Film show on the Forgotten Forests of Snowdonia and inter-active exhibition. Located a few miles SW of Bangor.

SD ♿ CP ♿ E ♿ RF ♿
C ⚹ S ⚹ WC ⚹ RFE ♿

BLAENAU FFESTINIOG

TOURIST INFORMATION CENTRE
Unit 3, High Street, Blaenau Ffestiniog LL41 3ES
Tel: (01766) 830360   Fax: (01766) 830360
Seasonal, in winter contact Betws-y-Coed.

ATTRACTION
LLECHWEDD SLATE CAVERNS
Blaenau Ffestiniog LL41 3NB
Tel: (01766) 830306   Fax: (01766) 831260
e-mail: llechwedd@aol.com
Discover the working conditions of Victorian slate mines where primitive tools were used to move millions of ton of rock. Surface exhibitions on mine tramways and slate mining, old smithy, slate mill and Victorian shops. All surface attractions, except Miners Arms, are accessible.
For the mine take the Miner's Tramway guided tour through an 1846 network of amazing man-made caverns of cathedral proportions, supplemented with tableaux and demonstrations of ancient mining

skills. Folding wheelchairs can be carried on the train, but transfer from wheelchair to train seat for journey and at several points underground is required.
NB: Entrance ramped at 1:9: Route to features is ramped at 1:10. The Deep Mine tour is not accessible.

SD ♿ CP ♿ E n/a RF ♿
C ♿ S ♿ WC ⚹ RFE n/a

DOLGELLAU
Quiet, historic market town with narrow streets once famed for the mining of Welsh gold. An excellent touring centre.

TOURIST INFORMATION CENTRE
Ty Meirion, Eldon Square, Dolgellau LL40 1PU
Tel: (01341) 422888   Fax: (01341) 422576

BUSES
Arriva Cymru: Tel: (01970) 617951
Some low floor buses.

CAR PARKS
Free unlimited orange badge parking.
Tel: (01341) 422341

WHEELCHAIR HIRE
British Red Cross: Tel: (01341) 422620

BED AND BREAKFAST
GRAIG-WEN HOUSE ♿
Arthog, Nr. Dolgellau LL39 1BQ
Tel: (01341) 250482   Fax: (01341) 250482
No. of Accessible Rooms: 1
Accessible Facilities: Lounge, Dining Room, Snooker Room. Set in 45 acres of woodland and pasture reaching down the spectacular Mawddach Estuary with views of surrounding mountains. Located five miles from Dolgellau and between there and Fairbourne on the A493.

SELF-CATERING
PEN Y LON ⚹
Pentre Bach Cottages, Llwyngwril, Dolgellau LL37 2JU
Tel: (01341) 250294   Fax: (01341) 250885
e-mail: smyth@pentrebach.com
web: www.pentrebach.com
No. of Accessible Units: 1
No. of Beds per Unit: 7 + cot

Old Welsh stone cottages in seaside village in the southern part of Snowdonia National Park. At the end of a 260m private, tree-lined drive, 12 miles from Dolgellau, with glorious views across Cardigan Bay to Lleyn Peninsula.

HARLECH

Small town on SW border of Snowdonia and a good base from which to explore the mountains inland. Against an amazing sea and mountain background, Harlech Castle is the epitomy of a medieval stronghold. It was erected as one of the Iron Ring of defences by Edward I in the late C13th.

TOURIST INFORMATION CENTRE
Gwyddfor House, High Street,
Harlech LL46 1DR
Tel/Fax: (01766) 780658
Seasonal, in winter contact Portmadog or Dolgellau.

MOTEL
ESTUARY MOTEL
Talsarnau, Harlech LL47 6TA
Tel: (01766) 771155   Fax: (01766) 771697
No. of Accessible Rooms: 10
Accessible Facilities: Lounge, Restaurant. Located three miles from the centre of Talsarnau and Portmeirion and four miles from Harlech.

SELF-CATERING
YSTUMOWERN FARM
Dyffryn Ardudwy, Nr. Harlech LL44 2DD
Tel: (01341) 247249   Fax: (01341) 247171
No. of Accessible Units: 1
Accessible Beds per Unit: 4
Accessible Facilities: Lounge, Dining Room, Kitchen. Farmhouse 5 miles from Harlech.

LLANBERIS

Lively mountain town and a popular touring centre at the foot of Snowdon, with two lakes and the craggy Llanberis Pass.

TOURIST INFORMATION CENTRE
41a High Street, Llanberis LL55 4UR
Tel: (01286) 870765   Fax: (01286) 871924
e-mail: llanberis.tic@gwynedd.gov.uk
Seasonal, in winter contact Caernarfon.

ATTRACTIONS
LLANBERIS LAKE RAILWAY
Gilfach Ddu, Llanberis LL55 4TY
Tel/Fax: (01286) 870549
e-mail: railway.freeserve.co.uk
Enjoy spectacular views of Snowdon and surrounding mountains. Starting at Gilfach Ddu station, the train takes about 40 minutes to run to Penllyn through Padarn Country Park and back with a short stop at Cei Llydan for sightseeing. Stop here for a picnic and catch a later train back to Llanberis.

SD   CP   E   RF
C   S   WC
RFE   TRAIN Specially adapted carriage to take 6 wheelchairs. Graded by WTB as accessible for unaccompanied wheelchair users.

SNOWDON MOUNTAIN RAILWAY
Llanberis LL55 4TY
Tel: (01286) 870223   Fax: (01286) 872518
For passengers with some limited mobility who can leave their wheelchairs, staff recommend these be left in Llanberis and use be made of the ones kept at the summit. Disembarkation at the summit is not possible for powered chairs.

SD   CP   E (Platform)   RF
C   S   WC
TRAIN – 2 trains able to accommodate either 2 manual or 1 powered wheelchair. Wheelchairs have to be carried from platform to carriage, but staff advise they will always help.

WELSH SLATE MUSEUM
Padarn Country Park, Llanberis LL55 4TY
Tel: (01286) 870630   Fax: (01286) 871906
Set among towering slate quarries, this is a living working site, a pocket of the past. There is a quarry workshop with demonstrations and the largest working waterwheel on mainland Britain. Plus spectacular 3-D presentation of life in the quarries, restored Chief Engineer's house and unique working slate incline.

SD   CP   E   RF
C   S   WC   RFE

PANT GLAS
Located on the SW edge of Snowdonia

HOTEL
HEN YSGOL OLD SCHOOL

Bwlch-Derwin, Pant Glas LL51 9EQ
Tel: (01286) 660701
e-mail: OldSchoolPantGlas@Talk21.com
No. of Accessible Rooms: 3
Accessible Facilities: Lounge, Dining Room, Gardens, Grounds. Historic country school built in 1858 now converted and retaining much of the traditional features. Situated on the NW boundary of the Snowdonia National Park, an ideal base for touring Snowdon and neighbouring area. Beaches of Criccieth and Pwllheli within 6-10 miles.

PORTHMADOG

Pretty town lying on the Glaslyn estuary on the Llyn Peninsula, designated an "Area of Outstanding Natural Beauty", with a number of beaches managed by the National Trust. The town has a fascinating maritime heritage and a lovely harbour.

TOURIST INFORMATION CENTRE
High Street, Porthmadog LL49 9LD
Tel: (01766) 512981   Fax: (01766) 515312
e-mail: porthmadog.tic@gwynedd.gov.uk

ATTRACTION
FFESTINIOG RAILWAY
Harbour Station, Porthmaddoc LL49 9NF
Tel: (01766) 512340   Fax: (01766) 514995
e-mail: info@festrail.demon.co.uk
web: www.festrail.co.uk
Famous railway with little steam-hauled narrow-gauge trains running along 13.5 miles main line in miniature from coastline at Porthmadog into the mountains at Blaenau Ffestiniog with wonderful views. Also on the sister railway between Caernarfon and Dinas, there are gentle pastoral views of the Menai Strait. Porthmadog and Blaenau Ffestiniog stations have ramped access routes and partially adapted WCs. Caernarfon and Dinas have ramped access. Coaches on some trains have extra wide doors (not electric chairs).

SD ♿   CP ♿   E ♿   RF ♿
C ♿   S ♿   WC 🚹

PWLLHELI

Historic market town, also on the Llyn Peninsula, has many buildings dating back to early C17th. It has a 420-berth marina and 5 miles of sand and shingle beaches.

TOURIST INFORMATION CENTRE
Min y Don, Sgwar yr Orsaf, Pwllheli. LL53 5HG
Tel: (01758) 613000   Fax: (01758) 701651
e-mail: pwllheli.tic@gwynedd.gov.uk

BED AND BREAKFAST
RHOSYDD   ♿
26 Glan Cymerau, Pwllheli LL53 5PU
Tel: (01758) 612956
No. of Accessible Rooms: 1
Accessible Facilities: Dining room. Detached bungalow situated close to beach, on outskirts of town.

SELF-CATERING
AFONWEN FARM   ♿ 🚹
Pwllheli LL53 6TX
Tel/Fax: (01766) 810939
No. of Accessible Units: 4
No. of Beds per Unit: 4 – 8
Accessible Facilities: Lounge, Kitchen, Games Room, Nature Trail around farm. Converted in 1995, 4 cottages and farm-house on owner's working farm between Snowdonia National park and Lyn Peninsula. Surrounded by farmland, lovely mountain views and within five minutes' of the beach.

CEFN COED   🚹
Chwilog, Pwllheli LL53 6NX
Tel: (01766) 810259

Full steam ahead for the top of Snowdon.

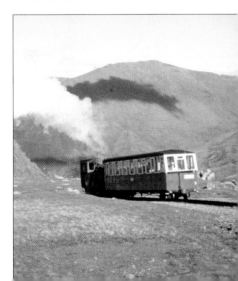

No. of Accessible Units: 1
No. of Beds per Unit: 6
Accessible Facilities: Lounge, Dining Room, Kitchen. C18th cottages on farm in quiet countryside with panoramic views of Cardigan Bay coast.

TRAWSFYNYDD
Located in heart of Snowdonia National Park midway between Dollgellau and Porthmadog.

BED AND BREAKFAST
OLD MILL FARMHOUSE
Trawsfynydd LL41 4UN
Tel/Fax: (01766) 540397
No. of Accessible Rooms: 1 Roll-in shower.
Accessible Facilities: Lounge, Dining Room, Garden. Holiday Care Award winning property, once the home of the village corn miller, dating back to early C18th. The farm land allows families plenty of open space and contact with safe friendly animals. Accommodation in converted old farm building adjacent to farmhouse, where breakfast is served.

TYWYN
Seaside resort on Cardigan Bay with important Christian monuments of St. Cadfan's Stone and Llanegryn Church. Located west of Dolgellau and Machynlleth at the SW tip of Snowdonia National Park.

TOURIST INFORMATION CENTRE
High Street, Tywyn LL36 9AD
Tel/Fax: (01654) 710070
e-mail: tywyn.tic@gwynedd.gov.uk
Seasonal, in winter contact Dolgellau.

ATTRACTION
TALYLLYN RAILWAY
Wharf Station, Tywyn LL36 9EY
Tel: (01654) 710472   Fax: (01654) 711755
Narrow gauge line using steam locomotives that opened in 1865 and runs inland from Tywyn on the mid Wales coast to Nant Gwernol. A journey of just under an hour, much of it within Snowdonia National Park with waterfalls at Dolgoch.
NB No road access at Nant Gwernol

terminus and so the main starting point is Abergynolwyn.

| SD [♿] | E [♿] | RFE [🚶] | C [🚶] |
| S [🚶] | WC [🚶] | RFE [♿] | |

TRAIN – entrance to compartment by ramp assisted by staff.

ISLE OF ANGLESEY
Web: www.anglesey.gov.uk

HOLYHEAD TOURIST INFORMATION CENTRE
The Kiosk, Stena Line, Terminal 1,
Holyhead LL65 1DR
Tel: (01407) 762622

CENTRE FOR INTEGRATED LIVING:
Tel: (01248) 750249
Information on most areas of transport.

ISLE OF ANGLESEY COUNTY COUNCIL
Tel: (01248) 752459

BUSES
Arriva Cymru: Tel: (01248) 750444

AMLWCH
Parys Mountain is the most spectacular hill in Anglesey, site of greatest copper mines in the world in the late C18th, with Amlwch as their port. Widened in the 1790s to make a harbour, the little port retains its late C18th appearance and is still used by various types of boat. The catholic church, Our Lady Star of the Sea, is built in the shape of an overturned boat, emphasising the area's seafaring tradition.

SELF CATERING
BEUDGWYN FARM
Carreglefyn, Almwich LL68 0RL
Tel: (02407) 711433
No. of Accessible Units: 1. Roll-in Shower
No. of Beds per Unit: 4 (1T,1D)
Accessible Facilities: Open plan Lounge/Diner/Kitchen.
Bluebell Cottage is newly converted and located in a rural setting on a farm full of domestic animals.

BEAUMARIS

Small town in glorious setting, overlooking the Menai Strait which is very broad at this point, the south shore rises to the mountains of Snowdonia. Popular with holidaymakers from late Georgian times it is an elegant resort with a pier, seafront green and brightly painted terraces facing the water.

HOTEL
THE BULKELEY HOTEL
Castle Street, Beaumaris LL58 8AW
Tel: (01248) 810415   Fax: (01248) 810146
web: www.consorthotels.com
No. of Accessible Rooms: Several
Accessible Facilities: Lounge, Restaurant. Built for the young Princess Victoria in 1832, retains the style and elegance. Very close to the beach and pier with views of Menai Straits to Snowdonia mountains.

BENLLECH

Popular holiday village above a sweeping bay on the east coast. Long and sandy beach for families with beach shops and cafes. Nearby cliffs rich in fossils.

BED AND BREAKFAST
BRYN MEIRION GUEST HOUSE
Amlwch Road, Benllech LL74 8SR
Tel: (01248) 853118
No. of Accessible Rooms: 6
Accessible Facilities: Lounge, Dining Room, Gardens. Panoramic views across the sea to Llandudno and Snowdonia mountains beyond. Family run guest house, set in lovely lawned gardens on fine coastal site on east coast of Anglesey. The owners, having worked in a residential school for children with disabilities, established this property to cater for all.

BRYNSIENCYN

Hamlet near shores of Menai Strait, looking across to Snowdonia.

ATTRACTION
ANGLESEY SEA ZOO
Brynsiencyn LL61 6TQ

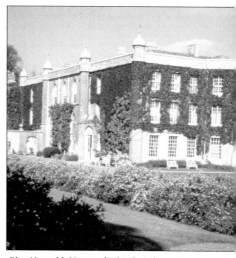

Plas Newydd. Home of Whistler's largest mural.

Tel: (01248) 430411   Fax: (01248) 430213
e-mail: FISHANDFUN@SEAZOO.demon.co.uk
web: www.nwi.co.uk/seazoo
Gaze at local creatures as they live and grow undisturbed in one of Britain's largest single underwater viewing stations. Wander through a shipwreck and a new exhibition on how pearls are bred and used. See, touch, smell and breathe the sea.

SD CP E RF
C S WC

LLANFAIRPWLL

It's compulsory to visit this village – Llanfairpwllgwyngyllgogerychwyrndrobwllllantysiliogogogoch – the longest name in Britain. It was a C19th hoax by a tailor from the Menai Bridge to attract tourists to the station. Get a souvenir platform ticket from James Pringle Weavers centre. Llanfair means St. Mary's.

TOURIST INFORMATION CENTRE
Station Site, Llanfairpwll LL61 5UJ
Tel: (01248) 713177   Fax: (01248) 715711

ATTRACTION
PLAS NEWYDD (NT)
Llanfairpwll LL61 6DQ
Tel: (01248) 714795   Fax: (01248) 713673

e-mail: ppnmsn@smtp.ntrust.ork.uk
C18th house with a mixture of classical and
Gothic architecture. Re-styled interior of
1930s, famous for Rex Whistler whose largest
wall painting is housed here plus an exhibition
about his work. Military museum with relics
of Battle of Waterloo and a fine garden.

SD   CP   E   RF
C [木]   S [&]   WC [木]

LLANGEFNI

County town of Angelesey standing on the
island's longest river, the Cefni. Many
leisure facilities and weekly open air
markets on Thursday and Saturdays. The
nearby Llyn Cefni reservoir offers trout
fishing and bird watching.

HOTEL
TRE-YSGAWEN HALL
Capel Coch, Llangefni LL77 7UR
Tel: (01248) 750750   Fax: (01248) 750035
No. of Accessible Rooms: 3
Accessible Facilities: Lounge, Restaurant.
Country house mansion, built in 1882, and
renovated in 1990. Set in the heart of a
3,000-acre estate

RED WHARF BAY

Superb sands make this one of Anglesey's
most popular beaches.

HOTEL
BRYN TIRION HOTEL
Red Wharf Bay, LL75 8RZ
Tel: (01248) 852366   Fax: (01248) 852013
e-mail: bthynysmon@aol.com
No. of Accessible Rooms: 1
Accessible Facilities: Lounge, Restaurant
Family run hotel enjoying superb views
over the bay.

SELF-CATERING
YR HEN YSGOL
Rhoscolyn, Nr. Trearddur Bay LL65 2RQ
Tel: (01407) 741593
No. of Accessible Units: 2
No. of Beds per Unit: 6
Accessible Facilities:
2 bungalows in unspoilt countryside, close
to beaches.

MERTHYR TYDFIL

High up the Taff Vale, for many years the
Iron Capital of the World, much of the
early industrial heritage remains. The last
foundry was shut down by British Steel in
1987, but this is still a proud, if rather
bleak town.

MERTHYR TYDFIL
TOURIST INFORMATION CENTRE
14A Glebeland Street,
Merthyr Tydfil CF47 8AU
Tel: (01685) 379884   Fax: (01685) 350043

PUBLIC TRANSPORT INFORMATION
Merthyr Tydfil County Borough Council,
Technical Services
Tel: (01685) 726256

BUSES
Stagecoach Red & White: Tel: (01685)
385539
Some low-floor buses.

TAXIS
A & P Cars: Tel: (01685) 374326
1 adapted vehicle.
First Class Cars: Tel: (01685) 373737
1 mini.

TRAINS
Valley Line: Special Needs:
Tel: (029) 20 449944
All trains have ramps – ring a few days
before travel – also provides park & ride.

CAR PARKS
Free parking. Tel: (01685) 726285

SHOPMOBILITY
St. Tydfil's Square, Shopping Centre,
Merthyr Tydfil
Tel/Fax: (01685) 373237
Minicom: (01685) 373400

HOTEL
TREGENNA HOTEL
Park Terrace, Merthyr Tydfil CF47 8RF
Tel: (01685) 723627   Fax: (01685) 721951
e-mail: treghotel@aol.com
No. of Accessible Rooms: 2 Accessible
Facilities: Lounge, Restaurant. Family run
and set in the heart of the National Park.

ATTRACTIONS

BRECON MOUNTAIN RAILWAY CO.
Plant Station, Merthyr Tydfil, CF48 2UP
Tel: (01685) 722988   Fax: (01685) 384854
Located 3 miles north of town. All- weather observation coaches behind vintage steam locomotive through beautiful scenery into the Brecon Beacons National Park along the full length of Taf Fechan Reservoir to Dol-y-Gaer.
Access positively described in literature.
Carriages: 1, specially designed to carry wheelchairs.

P & A [♿]   E [♿]   C tables not accessible
S [♿]   WC [♿]   Features: Platform [♿]

CYFARTHFA CASTLE MUSEUM and ART GALLERY
Brecon Road, Merthyr Tydfil   CF47 8RE
Tel/Fax: (01685) 723112
Gothic mansion built in 1825 with wonderful surviving gardens. Houses fine collection of decorative arts, archaeological and natural history items and social and industrial history of the region. Basement gallery has chairlift and wheelchair available at foot.

SD [♿]   CP [♿]   E [♿]   RF [♿]
S [♿]   WC [♿]   RFE [♿]

TREHARRIS
Located 8 miles from Merthyr Tydfil.

ATTRACTION

LLANCAIACH FAWR MANOR LIVING HISTORY MUSEUM
Plas Llancaiach Fawr, Nelson, Treharris CF46 6ER
Tel: (01443) 412248   Fax: (01443) 412688
Civil War period museum: 1645 invitation to meet the servants of the then Lord of the Manor, Colonel Edward Pritchard.
Access to ground floor only.

SD [♿]   CP [♿]   E [♿]   RF [♿]
C [♿]   S [♿]   WC [♿]   RFE [♿]

MONMOUTHSHIRE

ABERGAVENNY
One of the prettiest gateways to the Brecon Beacons with The Sugar Loaf, Blorenge and Skirrid Fawr mountains providing a dramatic backdrop to the town. This is a market town: Livestock on Tuesdays and crowded Market Hall on Tuesdays and Fridays. Fine parish church, St. Mary's, referred to as the Westminster Abbey of Wales for its amazing collection of beautifully carved tombs. A C19th hunting lodge in the Norman ruins of the castle is now home to the town's museum. Wales's oldest pub, The Skirrid Inn is here.

TOURIST INFORMATION CENTRE
Bus Station, Swan Meadow, Monmouth Road, Abergavenny NP7 5HH
Tel: (01873) 857588   Fax: (01873) 850217

PUBLIC TRANSPORT INFORMATION
Tel: (01495) 355444

BUSES
Stagecoach: Tel: (01633) 266336
Some low-loor buses.

TRAINS
Wales and West: Special Needs:
Tel: (0845) 3003005
Minicom: (0845) 7585469

CAR PARKS
Free three-hour parking in all council car parks and some on-street parking.

SELF-CATERING
LOWER GREEN FARM   [♿]
Llanfair Green, Crosh Ash,
Abergavenny NP7 8PA
Tel/Fax: (01873) 821219
No. of Accessible Units: 1. Shower
No. of Beds per Unit: 6
Accessible Facilities: Open plan Lounge/kitchen/diner.
Swallow Cottage is 1 of 2 converted barns on 170-acre farm, set in tranquil countryside. Guests are welcome to explore the farm and meet the farm animals.

ATTRACTION

ABERGAVENNY CASTLE AND MUSEUM
Castle Street, Abergavenny,
Monmouthshire NP7 5EE
Tel: (01873) 854282   Fax: (01873) 736004
Displays on the town's development and its surroundings. Almost every room in the Museum has steps to or from it and is not suitable for visitors who must remain in

their wheelchairs.

SD ♿   CP 🧍   E ♿   RF ♿
S ♿   WC 🧍   RFE 🧍

CHEPSTOW

Standing on the Monmouthshire/ Gloucestershire border, overlooking the lower reaches of the River Wye before it flows into the Severn. Mid C11th. castle, built after the Norman conquest, stands above a bend in the Wye. The castle is at the centre of many attractions in this walled town. There is a restored gatehouse and charming narrow streets lead to the castle.

TOURIST INFORMATION CENTRE
Castle Car Park, Bridge Street, Chepstow NP6 5EY
Tel: (01291) 623772   Fax: (01291) 628004

SELF-CATERING
BYRE COTTAGE   ♿
Cwrt-y-Gaer, Wolvesnewton, Chepstow NP6 6PR
Tel: (01291) 650700
No. of Accessible Units: 1
No. of Beds per Unit: 2 – 4
Accessible Facilities: Kitchen, Lounge, patio with furniture.
One of 3 stone cottages converted from farm buildings, in lovely location on the site of an ancient Welsh hill-top fort with 20 acres of woods and meadows.

ATTRACTION
CALDICOT CASTLE MUSEUM
Church Road, Caldicot, Nr Chepstow NP6 4HU
Tel: (01291) 420241   Fax: (01291) 420241
Well preserved Norman fortification, fully developed by late C14th and restored as Victorian family home. Set down is directly in front of Museum – route from CP to the entrance is very steep. Located just south of Chepstow at western end of Second Severn Crossing (M4).

SD ♿   CP n/a   E ♿   RF ♿
C ♿   S ♿   WC 🧍

MONMOUTH

Famous for its C13th gateway, on the Monnow Bridge, the only complete monument of its kind in Britain. There are well preserved Tudor and Georgian buildings

around Agincourt Square. High street connects here with narrow shopping lanes and courtyard eating areas. King Henry V was born at the town's castle in 1387, as was Sir Charles Rolls of Rolls-Royce fame.

TOURIST INFORMATION CENTRE
Shire Hall, Agincourt Square,
Monmouth NP5 3DY
Tel: (01600) 713899   Fax: (01600) 772794
Seasonal – winter contact Magor
Tel: (01633) 881122   Fax: (01633) 881985

SELF-CATERING
HARVEST HOME   ♿
The Hill, Bryngwyn, Raglan,
Nr. Monmouth NP5 2JH
Tel/Fax: (01291) 690007/691207
web: www.travel-uk.com
No. of Accessible Units: 1
No. of Beds per Unit: 2-4
Accessible Facilities: Lounge, Kitchen.
Set in lovely countryside with fine mountain and lovely garden views.
Located 7 miles from Monmouth.

TINTERN

"The most romantic valley in Wales" William Wordsworth. Riverside village in lovely stretch of Wye Valley.

HOTEL
THE ROYAL GEORGE HOTEL   🧍
Tintern NP6 6SF
Tel: (01292) 689205   Fax: (01291) 689448
No. of Accessible Rooms: 1
Accessible Facilities: Lounge, Restaurant, Bar. Built in 1598, converted in C17th to a coaching inn and extended and improved over the years into a 16-bedroom hotel. The ruins of Tintern Abbey (inaccessible) are a minute away as are the Forest of Dean and the River Wye. The hotel has an award-winning restaurant overlooking lovely gardens.

USK

At the heart of rural Monmouthshire this pretty town is famous for wonderful floral displays. A past winner of Britain in

Bloom and constant winner of Wales in Bloom. It also offers antique furniture shops, painted cottages and lovely pubs and restaurants. A great place to browse.

SELF-CATERING
THE PHEASANT PENS
Brace Farm, Llandenny, Nr. Usk NP5 1DN
Tel: (01291) 690216
No. of Accessible Units: 1
No. of Beds per Unit: 2-4
Accessible Facilities: Open plan Living room/Kitchen.
1 of 2 cottages converted from farm buildings on working farm. Situated in Usk Valley within easy reach of the Wye Valley.

ATTRACTION
GWENT RURAL LIFE MUSEUM
The Malt Barn, New Market Street, Usk NP5 1AU
Tel: (01291) 673777
The museum portrays life in the Welsh Border country from Victorian times until the end of WWII. All aspects of country life shown and explained with thousands of exhibits donated by local people over the past 30 years. Fascinating experience.

| SD- 🦽 | CP 🦽 | E 🦽 | RF 🦽 |
| S 🚹 | WC n/a | | |

NEATH AND PORT TALBOT

NEATH
Located where the Vale of Neath opens out into an industrial spread. Given a new look, the town is at its best in September at its annual fair, the oldest in Wales. There are ruins of its 1280-1330 abbey and boat trips on the spruced up canal.

BED AND BREAKFAST
CWNBACH COTTAGES 🦽
Cwmbach Road, Cadoxton, Neath SA10 8AH
Tel: (01639) 639825
No. of Accessible Rooms: 1
Accessible Facilities: Lounge, Dining Room. The Primrose Room (accessible) has its own car park and is next to Dining Room. Located on a hillside overlooking Neath and in a woodland area, six old miners' cottages converted. On the doorstep is Craig Gwladys Country Park,

Penscynor Wildlife Park and Aberdulais Falls.

ATTRACTION
ABERDULAIS FALLS (NT)
Aberdulais, Nr. Neath SA10 8EU
Tel: (01639) 636674   Fax: (01629) 645069
For over 300 years the Falls have powered the wheels of industry, grinding corn, refining copper and manufacturing tinplate. The Falls roar down the rock in a rustic landscape, surrounded by thick vegetation. Much loved by C18th and C19th landscape painters, including Turner. Since 1981 it has been cleared by the National Trust.

| SD 🦽 | CP 🦽 | E 🦽 | RF 🦽 | L 🦽 |
| C 🦽 | S 🦽 | WC 🚹 | RFE 🦽 | |

PORT TALBOT
One of the largest of Welsh towns, where the growing iron and copper industries flourished in the mid C19th. The port was extended in 1972 to allow for a deep-water harbour. The town is squeezed between the shore and rising hills, stretching for miles. This, with the chemical works to the west, complete a mainly industrial landscape.

PUBLIC TRANSPORT INFORMATION: Tel: (01792) 222718

TRAINS
First Great Western: Special Needs:
Tel: (0845) 7413775
Wales & West: Special Needs:
Tel: (0845) 3003005
Minicom: (0845) 7585469

SHOPMOBILITY
Unit 43, Aberavon Shopping Centre, Port Talbot
Tel: (01639) 894949   Fax: (01639) 646947

HOTEL
ABERAVON BEACH HOTEL 🦽
Port Talbot SA12 6QP
Tel: (01639) 884949   Fax: (01639) 897885
web: www.consorthotels.com/c161
No. of Accessible Rooms: 1
Accessible Facilities: Lounge, Restaurant,

Pool, Sauna, Spa. Modern hotel opposite wide sandy beach with fine views across Swansea Bay. All weather leisure centre

NEWPORT

Medieval cathedral and castle compete with Victorian architecture here: Roman walls and amphitheatre with modern developments. The most famous landmark, the Transporter Bridge, has been restored to working order.

TOURIST INFORMATION CENTRE
Museum and Art Gallery, John Frost Square, Newport NP9 1HZ
Tel: (01633) 842962   Fax: (01633) 222615

HOTELS
STAKIS NEWPORT
Chepstow Road, Langstone, Newport NP6 2LX
Tel: (01633) 413737   Fax: (01633) 413713
e-mail: reservations@stakis.co.uk
web: www.stakis.co.uk
No. of Accessible Rooms: 4
Accessible Facilities: Bar, Restaurant, Courtyard Garden.
Quality hotel located close to M4 (J24).

BEST WESTERN PARKWAY HOTEL AND CONFERENCE CENTRE
Cwmbran Drive, Cwmbran, Newport NP44 3UW
Tel: (01633) 871199   Fax: (01633) 869160
No. of Accessible Rooms: 3
Accessible Facilities: Lounge, Restaurant. Privately owned quality hotel, developed on a Mediterranean theme all 70 bedrooms enjoying Welsh countryside views. Located at M4 West (J25A), M4E (J26), between Newport and Cwmbran.

ATTRACTION
CAERLEON FORTRESS BATHS
High Street, Caerleon, Nr. Newport
Tel: (01633) 422578
An important Roman military base, Caerleon's Fortress Baths were excavated in the 1970s and show the most complete example of Roman Legionary bath building in Britain.

SD   CP   E ♿   RF ♿
C n/a   S ♿   WC n/a

PEMBROKESHIRE

PHYSICALLY IMPAIRED PEOPLE OF PEMBROKESHIRE ASSOCIATION
The Coach House, Bridgend Square
Haverfordwest SA61 2NO
Tel/Fax: (01437) 760999
Information and Advice plus Wheelchair Hire Scheme and RADAR toilet keys.

PEMBROKESHIRE/SNOWDONIA/ BRECON BEACONS TOURISM
19 Old Bridge, Haverfordwest SA61 2EZ
Tel: (01437) 760980
Fax: (01437) 764382
e-mail: tourism@pembrokeshire.gov.uk
web: pembrokshire.gor.ur

BONCATH
Small village in foothills of Preseli Mountains on edge of Pembrokeshire Coast National Park. Good centre for exploring southern Cardigan Bay and Teifi Valley.

SELF-CATERING
THE MEWS
Book through Holidays for You & Me.
Clynfyw, Abercych, Boncath
Tel/Fax: (01239) 841236
No. of Accessible Units: 1. Bath, Shower
No. of Beds per Unit: 6 + cot.
Accessible Facilities: Lounge, Dining Room, Kitchen, Fishing school with accessible pool 5 minutes drive, Accessible woodland trail now in planning stage. Conversion of part of original stable block of large country mansion within rural setting.

HAVERFORDWEST
Dominated by the ruins of its Norman Castle which was rebuilt during Georgian times, with little still standing. The coming of the railway destroyed much of its sea trade and in 1920 the last steamer sailed down the western Cleddar River. The town's maritime past is still evident in some old warehouses. Close by is the spacious sandy beach of Broad Haven.

PEMBROKESHIRE COAST NATIONAL PARK VISIT CENTRE
40 High Street, Haverfordwest
Tel: (01437) 760136

TOURIST INFORMATION CENTRE
19 Old Bridge Street, Haverfordwest
Tel: (01437) 763110   Fax: (01437) 767738

SELF-CATERING
KEESTON HILL COTTAGE
Keeston Kitchen, Keeston,
Haverfordwest SA62 6EJ
Tel: (01437) 710440   Fax: (01437) 710840
No. of Accessible Units: 1. Bath.
No. of Beds per Unit: 1d.1s.
Accessible Facilities: Living Room with galley-style Kitchen. Ground floor apartment in lovely converted cottage set in own large garden, set back from main Haverfordwest/St. David's road in quiet layby. 4 miles from Haverfordwest. Next door to family-run restaurant.

MILLMOOR FARM COTTAGES AND ROCKSDRIFT APARTMENTS 🦽
Broad Haven, Haverfordwest SA62 3JH
Tel: (01437) 781507   Fax: (01437) 781002
No. of Accessible Units: Millmoor – 2: Rocksdrift – 5
No. of Beds per Unit:
Millmoor – Granary, Stable, Milking Parlour, Calves Cot – each sleeps 6 + cot
Rocksdrift – 4 and 8 persons
Accessible Facilities: Lounge/Diner, Kitchen, Gardens
Located in heart of Pembrokeshire Coast National Park. Award winning property. Millmoor is group of typical stone cottages, 200m from the beach. The beach-side apartments at Rocksdrift are converted from C19th coach house and also have sea views.

ROSEMOOR HOUSE 🦽
Walwyn's Castle, Haverfordwest SA62 3ED
Tel: (01437) 781326   Fax: (01437) 781080
No. of Accessible Units: 1
No. of Beds per Unit: 2 - 10
Accessible Facilities: Lounge, Kitchen/Diner, Lawns facing west.
Ground floor of main house, owners living above: within grounds are other cottages

and all are surrounded by open country, trees and fields.

DREENHILL FARM 🚶
Dale Road, Haverfordwest SA62 3XG
Tel/Fax: (01437) 764494
No. of Accessible Units: 1
No. of Beds per Unit: 2. Shower.
Accessible Facilities: Living/Dining Room, Kitchen, Patio.
"Fledracks" is 1 of 2 self-contained properties attached to, and separated by, the main farmhouse. Situated in large gardens with fields and private nature trail. 120m from road. 2.5m from Haverfordwest.

ATTRACTION
SCOLTON MANOR MUSEUM VISITOR CENTRE
Spittal, Haverfordwest SA62 5QL
Tel: (01437) 731328   Fax: (01437) 731743
Exhibits in Victorian mansion and stables on history and natural history of the region and environmentally friendly visitor centre and 60 acres of grounds.

| SD ♿ | CP ♿ | E ♿ | RF ♿ |
| C ♿ | S 🚶 | WC ♿ | |

NARBETH
Small market town, convenient for beaches of Carmarthen Bay and resorts of Tenby and Saundersfoot. Many attractions nearby.

ATTRACTION
OAKWOOD PARK
Canaston Bridge, Narbeth SA67 8DE
Tel: (01834) 891373   Fax: (01834) 891380
e-mail: oakwoodltd@aol.com
web: www.oakwood-leisure.com
Theme park with numerous activities and rides, both undercover and outdoor. Includes Europe's largest wooden roller-coaster, pirate ship, boating lake, waterfall and bobsleigh rides amongst others.

SD ♿	CP ♿	E ♿	RF ♿
C- Restaurant 🚶	Acorn Tearoom ♿		
S ♿	WC ♿	RFE ♿	

PEMBROKE
A Norman town, still retaining an ancient street pattern and long burbage plots which run down to the last vestiges of the

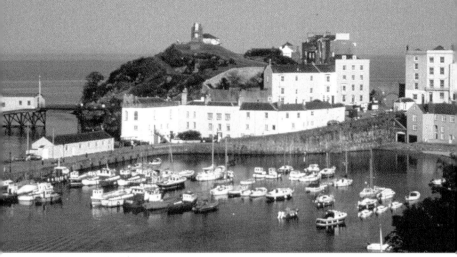

Picturesque Tenby harbour.

medieval walls. There is an imposing Norman castle, founded in 1090, one of the best-preserved in Britain. Pembroke was a Naval Dockyard until 1924.

TOURIST VISITOR CENTRE
Commons Road, Pembroke SA71 4EA
Tel: (01646) 622388 Fax: (01646) 621396
Seasonal, in winter contact Tenby.

BED AND BREAKFAST
ROSEDENE GUEST HOUSE
Hodgeston, Pembroke SA71 5JU
Tel: (01646) 672586 & (07775) 592407
No. of Accessible Rooms: 1
Accessible Facilities: Lounge, Dining Room, Garden, accessible by ramp. Charming property in peaceful village with private patio. Located midway between Tenby and Pembroke.

ST. DAVIDS
Tiny city, dominated by a fine cathedral on whose site as early as C6th a religious order was founded, the oldest cathedral settlement in Britain. The present building waqs completed in 1176. The city has many attractions relating to its coastal position, for, although a wild and remote spot, it is busy with more facilities than one would expect, the hub of activity is centred around the C14th market cross.

ATTRACTION
BISHOPS PALACE
St. Davids SA62 6PE
Tel: (01437) 720517
Sheltering in a grassy hollow this outstanding religious site, even in ruins conveys the affluence and power of the medieval church. This great palace in unequalled elsewhere in Wales. The Great Hall built, in early C14th, shows worldly life reflected in extravagance of architecture and lavish stone carvings. Ground floor at grass courtyard level, including 2 exhibition rooms, is accessible, the first floor is not.

SD | CP | E | RF
S | WC

ST. DAVID'S CATHEDRAL
The Close, St. Davids SA62 6PE
Tel: (01437) 720202 Fax: (01437) 721885
Varied architecture, built in the C12th and altered several times, including C20th extension. Fine ceilings and stone vaulting.

SD | CP | E | RF
S | WC

STACKPOLE (NT)
The old Home Farm, Stackpole SA71 5DQ
Tel: (01646) 661359 Fax: (01646) 661639
Stackpole Estate is set in an area of outstanding natural beauty and much of it is is designated as a Site of Special Scientific Interest. There are beaches, cliffs, limestone

grassland and dunes, lakes and woods. Wheelchair-accessible lakeside and woodland footpath and bird watching hide at the boat house, are shown clearly on the comprehensive map for visitors with disabilities. Strong companion pusher needed.

SD 🚹 CP 🚹 E 🚹 RF 🚹
C 🚹 S N/A WC 🚹

TENBY

Very popular holiday resort with pastel Georgian houses running down to lovely harbour and 3 great beaches. Medieval town walls are almost intact enfolding a maze of tiny streets and alleyways. Originally a fishing port, now offering much to see and many interesting excursions in the area.

TOURIST INFORMATION CENTRE
The Croft, Tenby SA70 8AP
Tel: (01834) 842402 Fax: (01834) 845439

HOTEL
GREENHILLS COUNTRY HOUSE HOTEL 🚹
St. Florence, Tenby SA70 8NB
Tel: (01834) 871291 Fax: (01834) 871948
No. of Accessible Rooms: 4
Accessible Facilities: Lounge, Restaurant, Pool, Sauna.
Lovely country house hotel in own grounds within floral award winning village. 3 miles from Tenby.

St. David's Cathedral.

ATLANTIC HOTEL 🚹
The Esplanade, Tenby SA70 7DU
Tel/Fax: (01834) 842881
web: smoothhound.co.uk/hotels/atlant1.html
No. of Accessible Rooms: 1
Accessible Facilities: Lounge, Restaurant.
Charming family-owned property fronted by lovely natural gardens with cliff top terraces and fine sea views.

SELF CATERING
HOMELEIGH COUNTRY COTTAGES 🚹
Red Roses, Whitland, Nr Tenby SA34 0PN
Tel: (01834) 831765
e-mail: homeleigh@talk21.com
web: www.ukworld.net/homeleigh
No. of Accessible units 3. Bath.
No of Beds per unit 6-8.
Accessible facilities – open plan.
Attractive cottages in peaceful Pembroke countryside in small village on A477, midway between St. Clears and Tenby.

ATTRACTION
MANOR HOUSE WILDLIFE PARK
St. Florence, Tenby SA70 8RJ
Tel/Fax: (01646) 651201
Central feature here is the Manor House itself, built in 1750s and now housing the Natural History Museum and the refreshment area. Wide collection of animals, birds, fish and reptiles, with bird of prey displays and snake handling. Go-karts, astroglide and remote boats and cars for children. Fine floral gardens.

SD 🚹 CP 🚶 E 🚹 RF 🚹
C 🚹 S 🚹 WC 🚶 RFE 🚹

387

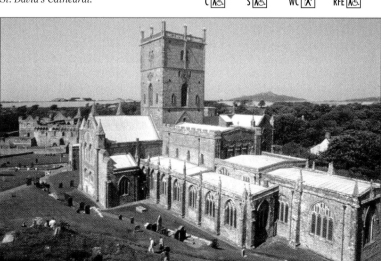

POWYS

ABECRAF
Located in the Upper Swansea Valley, on southern edge of Brecon Beacons National Park.

HOTEL
MAES-Y-GWERNEN HOTEL ♿
School Road, Abercraf,
Swansea Valley SA9 1XD
Tel: (01639) 730218   Fax: (01639) 730765
e-mail: maesyg@globalnet.co.uk
No. of accessible Rooms: 1
Accessible Facilities: Lounge, Restaurant, Sauna, Whirlpool, Bar, Conservatory, Gardens. Country hotel in private grounds, on the southern edge of the National Park, convenient for mountains and Gower coast.

ATTRACTION
CRAIG-Y-NOS COUNTRY PARK
Pen-y-cae, Nr. Abercraf,
Swansea Valley SA9 1GL
Tel/Fax: (01639) 730395
40 acres of countryside to enjoy in this lovely part of the upper Tawe valley. Access to Visitor Centre with displays and activity areas explaining what can be found, and accessible Welcome Point and map near parking area. Wheelchair available free of charge. Located north of Abercraf on A 4067.

SD ♿   CP ♿   E ♿   RF ♿
S ⚤   WC ⚤

BRECON
Fascinating medieval street plan still remains here, although many of the older houses are rebuilt or were given fashionable Georgian facades in the C18th and C19ths. Remains an important agricultural centre and good base for exploring the Brecon Beacons National Park.

TOURIST INFORMATION CENTRE
Cattle Market Car Park, Brecon LD3 9DA
Tel: (01874) 622485   Fax: (01874) 625256

BUSES
First Cymru: Tel: (01792) 580580
Some low-floor buses.

TAXIS
Wye Valley Taxis: Tel: (01982) 553142
1 adapted vehicle.

TRAINS
Valley Lines: Special Needs:
Tel: (029) 20 449944

CAR PARKS
Free unlimited parking in council car parks.
Tel: (01597) 826529

HOTEL
THE CASTLE OF BRECON ♿
The Castle Square, Brecon LD3 9DB
Tel: (01874) 624611   Fax: (01874) 623777
e-mail: hotel@castbrec.demon.co.uk
web: www.castbrec.demon.co.uk
No. of Accessible Rooms:
Accessible Facilities: Lounge, Restaurant
A listed building, originally a coaching inn in late C18th and one of the first hotels in Wales in early C19th. Occupying site and remains of Brecon Castle, it stands on a bluff of lands between two rivers, commanding fine views along valley of the River Usk, but 200m only from centre of town. Privately owned and managed.

BISHOPS MEADOW HOTEL ♿
Hay Road, Brecon LD3 9SW
Tel: (01874) 622051   Fax: (01874) 622428
No. of Accessible Rooms:12
Accessible Facilities: Restaurant.
Family-owned motel surrounded by lovely countryside with views of the Brecon Beacons.

ATTRACTION
BRECKNOCK MUSEUM
Captain's Walk, Brecon LD3 7DW
Tel: (01874) 624121   Fax: (01874) 611281
Exploration of area history with archaeological and historical artefacts, folklore and decorative arts.

SD ♿   CP ♿   E ♿ AT REAR
L ♿   S ⚤   WC ♿   RFE ⚤

BRECON BEACONS NATIONAL PARK AUTHORITY
7 Glamorgan Street, Brecon LD3 7DP
Tel: (01874) 624437   Fax: (01874) 622574
e-mail: Compuserve 100070,1353
The highest mountains in southern

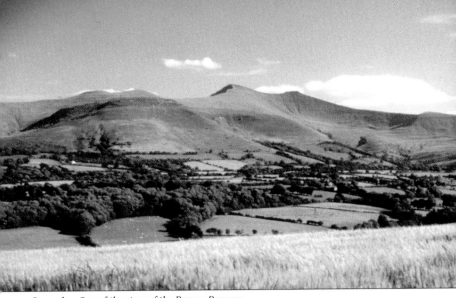

Pen-y-fan. One of the stars of the Brecon Beacons.

Britain, together with 500 square miles of the surrounding countryside, became a National Park in 1957. This is a landscape dominated by wildness, natural variety and farming tradition. It is a landscape of contrasts with open moorland and hidden waterfalls, windswept mountains and sheltered valleys, bustling market towns and isolated farmsteads. Welsh cultural traditions are very strong and the agricultural landscape is rich in wildlife habitats with a great variety of plants and animals. A strong sense of history pervades in the legacy of ancient monuments and buildings telling the story of the people who have lived and worked here during the past five thousand years.

NATIONAL PARK VISITOR CENTRE (MOUNTAIN CENTRE)
Libanus, Nr. Brecon LD3 8ER
Tel: (01874) 623366 Fax: (01874) 624515
The Mountain Centre, 5.5 miles south-west of Brecon is run so that visitors can enjoy the spectacular scenery, discover what to see and do in the area, learn about local features of interest and find out about the role of a National Park.

SD 🚹 CP 🚹 E 🚹 RF 🚹
C 🚹 S 🚹 WC 🚹

BUILTH WELLS
Small castle town on the banks of the Wye. Best known as home of the Royal Welsh Show, the country's largest agricultural event. There is no evidence of the spa which flourished in the C19th.

TOURIST INFORMATION CENTRE
The Groe Car Park. Builth Wells LD2 3BT
Tel: (01982) 553307
Seasonal, in winter contact Llandrindod Wells.

HOTELS
CAER BERIS MANOR HOTEL
Builth Wells LD2 3NP
Tel: (01982) 552601 Fax: (01982) 552586
No. of Accessible Rooms: 2. Roll-in Shower
Accessible Facilities: Lounge, Restaurant, Bar. Country house hotel situated in 27 acres of beautiful woodland on River Irfon.

PENCERRIG GARDENS HOTEL
Llandrindod Road, Builth Wells LD2 3TF
Tel: (01982)553266 Fax: (01982) 552347
No. of Accessible Rooms: 5
Accessible Facilities: Lounge, Restaurant. Reputedly of C15th origin, the property has grown from farmhouse to country house with many original, unique features retained. Large established gardens overlooking rolling hills of mid Wales.

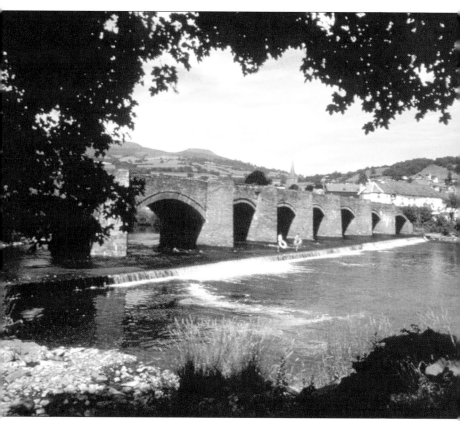

The age and style of bridges is a unique feature throughout Wales.

CRICKHOWELL

"The most cheerful-looking town I ever saw". Richard Fenton, 1804. Small and urban, little has changed since then with fine Crickhowell Bridge along the Usk and a square with The Bear, a Georgian inn.

TOURIST INFORMATION CENTRE
Beaufort Chambers, Beaufort Street,
Crickhowell NP8 1AA
Tel: (01873) 812105
Seasonal, in winter contact Brecon.

HOTEL
THE OLD RECTORY HOTEL 🚶
Llangattock, Crickhowell NP8 1PH
Tel/Fax: (01873 810373
No. of Accessible Rooms: 2
Accessible Facilities: Lounge, Restaurant,
Family owned and run 17th century building situated in a small hamlet. Set in 12 acres of grounds with 9-hole private golf course.

KNIGHTON

The town began as a Saxon settlement and is as old as Offa's Dyke, standing midway along its 172 miles of National Trail from Prestatyn to Chepstow. Now a market centre for the Tene Valley.

TOURIST INFORMATION CENTRE
Offas Dyke Centre, West Street,
Knighton LD7 1EW
Tel: (01547) 529424 Fax: (01547) 529427
e-mail: oda@offa.demon.co.uk

HOTEL
KNIGHTON HOTEL 🚶
Broad Street, Knighton LD7 1BL
Tel: (01547) 520530 Fax: (01547) 520529
No. of Accessible Rooms: 15
Accessible Facilities: Lounge, Restaurant.

LLANDRIDNOD WELLS

Elegant Victorian spa town where you can still take the waters at the Pump Room in Rock Park. It plays on its Victorian heyday with an annual Victorian Festival in August. A good touring centre for central Wales.

TOURIST INFORMATION CENTRE
Old Town Hall, Memorial Gardens,
Llandrindod Wells LD1 5DL
Tel: (01597) 822600

BUSES
Cross Gates: Tel: (01597) 851226
Some low-floor buses.

TAXIS
Adey's Taxis: Tel: (01597) 822118
1 adapted vehicle.
Martini Taxis: Tel: (01597) 823690
1 adapted vehicle.
Wye Valley Taxis: Tel: (01982) 553142
1 adapted vehicle.

TRAINS
Wales and West: Special Needs:
Tel: (0845) 3003005
Minicom: (0845) 7585469

Llandrindod Wells Station is accessible to wheelchairs by ramp access.

CAR PARKS
Free unlimited orange badge parking in council car parks.
Tel: (01597) 826529

HOTEL
THE BELL INN
Llanyre, Llandrindod Wells LD1 6DY
Tel: (01597) 823959   Fax: (012597) 825899
No. of Accessible Rooms: 1
Accessible Facilities: Lounge, Restaurant, During C17th and C18th, the hostelry provided stabling and nourishment for drovers, the original building being replaced by current stone building of 1890s. Now a charming country inn.

CORVEN HALL
Howey, Llandrindod Wells LD1 5RE
Tel: (01597) 823368
No. of Accessible Rooms: 1

Accessible Facilities: Lounge, Restaurant, Bar, Garden. Victorian country house in large grounds and peaceful setting.

ATTRACTION
GILFACH FARM NATURE RESERVE
St. Harmon, Rhayader,
Nr. Llandrindod Wells LD6 5LF
Tel: (01597) 870301   Fax: (01597) 823274
e-mail: radnorshirewt@cix.co.uk
Restored Welsh longhouse at the centre of a 418-acre nature reserve. Upland River, oak woodland meadows and upland moorland. Live film of wildlife from the reserve and history of Gilfach.

| SD ♿ | CP ♿ | E ♿ | RF ♿ |
| C ♿ | S ♿ | WC 🚶 | |

LLANFAIR CAEREINION

Tiny country town in which development has meant that the urban section of the railway, creeping past backyards and across roads, can never be linked to the main line.

ATTRACTION
WELSHPOOL and LLANFAIR LIGHT RAILWAY
The Station, Llanfair Caereinion SY21 0SF
Tel: (01938) 810441   Fax: (01938) 810861
8-mile trip through lovely scenery on narrow-gauge steam train. Many carriages and coaches from around the world on view. Two locations for boarding.

| SD ♿ | CP ♿ | E ♿ | RF ♿ |
| C ♿ | S ♿ | WC 🚶 | |

RFE ♿ Platform access via ramp

LLANGAMMARCH WELLS

Sleepy little town 185m. above sea level, renowned for fine trout fishing on River Irfon. Once a spa with water believed to cure gout and heart disease. Close to Epynt mountain.

HOTEL
THE LAKE COUNTRY HOUSE
Llangammarch Wells LD4 4BS
Tel: (01591) 620202   Fax: (01591) 620457
No. of Accessible Rooms: 2
Accessible Facilities: Lounge, Restaurant. Welsh country house furnished with antiques and set in 50 acres with sweeping

lawns, a par-3 golf course, croquet lawn, putting green, clay pigeon shooting, archery and tennis. Fishing close by.

MACHYNLLETH

Capital of the lower Dowey valley and surrounded by parkland rising into the hills of mid Wales. Busy and popular in summer. In 1404 Owain Glyn Dwr was crowned Prince of Wales here and held a parliament, though not in what is now called Parliament House, a good example of a late medieval town house.

TOURIST INFORMATION CENTRE
Canolfan Owain Glyndwr,
Machynlleth SY20 8EE
Tel: (01654) 702401   Fax: (01654) 703675

BED AND BREAKFAST
CWMDYLLUAN
Forge, Machynlleth SY20 8RZ
Tel: (01654) 702684   Fax: (01654) 700133
e-mail: dylluan@clara.co.uk
No. of Accessible Rooms: 3, Bath
Accessible Facilities: Lounge, Dining room
House built on elevated site in 1983,
standing in an acre of land in quiet country
location bordered by River Dulas. Forge is
a small village a mile from Machynlleth
along a quiet mountain road.

ATTRACTION
CELTICA
Y Plas, Aberystwyth Road,
Machynlleth SY20 8ER
Tel: (01654) 702702   Fax: (01654) 703604
e-mail: bryn@celtica.wales.com
Unique attraction relaying history of the
Celts, housed in restored mansion which
was once the country home of the Marquis
of Londonderry. The sights and sounds of
Wales' Celtic past are brought alive
through audio-visual technology as you
discover the Celtic settlement and the
Roundhouse where the characters tell
their own stories. An interpretative centre
with artefacts, photographs and books
gives insight into the Celtic way of life.

SD | CP | E | RF | L
C | S | WC | RFE

CENTRE FOR ALTERNATIVE TECHNOLOGY
Machynlleth SY20 9AZ
Tel: (01654) 702400   Fax: (01654) 702782
e-mail: cat@gn.apc.org
Web: www.foe.co.uk/CAT
Wales Tourism Award Winner. Seven acres
of environmental solutions to inspire,
inform and entertain. Tranquil organic
garden: transport maze: wind, water and
solar power displays: animals on smallholding: discover how to save energy –
and money!

SD | CP | E | RF
C | S | WC

YNYS-HIR RSPB RESERVE
Cae'r Berllan, Eglwysfach, Machynlleth
Tel: (01654) 781265   Fax: (01654) 781328
Although much of the reserve is
unsuitable for wheelchair access due to
the terrain, there is ramp overlooking the
estuary where visitors may drive down and
park, with good views of many of the
estuary birds, especially at high tide.
Please contact in advance for this facility.

SD | CP | E

NEWTOWN

Once the centre of Welsh flannel and
textiles industry and now the most
populous town in Powys with the best
shopping. The flourishing Tuesday market
has been active since 1279.

TOURIST INFORMATION CENTRE
The Park, Back Lane, Newtown SY16 2PW
Tel: (01686) 625580   Fax: (01686) 610065

PUBLIC TRANSPORT INFORMATION
Tel: (01597) 826678

BUSES
Arriva Cymru: Tel: (01492) 596969
No low-floor as yet.

TRAINS
Virgin Trains: Special Needs:
Tel: (0845) 7443366
Minicom: (0845) 7443367

CAR PARKS
Free unlimited Orange badge parking in

all council car parks
Tel: (01597) 826529

| SD ♿ | E ♿ | RF ♿ | L ♿ |
| S ♿ | WC 🚹 | | |

BED AND BREAKFAST
PEN-Y-GELLI 🚶
Wern Ddu Lane, Newton SY16 3AH
Tel/Fax: (016686) 628292
No. of Accessible Rooms: 2
Accessible Facilities: Lounge, Dining
Room, Evening meals are available,
Indoor Pool (accessible for visitors able to
walk a few steps). This guest house
overlooks open fields.

PRESTEIGNE
Located right on Herefordshire border and
seems rather English in character,
although it was the county town of
Radnorshire from the C16th-C19th. A
prosperous market town, it declined after
1899, but evidence of its importance is
shown in the large parish church, some
fine inns and the Venetian Gothic Market
Hall built in 1865. The streets are
Georgian in character with older
structures, possibly C17th.

TOURIST INFORMATION CENTRE
Shire Hall, Broad Street, Presteigne LD8 2AD
Tel: (01544) 260650   Fax: (01544) 260652

ATTRACTION
THE JUDGE'S LODGING
(as TIC above.)
The Old Shire Hall, now known as the
Judge's Lodging, is an elegant Victorian
building. Contrasting with the upstairs
grandeur of the judge's well furnished
lodging rooms and vast courtroom, were
the downstairs services or servants' hall,
kitchen and cells for prisoners awaiting
trial upstairs. After much research, repair
and restoration, the Shire Hall now
captures the Victorian heyday of a most
unusual household, by gaslight, lamp and
candle, for visitors to savour. Visitors are
accompanied by an audio-tour of voices
from the past as room by room, you hear
the inside story. A delightful and unique
museum. Entrance via a lift at the rear of
the building. Wheelchair lift takes 1 chair
and occupant and 1 other standing person.

WELSHPOOL
Attractive town with numerous half-
timbered buildings typical of upper
Severn Valley. The most unusual is the
hexagonal cockpit used until cockfighting
was outlawed in 1849. Nearby is Powis
Castle, built in C12th, and added to ever
since, plus lovely Glansevern Hall.

TOURIST INFORMATION CENTRE
Vicarage Garden, Church Street,
Welshpool SY21 7DD
Tel: (01938) 552043   Fax: (01938) 554038

SELF-CATERING
MADOG'S WELLS ♿
Llanfair Caereinion, Welshpool ST21 0DE
Tel/Fax: (01938) 810446
No. of Accessible Units: 1
No. of Beds per Unit: 5
Accessible Facilities: Lounge/Dining
Room, Kitchen, Games Room.
Small hill farm in quiet secluded valley.
Accessible bungalow adjacent to beamed
farmhouse in secluded valley. Watch the
birds from your breakfast table.

ATTRACTION
GLANSEVERN HALL GARDENS
Glansevern, Berriew, Welshpool SY21 8AH
Tel: (01686) 640200   Fax: (01686) 640829
18 acres, set in wider parkland and on
mostly level ground, and retaining warm
and intimate ambience of family garden.
Large number of unusual species of trees,
4 acre lake, profusely water, rock and rose
gardens and herbaceous borders and beds.

| SD ♿ | CP ♿ | E ♿ | RF 🚶 |
| C ♿ | S ♿ | WC 🚹 | |

RFE Garden – powered wheelchairs move more easily
over grass.

RHONDDA CYNON TAFF

PONTYPRIDD
Market town of substance on south outlet
of the Rhondda into the Taff Vale. The

393

river here is crossed by an elegant C18th bridge, and two fine chapels stand at the Bridgehead.

TOURIST INFORMATION CENTRE
Historical Centre, The Old Bridge,
Pontypridd CF37 3PE
Tel: (01443) 409512 Fax: (01443) 485565

HOTEL
HERITAGE PARK HOTEL
Coed Cae Road, Trehafod,
Nr. Pontypridd CF37 2NP
Tel: (01443) 687057 Fax: (01443) 687060
No. of Accessible Rooms: 1. Bath
Accessible Facilities: Restaurant, Lounge Bar.
Intimate and smallish hotel with large rooms
and attractive dining room situated in
Rhondda Valley just west of Pontypridd and
adjacent to the Heritage Park centre and
museum, 20 miles from Cardiff.

ATTRACTION
RHONDDA HERITAGE PARK
Lewis Merthyr Colliery, Coed Cae Road,
Trehafod, Nr. Pontypridd CF37 7NP
Tel: (01443) 682036 Fax: (01443) 687420)
e-mail: rhonpark@netwales.co.uk

It is hard now to imagine the impact coal had on Wales. This living history museum tells the story of coal mining in the valleys through visual and aural narrative in two winding houses and a ride down a shaft to the pit bottom guided by an ex-miner. There is a visitor centre with shop, indoor street reconstruction and art gallery and coffee shop on the first floor accessible by lift. Only area inaccessible is the final part of the mine tour, a simulated ride back to the surface. An excellent visit.

SD ♿   CP ♿   E ♿   RF ♿   L ♿
C ♿   S ♿   WC ♿   RFE ♿

SWANSEA

GOWER

The Gower Peninsular is 19 miles long, dipping into the Bristol Channel, with wonderful beaches and Britain's first designated "Area of Outstanding Natural Beauty" in 1957. The dramatic cliffs, sweeping marshlands and ancient farmland

Swansea Marina has all you would expect from a modern development.

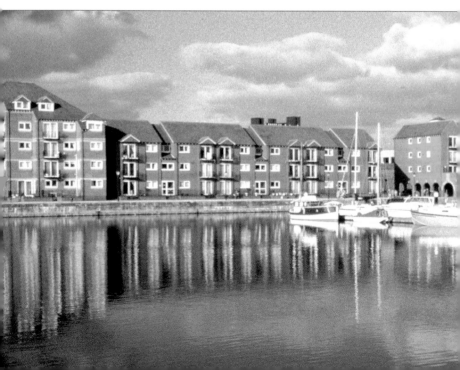

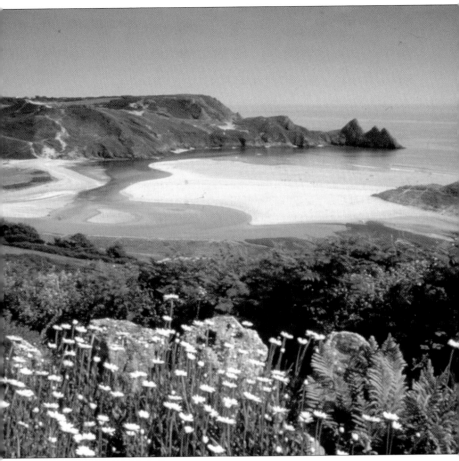

Stunning Three Cliffs Bay on the Gower Peninsular.

and commons, combine with glorious bays, Rhossili Bay, being notably spectacular.

ATTRACTION
GOWER HERITAGE CENTRE
Parkmill, Gower, Swansea SA3 2EM
Tel: (01792) 371206 Fax: (01792) 371471
e-mail: gower_heritage_centre@
compuserve.com

Located 8 miles from Swansea, the centre is based around a water-powered corn and saw mill complex with craft workshops. Farming museum, fishpond and animal farm, puppet theatre and picnic and adventure play areas. The mill was built around 1160AD by the Norman rulers of Gower, grinding corn to provide flour and foods for nearby Pennard Castle estate. It is a Grade II ancient monument and one of very few complete and working mills in Wales.

SD ♿	CP ♿	E ♿	RF ♿
C ♿	S ♿	WC ♿	

SWANSEA

Dramatically set in the crescent moon of Swansea Bay, Wales second largest city is modern and cosmopolitan, but with a splendid coastline, rural landscape and mountains. Fine shopping in The Quadrant and covered market. The bay is a fine natural harbour with busy docks and shipping lanes. An award-winning yachting marina has been created in the former south dock and there is a constant buzz of cafes, restaurants and pubs in the Maritime

Quarters. Much to see and do here.

TOURIST INFORMATION CENTRE
Rear of Grand Theatre, Westway,
Swansea SA1 3QG
Tel: (01792) 468321   Fax: (01792) 464602
Web: www.swansea.gov.uk
PUBLIC TRANSPORT INFORMATION
Tel: (01792) 636466

BUSES
First Cymru: Tel: (01792) 580580
Stagecoach: Tel: (01633) 266336

TAXIS
Data Cabs: Tel: (01792) 474747/545454
50 Adapted vehicles.
Yellow Cabs: Tel: (01792) 700400
1 adapted minibus.

TRAINS
First Great Western: Special Needs:
Tel: (0845) 7413775
Virgin Trains: Special Needs:
Tel: (0845) 7443366
Minicom: (0845) 7443367
Wales and West: Special Needs:
Tel: (0845) 3003005
Minicom: (0845) 7585469

CAR PARKS
Reduced charge for orange badge parking.
Tel: (01792) 636739

SHOPMOBILITY
12 St. David's Square, Swansea SA1 3LG
Tel: (01792) 461785   Fax: (01792) 636728

HOTELS
SWANSEA MARRIOTT
Maritime Quarter, Swansea SA1 3SS
Tel: (01792) 642020   Fax: (01792) 650345
No. of Accessible Rooms:1
Accessible Facilities: Lounge, Restaurant
Located on beach front, 5 minutes from
the town centre.

THE LAKESIDE (Hilton Associate)
Phoenix Way, Enterprise Park, Llansamlet,
Swansea SA7 9EG
Tel: (01792) 310330   Fax: (01792) 797535
No. of Accessible Rooms: 4

Accessible Facilities: Lounge, Restaurant,
Pool, Sauna.

ATTRACTIONS
SWANSEA MARITIME and INDUSTRIAL MUSEUM
Museum Square, Maritime Quarter,
Swansea SA1 1SN
Tel: (01782) 650351   Fax: (01782) 654200
e-mail:
swansea.maritime.museum@business.ntl.com
Selection of floating boats and displays
relating to the history of the Port of
Swansea, plus complete working woollen
mill. Also programme of temporary
exhibitions.

| SD | ♿ | | CP | ♿ | | E | ♿ | | RF | ♿ |
| C | 🚶 | | S | 🚶 | | WC | 🚶 | | | |

TORFAEN
BLAENAFON
A rather bleak village. 300m up on the
eastern rim of South Wales coalfield are 2
important sites which summarise much
of the regions' industrial history –
Blaenafon Ironworks and the Big Pit.

TOURIST INFORMATION CENTRE
Blaenafon Ironworks, North Street, Blaenafon
NP4
Tel: (01495) 792615
Seasonal, in winter contact Abergavenny.

ATTRACTION
BIG PIT MINING MUSEUM
Blaenafon NP4 9XP
Tel: (01495) 790311   Fax: (01495) 792618
e-mail: pwllmawr@aol.com
Closed as a working mine in 1980, but
visitors can don safety helmets and lamps
and go down the 300ft shaft to discover
what life was like. Pithead exhibition and
reconstructed miner's cottage also displayed.

SD	♿		CP	🚶		E	♿		RF	🚶
L	♿		C	♿		S	🚶		WC	🚶
RFE-	♿		Underground Tour							

CWMBRAN
Sixth largest town in Wales and the only
example of the comprehensively planned

new towns initiated after WWII. Designated a new town in 1949, it is unexciting architecturally with sweeping roads, housing neighbourhoods, industrial estates and pedestrianised shopping areas.

WYE VALLEY AND VALE OF USK TOURISM
Floor 6, County Hall, Cwmbran NP44 2XH
Tel: (01633) 644847   Fax: (01633) 644800
e-mail: mcc_tourism_@compuserve.com

ATTRACTION
GREENMEADOW COMMUNITY FARM
Greenforge Way, Cwmbran NP44 5AJ
Tel: (01633) 862202   Fax: (01633) 489332
Major farm attraction with milking demonstrations, tractor rides, farm and nature trails and adventure play area.

SD 🚹   CP 🚹   E 🚹   C 🚹
S 🚹   WC 🚹   RFE 🚹

PONTYPOOL
Easternmost of the Valleys towns, rather hilly. Considerable Italian influence from emigrants coming to South Wales in C19th.

ATTRACTION
VALLEY INHERITANCE MUSEUM AND COURTYARD ARTS
Park Buildings, Pontypool NP4 6JH
Tel: (01495) 752036   Fax: (01495) 752043
Housed in the Georgian stable block of the Hanbury mansion. Explore effects of man's relationship with the land and look at land formation from the primeval landscape to the hey-day of the coal industry.

SD 🚹   CP 🚹   E 🚹   C 🚹
S 🚹   WC 🚹

VALE OF GLAMORGAN

COWBRIDGE
Notable for good shopping, particularly fashion boutiques and a Tuesday cattle market which reinforces its agricultural traditions. Excellent centre for exploring the Vale, which has hamlets, thatched cottages and pubs.

HOTEL
JANE HODGE RESORT HOTEL 🚹
Grooms Holidays
Trerhyngyll, Nr. Cowbridge CF71 7TN
Tel: (01446) 772608   Fax: 901446) 775831
No. of Accessible Rooms: 39
Accessible Facilities: Lounge, Restaurant, Hydrotherapy Pool, Sauna, Whirlpool, Multi Gym, Sports Hall.
Located in quiet village, just outside Cowbridge, equidistant between Cardiff and Bridgend, and within the Gower Peninsula. Excellent facilities.

PENARTH
Genteel Victorian seaside resort with period charm and fine town houses built for ship owners and master mariners in the C19th. Describes itself as a "garden by the sea", with lovely sea views and lush green parks. No funfairs or "tat" usually associated with such resorts.

TOURIST INFORMATION CENTRE
The Esplanade, Penarth Pier,
Penarth CF64 3AU
Tel: (01222) 708849
Seasonal, in winter contact Cardiff.

ATTRACTION
COSMESTON COUNTRY PARK LAKES AND MEDIEVAL VILLAGE
Lavernock Road, Penarth CF64 5UY
Tel: (01222) 701678   Fax: (01222) 708686
Original village of Comeston decimated by first Great Plague of C14th. Strolls along wooden boardwalks through acres of parkland and 2 lovely lakes. Take a tour around the medieval village with costumed guides in the cottages, byres and barns, reconstructed on the site of an original C14th settlement. The boardwalks are inevitably slightly uneven and the surrounds of the cottages in the village are mainly uneven paving. Path to each individual building, but doorways are narrow.

SD 🚹   CP 🚹   E 🚹 (visitor centre)
RF 🚹   C 🚹   S 🚹
WC 🚹   visitor centre. 2 others on RADAR key
RFE 🚹

WREXHAM

Large, busy town which grew up around local coal and iron industries. Mineral-rich uplands enhanced its prosperity in C18th and C19th, but only Erdig remains. There is a fine parish church, St. Giles, with splendid 3-storey tower completed in 1506. Founder of Yale University, Elihu Yales, was born in Wrexham and is commemorated in St. Giles.

TOURIST INFORMATION CENTRE
Lambpit Street, Wrexham LL11 1WN
Tel: (01978) 292015   Fax: (01978) 292467

PUBLIC TRANSPORT INFORMATION
Tel: (01978) 363760

BUSES
Arriva Cymru: Tel: (01970) 617951 or (01492) 592111
Some low-floor buses.

TAXIS
Apollo Taxis: Tel: (01978) 262600
1 adapted vehicle.
Atax: Tel: (01978) 262380
3 adapted minibuses.
Prestige Taxis: Tel: (01978) 291999
2 adapted minibuses.
Wrexham Taxis: Tel: (01978) 357777
2 adapted minibuses.

TRAINS
Central Trains: Assistance:
Tel: (0845) 7056027
Web: www.centraltrains.co.uk
First North Western: Special Needs:
Tel: (0845) 6040231

CAR PARKS
Some unlimited orange badge parking
Tel: (01978) 292000

SHOPMOBILITY
21 Egerton Street, Wrexham LL11 1ND
Tel: (01978) 312390
Minicom: (01978) 262601

ATTRACTIONS
ALYN WATERS COUNTRY PARK
Mold Road, Gwersyllt, Wrexham LL11 4AG
Tel: (01978) 761222

Situated in the lovely Alyn Valley, the park is in 2 halves. Within the Gwersyllt half is the visitor centre with exhibitions on history and wildlife of the area and on the Llay side is a new cycle way with good access for wheelchair users. Located 3 miles north of Wrexham.

SD [access]   CP [access]   E [access]   S [access]
WC [access]   RFE [access] (Circular walk with disabled access – 500m. long)

BERSHAM HERITAGE CENTRE
Bersham, Wrexham LL14 4HT
Tel: (01978) 261529   Fax: (01978) 361703
The furnaces and foundries which produced cannons for the American War of Independence and cylinders for James Watt's steam engines are brought alive here in the story of this C18th ironworks. Limited access to actual ironworks.

SD [access]   CP [access]   E [access]   RF [access]
S [access]   WC [access]

TY MAWR COUNTRY PARK
Cae Gwilym Lane, Cefn Mawr,
Wrexham LL14 3PE
Tel: (01978) 822780
On the banks of the River Dee overlooking the Vale of Llangollen and the Pontcysyllte Aqueduct, this 35-acre grassland park offers a variety of wildlife plus rare breeds of sheep, donkeys, ponies and goats. Farmed organically Ty Mawr still manages hay meadows along the river in the traditional way. Informative visitor centre and surfaced paths for easier access. Great for picnics or barbecues – hire a barbie from the visitor centre.

SD [access]   CP [access]   E [access]   RFE [access]
S [access]   WC [access]   RFE [access]

SPORTING VENUE
BANGOR-ON-DEE RACECOURSE
Bangor-on-Dee, Wrexham LL13 0DA
Tel: (01978) 780323   Fax: (01978) 780985
CP [access]   No road or public CP nearby
RE [access]   ED [access]   INT [access]
WC [access] (1 adapted WC in each toilet block – 6 in total)
SS – Viewing platform for wheelchairs   B/R [access]

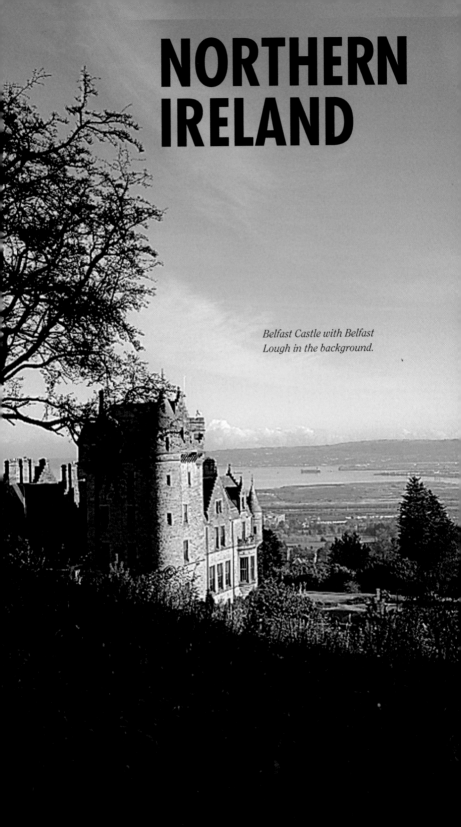

NORTHERN IRELAND

Belfast Castle with Belfast Lough in the background.

TOURIST BOARDS

NORTHERN IRELAND TOURIST BOARD
St. Anne's Court, 59 North Street,
Belfast, Co. Antrim BT1 1NB
Tel: (028) 90 246609   Fax: (028) 90 240960
Minicom: (028) 90 233228
e-mail: nitb@nics.gov.uk

DISABILITY ORGANISATIONS
ASSOCIATION FOR SPINA BIFIDA &
HYDROCEPHALUS (ASBAH)
Graham House, Knockbracken Healthcare Park,
Saintfield Road, Belfast BT8 8BH
Tel: (028) 90 798878
Similar to ASBAH in introduction

DISABILITY ACTION (HEAD OFFICE)
2 Annadale Avenue, Belfast BT7 3JH
Tel: (028) 90 491011   Fax: (028) 90 491627
This organisation works to ensure that
people with disabilities attain their full
rights as citizens. Currently very involved in
accessible transport. Will supply
information as required.
Publishes *Getting Out and About*.

IRISH DISABLED FLY FISHING ASSOCIATION
6 Old Park Drive, Ballymena,
Co. Antrim BT42 1BG
Tel: (028) 256 42539

NORTHERN IRELAND PARAPLEGIC ASSOCIATION
c/o Disability Action (see above)

NORTHERN IRELAND REGIONAL ACCESS
COMMITTEE
c/o Disability Action (see above)

PHAB NORTHERN IRELAND
Mourne Villa, Knockbracken Healthcare Park,
Belfast BT8 8BH
Tel: (028) 90 796565   Fax: (028) 90 796070
Web: www.phabni.dnet.co.uk/
Provides range of services to encourage
those with disabilities to achieve equal
opportunities, including fully accessible
residential activity centre in Ballinran, Co.
Down.

ACCESSIBLE TRANSPORT
DOE Transport (Policy and Support) Division
12th Floor, River House, 48 High Street,

Belfast BT1 2AR
Tel: (028) 90 251300   Fax: (028) 90 257333
e-mail: tpsd@nics.gov.uk

TRANSLINK
Integrated public transport operations of
Citybus, NI Railways and Ulsterbus.
web: www.translink.co.uk
    www.citybus.co.uk
    www.ulsterbus.co.uk
    www.nirailways.co.uk

COUNTY ANTRIM

BALLYCASTLE
Lying at the heart of the Causeway Coast
and renowned as the site of the Ould
Lammas Fair, Ballycastle has been
designated an architectural conservation
area. A medium sized resort town with an
attractive harbour and central sandy beach.

TOURIST INFORMATION CENTRE
Sheskburn House, 7 Mary Street,
Ballycastle BT54 6QH
Tel: (028) 207 62024   Fax: (028) 207 62515
e-mail: tourism@moyle-council.org

HOTEL
MARINE HOTEL
North Street, Ballycastle BT54 6BN
Tel: (028) 207 62222   Fax: (028) 207 69507
No. of Accessible Rooms: 2
Accessible Facilities: Restaurant, Bar.
Attractive hotel on the sea front,
overlooking a fine bay across to Rathlin
Island and the Scottish Isles.

BALLYCLARE
Inland from Larne on A8.

BED AND BREAKFAST
RUA-WAI FARM
149 Templepatrick Road, Ballyclare BT39 9RW
Tel: (028) 93 352417
No. of Accessible Rooms: 3
Accessible Facilities: Dining Room.
Bungalow with large garden on 20 acre
horse farm, 2 miles from Ballyclare.

BALLYGALLEY

On the Antrim coast, a few miles north of Larne.

BED AND BREAKFAST
CAIRNVIEW
13 Croft Heights, Ballygalley BT40 2QS
Tel: (028) 28 583269
No. of Accessible Rooms: 1
Accessible Facilities: Dining Room, Lounge.
Modern house in quiet residential area of
Ballygalley with fine views.

BALLYMENA

Prosperous town surrounded by some of the
richest farmland in Northern Ireland. Good
Saturday livestock market. Close by is
Gracehill, a small Moravian settlement with
some C18th buildings still standing.

TOURIST INFORMATION CENTRE
13-15 Bridge Street, Ballymena BT43 5EJ
Tel: (028) 256 44111   Fax: (028) 256 46296

HOTELS
TULLYGLASS HOUSE HOTEL
178 Galgorm Road, Ballymena BT42 1HJ
Tel: (028) 256 52639   Fax: (028) 256 46938
No. of Accessible Rooms: 1. Shower
Accessible Facilities: Lounge, Restaurant,
Bar. Converted period house set in private
own grounds on outskirts of town.

CAIREAL MANOR GUEST HOUSE
90 Glenravel Road, Martinstown,
Ballymena BT43 6QQ
Tel/Fax: (028) 217 58465/58344/58221
No. of Accessible Rooms: 2. Shower
Accessible Facilities: Lounge, Dining Room
Detached villa located on A43 gateway to
the Glen of Glenariffe, within 15 minutes
drive of Ballymena and surrounded by
lovely countryside.

GALGORM MANOR
136 Fenaghy Road, Ballymena BT42 1EA
Tel: (028) 25 881001
Fax: (028) 25 880080
No. of Accessible Rooms: 1.
Accessible Facilities: Restaurant. C19th
gentleman's residence in 85 acres with
various activities on site including fishing.

BALLYMONEY

Busy town in the Bann Valley.

TOURIST INFORMATION CENTRE
Riada House, 14 Charles Street,
Ballymoney BT53 6DZ
Tel: (028) 276 62280   Fax: (028) 276 65150

BED AND BREAKFAST
GLEN LODGE
93a Frocess Road, Ballymoney BT53 7EJ
Tel: (028) 276 63800
No. of Accessible Rooms: 1
Accessible Facilities: Dining room/Lounge.
Modern detached chalet bungalow with
spacious gardens.

MOUNTVIEW HOUSE
23 Carrowcroey Road, Armoy,
Ballymoney BT53 8UH
Tel: (028) 276 51402
No. of Accessible Rooms: 1. Shower
Accessible Facilities: Lounge, Dining Room.
Large farmhouse on working farm situated
close to Causeway Coast.

ATTRACTION
BANVARDEN GARDENS
Benvarden, Dervock, Ballymoney, BT53 6NN
Tel: (028) 276 41331   Fax: (028) 276 41955
2-acre walled garden ranging from rose beds
to kitchen garden, the grounds stretching
down to a river bank and Woodland Pond.
Cobbled Stable Yard contains stables, coach
and cart houses and tea room.

LESLIE HILL OPEN FARM
Ballymoney BT53 6QL
Tel/Fax: (028) 276 66803
An C18th estate with lovely grounds.
Extensive collection of rare breeds, poultry,
horsedrawn machinery, museum, working
forge and walled garden.

BELFAST

Only city in Ireland to experience the full
force of the Industrial Revolution and its
ship-building, rope-making and tobacco

industries caused massive rise in population by the end of WW1. The legacy of imposing buildings is still evident, although the Troubles and industrial decline have damaged economic lift. Still a handsome city.

BELFAST VISITOR AND CONVENTION BUREAU
Floor 4, Albany House, 73-75 Great Victoria Street, Belfast BT2 7AF
Tel: (028) 90 239026   Fax; (028) 90 249026
web: www. belfastvisitor.com

TOURIST INFORMATION CENTRE
St. Anne's Court, North Street, Belfast BT1 1NB
Tel: (028) 90 246609
DOE Transport (Policy and Support) Division
12th Floor, River House, 48 High Street,
Belfast BT1 2AR
Tel: (028) 90 257312   Fax: (028) 90 257333
e-mail: tpsd@nics.gov.uk

BUSES
Translink (Citybus, NI Rail, Ulsterbus -latter does not operate in Belfast City)
New buses have been fitted with ramps and low-floor level wheelchair accessibility/

Citybus: Tel: (028) 90 246485
NI Rail: Tel: (028) 90 899411
Ulsterbus: Tel: (028) 90 33300
Centrelink: Every 15 minutes. Low-floor buses.

TAXIS
For all queries call: (028) 90 491011
Community Black Taxis, London style, operate in certain areas of Belfast and Londonderry - not all are accessible. This is a bus type of service. Public hire taxis in Belfast are identified by a yellow plate at the rear and front of the vehicle. Private hire taxis are identified by a roof sign with white front panel and a green licence disc on the windscreen.

TRAINS
NI Railways
Central Station, Belfast BT1 3PB
Enquiries: Tel: (028) 90 899411
or (01849) 429185
Wheelchair users well catered for with dedicated space in carriage plus call button facilities. Ramps available. One carriage in each train has space set aside for wheelchairs users.

The glittering lights of nightime Belfast Waterfront complex.

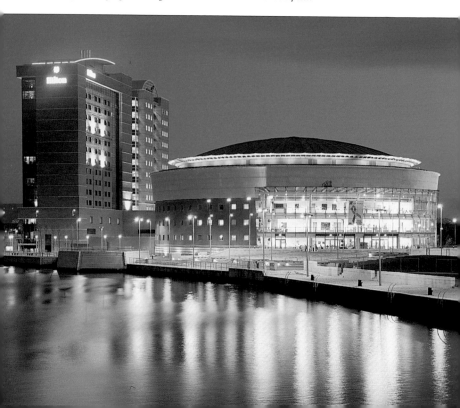

SHOPMOBILITY
Unit 26, Victoria Centre, Victoria Square,
Belfast BT1 4TL
Tel: (028) 90 808090   Fax: (028) 90 808099

HOTEL
ALDERGROVE AIRPORT HOTEL
Belfast International Airport, Crumlin,
Belfast BT29 4ZY
Tel: (028) 94 422033   Fax: (028) 94 423500
No. of Accessible Rooms: 3
Accessible Facilities: Lounge, Restaurant.
Modern airport hotel.

BALMORAL HOTEL
Blacks Road, Dunmurry, Belfast BT10 0ND
Tel: (028) 90 301234   Fax: (028) 90 601455
No. of Accessible Rooms: 8
Accessible Facilities: Lounge, Restaurant.
Modern purpose-built hotel in its own
grounds three miles from the centre of
Belfast, adjacent to the M1 motorway

HASTINGS EUROPA HOTEL
Great Victoria Street, Belfast BT2 7AP
Tel: (028) 90 327000   Fax: (028) 90 327800
e-mail: res.eur@hastingshotels.com
web: www.hastingshotels.com
No. of Accessible Rooms: 2
Accessible Facilities: Lounge, Restaurants
2.
Quality hotel situated in the heart of the
city on the Golden Mile.

HOLIDAY INN EXPRESS
106 University Street, Belfast BT7 1HP
Tel: (028) 90 311909   Fax: (028) 90 311910
e-mail: express@holidayinn-ireland.com
web: www.holidayinn-ireland.com
No. of Accessible Rooms: 6
Accessible Facilities: Lounge, Restaurant.
Business hotel situated 1km from the city
centre. All bedrooms fitted with
workstations and computer points.

STORMONT HOTEL
Upper Newtownards Road, Belfast BT4 3LP
Tel: (028) 90 658621   Fax: (028) 90 480240
e-mail: res.stor@hastingshotels.com
web: www.hastingshotels.com
No. of Accessible Rooms: 1
Accessible Facilities: Lounge, Restaurants
2, Bar. Quality modern hotel located

opposite the Parliament Buildings, 4 miles
east of the city centre.

JURYS BELFAST INN
Fisherwick Place, Gt. Victoria Street,
Belfast BT2 7AP
Tel: (028) 90 533500   Fax: (028) 90 533511
No. of Accessible Rooms: 1. Roll-in Shower
Accessible Facilities: Lounge, Restaurant,
Bar. Modern hotel in city centre adjacent to
the Opera House. All public areas are level,
carpeted and wide with much natural light.
Bedrooms are notably spacious. Room 104
(accessible) on the first floor is accessed by
an accessible lift. There are 4 other semi-
accessible rooms.

THE McCAUSLAND HOTEL
34-38 Victoria Street, Belfast BT1 3EH
Tel: (028) 90 220200   Fax: (028) 90 220220
e-mail: info@mccauslandhotel.com
No. of Accessible Rooms: 3
Accessible Facilities: Restaurant
Formerly 2 warehouses designed in
Italianate classical style in the 1850s, and
opened late 1999 as a prestigious 60-
bedroom hotel. Original cast-iron pillars,
high arched ceilings and oak beams have all
been retained.

BED AND BREAKFAST
GREENWOOD HOUSE
25 Park Road, Belfast BT7 2FW
Tel: (028) 90 202525   Fax: (028) 90 202530
e-mail: greenwood.house@virgin.net
No. of Accessible Rooms: 1
Accessible Facilities: Lounge, Dining Room.
The house faces a quiet park with paved paths.

ATTRACTIONS
BELFAST ZOO
Antrim Road, Belfast BT36 7PN
Tel: (028) 90 776277   Fax: (028) 90 370578
50-acre zoo with award-winning primate
house, penguin enclosure and free-flight
aviary. Red pandas and rare spectacled bears,
free-ranging lemurs and an African
enclosure also. As an outdoor facility, levels
do vary and some are hilly

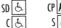

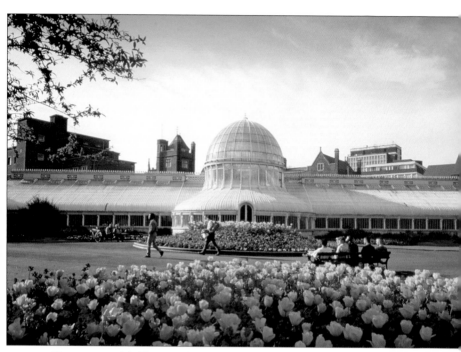

Warm up on a visit. The tropical house at the Botanic Gardens.

BOTANIC GARDENS
Stranmillis Road BT7 1JB
Tel: (028) 90 324902   Fax: (028) 90 237070
A rose garden, colourful herbaceous and
shrub borders and children's playground are
complimented by the Tropical Ravine House
and the Palm House.

SD ♿   CP ♿   E ♿   RF (Ravine) ♿
L 🚹   C ♿   S ♿
WC: (Museum/Bowling Green) 🚹
RFE: (Palm House/Ravine) ♿

LAGAN LOOKOUT VISITOR CENTRE
1 Donegall Quay, Belfast BT1 3EA
Tel: (028) 90 315444   Fax: (028) 90 311955
Tells story of the important role of the River
Lagan in Belfast's development via models,
interactive displays and videos.

SD ♿   CP ♿
E ♿ (warning -very long ramp at 1:11)
L ♿   WC 🚹

ULSTER MUSEUM
Within, but separate from, the Botanic Gardens
Tel: (028) 90 383000   Fax: (028) 90 383003
web: www.ulstermuseum.org.uk
Collection of fine and decorative arts,

archaeology, local history and natural
sciences.

SD ♿   CP 🚹   E ♿   RF ♿   L ♿
C ♿   S ♿   WC ♿   RFE ♿

BUSHMILLS
Small town with an attractive square and
fine River, but its main claim to fame is
whiskey.

TOURIST INFORMATION CENTRE
See Giant's Causeway Visitor Centre
(page 405).

BED AND BREAKFAST
VALLEY VIEW   ♿
6a Ballyclough Road, Bushmills BT57 8TU
Tel/fax: (028) 207 41608/41319
e-mail: valerie.mcfall@btinternet.com
No. of Accessible Rooms: 1
Accessible Facilities: Lounge, Dining Room
Comfortable family-run country house
overlooking the Bush River Valley and
Antrim Mountains.

BROWN'S COUNTRY HOUSE

174 Ballybogey Road, Bushmills BT52 2LP
Tel: (028) 207 32777 Fax: (028) 207 31627
No. of Accessible Rooms: 3
Accessible Facilities: Lounge, Restaurant
Attractive property with long established
reputation for fine food. Close to Giant's
Causeway.

THE POACHERS REST

11 Cozies Road, Castlecatt, Bushmills BT57 8YG
Tel: (028) 207 42125
No. of Accessible Rooms: 1
Accessible Facilities: Lounge, Dining Room.
Very quiet location 2.5 miles from
Bushmills and close to Bushmills Distillery
and Giants Causeway.

SELF-CATERING
BALLYLINNEY COTTAGES

1Giants Causeway, Bushmills BT57 8SU
Tel/Fax: (028) 207 31683
No. of Accessible Units: 1. Roll-in Shower
No. of Beds per Unit: 6
Accessible Facilities: Lounge, Dining Room,
Kitchen. Weirs Snout is one of six quality
self-contained cottages set alongside the
Laverty farm. Cottages are grouped
together around landscaped garden. Fine
views over the Causeway, sleepy seaside
village of Portballintrae and the Donegal
Coastline beyond. Located a mile from
Bushmills.

ATTRACTION
THE OLD BUSHMILLS DISTILLERY CO.

Bushmills BT57 8XH
Tel: (028) 207 31521 Fax: (028) 207 31339
web: www.bushmills.com
World's oldest licensed whiskey distillery to
which James I granted the original license
in 1608. For over four centuries the art of
distillation has been passed down through
the generations. The tour is not accessible,
but an excellent video is shown in the
accessible viewing room, where chairs are
moveable, will allow those in wheelchairs to
gain some sense of the distillery tour,
joining up with able-bodied friends at the
shop afterwards. From the visitor centre to
the shop there's a downward gradient of
1:15, staff will assist.

SD n/a   CP [&]   E [&] Visitor Centre

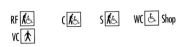
RF [&]   C [&]   S [&]   WC [&] Shop
VC [&]

GIANT'S CAUSEWAY VISITOR CENTRE

44 Causeway Road, Bushmills BT57 8SU
Tel: (028) 207 31855 Fax: (028) 207 32537
Unique rock formations stand as natural
rampart against ferocity of Atlantic storms.
The rugged hexagonal symmetry of the
columns is amazing. Now generally
accepted that the Causeway was a result of
intense volcanic activity which took place
when continents were separating and
oceans forming some 60 million years ago.
VC has shops, WC, café, video cinema and
exhibition. The Ulster Bus or Translink Bus
taking visitors down to the Causeway from
the VC, 0.75 mile, has space for one
wheelchair at the rear, but no actual
tailgate lift. During our visit, some visitors
in wheelchairs were pushed down by
companions and bused back.

SD [&]   CP [&]   E [&]   RF [&]
C [&]   S [&]   WC [&]
RFE [&] Causeway Bus

CARNLOUGH

Long farmed area with dry-stone walls,
located at the foot of the Glencoy. Good
base for touring the Glens, particularly
Garron Moor, and Giant's Causeway, with a
fine sandy beach and delightful harbour.

HOTEL
THE LONDONDERRY ARMS HOTEL

20 Harbour Road, Carnlough BT44 0EU
Tel: (028) 28 885255 Fax: (028) 28 885263
e-mail: lda@glensofantrim.com
No. of Accessible Rooms: 1
Accessible Facilities: Lounge, Restaurant
Family run hotel, built in 1848, once
owned by Sir Winston Churchill.

BED AND BREAKFAST
BETHANY HOUSE

5 Bay Road, Carnlough, BT44 0HQ
Tel: (028) 28 885667
No. of Accessible Rooms: 1
Accessible Facilities: Lounge, Dining Room.
Detached house in the centre of the village
with good sea views.

CARRICKFERGUS

The town grew up around the massive castle begun in 1180, which, sadly, due to an entrance ramped at a gradient of 1:7, is not accessible. Worth viewing from the harbour.

TOURIST INFORMATION CENTRE
Knight Ride Centre, Heritage Plaza,
Carrickfergus BT38 7DQ
Tel: (028) 93 366455
Fax: (028) 93 350350

BED AND BREAKFAST
HILLCREST
66 Bellahill Road, Carrickfergus BT38 9DB
Tel/Fax: (028) 93 367342
No. of Accessible Rooms: 2
Accessible Facilities: Lounge, Dining Room.
Large, modern bungalow set in its own grounds of five acres with extensive landscaped gardens. Rural location overlooking Belfast Lough, three miles from Carrickfergus, 15 from Belfast. Good base for touring Antrim Glens and coast.

ATTRACTION
KNIGHT RIDE
The Heritage Plaza, Antrim Street,
Carrickfergus BT38 7DG
Tel: (028) 93 366455
Fax: (028) 93 350350
Accessible trip through time, experiencing over 1,000 years of the town's stormy history, see, feel and smell the past of one of Ulster's liveliest towns.

SD CP E S
WC L

Features: Knight Ride: In a wheelchair enter the shop and go up to the Ride via the lift. Technician will put you, in your chair, into a specially designed helmet/car to enjoy the ride.

CUSHENDALL

Attractive village in the Heart of the Glens of Antrim between the hills and the sea of Moyle. Located at the bottom of Ballyeamon, on of the nine glens. One of the first villages in Northern Ireland to be declared a Conservation Area it has retained its character and charm.

BED AND BREAKFAST
THE MEADOWS
79-81 Coast Road, Cushendall BT44 0QW
Tel: (028) 217 72020
No. of Accessible Rooms: 1. Shower
Accessible Facilities: Lounge, Dining Room
Detached house on Larne side of town.

THE BURN
63 Ballyeamon Road, Cushendall BT44 0SN
Tel: (028) 217 71733   Fax: (028) 217 46111
Theburn@ireland-holidays.net
N. of Accessible Rooms: 2
Accessible Facilities: Lounge, Dining Room, Bar. Detached bungalow a mile from Cushendall.

CULLENTRA HOUSE
16 Cloughs Road (off Gault's Road),
Cushendall BT44 0SP
Tel/Fax: (028) 217 71762
e-mail: cullentra@ireland-holidays.net
No. of Accessible Rooms: 1. Bath
Accessible Facilities: Lounge, Dining Room
Award-winning country guesthouse with fine scenery of Antrim coast, overlooking the sea of Moyle with views of Scottish hills in the background.

GARRON VIEW
14 Cloghs Road, Cushendall BT44 0SP
Tel: (02821) 771018
No. of Accessible Rooms: 3
Accessible Facilities: Lounge, Dining Room
Working farm situated just off main road outside village. Fine views of Red Bay and Garron Point.

CUSHENDUN

At the foot of the River Dun and at the mouth of Glendun, the village has unique Cornish architecture and is an area of outstanding beauty. The heart of the village is rather a surprise with its main street of whitewashed dwellings, a shop, teahouse and pub (reputedly the smallest in Ireland). The street continues across the bridge over the River Dun. Long attracted many of Irelands' best known artists.

BED AND BREAKFAST
CLONEYMORE BED & BREAKFAST

103 Knocknacarry Road,
Cushendun BT44 0NT
Tel: (028) 25 61443
e-mail: CDDA@antrim-glens.demon.co.uk
No. of Accessible Rooms: 1. Roll-in Shower
Accessible Facilities: Lounge, Dining Room.
Attractive old house, family owned, in lovely
surroundings.

ISLANDMAGEE

The 'island' is eight miles long, joined to the
mainland by attractive raised causeway
(B90). Ragged cliffs look east toward
Scotland, whilst west faces the sheltered
water of Lough Larne with sandy beaches.
Scattered farms and quiet lanes combine
with old world charm on this peninsula
where local communities are proud of
seafaring and farming traditions. Much to
see and do here.

BED AND BREAKFAST
HILL VIEW   🧍
30 Middle Road, Islandmagee BT40 3SL
Tel: (028) 93 372581
No. of Accessible Rooms: 3. Bath
Accessible Facilities: Lounge.
Modern, attractive house with fine
countryside views.

LARNE

Not the prettiest of towns, but it does lie on
the threshold of the fine Antrim coastline.
The sheltered waters of Larne Lough have
been a landing point for 9,000 years, most
recently in 1914 when the UVF landed a
huge cache of German arms here during its
campaign against Home Rule.

TOURIST INFORMATION AND
INTERPRETIVE CENTRE
Narrow Gauge Road, Larne BT40 1XB
Tel/Fax: (028) 28 260088
e-mail: mail@larne-bc.com

HOTEL
MAGHERAMORNE HOUSE HOTEL   🧍
59 Shore Road, Magheramorne,
Larne BT40 3HW
Tel: (028) 28 279444 Fax: (028) 28 260138
No. of Accessible Rooms: 2

Accessible Facilities: Lounge, Restaurant
Originally the stately home of the first
Baron Magheramorne, the great uncle of
former Lord Chancellor, Lord Hailsham. Set
in 43 acres of lovely grounds, overlooking
Larne Lough, the hotel recreates the world
of the 1880s when the house was built.

BED AND BREAKFAST
CAIRNVIEW   🧍
13 Croft Heights, Ballygalley, Larne BT40 2QS
Tel: (028) 28 583269   Fax: (028) 28 583269
No. of Accessible Rooms: 1. Bath
Accessible Facilities: Lounge, Dining Room.
Ulster Guesthouse of the Year 1998.
Lovely modern house 4 miles north of Larne
in village of Ballygalley.

ATTRACTIONS
CARRFUNNOCK COUNTRY PARK
Coast Road, Larne
Tel: (028) 28 270541
Beautiful woodland and fine gardens with
unique collection of sundials and maze in
the shape of N.I. Superb children's activity
centre.

| SD ♿ | CP ♿ | E ♿ | C ♿ |
| S ♿ | WC 🧍 | RFE ♿ | |

LARNE INTERPRETIVE CENTRE (see TIC)
Story of the building of the Antrim Coast
Road.

LISBURN

Located in the Lagan Valley, this was an
important centre for linen-making during
C18th, established in Lisburn by Louis
Cromell a French Hugenot and refugee. He is
buried in the planters gothic cathedral here.

TOURIST INFORMATION CENTRE
Irish Linen Centre and Lisburn Museum, Market
Square, Lisburn BT28 1AG
Tel: (028) 92 660038

BED AND BREAKFAST
HILLTOP   🧍
60 Tullyard Road, Drumbo, Lisburn BT27 5JN
Tel: (028) 92 826021 Fax: (028) 92 826061)
No. of Accessible Rooms: 1
Accessible Facilities: Lounge, Dining Room.
Modern bungalow off Hillhall Road.

ATTRACTION
IRISH LINEN CENTRE AND LISBURN MUSEUM
Market Square, Lisburn BT28 1AG
Tel: (028) 92 663377   Fax: (028) 92 672624
Follow the history of linen from C17th: visit
a spinner's cottage: see and hear Victorian
mill girls: watch damask linen being
prepared in the traditional way: learn how
linen was made from flax and watch
spinning – and more. Truly fascinating.

SD 🚲   CP 🚲   E 🚲   RF 🚲
L 🚲   C 🚲   S 🚲   WC 🚲

NEWTOWNABBEY
Located seven miles north of Belfast, major
site for out of town shopping with huge
mall, on main road between Glengormley
and Templepatrick. Known for Ballyclare
May Fair, traditionally a hiring fare for the
farming community, and still renowned as a
horse fair.

NEWTOWNABBEY LEISURE AND TECHNICAL SERVICES DEPT.
Glenmount, 49 Church Road,
NewtownAbbey BT36 7LG
Tel: (028) 90 868751   Fax: (028) 90 365407

HOTEL
CORR'S CORNER HOTEL 🚲
315 Ballyclare Road, NewtownAbbey BT36 4TQ
Tel: (028) 90 849221   Fax: (028) 90 832118
No. of Accessible Rooms: 1
Accessible Facilities: Restaurant
Originally opened in 1919 as a bar for
travellers between Belfast and the coast and
more recently a roadhouse. In mid 1997 30
bedrooms were added, making this a small,
comfortable property. Family-owned and
operated.

CHIMNEY CORNER HOTEL 🚶
630 Antrim Road, NewtownAbbey BT36 4RH
Tel: (028) 90 844925   Fax: (028) 90 844352
No. of Accessible Rooms: 1
Accessible Facilities: Lounge, Restaurant,
Garden. Located on main road from
Glengormley to Templepatrick.

PORTRUSH
A rather brash resort with an abundance of
souvenir shops and amusement arcades.

TOURIST INFORMATION CENTRE
Dunluce Centre, Sandhill Drive, Portrush
Tel: (028) 70 823333   Fax: (028) 70 822256

HOTEL
MAGHERABUOY HOUSE HOTEL 🚶
41 Magheraboy Road, Portrush BT56 8NX
Tel: (028) 70 823507   Fax: (028) 70 824687
e-mail:
administration@magherabuoy.freeserve.co.uk
No. of Accessible Rooms: Unknown
Accessible Facilities: Breakfast room, Dining
Room. The hotel overlooks the Atlantic
Ocean and is a short distance from the
Giant's Causeway.

BED AND BREAKFAST
DUKES LODGE
6 - 7 Kerr Street, Portrush BT56 8DG
Tel/Fax: (028) 70 824159
No. of Accessible Rooms: 1
Accessible Facilities: Dining Room, 2
Lounges, Lift. House along the seafront
beside Barrys and the train/bus station.

HAYESBANK KANTARA 🚶
5/6 Ramore Avenue, Portrush BT56 8BB
Tel: (028) 70 823823   Fax: (028) 70 822741
No. of Accessible Rooms: 1. Bath, First floor,
accessible by chair lift.
Accessible Facilities: Dining Room
Family run guest house in pleasant area
overlooking bowling greens and convenient
to amenities.

ISLAY-VIEW 🚶
36 Leeke Road, off Ballymagarry Road,
Portrush BT56 8NH
Tel: (028) 70 823220
No. of Accessible Rooms: 1. Bath.
Accessible Facilities: Open plan Lounge/Dining
Room. Chalet bungalow on a working
farm, convenient for Giant's Causeway.

ATTRACTION
THE DUNLUCE CENTRE
10 Sandhill Drive, Portrush BT56 8BF
Tel: (028) 70 824444   Fax: (028) 70 822256
Fine inter-active hi-tec family entertainment.

SD 🚲   CP 🚲   E 🚲   C 🚶
S 🚲   WC 🚶   RFE 🚲

TEMPLEPATRICK
ATTRACTION
PATTERSON'S SPADE MILL (NT)
751 Antrim Road, Templepatrick BT38 9AP
Tel/Fax: (028) 94 433619
Only surviving water-driven spade mill in
Ireland. Restored by National Trust and
back in production.

SD [♿]   CP [♿]   E [♿]   RF [♿]
WC [🚹]   RFE [♿]

COUNTY ARMAGH

ARMAGH
One of Ireland's oldest cities, dating back
to the age of St. Patrick in the C5th.
Narrow streets in the centre follow the
ditches which once ringed the church,
founded by the saint in 455AD. There are 2
cathedrals, both called St. Patrick's, one
catholic, one protestant, sitting on
opposing hills. The elegant mall
surrounding a peaceful park, is full of
dignified Georgian houses.

TOURIST INFORMATION CENTRE
Old Bank Buildings, 40 English Street, Armagh
Tel: (028) 37 521800   Fax: (028) 37 528329

BUSES
Ulsterbus: Tel: (028) 37 522266

BED AND BREAKFAST
HILLVIEW LODGE   [🚹]
33 Newtownhamilton Road, Armagh BT60 2PL
Tel: (028) 37 522000   Fax: (028) 37 528276
e-mail: alice@hillviewlodge.com
web: www.hillviewlodge.com
No. of Accessible Rooms: 1
Accessible Facilities: Lounge, Dining Room
Set in rolling hills, enjoying lovely rural
location, 1 mile from Armagh.
Guesthouse of the Year Finalist 1998.

NI EOGHAIN LODGE   [🚹]
32 Ennislare Road, Armagh BT60 2AX
Tel/Fax: (028) 37 525633
No. of Accessible Rooms: 3
Accessible Facilities: TV Lounge, Dining
Room. Farmhouse set amid award-winning
gardens, located two miles off A29
Keady/Armagh road.

ATTRACTION
ARMAGH COUNTY MUSEUM
The Mall East, Armagh BT61 9BE
Tel: (028) 37 523070   Fax: (028) 37 522631
Located on the Mall, an area of urban
parkland in the city centre this is the oldest
County museum in Ireland with a distinctive
Greek classical design although built in 1834.
Extensive collection of artefacts include
military costumes, ceramics, natural history
specimens, railway material and historic
household items. Ever changing temporary
exhibitions.

SD [♿]   CP n/a – Street parking only, very close.
E [♿]   RF [♿]   L [♿]   S [♿]   WC [♿]

ARMAGH PLANETARIUM
College Hill, Armagh BT61 9DB
Tel: (028) 37 524725   Fax: (028) 37 526187
Multimedia Star-Show with 3-D effects and
tour of the Hall of Astronomy and
Eartharium, Weather Room and School's
Internet Centre.

SD [♿]   CP [🚹]   E [♿] (Main E. has disabled lift)
RF [♿]   C [🚹]   S [♿]   WC [🚹]   RFE [🚹]

THE NAVAN CENTRE
81 Killylea Road, Armagh BT60 4LD
Tel: (028) 37 525550   Fax: (028) 37 522323
e-mail: navan@anterprise.net
Navan Fort is a famous Celtic site: seat of
ancient Kings of Ulster. The Centre tells the
history and archaeology of the fort in superb
visual interactive display. NB: Access to
Navan Fort Ancient Monument is difficult
for wheelchairs.

SD [♿]   CP [♿]   E [♿]   RF [♿]
C [♿]   S [♿]   WC [🚹]

PALACE STABLES HERITAGE CENTRE
The Palace, Demesne, Armagh BT60 4EL
Tel: (028) 37 529629   Fax: (028) 37 529630
Housed in Georgian stables and courtyard
where visitors can experience stable life in
the C18th via life-like models, audio-
commentary and colour murals.

SD [♿]   CP [♿]   E [♿]   RF [♿]   L [♿]
C [🚹]   S [♿]   WC [♿]   RFE [♿]

SAINT PATRICK'S TRIAN VISITOR COMPLEX
40 English Street, Armagh BT61 7BR
Tel: (028) 37 521801   Fax: (028) 37 510180
Name derives from three distinct districts or

Trians - here there are three major exhibitions. The Armagh Story with AV presentation: exhibition on Saint Patrick and the Land of Lilliput where adventures of Gulliver are narrated, Jonathan Swift having spent time in Armagh. Much to see.

SD ♿ CP ♿ E ♿ RF ♿
L ♿ C ♿ S ♿ WC ♿

CRAIGAVON

Located in the NE area of the County, this is a new town, not beautiful, but with two large artificial lakes and close to Lough Neagh.

LOUGH NEAGH DISCOVERY CENTRE
Oxford Island National Nature Reserve,
Nr. Craigavon BT66 6NJ
Tel: (028) 38 322205 Fax: (028) 38 367438
History and wildlife of the Lough through audio-visual shows, interactive games and exhibitions and then experience it all for yourself.

SD ♿ CP ♿ E ♿ RF ♿
C ♿ S ♿ WC ♿

NEWRY

Old prosperous town on the River Clanrye with imposing houses and public buildings. Newry Canal, the oldest in Britain, now well stocked with fish.

TOURIST INFORMATION CENTRE
Town Hall, Newry BT35 6HR
Tel: (028) 302 68877 Fax: (028) 302 68833

BED AND BREAKFAST
GREEN VALE
141 Longfield Road, Forkhill, Newry BT35 9SD
Tel: (028) 30 888314
No. of Accessible Rooms: 2
Accessible Facilities: Lounge, Dining Room.
Bungalow on farm, 1.5 miles from Forkhill.

PORTADOWN

Old linen town in the industrial NE area of the county. Close to Lough Neagh and the river Bann.

HOTEL
SEAGOE HOTEL
Upper Church Lane, Portadown BT63 5JE
Tel: (028) 38 333076

Fax: (028) 38 350210
No. of Accessible Rooms: 2. Bath
Accessible Facilities: Restaurant, Bar.
Situated close to Lough Neagh.
Contemporary 34 bedroom hotel in attractive grounds.

COUNTY DOWN

BALLYNAHINCH
BED AND BREAKFAST
NUMBER THIRTY
30 Mountview Road,
Ballynahinch BT24 8JR
Tel: (028) 97 562956
No. of Accessible Rooms: 1. Bath
Accessible Facilities: Dining Room
Modern chalet bungalow situated in quiet country area overlooking the Mournes.

BANBRIDGE

Main gateway to the famous Mourne Mountains, with a great hill on the south of the river Bann. In 1834 the main street of Banbridge was divided into 3 sections with an underpass cut out in the middle to lower the hill and a bridge built over the gap.

GATEWAY TOURIST INFORMATION CENTRE
200 Newry Road, Banbridge
Tel: (028) 406 23322

BED AND BREAKFAST
MOURNEVIEW
32 Drumnascamph Road, Laurencetown,
Banbridge BT63 6DU
Tel: (028) 406 26270
Fax: (028) 406 24251
e-mail: N.W.79@dial.pipex.com
No. of Accessible Rooms: 4
Accessible Facilities: Lounge, Dining Room.
Detached bungalow 2 miles from Banbridge.

BANGOR

Resort town with modern marina and well known yacht clubs. A little south of the town is Donaghadee from where boats sail to the uninhabited Copeland Islands.

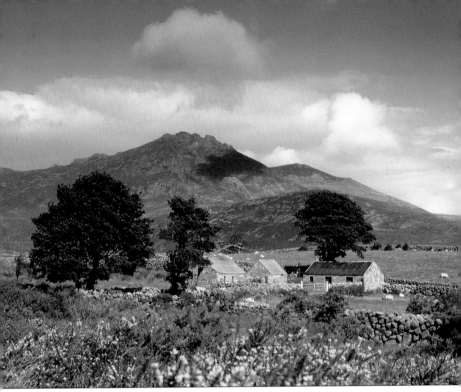

The Mountains of Mourne. You can almost taste the Guinness!

TOURIST INFORMATION CENTRE
Tower House, 34 Quay Street, Bangor BT20 5ED
Tel: (028) 91 270069   Fax: (028) 91 274466

BUSES
Ulsterbus: Tel: (028) 91 271143
Majority of buses in Co. Down are NOT
wheelchair accessible, the fleet is being
renewed. Call Ulsterbus before travelling.

RAIL
NI Railways, Bangor Rail Station,
Abbey Street, Bangor
Tel: (028) 91 270141
One carriage on each train is wheelchair
accessible and has ramps.

SHOPMOBILITY
55-59 The Arcade, High Street,
Bangor BT20 5BE
Tel: (028) 91 456586

HOTELS
CLANDEBOYE LODGE HOTEL
10 Estate Road, Clandeboye, Bangor BT19 1UR

Tel: (028) 91 852500   Fax: (028) 91 852772
e-mail: consorthotels@compuserve.com
web: www.consorthotels.com
No. of Accessible Rooms: 2
Accessible Facilities: Lounge, Restaurant,
Lift. Set in woodland overlooking
Clandeboye Estate. Furnished and decorated
to reflect relaxed rural setting. 3 miles from
Bangor,11 from Belfast.

MARINE COURT HOTEL
The Marina, 18-20 Quay Street,
Bangor BT20 5ED
Tel: (028) 91 451100   Fax: (028) 91 421200
No. of Accessible Rooms: 1. Shower
Accessible Facilities: Lift, Lounge,
Restaurant, Pool, Sauna, Spa.
Purpose-built hotel in centre of Bangor with
seafront location overlooking Marina.

CASTLEWELLAN
Hill top market town in foothills of the
Mournes with 2 large market places. The
town is surrounded by private woods.

BED AND BREAKFAST
TREETOPS
39 Circular Road, Castlewellan BT31 9ED
Tel: (028) 437 78132
No. of Accessible Rooms: 1
Accessible Facilities: Dining Room.
Two-storey modern house set in spacious
gardens.

SELF-CATERING
COAST VIEW COTTAGE
41 Ballywillwill Road, Castlewellan BT31 9LF
Tel: (028) 437 78006
e-mail: murray@unite.co.uk
No. of Accessible Units: 1
No. of Beds per Unit: 4
Accessible Facilities:
Charming cottage with stunning views from
Mountains of Mourne to Belfast Lough.

COMBER
A pleasant town with a prominent statue of
Robert Gillespie, Ulster military hero in
Indian campaigns.

BED AND BREAKFAST
THE OLD SCHOOLHOUSE INN
100 Ballydrain Road, Castle Espie,
Comber BT23 6EA
Tel: (028) 97 541182   Fax: (028) 97 542583
No. of Accessible Rooms: 12
Accessible Facilities: Lounge, Dining Room.
The last bell rang in the playground 14 years
ago. Now a guest house and restaurant in a
rural location, three miles from Comber.

ATTRACTION
THE WILDFOWL AND WETLANDS TRUST
Castle Espie, Ballydrain Road, Comber BT23 6EA
Tel: (028) 91 874146   Fax: (028) 91 873857
Home to Ireland's largest collection of ducks,
geese and swans. Three hides, landscaped
gardens and 30 acres of woodland to explore.

SD		CP		E		RF	
C		S		WC		RFE	

GREYABBEY
Located on the shore of Strangford Lough,
where in Norman times, the monks were
encouraged to build in the glorious scenery.
GreyAbbey has one of the most complete

Cistercian Abbeys in Ireland.

BED AND BREAKFAST
BRIMAR
4 Cardy Road, GreyAbbey BT22 2LS
Tel/Fax: (028) 427 88681
No. of Accessible Rooms: 2
Accessible Facilities: Lounge, Dining Room.
Detached property close to town centre.

HOLYWOOD
History dates back to 700AD, when
townland of Balleyderry (town of the
wood), was renamed by the Normans to
Sanctus Boscus – the Holy Wood. Situated
on shores of Lough Belfast with good
restaurants, pubs and excellent shopping.
High street has one of few remaining
Maypoles in Ireland -a ship's mast
presented to the town by grateful Dutch
sailors after a shipwreck.

BED AND BREAKFAST
ARDSHANE COUNTRY HOUSE
5 Bangor Road, Holywood BT18 0NU
Tel: (028) 90 422044   Fax: (028) 90 427506
No. of Accessible Rooms: 2
Accessible Facilities: Lounge, Dining Room.
Built at turn of C19th on 800-year-old
camp site of King John's army as it
marched through Ireland. Ardshane means
Hill of John. Guest house on the outskirts
of the town amidst mature gardens and
glens. Main reception area restored to
reflect living styles of 1902 and the
Victorian theme includes staff uniforms.

ATTRACTION
ULSTER FOLK AND TRANSPORT MUSEUM
Cultra, Holywood BT18 0EU
Tel: (028) 90 428428   Fax: (028) 90 427925
e-mail: uftm@nidex.com
web: www.nidex.com/uftm
Irish Railway Collection, Transport and
Folk Galleries, Town and Rural Areas.
Many exhibition galleries are ramped
throughout: buildings in the open-air
museum are all original, brought from
original locations and re-erected in the
Museum – their interiors therefore are
inaccessible. Given the nature of the
museum, distances involved and some

gradients on the site, DISABLED VISITORS MAY GO ROUND THE OPEN-AIR MUSEUM BY CAR, AFTER 3PM. The Transport Museum covers many aspects including the Titanic exhibition and the Irish Railway collection.

SD   CP   E   RF   S

WC   Irish Railway Collection & Road Transport Galleries:

RF   C   WC   Folk Galleries:

RF   S   WC

KILKEEL

Busy, prosperous town and fishing port, home to the coast's main fishing fleet. Built on the site of a prehistoric fort, the ruins of a C14th castle stand in the square located in the heart of the Mourne Mountains, there are great views of coastal and mountain scenery on the Spelga Pass towards Hilltown.

TOURIST INFORMATION CENTRE
6 Newcastle Street, Kilkeel BT34 4AF
Tel/Fax: (028) 417 62525

HOTEL
KILMOREY ARMS
41-43 Greencastle Street, Kilkeel BT34 4BH
Tel: (028) 417 62220   Fax: (028) 417 65399

No. of Accessible Rooms: 2
Accessible Facilities: Lounge, Restaurant.
Original building 250 years old. Located in the town centre .

BED AND BREAKFAST
SHARON FARM
6 Ballykeel Road, Ballymartin,
Nr. Kilkeel BT34 4PL
Tel: (028) 417 62521
No. of Accessible Rooms: 1. Bath
Accessible Facilities: Lounge, Dining Room.
Modern bungalow situated on outskirts of Ballymartin, with lovely sea and mountain views.

HILL VIEW BED AND BREAKFAST
18 Bog Road, Attical, Kilkeel BT34 4HT
Tel: (028) 417 64269
No. of Accessible Rooms: 2
Accessible Facilities: Lounge, Dining Room.
Farmhouse located in the Morne countryside.

LISBURN

BED & BREAKFAST
BROOK LODGE
79 Old Ballynahinch Road, Lisburn BT27 6TH
Tel: (028) 92 638454

Strangford Lough.

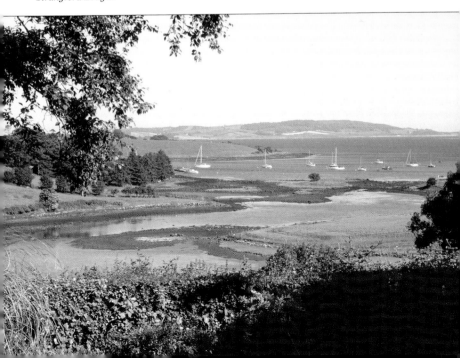

No. of Accessible Rooms: 1.
Accessible Facilities: Dining Room
Modern guest house on 65-acre mixed farm
with views of Dromara Hills and Mourne
Mountains. 5 miles from Lisburn.

NEWCASTLE

Attractive, lively town and a popular resort
since the early C19th, Newcastle's promenade
overlooks golden beaches and rolling hills.
Close by is forest park of Tullmore.

TOURIST INFORMATION CENTRE
Annesley Mansions, Central Promenade,
Newcastle BT33 0AA
Tel: (028) 437 22222   Fax: (028) 437 22400

HOTELS
BURRENDALE HOTEL and COUNTRY CLUB
51 Castlewellan Road, Newcastle BT33 0JY
Tel: (028) 437 22599   Fax::(028) 437 22328
No. of Accessible Rooms: 12
Accessible Facilities: Lounge, Bar, Restaurant
(2), Country Club with poolside lift for pool
and jacuzzi. The hotel provides excellent
guide to its facilities for disabled guests.
Delightful, modern hotel located between
Mourne Mountains and Irish Sea, one hour
from Belfast and close to Newcastle.

HASTINGS SLIEVE DONARD HOTEL
Downs Road, Newcastle BT33 0AH
Tel: (028) 437 23681   Fax: (028) 437 24830
e-mail: res.sdh@hastingshotels.com
web: www.haatingshotels.com
No. of Accessible rooms: 4. Bath.
Accessible Facilities: Lounge, Restaurant
Quality hotel in 6 acres of grounds leading
to beach. Close to Tullymore Forest Park.

BED AND BREAKFAST
MOURNE VIEW HOUSE
16 off Main Street, Dundrum,
Nr. Newcastle BT33 0LU
Tel: (028) 437 51457
No. of Accessible Rooms: 1
Accessible Facilities: Dining Room
Cottage-style property situated in its own
grounds. Located just off the main
Dundrum street at the entrance to the Quay.
4 miles from Newcastle.

NEWTOWNARDS

Popular for medievalists, there is an
impressive town square. Best known as
home of Mt. Stewart.

TOURIST INFORMATION CENTRE
31 Regent Street, Newtownards BT23 4AD
Tel: (028) 91 826846   Fax: (028) 91 826681

BED & BREAKFAST
ERNSDALE
120 Mountstewart Road, Carrowdore,
Newtownards BT22 2ES
Tel: (028) 91 861208
No. of Accessible Rooms: 3. Bath
Accessible Facilities: Dining Room.
Working farm located close to
Mountstewart House. 6.5 miles from town.

17 BALLYROGAN ROAD
Newtownards BT23 4ST
Tel: (028) 91 811693
No. of Accessible Rooms: 1
Accessible Facilities: Dining Room.
Chalet bungalow in rural setting
convenient for Ards Peninsula, and
situated off old Belfast/Newtownards road.

SELF-CATERING
BEECH COTTAGE
20 Mountstewart Road, Newtownards
Tel/Fax: (028) 91 88357
No. of Accessible Units: 1
No. of Beds per Unit: 1 -double
Accessible Facilities: Lounge, Dining
Room, Kitchen. Quiet rural setting 2.5
miles from Restaurant, pub and groceries.

ATTRACTION
MOUNT STEWART HOUSE AND GARDENS (NT)
Portaferry Road, Newtownards BT22 2AD
Tel: (028) 91 88387   Fax: (028) 91 88569
e-mail: umsest@smtp.ntrust.org.uk
umsest@smtp.ntrust.org.uk
Charming C18th house with C19th
additions, the childhood home of Lord
Castlereagh and famous for its fine garden.
Wheelchairs and 2 self-drive buggies
available.

SD   CP   E   RF
C   S   WC

SOMME HERITAGE CENTRE
233 Bangor Road, Newtownards BT23 7PH
Tel: (028) 91 823202

Examines Irelands' contribution to WW1
through 10th & 16th (Irish) Divisions and
36th (Ulster) Division. Reconstructed trench
system, museum and audio-visual recreation
of the Battle of the Somme.
Café opening this year.

SD [&] CP [&] E [&] RF [&]
C [Å] S [&] WC [Å]

PORTAFERRY

Conservation village with brightly painted
houses on the shores of Strangford Lough,
one of the most important marine sites in
Europe. On the waterfront look across to
Strangford village.

TOURIST INFORMATION CENTRE
The Stables, Castle Street, Portaferry BT22 1NZ
Tel: (028) 427 29882   Fax: (028) 427 29822
(Seasonal)

BED AND BREAKFAST
THE NARROWS   [&]
8 Shore Road, Portaferry BT22 1JY
Tel: (028) 427 28148   Fax: (028) 427 28105
e-mail: the.narrows@dial.pipex.xom
web:
www.nova.co.uk,/nova/strngfrd/narrow1/htm
No. of Accessible Rooms: 8
Accessible Facilities: Lounge, Dining Room,
Sauna. National Holiday Care Award Winner
1996. Highest proportion of accessible
bedrooms of any small mainstream hotel in
UK. Seafront location, all rooms having
wonderful views of Strangford Lough,
Ireland's first Marine Nature Reserve.
Exceptional variety of marine life and
colonies of common seals.

ATTRACTION
EXPLORIS
The Ropewalk, Castle Street, Portaferry, BT22 1NZ
Tel: (028) 427 728062   Fax: (028) 427 728396
web: www.globegateway.com/ards
Aquarium with Open Sea Tank, Shoal Ring.
Journey from Strangford Lough through the
neck of the Lough – the Narrows.

SD [&] CP [&] E [&] RF [&] L [&]
C [&] S [Å] WC [&] RFE [Å]

SAINTFIELD
ATTRACTION
ROWALLANE GARDEN (NT)
Saintfield BT24 7LH
Tel: (028) 97 510131   Fax: (028) 97 511242
e-mail: liroest@smtp.ntrust.org.uk
21 hectare shrub and tree garden containing
many exotic species from around the world.
Fine displays of azaleas and rhododendrons .
Accessed by compacted gravel or mown
grass paths. Some area undulating

SD [&] CP [&] E [&] RF [&]
C- [&] WC [&] RFE [Å]

COUNTY FERMANAGH

FERMANAGH TOURIST INFORMATION CENTRE
Wellington Road, Enniskillen BT74 7EF
Tel: (028) 66 323110   Fax: (028) 66 325511
web: www.lakelands.net

BELLEEK

Northern Ireland's most westerly village,
close to Lower Lough Erne. Famous for its
pottery.

BED AND BREAKFAST
RIVERSIDE GUEST HOUSE   [&]
601 Loughshore Road, Drumbadreevagh,
Belleek BT93 3FT
Tel: (028) 686 58649
No. of Accessible Rooms: 1. Shower
Accessible Facilities: Lounge, Dining Room
Large bungalow with conservatory and
garden a mile from Belleek on A46 Shore
Road. Convenient for Pottery, River Erne,
Lough Melvin and Donegal beaches.

ATTRACTION
BELLEEK POTTERY VISITOR CENTRE
Tel: (028) 686 59300   Fax: (028) 686 58625
e-mail: info@belleek.ie
Lining walls of reception in Centre are
photographs telling the Belleek story since
its establishment in 1857. Museum contains
some pieces dating back over 100 years: AV
theatre presentation takes you through
production process, followed by 20 minute
tour, all on one level. Visit the Casting and
Fettling Shops, and Flowering rooms and

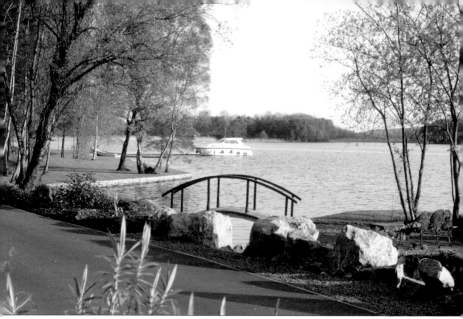

Cruising on Lough Erne.

see craftsmen design, mould and shape the intricate basketware. Quite fascinating.

SD   CP   E   RF
C   S   WC   RFE-TOUR

DERRYGONNELLY
BED AND BREAKFAST
NAVAR GUEST HOUSE
Derryvarey, Derrygonnelly BT93 6HW
Tel: (028) 686 41384
No. of Accessible Rooms: 5. Bath
Accessible Facilities: Lounge, Dining Room.
(1 step at front entrance). Modern bungalow
on working farm, in rural setting close to
Loughs Melvin and Erne. Located 1.5 miles
from Derrygonnelly toward Eniskillen.

ENNISKILLEN
Dominated by its C15th castle, the town
appears initially medieval, but modern
buildings rather spoil the illusion. Before
the plantation, the Maguires ruled this
lakeland area. The centre of Enniskillen is
rather a jumble, with a winding main street
and an old buttermarket, known for hand-
crafted goods. The centre occupies an island
between Upper and Lower Lough Erne. The
C17th. Church of Ireland cathedral was reconstructed in C19th.

TOURIST INFORMATION CENTRE
Wellington Road, Enniskillen
Tel: (028) 66 323110

BUSES
Ulsterbus: Tel: (028) 66 322633

HOTEL
KILLYHEVLIN HOTEL
Dublin Road, Enniskillen BT74 6RW
Tel: (028) 66 323481   Fax: (028) 66 324726
e-mail: rodney@eastnet.co.uk
web: www.killhevlin.com
No. of Accessible Rooms: 1
Accessible Facilities: Lounge, Restaurant
Family run hotel situated on the shores of
beautiful Lough Erne, in extensive
grounds. 05.miles from town centre.

BED AND BREAKFAST
BRINDLEY GUEST HOUSE
Tully, Killadeas, Enniskillen BT94 1RE
Tel: (028) 66 28065
No. of Accessible Rooms: 3
Accessible Facilities: Lounge, Dining Room.
Modern property with fine views over Lower
Lough Erne.

LACKABOY FARM HOUSE
Tempo Road, Enniskillen BT74 6EBA
Tel: (028) 66 322488

No. of Accessible Rooms: 1.
Accessible Facilities: Lounge, Dining Room.
60-acre dairy farm, 2 miles from
Enniskillen centre and close to Castle
Coole.

THE POINT
Tempo Road, Enniskillen BT
Tel: (028) 66 323595
No. of Accessible Rooms: 1
Accessible Facilities: Lounge, Dining Room
Spacious modern house located 1 mile
outside town boundary.

SELF-CATERING
BELMORE COURT MOTEL
Tempo Road, Enniskillen BT74 6HX
Tel: (028) 66 326633
Fax: (028) 66 326362
e-mail: book@motel.co.uk
web: www.motel.co.uk
No. of Accessible Units: 1. Shower
No. of Beds per Unit: 2
Accessible Facilities: Kitchenette. Quality
apartments situated on the edge of town, at
junction of Dublin and Temp roads, close
to main amenities.

ATTRACTIONS
CASTLE COOLE (NT)
Dublin Road, Enniskillen BT74 6JY
Tel: (028) 66 322690   Fax: (028) 66 325665
e-mail: UCASCO@smtp.ntrust.org.uk
One of finest neo-classical buildings in
Britain, built between 1789/95 by architect
James Wyatt, with wonderful plasterwork
ceilings and superb Regency furniture.
Outside lawns slope gently toward Lough
Coole. WARNING: Entrance is ramped at
1:5, but staff are vvery caring and an
electric buggy is OK - otherwise, make sure
you have a very strong pusher!

SD ♿   CP ♿   E n/a (see above)
RF ♿   C ♿   S ♿   WC ♿

ENNISKILLEN CASTLE
Castle Barracks, Enniskillen BT74 7HL
Tel: (028) 66 325000   Fax: (028) 66 327342
Three-storey keep surrounded by huge
barracks with C17th water gate, which
houses two museums and a heritage
centre. Exhibits on Royal Enniskillen

Fusiliers regiment and area antiquities.
SD ♿   CP ♿   E ♿   RF ♿
L ♿   S ♿   WC ♿   RFE ♿

ADAPTIVE CRUISERS
ERINCURRACH CRUISERS
Blaney, Enniskillen BT93 7EQ
Tel: Office: (028) 66 641507
Marina: (028) 66 641737
Fax: (028) 66 641734
Accessible Cruiser Class: Blaney
No. of Accessible Cruisers: 1
No. of Berths: 6
Sedan style cruiser specially adapted for access
to wheelchairs to all compartments via
interior lifts. Explore the waterways and lakes
of the Lough Erne and River Shannon systems.

FLORENCECOURT
ATTRACTION
MARBEL ARCH CAVES/
CUILCAGH MOUNTAIN PARK
Marlbank Scenic Loop, Florencecourt BT92 1EW
Tel: (028) 66 348855   Fax: (028) 66 348928
The Caves are unsuitable for wheelchair
users, but Reception/Exhibition building is
accessible with audio-visual facility.
SD ♿   CP ♿   E ♿   RF ♿
L ♿   C ♿   S ♿   WC ♿

GARRISON
Charming village on shores of Lough Melvin

BED AND BREAKFAST
LOUGH MELVIN HOLIDAY CENTRE
Garrison BT93 4FG
Tel: (028) 686 58142   Fax: (028) 686 58719
No. of Accessible Rooms: 1
Accessible Facilities: Dining Room, TV
Lounge. Modern holiday centre on the
shores of Lough Melvin, central to the
county's top attractions with quality
restaurant and coffee shop on site. Caters for
range of activities that include accessible
boating on the Lough.

KESH
Busy little fishing village where one can
learn the old skills of spinning and weaving
nearby at Ardress.

417

BED AND BREAKFAST
DRUMRUSH LODGE ⬚
Drumrush, Kesh
Tel: (028) 686 31578
No. of Accessible Rooms: 1
Accessible Facilities: Lounge, Dining Room.
Purpose built complex overlooking Muckross
Bay in Lower Lough Erne beside marina.

CLAREVIEW ⬚
Scenic Route, 85A Crevenish Road,
Kesh BT93 1RQ
Tel: (028) 686 31455
e-mail: kesh@clareview.swinternet.co.uk
No. of Accessible Rooms: 2. Bath
Accessible Facilities: Lounge, Dining Room.
Modern bungalow on elevated site on scenic
route between Kesh and Castle Archdale
with fishing and boating close by.

LISNASKEA
Interesting market town with restored
market cross and ruined C17th castle in the
town centre.

SELF-CATERING
SHARE HOLIDAY VILLAGE ⬚
Smith's Strand, Lisnaskea BT92 0EQ
Tel: (028) 207 22122   Fax: (028) 207 21893
e-mail: share@dnet.co.uk
web: www.sharevillage.org
No. of Accessible Chalets: 17
No. of Accessible Guesthouse Rooms: 6
Charity promoting integration between able-
bodied people and those with special needs.
The village is a lakeside activity centre with
purpose-built accommodation for use by
physically challenged guests. Wide range of
outdoor sports and wheelchair accessible
coaches for trips to local places of interest.

NEWTOWNBUTLER
Located on Upper Lough Erne

ATTRACTION
CROM ESTATE (NT)
Newtownbutler BT92 8AP
Tel/Fax: (028) 66 38118
e-mail: cromw@smtp.ntrust.org.uk
An important conservation area with
woodland, parkland and wetland on the

shores of Upper Lough Erne. Wheelchair
and self-drive buggy available.

SD ⬚	CP 🚶	E ⬚	RF ⬚
C ⬚	S ⬚	WC 🚶	RFE 🚶

COUNTY LONDONDERRY

AGHADOWEY
Located a few miles south of Coleraine and
10 miles from the coast.

HOTEL
BROWN TROUT GOLF AND COUNTRY INN ⬚
209 Agivey Road, Aghadowey BT51 4AD
Tel: (028) 70 868209
Fax: (028) 70 868878
e-mail: billohara@aol.com
No. of Accessible Rooms: several
Accessible Facilities: Lounge, Bar,
Restaurant (accessed by stair lift). Situated
on banks of River Agivey, one of the
country's oldest hostelries. A family affair,
the first record dating from 1817, this is a
charming property, the first golf hotel in
Northern Ireland. Owner's sister, returning
to help with staff training and catering, used
to be with London Tara Hotel, well-known
for its facilities for disabled guests.

COLERAINE
Home to the Coleraine campus of the
University of Ulster, with the ambience of a
university town. Founded by St. Patrick, most
of the town was developed by the Irish
Society of London. The river Bann runs
through the centre, and a rare collection of
daffodils and narcissi bloom here in late April.

TOURIST INFORMATION CENTRE
Railway Road, Coleraine
Tel: (028) 703 44723
Fax: (028) 703 51756

CAUSEWAY COAST AND GLENS
11 Lodge Road, Coleraine,
Co. Londonderry BT52 1LU
Tel: (028) 70 327720
Fax: (028) 70 327719
e-mail: causewayandglens@breathemail.net

HOTEL
BOHILL HOTEL & COUNTRY CLUB 🚶
69 Cloyfin Road, Coleraine BT52 2NY
Tel: (028) 703 44406 Fax: (028) 703 55873
No. of Accessible Rooms: 36
Accessible Facilities: Lounge, Restaurant,
Gardens, Grounds.
Modern hotel with chalet type rooms.

BED AND BREAKFAST
COOLBEG ♿
2e Grange Road, Coleraine BT52 1NG
Tel: (028) 703 44961 Fax: (028) 703 43278
No. of Accessible Rooms: 2
Accessible Facilities: Lounge, Dining Room,
Garden access. Modern bungalow situated in
quiet residential area. Surrounding area is
flat and town centre under a mile. Plenty of
Restaurants and eating places in the area.

THE LODGE HOTEL AND TRAVELSTOP 🚶
Lodge Road, Coleraine BT52 1NF
Tel: (028) 703 44848 Fax: (028) 70354555
e-mail: info@thelodgehotel.com
web: www.thelodgehotel.com
No. of Accessible Rooms: 2
Accessible Facilities: Restaurants (2)
Accessible rooms in Travelstop adjacent
main hotel with facilities available. Located
0.5 mile from town centre and close to
Giant's Causeway and Mussendum Temple -
1770s, maintained by National Trust with
cliff top views.

SELF-CATERING
KINGS COUNTRY COTTAGES ♿
"Ballyvennox" 66 Ringrash Road, Macosquin,
Coleraine BT51 4LJ
Tel/Fax: (028) 703 51367
No. of Accessible Units: 1. Roll-in Shower
No, of Beds per Unit: 6
Accessible Facilities: Lounge, Kitchen
1 of 4 cottages in quiet farmyard setting, in
village just south-west of Coleraine.

KILREA
In the Bann Valley on B64 between
Coleraine and Maghera, before the Bann
broadens out into Loch Beg and then Loch
Neagh. Attractive farming landscape, highly
cultivated.

BED AND BREAKFAST
PORTNEAL LODGE ♿
75 Bann Road, Kilrea BT51 5RX
Tel: (028) 295 41444 Fax: (028) 295 41424
No. of Accessible Rooms: 1.Bath
Accessible Facilities: Dining room.
Homely b & b situated in seven acres of
woodland overlooking a stretch of the Lower
Bann River, very close to town. Evening meals
available. Known for coarse and game angling.

LIMAVADY
Largely of modern character but some
Georgian evidence in early streets.
Beautifully located in the Roe Valley with
glorious mountain landscapes to the north
and south-east.

TOURIST INFORMATION CENTRE
Council Offices, 7 Connell Street, Limavady
Tel: (028) 777 22226 Fax: (028) 777 22010

HOTEL
GORTEEN HOUSE HOTEL ♿
187 Roe Mill Road, Limavady BT49 9EX
Tel: (028) 777 22333
No. of Accessible Rooms: 6. Shower
Accessible Facilities: Lounge, Restaurant, Bar.
Former 18th century residence located on
outskirts of the town, close to Derry Airport.

RADISSON ROE PARK HOTEL & GOLF RESORT ♿
Roe Park, Limavady BT49 9LB
Tel: (028) 777 22222
Fax: (028) 777 22313
e-mail: reservation@radisson.nireland.com
No. of Accessible Rooms: 1
Accessible Facilities: Lounge, Restaurants
(2). Quality hotel set within private 18-hole
golf course and surrounded by lovely tranquil
countryside of Roe Valley Country Park.

BED AND BREAKFAST
THE POPLARS 🚶
352 Seacoast, Limavady BT49 0LA
Tel: (028) 777 50360
No. of Accessible Rooms: 1. Bath
Accessible Facilities: Dining Room.
Evening Meal available. Detached modern
farm bungalow in mature gardens with good
views of Donegal Hills. Close to Benone
Strand, 6 miles from Limavady.

419

(LONDONDERRY) DERRY

Derry is the only completely walled city in Ireland. Developed by the City of London in the early C17th, it took on the London prefix and the city's walls and inner city were the showpiece development of the Plantation era in Ulster. There are many Georgian streets, some fine buildings, including St. Columb's Cathedral of 1633 (sadly not very accessible) and the lavish neo-Gothic Guildhall.

VISITOR AND CONVENTION BUREAU
44 Foyle Street, Derry BT48 6AT
Tel: (028) 71 377577   Fax: (028) 71 377992
e-mail: info@derryvisitor.com
web: www.derryvisitor.com

TOURIST INFORMATION CENTRE
Bishop Street, Derry
Tel: (028) 71 267284

BUSES
Ulsterbus: Tel: (028) 90 333000
10 low-floor buses for city service wheelchair assisted access.
Translink (Citybus, NI Rail, Ulsterbus)
New buses have been fitted with ramps and low-floor level wheelchair accessibility.
Citybus: Tel: (028) 90 246485
NI Rail: Tel: (028) 90 899411
Ulsterbus: Tel: (028) 90 33300

TAXIS
For all queries call: (028) 90 491011
Community Black Taxis -London style- operate in certain areas of Belfast and Londonderry – not all are accessible. This is a bus type of service. Public hire taxis in Belfast identified by yellow plate at rear and front of vehicle. Private hire taxis identified by car roof sign with white front panel and green licence disc on windscreen.

RAIL
NI Railways: Tel: (028) 71 342228
Ramps available and one carriage in each train is wheelchair accessible. 24 hour notice to book assistance.

HOTEL
WATERFOOT HOTEL & COUNTRY CLUB
14 Clooney Road, Londonderry BT47 1TB
Tel: (028) 71 345500   Fax: (028) 71 311006

No. of Accessible Rooms: 2
Accessible Facilities: Dining Room, Bar (2 steps). Lovely hotel situated at eastern end of the Foyle Bridge with fine views of both the River and Co. Donegal

ATTRACTION
FOYLE VALLEY RAILWAY MUSEUM
Foyle Road Station, Londonderry BT48 6SQ
Tel: (028) 71 265234
Londonderry was once the meeting point of 4 railway systems and this museum hosts fine collection of relics from the past. Majestic steam locomotives, railcars and wagons with hands-on activities. Ramp onto train.

PORTSTEWART

Originally popular with the Victorian middle-classes, this seaside resort remains rather sedate. It has a long crescent-shaped seafront promenade and west of the town is the Strand, a fine long sandy beach protected by the National Trust.

BED AND BREAKFAST
NORTHGATE
13 Old Coach Road, Portstewart BT55 7BX
Tel: (028) 70 832497
No. of Accessible Rooms: 1. Shower
Accessible Facilities: Lounge, Dining Room. Quiet family run home overlooking lovely sea views and golf course with small garden.

COUNTY TYRONE

BERAGH
BED AND BREAKFAST
MON ABRI
14 Moylagh Road, Beragh BT79 0TQ
Tel: (028) 807 58224
No. of Accessible Rooms: 1
Accessible Facilities: Lounge, Dining Room. Modern bungalow in country location, half a mile from the village on B46 Beragh to Fintona road and 7 miles from Omagh.

CLOGHER

Small cathedral town in Clogher Valley, an

area of quiet lanes and woodlands. Known for largest annual one-day show in Ireland, Clogher Valley Agricultural Show in Augher and in Clogher the William Carleton Summer School, a five-day arts event. Several places of interest nearby.

BED AND BREAKFAST
CORCIK HOUSE
20 Corick Road, Clogher BT76 0BZ
Tel: (028) 855 48216   Fax: (028) 855 49531
No. of Accessible Rooms: 1
Accessible Facilities: Lounge, Dining Room
Charmingly restored 10-bedroomed C17th William and Mary house set in 20 acres of gardens overlooking River Blackwater. Tower and Garden Front added in 1863. Located 0.5 mile off main A4 Belfast to Enniskillen road between village of Augher and Clogher.

COOKSTOWN
Well known for its stately central thoroughfare 2km long and totally straight. A C17th Plantation town, the countryside around is rich in Neolithic and early Christian monuments.

TOURIST INFORMATION CENTRE
48 Moleworth Street, Cookstown BT80 4DL
Tel: (028) 867 66727 (Seasonal)
(028) 867 62205 (all year-Council offices)

HOTEL
GLENAVON HOUSE HOTEL
52 Drum Road, Cookstown BT80 8JQ
Tel: (028) 867 64949   Fax: (028) 867 64396
No. of Accessible Rooms: 1
Accessible Facilities: Lounge, 1 Restaurant (the other not accessible). Situated on the outskirts of town in nine acres of mature gardens. Located at the foot of the Sperrins.

TULLYLAGAN COUNTRY HOUSE
40b Tullylagen Road, Cookstown BT80 8UP
Tel: (028) 867 65100   Fax: (028) 867 61715
No. of Accessible Rooms: 2
Accessible Facilities: Restaurant, Lounge. Early C19th property in style of late Georgian classic villa. Rural setting in 30 acres of mature grounds with Tullylagan River flowing through the estate. Located midway between Dungannon and Cookstown.

ATTRACTION
DRUM MANOR FOREST PARK
Oaklands, Cookstown
Tel: (028) 87 759311   Fax: (028) 87 759181
Small, yet varied and attractive, forest estate with Butterfly Garden with wide variety of wildflower and shrubs specially grown to attract native butterflies. High fertility of soil means wide tree variety can be grown. 4 Wayside Trails, No.2 being an Adapted trail of 0.8 mile – gentle trail following promenade path to Butterfly Gardens, continuing to half-way picnic table and view point with easy return to car park. Car parking, with excellent spacing, is 400m from entrance.

| SD | CP n/a | E | RF |
| C | S n/a | WC | RFE |

KINTURK CULTURAL CENTRE
7 Kinturk Road, Cookstown
Tel: (028) 867 36512

| SD | CP | E | RF |
| L- | C | S | |

DUNGANNON
Hilly location and site of government of the O'Neill dynasty from C14th until Plantation. The town's Royal School, opened in 1614, claims to be the oldest in Northern Ireland. Originally known for its linen manufacture, the best known factory now is Tyrone Crystal.

TOURIST INFORMATION CENTRE
190 Ballgawley Road, Dungannon BT70 1TF
Tel: (028) 87 767359   Fax: (028287) 767911

HOTEL
COHANNON INN & AUTO LODGE
212 Ballynakilly Road, Dungannon BT71 6HJ
Tel: (028) 87 722215   Fax: (028) 87 752217
No. of Accessible Rooms: 1
Accessible Facilities: Restaurant
Located at the A45 Filling Station, convenient to M1 Motorway (J.14), close to Lough Neagh and Sperrins foothills.

ATTRACTION
US GRANT ANCESTRAL HOMESTEAD
Dergenagh Road, Dungannon BT70 1TW
Tel: (028) 855 57133   Fax: (028) 855 767911
Ancestral homestead of Ulysses S. Grant,

421

18th President of the USA, restored to appearance of C19th Irish smallholding. Visitor Centre offers exhibitions on American Civil War and Ulster Scots Plantation.

SD | CP | E | RF
C | S | WC | RFE

FIVEMILETOWN

Deep in the heart of the Clogher Valley, surrounded by fine lakelands.

HOTEL
VALLEY HOTEL
60 Main Street, Fivemiletown BT75 0PW
Tel: (028) 895 21505   Fax: (028) 895 21588
No. of Accessible Rooms: Several, accessible by Lift. Accessible Facilities: Lounge (2 steps), Restaurant, Bar. Well established family run hotel in town centre.

OMAGH

Capital of Tyrone, separated from Cookstown by the Black Bog, a nature reserve, which explains the turfcraft (compressed and heated peat) souvenirs available here. Lovely twin-spired church. Good for fishing on the Camowen and Owenreach Rivers.

TOURIST INFORMATION CENTRE
1 Market Street, Omagh BT78 1EE
Tel: (028) 82 247831

BUSES
Ulsterbus: Tel: (028) 82 242711

BED AND BREAKFAST
GREENMOUNT LODGE COUNTRY HOUSE
58 Greenmount Road, Gorlaclare,
Omagh BT79 0YE
Tel: (028) 82 841325 Fax: (028) 82 840019
No. of Accessible Rooms: 1
Accessible Facilities: Lounge, Dining Room. Former C18th estate building which was rebuilt in 1970.

ATTRACTIONS
ULSTER-AMERICAN FOLK PARK
Mellon Road, Castletown, Omagh BT78 5QY
Tel: (028) 82 243292
Fax: (028) 82 242241
e-mail: mail@folkpark.com

Outdoor museum tracing Ulster's links with USA and emigration during C18th and C19th. 70-acre site divided into old and New Worlds, the former centred around restored farmhouse of Thomas Mellon, who emigrated to Pennsylvania in 1818, and the latter around log houses and outbuildings. Visitor Centre with exhibitions, AV presentations and Emigration Gallery complete with dockside buildings and emigrant ship. A must.

SD | CP | E | RF
C | S | WC | RFE

THE ULSTER HISTORY PARK
Cullion, Omagh BT79 7SU
Tel: (028) 82 648188   Fax: (028) 82 1648011
e-mail: tourism@omagh.gov.uk
Access Award-winning museum with excellent visitor centre including accessible exhibition area, telling of first 10,000 years of Irish history with displays and video.
EXTERIOR – Neolithic section with uneven, steep gravel paths – is not accessible. Plantation is accessible with reconstructed houses and exhibition telling of first settlers. Fascinating.

SD | CP | E | RF | Visitor Centre
C | S | WC

STRABANE

Bustling border town where the River Finn joins the River Foyle. Birthplace of John Dunlap, printer of the American Declaration of Independence. East of the town one passes into the lovely Tyrone Hills.

TOURIST INFORMATION CENTRE
Abercorn Square, Strabane BT82 8AE
Tel: (028) 71 883735 (Seasonal)
(028) 71 382204 (all year-Council offices).

BED AND BREAKFAST
HOLLYBUSH
421a Victoria Road, Ballymagorry,
Strabane BT82 0AT
Tel: (028) 71 382370
No. of Accessible Rooms: 2. Bath
Accessible Facilities: Lounge, Dining Room. Adjacent accessible restaurant.
Chalet-style bungalow with large garden behind Ballymagorry Arms in village centre.

Against each town are letters relating to the following facilities:
A: Accommodation   B: Attraction   C: Tourist Information Centre   D: Transport Information   E: Theatre   F: Sports
The bold figure at the end of each line denotes the page on which the town will be found.

Against each town are letters relating to the following facilities:
A: Accommodation   B: Attraction   C: Tourist Information Centre   D: Transport Information   E: Theatre   F: Sports
The bold figure at the end of each line denotes the page on which the town will be found.

Against each town are letters relating to the following facilities:
A: Accommodation   B: Attraction   C: Tourist Information Centre   D: Transport Information   E: Theatre   F: Sports
The bold figure at the end of each line denotes the page on which the town will be found.

Against each town are letters relating to the following facilities:
A: Accommodation   B: Attraction   C: Tourist Information Centre   D: Transport Information   E: Theatre   F: Sports
The bold figure at the end of each line denotes the page on which the town will be found.

Against each town are letters relating to the following facilities:
A: Accommodation   B: Attraction   C: Tourist Information Centre   D: Transport Information   E: Theatre   F: Sports
The bold figure at the end of each line denotes the page on which the town will be found.

Against each town are letters relating to the following facilities:
A: Accommodation B: Attraction C: Tourist Information Centre D: Transport Information E: Theatre F: Sports
The bold figure at the end of each line denotes the page on which the town will be found.